Rehabilitative Surgery

Andrew I. Elkwood
Matthew Kaufman • Lisa F. Schneider
Editors

Rehabilitative Surgery

A Comprehensive Text for an
Emerging Field

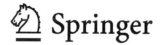 Springer

Editors
Andrew I. Elkwood
Institute for Advanced Reconstruction
The Plastic Surgery Center
Shrewsbury, NJ
USA

Lisa F. Schneider
Institute for Advanced Reconstruction
The Plastic Surgery Center
Shrewsbury, NJ
USA

Matthew Kaufman
Institute for Advanced Reconstruction
The Plastic Surgery Center
Shrewsbury, NJ
USA

ISBN 978-3-319-41404-1   ISBN 978-3-319-41406-5   (eBook)
DOI 10.1007/978-3-319-41406-5

Library of Congress Control Number: 2017936881

Printed on acid-free paper

This Springer imprint is published by Springer Nature
The registered company is Springer International Publishing AG
The registered company address is: Gewerbestrasse 11, 6330 Cham, Switzerland

We dedicate this book to our teachers, who gave us the tools and insight to innovate, and to our spouses, whose support makes everything possible.

Preface

The paralyzed or severely neurologically impaired patient is one of the greatest challenges in long-term chronic care that we face as clinicians, whether we are occupational therapists or orthopedists or physiatrists or surgeons. Because of the complexity of their treatment and the severity of their injury, these patients may be viewed as a hopeless cause for many physicians, especially surgeons. Optimization of their care – and potentially improvement in quality and length of life – requires a complex and delicate interaction between multiple surgical and medical specialties across disciplines and time.

The current state of rehabilitative medicine works to maximize patient function as well as manage the lifelong maintenance required to continue that level of function. Although surgery has always been part of the treatment of the paralyzed patient, it may be seen as an afterthought or the modality of last resort for the rehabilitation community or even surgeons who have little experience taking care of these patients. Once surgery is considered, the procedures needed to care for these patients and improve their lives often exist at the margins of existing surgical specialties or at the junction of multiple disciplines, performed haphazardly without a unified understanding of a comprehensive treatment approach. These procedures and their context may be difficult to understand, requiring familiarity with different interlocking yet distinct specialties, making approaching this topic particularly daunting for the student of any field.

We introduce the new field of rehabilitative surgery, a unique designation combining state-of-the-art surgeries from multiple surgical specialties in order to reimagine our approach to these patients. In this text, *Rehabilitative Surgery: A Comprehensive Text for an Emerging Field*, we present a completely different framework for understanding, coordinating, and providing treatment for the paralyzed or severely neurologically impaired patient. Contrary to the traditional approach of rehabilitative medicine, surgery is in fact a critical component of the care of the chronically impaired patient and may create opportunities to change their everyday life in a profound way by creating a new baseline of functional status.

We believe that much of the resistance to the surgical treatment of these patients arises from a lack of understanding of how even some straightforward interventions, performed in a coordinated way, can dramatically improve a patient's life. Patients who can now move a joystick on a wheelchair or feed themselves again often have profound appreciation for this incremental increase in independence, a small but significant liberation from the prison of paralysis.

This compendium represents the first interdisciplinary text for the emerging field of rehabilitative surgery, synthesizing various perspectives into a cornerstone for the rehabilitation field. The text is designed for both surgical and nonsurgical readers. An expert has written each evidence-based chapter with concise and straightforward explanations for clinicians who have no previous experience in that specialty. Specific descriptions of surgical procedures are included as well as surgical videos that can be accessed from the companion website.

Every major aspect of the reconstructive surgical treatment of these patients has been considered from a multidisciplinary vantage point, including orthopedic surgery, plastic surgery, neurosurgery, general surgery, and otolaryngology. We clearly describe and evaluate the most up-to-date and evidence-based surgeries that are currently standard of care including treatment of pressure sores, placement of feeding tubes, and upper extremity interventions to improve function and hygiene. As international leaders in the field of nerve reanimation surgery, we describe our cutting-edge protocols for the surgical treatment of severe nerve injuries, spinal cord injury (SCI) and stroke, or cerebrovascular accidents (CVA). We provide the first description and evidence for phrenic nerve repair to assist weaning paralyzed patients from their ventilators. This includes an exciting subset of patients with amyotrophic lateral sclerosis (ALS), who have shown benefit from phrenic nerve reconstruction in conjunction with nerve stimulation. These patients need our help. It falls on us – their clinicians and caretakers – to do everything we can to maximize their function to help them live as well and as independently as possible.

Shrewsbury, NJ   Andrew I. Elkwood
                                                                     Matthew Kaufman
                                                                     Lisa F. Schneider

Foreword

The explosion of medical/surgical knowledge and the introduction of complex treatment protocols dictated the need for the development of interdisciplinary teams.[1] The day of the physician working alone in a single office became an anachronism.

As superbly illustrated in *Rehabilitative Surgery*, the concept of the truly functional interdisciplinary team is an absolute necessity in modern clinical practice. The surgeon's role is no longer limited to a defined period in the operating room, but, equally as important, it is also defined by the extra-operating periods of the working week – meeting jointly with colleagues and evaluating patients with their clinical problems, developing treatment protocols, providing postoperative care and rehabilitation, and, hopefully, participating in designing well-controlled outcome studies.

The benefits of the clinical team are obvious. First of all, it provides optimal patient care – the primary requisite of clinical medicine. In addition, it promotes patient/family education. For the participating clinician, membership in a clinical team ensures exposure to cutting-edge care and enormous opportunities for learning from members from other disciplines, i.e., "cross-fertilization." New treatment programs can be undertaken and research protocols developed. The clinical gains from these joint efforts can be exponential and can result in paradigm shifts in clinical care. In the process, lifelong friendships are formed within the team.

To paraphrase Gertrude Stein, "A team is not a team, is not a team...." Not all teams are functional, and as in athletics, one can ask what distinguishes a truly successful, winning team. I believe it comes down to the commitment of the individual member – a dedication to the patient; a desire to learn from each other; a reliability or accountability; an open-mindedness with an ability to abandon old, unproven dogma; and an enthusiasm for advancing the clinical field.

The original version of this book was revised. An erratum to this chapter can be found at (DOI 10.1007/978-3-319-41406-5_28).

[1] I prefer the term interdisciplinary to multidisciplinary, as the former implies clinicians from different specialties *working together* as compared to clinicians from different specialties existing together (multidisciplinary)

As one reviews the list of authors and their clinical backgrounds, as well as the wide variety of subjects covered, one cannot help but question the legitimacy of age-old "specialty" designations. In many ways, they appear as anachronistic as the medieval guilds. Clinicians today identify themselves as belonging to clinical teams treating specific conditions of common interest. The opportunities and advances in health care have broken down the walls of "specialty" isolation and narrow-mindedness.

The editors and authors of Rehabilitative Surgery, in their organization and presentation of content, superbly direct the reader to the new world of health care organized to address and care for individual patient health problems.

Joseph G. McCarthy, MD
NYU School of Medicine, New York, NY, USA

Director Emeritus of the Institute of Reconstructive
Plastic Surgery, NYU Langone Medical Center,
New York, NY, USA

Lawrence D. Bell,
Professor Emeritus
NYU School of Medicine, New York, NY, USA

Director Emeritus of the Institute of Reconstructive
Plastic Surgery, NYU Langone Medical Center,
New York, NY, USA

Helen Kimmel,
Professor Emeritus of Plastic Surgery
NYU School of Medicine, New York, NY, USA

Director Emeritus of the Institute of Reconstructive
Plastic Surgery, NYU Langone Medical Center,
New York, NY, USA

Acknowledgments

We gratefully acknowledge the dedication of Catarina Martins and Kristie Rossi, whose tireless work made this manuscript a reality.

We also gratefully acknowledge our illustrator, Jeannine Sico, whose skill and vision are without equal.

Contents

Contributors

Hamid Abdollahi, MD The Plastic Surgery Center, Institute for Advanced Reconstruction, Shrewsbury, NJ, USA

A. Ashinoff, MD The Plastic Surgery Center, Institute for Advanced Reconstruction, Shrewsbury, NJ, USA

Azra Ashraf, MD Private Practice, Shrewsbury, NJ, USA

Patricia Ayoung-Chee, MD Division of Trauma, Emergency Surgery and Surgical Critical Care, Department of Surgery, NYU School of Medicine, New York, NY, USA

Melissa Baldwin, MD General Surgery, NYU School of Medicine, New York, NY, USA

Howard Bar-Eli, MD Rutgers Robert Wood Johnson Medical School, New Brunswick, NJ, USA

Thomas Bauer, MD Jersey Shore University Medical Center, Neptune, NJ, USA

W. Hugh Baugher, MD The Curtis National Hand Center, MedStar Union Memorial Hospital, Baltimore, MD, USA

D.J. Brown, MD, MPH Department of Surgery, Rutgers Robert Wood Johnson Medical School, New Brunswick, NJ, USA

John Cece, BAS The Plastic Surgery Center, Institute for Advanced Reconstruction, Shrewsbury, NJ, USA

Andrew I. Elkwood, MD, MBA The Plastic Surgery Center, Institute for Advanced Reconstruction, Shrewsbury, NJ, USA

David Estin, MD Neurosurgeons of New Jersey, West Long Branch, NJ, USA

Christopher L. Forthman, MD The Curtis National Hand Center, MedStar Union Memorial Hospital, Baltimore, MD, USA

Jan Fridén, MD, PhD Department of Hand Surgery, Swiss Paraplegic Centre, Nottwil, Switzerland

Centre for Advanced Reconstructions of Extremities (C.A.R.E.) and Department of Hand, Institute of Clinical Sciences, Sahlgrenska University Hospital, Goteborg, Sweden

Andreas Gohritz, MD Department of Hand Surgery, Swiss Paraplegic Centre, Nottwil, Switzerland

Department of Plastic, Reconstructive and Aesthetic Surgery, Hand Surgery, University Hospital, Basel, Switzerland

Neil R. Holland, MBBS, MBA, FAAN Neurology, Geisinger Health System, Danville, PA, USA

Medicine (Neurology), Commonwealth Medical College, Scranton, PA, USA

Hilton M. Kaplan, MBBCh, FCSSA, PhD Rutgers, The State University of New Jersey, New Brunswick, NJ, USA

Ryan D. Katz, MD The Curtis National Hand Center, MedStar Union Memorial Hospital, Baltimore, MD, USA

Matthew Kaufman, MD, FACS The Plastic Surgery Center, Institute for Advanced Reconstruction, Shrewsbury, NJ, USA

I. David Kaye, MD Division of Spine Surgery, The Rothman Institute at Thomas Jefferson University Hospital, Philadelphia, PA, USA

Matthew Klein, MD Monmouth Pain Care, Long Branch, NJ, USA

Sean Li, MD Interventional Pain Physician, Premier Pain Centers, Shrewsbury, NJ, USA

Timothy Link, MD Neurosurgeons of New Jersey, West Long Branch, NJ, USA

Todd A. Linsenmeyer, MD Kessler Institute for Rehabilitation, West Orange, NJ, USA

Jonathan Lustgarten, MD Neurosurgeons of New Jersey, West Long Branch, NJ, USA

Mary Massery, PT, DPT, DSc Massery Physical Therapy, Glenview, IL, USA

Kenneth R. Means, MD The Curtis National Hand Center, MedStar Union Memorial Hospital, Baltimore, MD, USA

Henry Moyle, MD Neurosurgeons of New Jersey, West Long Branch, NJ, USA

Ty Olson, MD, FACS Monmouth Medical Center, Long Branch, NJ, USA

Columbia University Medical Center, New York, NY, USA

Raymond P. Onders, MD Department of Surgery, University Hospitals Case Medical Center, Case Western Reserve University School of Medicine, Cleveland, OH, USA

Leo R. Otake, MD, PhD Assistant Clinical Professor, Plastic Surgery, Yale School of Medicine, St. Francis Medical Center, Hartford, CT, USA

H. Leon Pachter, MD Department of Surgery, NYU School of Medicine, New York, NY, USA

Peter G. Passias, MD Division of Spinal Surgery, NYU School of Medicine, New York, NY, USA

Tushar Patel, MD The Plastic Surgery Center, Institute for Advanced Reconstruction, Shrewsbury, NJ, USA

David Polonet, MD Jersey Shore University Medical Center, Neptune City, NJ, USA

Rutgers Robert Wood Johnson Medical School, New Brunswick, NJ, USA

Matthew Pontell, MD Department of Surgery, Drexel University College of Medicine, Philadelphia, PA, USA

Richard J. Redett, MD Department of Plastic and Reconstructive Surgery, Brachial Plexus Clinic at Kennedy Krieger Institute, Johns Hopkins Medical Institutions, Baltimore, MD, USA

Michael I. Rose, MD The Plastic Surgery Center, Institute for Advanced Reconstruction, Shrewsbury, NJ, USA

Adam Saad, MD The Plastic Surgery Center, Institute for Advanced Reconstruction, Shrewsbury, NJ, USA

Justin M. Sacks, MD, FACS Department of Plastic and Reconstructive Surgery, Johns Hopkins School of Medicine, Baltimore, MA, USA

Vascularized Composite Allograft Transplant Laboratory, Carey School of Business, Johns Hopkins Outpatient Center, Johns Hopkins University, Baltimore, MA, USA

Lisa F. Schneider, MD The Plastic Surgery Center, Institute for Advanced Reconstruction, Shrewsbury, NJ, USA

Keith A. Segalman, MD The Curtis National Hand Center, MedStar Union Memorial Hospital, Baltimore, MD, USA

Peter S. Staats, MD, MBA Interventional Pain Physician, Premier Pain Centers, Shrewsbury, NJ, USA

Istvan Turcsányi, MD Department of Orthopaedics, Szabolcs-Szatmár-Bereg County Hospitals and University Hospital, Nyiregyhaza, Hungary

Jonathan Weiswasser, MD The Plastic Surgery Center, Institute for Advanced Reconstruction, Shrewsbury, NJ, USA

Eric G. Wimmers, MD The Plastic Surgery Center, Institute for Advanced Reconstruction, Shrewsbury, NJ, USA

Raymond A. Wittstadt, MD The Curtis National Hand Center, MedStar Union Memorial Hospital, Baltimore, MD, USA

Victor W. Wong, MD Department of Plastic and Reconstructive Surgery, Johns Hopkins Medical Institutions, Baltimore, MD, USA

Wise Young, MD, PhD Rutgers, The State University of New Jersey, New Brunswick, NJ, USA

Deborah Yu, MD The Plastic Surgery Center, Institute for Advanced Reconstruction, Shrewsbury, NJ, USA

Part I

Introduction

Introduction to Rehabilitative Surgery

1

Andrew I. Elkwood, Matthew Kaufman,
and Lisa F. Schneider

The paralyzed or severely neurologically impaired patient is one of the greatest challenges in long-term chronic care that we face as clinicians, whether we are therapists or neurologists, physiatrists, or surgeons. Because of the complexity of their treatment and the severity of their injury, these patients may be viewed as a hopeless cause for many physicians, especially surgeons. Optimization of their care – and potentially improvement in quality and length of life – requires a complex and delicate interaction between multiple surgical and medical specialties across disciplines and time.

The current state of rehabilitative medicine works to maximize patient function as well as manage the lifelong maintenance required to continue that level of function. Although surgery has always been part of the treatment of the paralyzed patient, it may be seen as an afterthought or the modality of last resort for the rehabilitation community or even surgeons who have little experience taking care of these patients. Once surgery is considered, the procedures needed to care for these patients and improve their lives often exist at the margins of existing surgical

specialties or at the junction of multiple disciplines, performed haphazardly without a unified understanding of a comprehensive treatment approach. These procedures and their context may be difficult to understand, requiring familiarity with different interlocking yet distinct specialties, making approaching this topic particularly daunting for the student of any field.

We introduce the new field of rehabilitative surgery, a unique designation combining state-of-the-art surgeries from multiple surgical specialties in order to reimagine our approach to these patients. In this text, *Rehabilitative Surgery: A Comprehensive Text for an Emerging Field*, we present a completely different framework for understanding, coordinating, and providing treatment for the paralyzed or severely neurologically impaired patient. Contrary to the traditional approach of rehabilitative medicine, surgery is in fact a critical component of the care of the chronically impaired patient and may create opportunities to change their everyday life in a profound way by creating a new baseline of functional status.

We believe that much of the resistance to the surgical treatment of these patients arises from a lack of understanding of how even some straightforward interventions, performed in a coordinated way, can dramatically improve a patient's life. Patients who can now move a joystick on a wheelchair or feed themselves again often have profound appreciation for this incremental increase in independence, a small but significant liberation from the prison of paralysis.

A.I. Elkwood, MD, MBA (✉)
M. Kaufman, MD, FACS • L.F. Schneider, MD
The Plastic Surgery Center, Institute for Advanced Reconstruction, 535 Sycamore Ave, Shrewsbury, NJ 07702, USA
e-mail: aelkwoodmd@theplasticsurgerycenternj.com; mkaufmanmd@theplasticsurgerycenternj.com; lschneidermd@theplasticsurgerycenternj.com

© Springer International Publishing Switzerland 2017
A.I. Elkwood et al. (eds.), *Rehabilitative Surgery*, DOI 10.1007/978-3-319-41406-5_1

This compendium represents the first interdisciplinary text for the emerging field of rehabilitative surgery, synthesizing various perspectives into a cornerstone for the rehabilitation field. The text is designed for both surgical and nonsurgical readers. An expert has written each evidence-based chapter with concise and straightforward explanations for clinicians who have no previous experience in that specialty. Specific descriptions of surgical procedures are included as well as surgical videos that can be accessed from the companion website.

Every major aspect of the reconstructive surgical treatment of these patients has been considered from a multidisciplinary vantage point, including orthopedic surgery, plastic surgery, neurosurgery, general surgery, and otolaryngology. We clearly describe and evaluate the most up-to-date and evidence-based surgeries that are currently standard of care including treatment of pressure sores, placement of feeding tubes, and upper extremity interventions to improve function and hygiene. As international leaders in the field of nerve reanimation surgery, we describe our cutting-edge protocols for the surgical treatment of severe nerve injuries, spinal cord injury (SCI), and stroke or cerebrovascular accidents (CVA). We provide a description and evidence for phrenic nerve repair to assist weaning paralyzed patients from their ventilators. Furthermore, there is the exciting potential for diaphragm muscle replacement using innervated, vascularized muscle transfers to overcome severe denervation atrophy as a result of prolonged ventilator dependency.

These patients need our help. It falls on us – their clinicians and caretakers – to do everything we can to maximize their function to help them live as well and as independently as possible.

Hamid Abdollahi and Deborah Yu

Surgical Metabolism and Nutrition in the Surgical Patient

Once an injury is sustained, the body's metabolism shifts toward a state with higher metabolic expenditure. Understanding the changes that occur in amino acid, carbohydrate, and lipid metabolism allows the physician and care team to provide optimal nutritional support for the surgical patient [1]. In a healthy adult, approximately 22–25 kcal/kg per day are required to maintain basic metabolic needs. This requirement can increase to up to 40 kcal/kg in patients that have undergone severe stress and injury [1] (Table 2.1). This stress response is triggered by the release of catecholamines and sympathetic activation. Furthermore, during the fasting state, a significant amount of protein is used to provide the substrate for gluconeogenesis in the liver leading to muscle wasting as the body enters a catabolic state [2]. The magnitude of protein catabolism is directly proportional to the severity of the injury with even elective operations and minor injuries leading to decreased protein synthesis and protein breakdown [3]. Nutritional deficits can lead to impairment of the immune system, poor tissue repair and healing, loss of muscle function, and overall increase in complications.

The goal for nutritional support in a surgical patient is to prevent and reverse the catabolic state associated with injury. It is of crucial importance to evaluate each patient's nutritional status prior to and after any surgical intervention to optimize the success of the treatment. While a detailed physical exam is extremely useful to determine nutritional status, certain lab values are helpful in establishing objective values. These studies include albumin, pre-albumin, and transferrin levels. Concentrations of serum albumin less that 3.0 g/dl are an indicator of malnutrition. Albumin has a half-life of 14–18 days, demonstrating the patient's recent nutritional status, whereas pre-albumin (half-life 3–5 days) and transferrin (half-life 7 days) may show more rapid changes in nutritional status. These serum markers can guide clinical decisions and serve as a benchmark for nutritional optimization. Furthermore, an individual's energy requirements can be measured by indirect calorimetry and trends in serum markers as well as estimated from urinary nitrogen excretion [4]. In addition to supplying sufficient calories and protein to prevent the catabolic state and allow for protein synthesis and tissue repair, some patients may require essential vitamin and mineral supplementation.

In terms of nutritional supplementation, enteral feeding is preferred over parenteral, not only based on the cost and avoidance of vascular

H. Abdollahi, MD • D. Yu, MD (✉)
The Plastic Surgery Center, Institute for Advanced Reconstruction, 535 Sycamore Ave, Shrewsbury, NJ 07702, USA
e-mail: habollahimd@theplasticsurgerycenternj.com; dyumd@theplasticsurgerycenternj.com

© Springer International Publishing Switzerland 2017
A.I. Elkwood et al. (eds.), *Rehabilitative Surgery*, DOI 10.1007/978-3-319-41406-5_2

Table 2.1 Caloric adjustments above basal energy expenditure in hypermetabolic conditions

Condition	kcal/kg/day	Adjustment above baseline energy expenditure	Grams of protein/kg/day
Normal	25	1	1
Mild stress	25–30	1.2	1.2
Moderate stress	30	1.4	1.5
Severe stress	30–35	1.6	2
Burns	35–40	2	2.5

access-associated complications but also for the benefits attained from feeding the intestine directly [5]. There are numerous routes for enteral feeding including temporary ones such as Dobhoff tubes to more permanent methods that involve surgical placement of feeding tubes (Table 2.2). Using the gastrointestinal tract prevents diminished secretory IgA production, bacterial overgrowth, and altered mucosal defenses associated with parenteral nutrition.

Patients that benefit from nutrition supplementation are those that have poor preoperative nutritional statuses [6, 7]. Healthy patients without malnutrition undergoing elective surgery can tolerate partial starvation for up to 10 days before any clinically significant protein catabolism occurs. However, in the critically ill patient, early enteral feeding has become the standard of care and has been shown to reduce both morbidity and mortality [8]. Furthermore, early intervention with supplement nutrition is favored for patients who show preoperative protein-calorie malnutrition (Table 2.3).

Indications for parenteral nutrition are limited to patients that have a contraindication in using the gastrointestinal tract or have failed enteral supplementation. It comes in two forms: total parenteral nutrition (TPN) and peripheral parenteral nutrition (PPN). TPN requires central venous access because it has a high osmolarity from high dextrose content, whereas PPN can be administered through the peripheral intravenous line because of much lower dextrose and protein concentrations. Some nutrients cannot be concentrated into the small volumes required for PPN, thereby making it inappropriate for patients with severe malnutrition [1]. PPN can be considered if central access is unavailable or it is used to augment oral nutrition. It should only be used for

Table 2.2 Common feeding routes

Access option	Comments
Nasogastric tube	Only for short-term use, increase risk of aspiration, frequently dislodged
Dobhoff tube	May use slightly longer than NG tube, although it is a temporary feeding route. Decrease risk of aspiration due to post-pyloric placement. More challangening to place than NG tube. Easily dislodged
Percutaneous endoscopic gastrostomy (PEG)	Placed via endoscope, can be used for longer periods of time. Aspiration risks due to pre-pyloric placement. Can have complications related to placement and site leaks
Surgical gastrostomy	Requires surgery, procedure may allow placement of extended duodenal/jejunal feeding port which allow for gastric decompression and post-pyloric feeding
Fluoroscopic gastrostomy	Blind placement using needle and T-prongs to anchor to the stomach, can thread smaller catheter through gastrostomy into duodenum/jejunum under fluoroscopy
PEG-jejunal tube	Jejunal placement with regular endoscope is operator dependent, jejunal tube often dislodges retrograde, two-stage procedure with PEG placement, followed by fluoroscopic conversion with jejunal feeding tube through PEG
Surgical jejunostomy	Requires surgery, allows for post-pyloric feeds, less risk of aspiration

short periods after which TPN should be considered. Complications related to parenteral nutrition include sepsis from catheter site infection, cholestasis and gallstone formation as well as intestinal atrophy leading to impaired gut immunity, bacterial overgrowth, and reduced IgA production [1]. The best way to avoid these complications is to feed enterally whenever possible.

Table 2.3 Comparison of tube feed products

Product	Caloric density (kcal/ml)	Protein (%kcal)	Features
Crucial	1.5	25	Promotes absorption and tolerance in critically ill patients with GI dysfunction
Diabetisource AC	1.2	20	For patients with diabetes or stress-induced hyperglycemia
Glucerna 1.2	1.2	20	Nutrition for glycemic control
Impact	1	22	Supports immune defense in patients at risk for infections
Jevity 1.2	1.2	18.5	18 g of dietary fiber/L
Optimental	1	20.5	For malabsorptive conditions
Pivot 1.5	1.5	25	Very high-protein calorically dense for metabolic stress
Peptamen 1.5	1.5	18	High-caloric GI formula
Perative	1.3	20.5	Peptide-based semi-elemental protein for easier absorption
Promote	1	25	For patients with lower calorie needs but higher protein needs

Table was adapted from the original and provide the full AMA citation, used by permission

Inflammation and Injury

In order to provide the optimal care and surgical treatment, we must approach and understand the patient on a variety of levels, whether it is related to the molecular level of injury and its related systemic response or to the metabolism involved in healing. All aspects must be considered to achieve the best outcome. Injury to the patient results in an inflammatory process that is triggered on a local level. Inflammation describes the process in which fluid and circulating leukocytes accumulate in the extravascular tissue [1]. It describes not only the localized effects but also the triggered systemic response. The inflammatory response is closely associated with healing and repair and therefore closely interrelated to every aspect of surgery.

Inflammation is fundamentally a protective response that allows for removal of harmful agents and cellular debris as well as repair damage. However, excess inflammation can be pathological and harmful. The initiation, maintenance, and termination of inflammation are highly complex and coordinated process mediated by a myriad of cells as well as cytokines.

Cytokines mediate a broad range of cellular activities and function locally at the site of injury to promote wound healing and eradicate infection [8–12]. Cytokines can have both proinflammatory and anti-inflammatory actions, and their balance is a well-coordinated system. Some of the important cytokines involved in this process include tumor necrosis factor (TNF), interleukins, and interferon.

The release of cytokines from damaged cells not only plays a role on a local level but also can trigger a systemic response. This can induce a response from the central nervous system via the hypothalamic-pituitary-adrenal axis in the form of released hormones [1]. The two principle hormones that are involved are glucocorticoids and catecholamines. During injury, there is an increase in the production of cortisol, which plays an important role in decreasing the inflammatory process and limiting the harmful aspect of inflammation [13–15]. Catecholamine release in the form of epinephrine and norepinephrine activates increased cellular metabolism throughout the body and mobilization of glucose via glycogenolysis, gluconeogenesis, lipolysis, and ketogenesis. The catecholamine release also helps to reestablish and maintain homeostasis [16]. Critically ill patients who suffer from severe stress often have insulin resistance leading to hyperglycemia [17]. Hyperglycemia during these periods often leads to increased morbidity and mortality. Tight management of blood sugars has been shown to decrease complications [18].

Wound Healing

All tissue heals in four divided phases, which can overlap. These four phases are (1) hemostasis/inflammation, (2) cellular migration, (3) proliferation, and (4) remodeling. The first step in the process consists of the initial injury leading to a disruption of tissue integrity. This triggers platelet aggregation in order to form a clot and the release of a variety of growth factors and cytokines from the platelet granules. Furthermore, the fibrin clot serves as the scaffold for the migration inflammatory cells, including polymorphonuclear leukocytes (neutrophils) and monocytes [19].

Neutrophils are the first cells to enter the wound and peak at 24–48 h. Their role is to remove bacteria and tissue debris as well as to release further inflammatory cytokines (Fig. 2.1). Following the

neutrophils, the second kind of inflammatory cell to migrate to the wound is the macrophage. These cells have the highest concentration in the wound at 48–96 h and participate in wound debridement as well as the release of further cytokines and growth factors, which regulate cell proliferation, matrix deposition, and angiogenesis [20, 21].

The proliferative phase occurs from day 4 to 12. It is during this time that tissue continuity is reestablished. Fibroblasts are the main cell involved during this phase. The fibroblasts produce collagen and participate in wound contraction. Endothelial cells are also present and partake in angiogenesis. Collagen formation plays an important role in the maturation of the wound. Initially, there is a predominance of type III collagen, which is eventually transformed into type I during the remodeling phase [19].

Maturation and remodeling begin during the fibroblastic phase, characterized by collagen breakdown and reorganization. Several weeks after the injury, the wound reaches a plateau of collagen quantity, while the tensile strength of the wound continues to increase for several

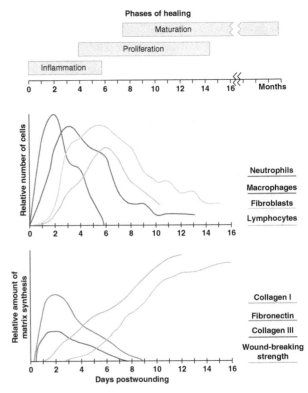

Fig. 2.1 The cellular, biochemical, and mechanical phases of wound healing (From Wound Healing Schwartz's principles of surgery, 10e, 2014)

months [22]. Scars can take up to 1 year to fully mature, but the strength of the scar never reaches their pre-injury state, usually only approaching 80% of its former state.

Epithelialization of the wound occurs within 1 day after injury. Cells at the edge of the wound proliferate and migrate until the defect is bridged. This process occurs through a loss of contact inhibition of the cells [23–26]. Re-epithelialization is complete within 48 h after incised wounds but may take significantly longer time for larger wounds.

There are certain factors that affect wound healing that one has to be cognizant of in order to counteract them. Low-oxygen states that are found in hypoxia stemming from peripheral vascular disease, radiation-induced injury, or anemia can have poor outcomes on wound healing. Fibroplasia and collagen synthesis are both decreased in hypoxic wounds. Patients that may suffer from these conditions benefit by increasing the oxygen tension in the tissue, whether it is through revascularization procedures or treatment with hyperbaric oxygen.

Steroids can also have a deleterious impact on wounds. They reduce collagen synthesis and wound strength via inhibition of the inflammatory phase of wound healing [27]. Furthermore, they hinder epithelialization and wound contraction. Vitamin A has been shown to have positive effects in mitigating the harm caused by steroids [28]. In addition, metabolic disorders can cause an increase in wound problems, with diabetes mellitus being the most common disorder encountered. Hyperglycemic states can cause decrease in inflammation, angiogenesis, and overall collagen synthesis. Patients with diabetes often suffer from vascular disorders leading to hypoxemia, confounding the problems [29]. Aggressive glycemic control can improve outcomes.

Surgical Technique

Antiseptic Technique

There are several antiseptics used to clean the skin preoperatively. A review of the current literature has demonstrated that preoperative skin with 0.5% chlorhexidine in methylated spirits was associated with lower rates of surgical-site infections following clean surgery than alcohol-based povidone-iodine paint [30]. In the Dumville et al. review, no other comparisons of skin antiseptic techniques showed statistically significant differences in surgical-site infection rates [30].

Sutures

Types

There are several types of suture materials currently manufactured. The choice of suture depends on several factors, including the amount of tension on the wound, the number of layers of closure, the depth of suture placement, the anticipated amount of edema, and the anticipated timing of suture removal [31]. The size of the suture material represents the diameter of the suture material [31]. The higher number prior to the 0, the smaller the suture. For example, 5–0 suture is smaller than 2–0 suture. If the suture does not have a "0" in the size, then the size correlates with the increasing number, i.e., size 2 suture is larger than size 1, which is larger than 0 or 2–0. The smaller the diameter of the suture, the less the tensile strength [31].

The next characteristic that must be chosen is the use of braided or multifilament suture versus single-stranded/monofilament suture. Monofilament suture encounters less resistance in the tissue and also is less likely to harbor infection-causing organisms [31]. Crushing or clamping of this suture can break or weaken the suture [31]. One must take care in tying knots with this suture as the knots can slip. Multifilament sutures are composed of several strands braided together, affording greater tensile strength and flexibility [31]. Published data have shown that absorbable braided suture has statistically significant bacterial adherence versus all other sutures [32].

Finally, the surgeon must choose between absorbable and nonabsorbable suture materials. Absorbability is classified according to the suture degradation properties [31]. Sutures that lose their tensile strength within 60 days, undergoing rapid degradation in tissues, are categorized as absorbable sutures [31]. Sutures that maintain their tensile strength greater than 60 days are considered nonabsorbable sutures [31]. Nonabsorbable sutures are not digested by the body's enzymes or hydrolyzed in the body's tissues [31]. Instead, these sutures are walled off by the body's fibroblasts [31]. These sutures are usually used in deep layers, but when used for skin closure, they must be removed postoperatively [31] (Table 2.4).

Techniques

There are several suturing techniques (Fig. 2.2). Interrupted sutures are the ones where the suture only passes across the defect or closure line once. Running or continuous sutures are the ones where

Table 2.4 Absorbable and nonabsorbable sutures

Absorbable sutures

Suture	Absorption rate
Plain gut	Absorbed by proleolytic enzymatic digestive process
Chromic gut	Absorbed by proleolytic enzymatic digestive process
Polyglactin 910 rapide (Vicryl RAPIDE)	Absorbed by hydrolysis. Essentially complete at 42 days
Poliglecaprone 25 (Monocryl)	Absorbed by hydrolysis. Complete at 91–119 days
Polyglactin 910 plus antibacterial (Vicryl Plus)	Absorbed by hydrolysis. Essentially complete at 56–70 days
Polyglactin 910 (Vicryl)	Absorbed by hydrolysis. Essentially complete at 56–70 days
Polydioxanone (PDS)	Absorbed by slow hydrolysis. Minimal until 90th day. Essentially complete by 6 months

Nonabsorbable sutures

Suture	Absorption rate
Silk	Gradual encapsulation by fibrous connective tissue
Stainless steel	Nonabsorbable
Nylon (monofilament and braided) (Ethilon and Nurolon)	Gradual encapsulation by fibrous connective tissue
Polyester fiber (Mersilene, Ethibond)	Gradual encapsulation by fibrous connective tissue
Polypropylene	Nonabsorbable

Adapted from Dunn [31]

one suture is used to close a larger area rather than several separate ones. There are also mattress sutures (vertical and horizontal) that are used to distribute tension of the suture over a greater area and help evert the wound edges to allow for an improved closure. Sutures are also described by what layer they close. Deep dermal sutures approximate the deep layer of the dermis and subcuticular sutures approximate the epidermal-dermal junction.

Complications

If sutures are left in for a prolonged period of time, "railroad track" marks can form from the suture exit holes. In cosmetically sensitive areas, sutures are removed 5–7 days after placement to avoid such types of scarring. Some sutures cause a localized reaction and small "suture abscesses" develop at the site of a suture knot. In this situation, a small pustule, about 1 mm in diameter, will form and can be easily drained with a sterile needle. These suture abscesses do not need to be treated with antibiotics. Usually, removal of the inciting agent (the suture knot) and/or drainage of the pustule is the complete treatment.

Drains

Drains are used to evacuate fluid from a potential space. That space is the result of removal of the tissue that once occupied that area or from the separation of the layers during the course of the operation. There are several types of drains (Fig. 2.3), but they perform a similar function, removing fluid through negative pressure. They are a closed suction system. They will not prevent drainage from occurring, but drains will allow the egress of fluid. Drains are usually not removed until the fluid that is draining is less than 30 ml over a 24-h period.

Surgical Complications

Infections

Surgical infections can occur for several reasons. There are several risk factors for surgical-site

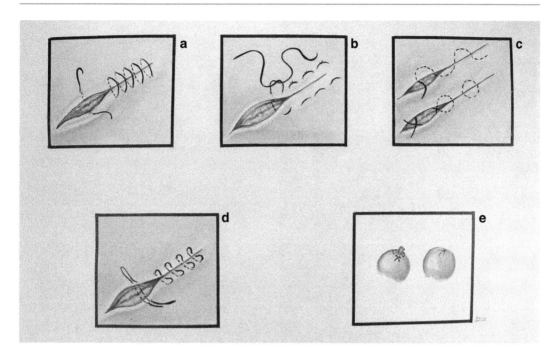

Fig. 2.2 Illustrations of various sutures. (**a**) Running suture or "baseball" suture. (**b**) Horizontal mattress suture. (**c**) Subcuticular suture. (**d**) Vertical mattress suture. (**e**) Purse string suture

infections. In the plastic surgery literature, risk factors for surgical-site infections were age greater than or equal to 50 years, body mass index greater than or equal to 30 kg/m², or operative time greater than 4.25 h [33]. After clean spinal operations, multiple other factors were noted for increased risk of surgical-site infections: trauma, a past history of diabetes, smoking, being confined to bed, in the perioperative period, mean blood sugar levels above 120 mg/dl, longer lengths of incisions, and longer hospital stay [34]. Simple skin erythema or cellulitis can often be treated with intravenous or oral antibiotics. Deeper infections or abscesses must be drained in addition to the use of antibiotics.

Wound infections manifest as erythema of the wound edges and warmth. The erythema is not isolated to around the suture exit sites, which is a normal inflammatory reaction to sutures, but instead, the erythema is in a non-patterned distribution. If the erythema is in a discrete shape or distribution, suspicion should be raised for a contact dermatitis or other allergic reaction to a product being utilized on the skin.

In the cases of an abscess, there will often be edema and thinning of the skin over the collection. The area will be fluctuant as the fluid deep to the skin is trying to drain itself. Eventually, some abscesses will spontaneously drain. The difference between a seroma and an abscess is the fluid that the cavity contains. Seromas contain serous, straw-colored to amber-colored fluid versus purulent, thick material of abscesses. Occasionally, the fibrinous exudate of a wound is mistaken for purulence. Fibrinous exudate is typically adherent to a wound edge or base, whereas purulence can be easily wiped off with a gauze or a glove. Pus also has a foul odor that fibrinous exudate may not have.

With surgical-site or wound infections, patients may become febrile and/or develop leukocytosis. Deeper infections may not be readily apparent on the skin surface, so often additional imaging must be obtained. Ultrasonography is the least invasive technique to diagnose a deeper collection. Computed tomography (CT) scans are useful in cases to distinguish the exact location and accessibility should the collection need to be

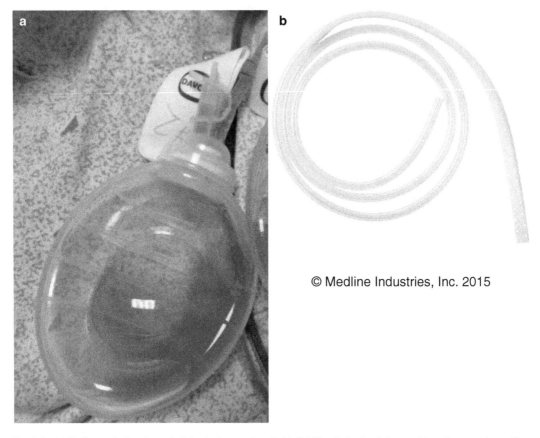

© Medline Industries, Inc. 2015

Fig. 2.3 (**a**) Bulb attached to the end of the drain to collect fluid. (**b**) Flat drain that is inserted into the wound to collect fluid

percutaneously drained. CT scans are also useful as oral contrast can be given to see if the collection has a connection to the bowel. Finally, magnetic resonance imaging (MRI) is useful in diagnosis of osteomyelitis, particularly in relation to the bone within a decubitus ulcer.

Hernias

A hernia is a defect in the fascia. Hernias develop from previous incisions or from a weakening of the fascia over time. Incisional abdominal hernias occur from the acute separation of the sutured abdominal walls in less than 1 % of the time or from chronic wound dehiscence in greater than 20 % of the time [35]. Incisional hernias are recognized more now with increased imaging

postoperatively and increased long-term follow-up [35]. There are two categories of factors that can affect incisional hernia development: surgical technique (type of incision, suture material, and suture technique) and patient-related factors (age, gender, comorbidities, exogenous toxins, and hereditary connective disease) [35]. Patients may present with a history of a bulge that is exacerbated with exercise or coughing and relieved after ceasing the activity [35]. Hernias become problematic when they become symptomatic. Symptoms of hernias include pain, change in bowel habits (constipation or diarrhea), or nausea and vomiting. Tissue such as fat, omentum, and bowel can protrude through the defect, become strangulated by the narrow opening, and become ischemic. Ultrasonography can be a helpful diagnostic tool, especially since it is noninvasive and less expensive [35]. CT or MRI scan is useful for complicated hernias or large abdominal wall defects and may be obtained preoperatively for surgical planning [35].

There is no set defect size at which incisional hernias or hernia should be repaired [35]. Once hernias become symptomatic, it is recommended that they be repaired. If the edges of the fascia in a hernia defect can be approximated without tension, then that is the initial procedure performed. Sometimes mesh, either biologic or prosthetic, is used to reinforce the closure to prevent recurrence. In some cases, the two edges of fascia can be approximated only after relaxing incisions are made lateral to the defect. In the abdomen, this procedure is called component separation, where incisions are made in the external oblique aponeurosis just lateral to the rectus [36]. In some cases, the two edges of fascia cannot be approximated, and mesh is used to bridge the defect.

Fistulas

Fistulas are epithelialized tracts that are abnormal between two epithelialized organs. The communication occurs between the gastrointestinal tract and adjacent organs in an internal fistula, whereas an external fistula describes a communication from the GI tract to the skin. Furthermore, fistulas can be categorized by the amount of their daily output. Low-output fistulas drain less than 200 cc of fluid per day compared to high-output fistulas, which drain greater than 500 cc of fluid. Their clinical manifestation can very dependent on which structures are involved such as recurrent urinary tract infection in the enterovesicular fistula and skin breakdown and excoriation in enterocutaneous fistulas. In addition, the degree of output can lead to dehydration, electrolyte imbalances, as well as malnutrition [37].

The majority of enterocutaneous fistulas arise from iatrogenic causes, with the remainder occurring as a manifestation of underlying Crohn's disease or cancer. Fistulas tend to remain open for several reasons: presence of a foreign body, radiation, infection, epithelialization, neoplasms,

or distal obstruction. All of these causes prevent normal healing of a wound. They are best diagnosed with imaging using CT scans with enteral contrast, small bowel studies with follow through, as well as fistulagrams.

In order to fix a fistula, the source must be identified to prevent recurrence. Prior to any intervention, the patient must be optimized in terms of nutrition and fluid as well as treatment of any underlying infections. Initial conservative measures are implemented to increase the chance for spontaneous closure; these include bowel rest with parenteral nutrition as well as treatment with octreotide to decrease the daily output. If conservative methods fail, surgical intervention may be required. In surgical treatment the fistula tract must completely excised in order to allow fresh adjacent tissue to approximate and close down the space [38, 39].

Marjolin's Ulcer

Nonhealing wounds should be investigated for causes of nonhealing, such as long-standing steroid use, diabetes, and infection. If a nonhealing wound is excised or debrided, the specimen should be sent for pathology as malignancy can develop within these wounds [40, 41]. Marjolin's ulcer is a rare but aggressive malignancy seen in previously traumatized and chronically inflamed skin [41]. One study reported that the majority of these squamous cell cancers were within burn scars [40]. Risk factors for the development of neoplasms after burns are healing by secondary intention, nonhealing wounds, and fragile, ulcerated scars [41]. Two variants of Marjolin's ulcers have been described: acute and chronic [41]. Acute degeneration occurs within a year with chronic degeneration after 1 year [41]. In the chronic type, the average time to malignant transformation is 35 years [41]. The most common histological type seen in Marjolin's ulcers is squamous cell carcinoma, but many different cell types can be seen [41]. Treatment of these lesions is radical excision [41]. Kerr-Valentic et al. argue the malignant degeneration can be preventable if early wound coverage is undertaken [40].

References

1. Corbett SA. Systemic response to injury and meta-bolic support. In: Brunicardi F, Andersen DK, Billiar TR, Dunn DL, Hunter JG, Matthews JB, Pollock RE, editors. Schwartz's principles of surgery. 10th ed. New York: McGraw-Hill; 2014.
2. Mitch WE, Price SR. Mechanisms activating proteolysis to cause muscle atrophy in catabolic conditions. J Ren Nutr. 2003;13:149–52.
3. Long CL, Schaffel N, Geiger J, et al. Metabolic response to injury and illness: estimation of energy and protein needs from indirect calorimetry and nitrogen balance. J Parenter Enteral Nutr. 1979;3:452.
4. Vidal-Puig A, O'Rahilly S. Metabolism. Controlling the glucose factory. Nature. 2001;413:125–6.
5. Heslin MJ, Brennan MF. Advances in perioperative nutrition: cancer. World J Surg. 2000;24:1477–85.
6. Heslin MJ, Latkany L, Leung D, et al. A prospective, randomized trial of early enteral feeding after resection of upper gastrointestinal malignancy. Ann Surg. 1997;226:567–77.
7. Abunnaja S, Cuviello A, Sanchez JA. Enteral and parenteral nutrition in the perioperative period: state of the art. Nutrients. 2013;5:608–23.
8. Khalil AA, Hall JC, Aziz FA, Price P. Tumour necrosis factor: implications for surgical patients. ANZ J Surg. 2006;76:1010–6.
9. Dinarello CA. Interleukin-1 in the pathogenesis and treatment of inflammatory diseases. Blood. 2011;117:3720–32.
10. Stylianou E, Saklatvala J. Interleukin-1. Int J Biochem Cell Biol. 1998;30:1075–9.
11. Jawa RS, Anillo S, Huntoon K, Baumann H, Kulaylat M. Interleukin-6 in surgery, trauma, and critical care part II: clinical implications. J Intensive Care Med. 2011;26:73–87.
12. Rauch I, Muller M, Decker T. The regulation of inflammation by interferons and their STATs. JAKSTAT. 2013;2:e23820. 1–13.
13. Heitzer MD, Wolf IM, Sanchez ER, Witchel SF, DeFranco DB. Glucocorticoid receptor physiology. Rev Endocr Metab Disord. 2007;8:321–30.
14. Silverman MN, Sternberg EM. Glucocorticoid regulation of inflammation and its functional correlates: from HPA axis to glucocorticoid receptor dysfunction. Ann N Y Acad Sci. 2012;1261:55–63.
15. Hardy RS, Raza K, Cooper MS. Endogenous glucocorticoids in inflammation: contributions of systemic and local responses. Swiss Med Wkly. 2012;142:w13650.
16. Wong DL, Tai TC, Wong-Faull DC, et al. Epinephrine: a short- and long-term regulator of stress and development of illness: a potential new role for epinephrine in stress. Cell Mol Neurobiol. 2012;32:737–48.
17. Van den Berghe G. How does blood glucose control with insulin save lives in intensive care? J Clin Invest. 2004;114:1187–95.
18. Sung J, Bochicchio GV, Joshi M, Bochicchio K, Tracy K, Scalea TM. Admission hyperglycemia is predictive of outcome in critically ill trauma patients. J Trauma. 2005;59:80–3.
19. Barbul A, Efron DT, Kavalukas SL. Wound healing. In: Brunicardi F, Andersen DK, Billiar TR, Dunn DL, Hunter JG, Matthews JB, Pollock RE, editors. Schwartz's principles of surgery. 10eth ed. New York: McGraw-Hill; 2014.
20. DiPietro LA. Wound healing: the role of the macrophage and other immune cells. Shock. 1995;4:233.
21. Zabel DD, Feng JJ, Scheuenstuhl H, et al. Lactate stimulation of macrophage-derived angiogenic activity is associated with inhibition of poly(ADP-ribose) synthesis. Lab Invest. 1996;74:644.
22. Levenson SM, Geever EF, Crowley LV, et al. The healing of rat skin wounds. Ann Surg. 1965;161:293.
23. Stenn KS, Depalma L. Re-epithelialization. In: Clark RAF, Hensen PM, editors. The molecular and cellular biology of wound repair. New York: Plenum; 1988. p. 321.
24. Johnson FR, McMinn RMH. The cytology of wound healing of the body surface in mammals. Biol Rev. 1960;35:364.
25. Woodley DT, Bachman PM, O'Keefe EJ. The role of matrix components in human keratinocyte re-epithelialization. In: Barbul A, Caldwell MD, Eaglstein WH, et al., editors. Clinical and experimental approaches to dermal and epidermal repair. Normal and chronic wounds. New York: Wiley-Liss; 1991. p. 129.
26. Lynch SE. Interaction of growth factors in tissue repair. In: Barbul A, Caldwell MD, Eaglstein WH, et al, editors. Clinical and experimental approaches to dermal and epidermal repair. Normal and chronic wounds. New York: Wiley-Liss; 1991:341.
27. Ehrlich HP, Hunt TK. Effects of cortisone and Vitamin A on wound healing. Ann Surg. 1968;167:324.
28. Anstead GM. Steroids, retinoids, and wound healing. Adv Wound Care. 1998;11:277.
29. Yue DK, McLennan S, Marsh M, et al. Effects of experimental diabetes, uremia, and malnutrition on wound healing. Diabetes. 1987;36:295.
30. Dumville JC, McFarlane E, Edwards P, et al. Preoperative skin antiseptics for preventing surgical wound infections after clean surgery. Cochrane Database Syst Rev. 2015;(4):CD003949.
31. Dunn DL. Ethicon wound closure manual. Ethicon, Inc. Somerville, NJ; 2005.
32. Masini BD, Stinner DJ, Waterman SM, et al. Bacterial adherence to suture materials. J Surg Educ. 2011;68:101–4.
33. Wincour S, Martinez-Jorge J, Habermann E, et al. Early surgical site infection following tissue expander breast reconstruction with or without Acellular Dermal Matrix: National Benchmarking Using National Surgical Quality Improvement Program. Arch Plast Surg. 2015;42:194–200.

34. Saeedinia S, Nouri M, Azarhomayoun A, et al. The incidence and risk factors for surgical site infection after clean spinal operations: a prospective cohort study and review of the literature. Surg Neurol Int. 2015;6:154.

35. Schumpelick V, Junge K, Klinge U, et al. Incisional hernia: pathogenesis presentation and treatment. Dtsch Arztebl. 2006;103:A2553–8.

36. Heller L, McNichols CH, Ramirez OOM. Component separations. Semin Plast Surg. 2012;26:25–8.

37. Tavakkoli A, Ashley SW, Zinner MJ. Small intestine. In: Brunicardi F, Andersen DK, Billiar TR, Dunn DL, Hunter JG, Matthews JB, Pollock RE, editors. Schwartz's principles of surgery. 10th ed. New York: McGraw-Hill; 2014.

38. Chamberlain RS, Kaufman HL, Danforth DN. Enterocutaneous fistula in cancer patients: etiology, management, outcome, and impact on further treatment. Am Surg. 1998;64:1204–11.

39. Owen RM, Love TP, Perez SD, et al. Definitive surgical treatment of enterocutaneous fistula: outcomes of a 23-year experience. Arch Surg. 2012;15:1–9.

40. Kerr-Valentic MA, Samini K, Rohlen BH, et al. Marjolin's ulcer: modern analysis of an ancient problem. Plast Reconstr Surg. 2009;123:184–91.

41. Copcu E. Marjolin's ulcer: a preventable complication of burns? Plast Reconstr Surg. 2009;124:156e–64.

42. Collins N. Nutrition 411: selecting the right tube feeding formula. Ostomy Wound Manag. 2011;57:2.

Part II

Anesthesia

Matthew Klein

Introduction

The field of rehabilitative surgery has grown considerably over the past decade. Care of the neurologically injured patient previously entailed providing support and comfort care. We now aim to restore functionality for these patients and repair their injuries. Patients with brain and spinal cord injury (SCI) have unique challenges because of their injuries. This chapter will discuss the anesthetic management of these patients, including preoperative evaluation and preparation, intraoperative management, and postoperative care, including acute pain management.

SCI is associated with reduced life expectancy among survivors. Mortality is highest in the first year. After the first year, life expectancy is approximately 90% of normal [1–3]. Higher level of injury, i.e., cervical or high thoracic, and advanced age are negative risk factors. The most common causes of death are pulmonary complications followed by cardiovascular events [1, 2]. The rate of suicide is also higher than in the general population [3].

Autonomic Dysreflexia

Autonomic dysreflexia (AD), seen in SCI above T6, is a manifestation of the loss of coordinated autonomic response to stimuli on cardiac function and vascular tone [4, 5]. Exaggerated sympathetic response to stimulation below the level of the injury leads to diffuse vasoconstriction and hypertension. A compensatory parasympathetic response above the level of the injury leads to vasodilation and bradycardia. This does not allow for enough "runoff" to reduce elevated blood pressure. Lesions lower than T6 do not have this problem as the neurologically intact splanchnic vascular bed provides compensatory dilatation. Although any stimulation below this level can cause this syndrome, typical sources include bladder distention, stool impaction, pressure ulcers, bone injury, or even positioning on the operating room (OR) table [6]. It can also complicate the peripartum period.

Symptomatic manifestations include headache, diaphoresis, elevated blood pressure, flushing, nausea, and blurred vision. Severity ranges from asymptomatic to severe cardiac and/or neurological events. The higher the level of SCI is, the greater the frequency and severity of the attacks. Acute management of AD attacks involves:

1. Monitoring blood pressure (BP) and heart rate (HR).
   - Prompt reduction in BP and correction of HR abnormalities with short-acting agents

M. Klein, MD
Monmouth Pain Care, 279 Third Avenue, Suite 601, Long Branch, NJ 07740, USA
e-mail: mskleinmd@yahoo.com

© Springer International Publishing Switzerland 2017
A.I. Elkwood et al. (eds.), *Rehabilitative Surgery*, DOI 10.1007/978-3-319-41406-5_3

- Common agents include:
  - Nitrates (1″ Nitropaste®)
  - Enalapril (1.25 mg IV)
  - Sublingual nifedipine (10 mg)
  - IV hydralazine (10 mg)
2. Reverse Trendelenburg positioning (placing the head of the bed below the foot) to induce orthostatic hypotension.
3. Look for and correct noxious stimuli.

Preoperative Evaluation

As with all patients, preoperative evaluation begins with a systemic analysis, with special emphasis on the areas of increased risk in SCI (Table 3.1). These patients may have been disabled for many years, requiring an anesthesiologist to have a higher level of vigilance for earlier onset of disease states. SCI patients often have undergone multiple surgical procedures to address urological issues. Integument and gastrointestinal pathology may occur at a higher rate than in the general population.

Cardiovascular System

Patients with high spinal lesions lack innervation to the sympathetic splanchnic outflow. Lack of basal sympathetic tone to peripheral blood vessels results in vasodilation and postural hypotension. This is modulated over time by an increase in the renin–angiotensin system compensation resulting in a higher capacitance vessel tone. Intravascular volume is often decreased in these patients, and it is critical to ensure adequate volume resuscitation prior to induction of anesthesia. In addition, they have inadequate norepinephrine release that often magnifies the hypotension on induction.

Table 3.1 Expected functional recovery following complete spinal cord injury by spinal level

Spinal level	Activities of daily living	Mobility/locomotion
C1–C4	Feeding possible with balanced forearm orthoses Computer access by tongue, breath, voice controls Weight shifts with power tilt and recline chair Mouth stick use	Operate power chair with tongue, chin, or breath controller
C5	Drink from cup, feed with static splints and setup Oral/facial hygiene, writing, typing with equipment Dressing upper body possible Side-to-side weight shifts	Propel chair with hand rim projections short distances on smooth surfaces Power chair with hand controller
C6	Feed, dress upper body with setup Dressing lower body possible Forward weight shifts	Bed mobility with equipment Level surface transfers with assistance Propel indoors with coated hand rims
C7	Independent feeding, dressing, bathing with adaptive equipment, built-up utensils	Independent bed mobility, level surface transfers Wheelchair use outdoors (power chair for school or work)
C8	Independent in feeding, dressing, bathing Bowel and bladder care with setup	Propel chair, including curbs and wheelies Wheelchair-to-car transfers
T1	Independent in all self-care	Transfer from floor to wheelchair
T2–L1		Stand with braces for exercise
L2		Potential for swing to gait with long leg braces indoors Use of forearm crutches
L3		Potential for community ambulation Potential for ambulation with short leg braces
L4–S1		Potential for ambulation without assistive devices

This article was published in Randall [24]. Copyright 2000 Elsevier

As mentioned above, lesions above T6 interrupt the cardiac accelerator fibers resulting in bradycardia and a diminution in inotropy. As a result, patients present with high vagal tone with conduction defects, heart block, and arrhythmias. A preoperative electrocardiogram (ECG) should be routine regardless of the patient's age.

Respiratory System

Respiratory compromise is common not only in patients with lesions above C6, the level of innervation of the diaphragm, but in those with thoracic lesions as well. In thoracic lesions, abdominal muscle activity may be absent and intercostal activity, minimal. This impairs coughing, deep breathing, and clearing secretions [7]. Upper accessory muscles, e.g., the sternocleidomastoid and trapezius, may play a larger role in breathing. Gastric and bowel distention from autonomic dysfunction may further impair diaphragmatic excursion and increase atelectasis, as well as increased risk of regurgitation and aspiration. Kyphoscoliosis, an abnormal curvature of the spine in both a coronal and sagittal plane, is common in these patients and may aggravate these issues. Pulmonary function tests (PFTs) often show a decrease in vital capacity, functional residual capacity, and expiratory flows as well as a decrease in PaO_2 and increase in dead space and $PaCO_2$ secondary to the increase in atelectasis. Management may include placement of a nasogastric tube to decompress bowel, chest physiotherapy, and tracheal suctioning.

Genitourinary System

Chronic infection and colonization of the urinary tract develops early in the spinal cord-injured patient. Chronic infection leads to proteinuria, hypocalcemia, and renal insufficiency. A main cause of death in chronic spinal cord lesion patients is renal failure [8]. Patients also develop amyloidosis and hypoalbuminemia secondary to albuminuria. This can lead to significant peripheral edema and skin breakdown. These patients often need prophylactic corticosteroid administration secondary to adrenal cortical dysfunction. Adrenocorticotropic hormone (ACTH) levels can be measured to assist in monitoring adrenal function [11].

Chronic renal insufficiency also leads to a decrease in hemopoietin hormone production causing chronic anemia. This may require blood transfusions prior to surgery. The resultant renal insufficiency can also result in electrolyte and acid–base imbalances often exacerbated by treatment for constipation with enemas, diuretics for peripheral edema, and low-salt diets.

Calcium and potassium imbalances can put the patient at risk for cardiac arrhythmias if not corrected preoperatively [9].

Musculoskeletal System

SCI patients develop osteoporosis and muscle wasting very quickly after injury [10]. Hypocalcemia from renal insufficiency accelerates mobilization of calcium from bones resulting in a high propensity for pathologic fractures from simple movement or positioning on an operating room table. Pressure injury to the skin below the level of the SCI occurs commonly. Decubitus ulcers can develop after 2 h of continuous pressure on a skin area. The chronic anemia and hypoalbuminemia of renal insufficiency make para- and quadriplegic patients even more susceptible to this kind of injury. Secondary osteomyelitis develops at these areas, particularly the ischium, sacrum, and heels. Ulceration at the site of possible injection, fever, elevated white count, or untreated infection are contraindications to regional anesthetic block [11]. Skeletal muscle spasm can also occur after a stimulus below the level of the spinal cord lesion. This involves a spinal reflex arc. This can occur intraoperatively and interfere with the surgical procedure.

Thermal Regulation

The SCI patient is poikilothermic, having a body temperature that varies with the temperature of the surroundings below the level of the spinal cord injury with loss of autonomic control cutaneous vasoactivity, sweating, and shivering. These patients are particularly susceptible to the changes in ambient temperature in an OR. They are not able to efficiently get rid of heat in a warm OR or develop hypothermia quickly in a cold OR [12].

This requires close monitoring of temperature with either an esophageal or bladder temp probe. Forced air warmers and warmed intravenous (IV) fluids should be immediately available.

Psychological Issues

Depression is common in these patients, particularly at the time of the acute lesion. Emotional strains are compounded by the work of rehabilitation economic pressures and recognition of their permanent handicap. Frequently, these problems are compounded by alcohol and drug dependence. It is important to elicit any drug or alcohol use in the preoperative interview as well as any herbal or homeopathic remedies [13].

Intraoperative Considerations

Intraoperative Monitoring

Routine monitoring, including ECG, BP, pulse oximetry, and EtCO$_2$, as well as temperature measurement, should be used on all cases. A urinary catheter is necessary as these patients have no control of bladder function. More invasive monitors, including intra-arterial monitors, should be used if there are expected fluid shifts, a prolonged case, or a patient with a history of severe autonomic hyperreflexia because blood pressure changes may be unpredictable. This also allows for regular measurement of hematocrit, electrolytes, and arterial blood gases.

Central venous pressure monitoring also is recommended when significant fluid shifts are expected because urine output in these patients is not always a good marker of fluid status. It also allows for vasoactive drugs to be given directly into the central circulation to treat episodes of hyper- and hypotension.

Anesthetic Considerations

Patients with SCI require anesthesia for procedures because of the occurrence of autonomic hyperreflexia in otherwise insensitive areas (Box 3.1). It is not recommended to perform surgery on these patients, including common urinary tract work (calculi, fistulas, or bladder work), debridement of decubitus ulcers, or even minor procedures, without an anesthetic that blocks reflexes at the spinal cord level. An episode of hyperreflexia can provoke life-threatening hypertension and bradycardia. Furthermore, topical anesthesia does not block afferent transmission to the spinal cord. Attempting to perform a procedure under inadequate, local anesthesia in a patient with SCI may be extremely dangerous and should not be attempted [14].

General Anesthesia

Induction

Induction of anesthesia in these patients is full of challenges. Not enough anesthesia can induce a hyperreflexic crisis, but too much and profound hypotension and tachycardia ensues. A slow and gentle induction in these patients is required along with the availability of agents to treat wide swings in blood pressure. It is often valuable to monitor BP with an arterial line in these patients so beat-to-beat changes can be treated quickly. Direct-acting agents, like epinephrine, norepinephrine, and phenylephrine, and adequate fluid

> **Box 3.1: Common Symptoms and Signs of AD**
> - Headache
> - Hypertension (note: comparatively low-resting blood pressure in SCI)
> - Flushing/blotching of skin above level of injury
> - Sweating above level of injury
> Reproduced from *Autonomic dysreflexia: a medical emergency*, J Bycroft, I S Shergill, E A L Choong, N Arya, P J R Shah, 81, p. 232–235, 2004

resuscitation should be used. Indirect-acting agents such as ephedrine should be avoided [15]. Depolarizing paralytics, e.g., succinylcholine, should not be used in the first 18 months after injury, as it can cause release of large amounts of potassium into the bloodstream causing ventricular fibrillation. A defasciculating dose does not mitigate this risk. Non-depolarizing agents should be used exclusively in these patients [16].

These patients remain at high risk of aspiration during anesthesia and should always be considered "a full stomach." As discussed earlier, they often do not have adequate respiratory function and reserve and, under anesthesia, are unable to develop adequate inspiratory pressures. For this reason, laryngeal mask airways should be avoided. Endotracheal intubation is the preferred method of protecting the airway. A rapid sequence induction with a non-depolarizing agent, Sellick maneuver (cricoid pressure), and preoxygenation is standard. Awake intubation is an option in patients with an unstable neck or a fixed and fused spine. Newer intubation tools such as video laryngoscopes also have a role. Asleep intubation with a fiberoptic scope is another safe and useful way to secure the airway. The key is a thorough and careful airway examination.

Maintenance

Inhalational anesthetics, particularly agents such as desflurane and sevoflurane, allow for careful titration to stimulus. Maintaining adequate levels of anesthesia allows for attenuation of hypertensive response to stimulus. This often means keeping the patient "deep" until the end of the operation. The choice of inhalational anesthetic is dependent on the underlying hemodynamics of the patient and comorbidities. Renal disease is common in patients with SCI; avoiding sevoflurane in these patients would be appropriate. On the other hand, desflurane can cause tachycardia in therapeutic doses, making hemodynamic control more difficult. Narcotics should be used judiciously in these patients both intra- and postoperatively as they contribute to ileus, which is already common in these patients. One approach to pain management is the use of multimodal therapy, including intravenous (IV) nonsteroidal anti-

inflammatory drugs, IV acetaminophen, steroids, gabapentins, and judicious use of narcotics.

This helps speed return of bowel function and prevention of ileus.

Use of non-depolarizing muscle relaxants is important to prevent mass muscle reflex occurring during abdominal surgery and facilitates mechanical ventilation in a patient with limited functional reserve capacity. This helps with pulmonary toilet and helps to prevent hypercarbia, atelectasis, and respiratory fatigue in patients with limited reserve [17]. However, mechanical ventilation causes diminished preload by impeding venous return to the heart contributing to the hypotension from the inhalation anesthetics. This is best treated with increased fluids and repairing preload [18].

Increased bleeding is noted in these patients, even in the face of normal clotting parameters. This may be related to the loss of sympathetic tone in arterioles and smaller venules. Hypertensive responses will increase this bleeding, and early transfusion is recommended [13]. Integument protection and temperature control are also critical in these patients. They are far more prone to decubitus ulcers and skin degradation or abrasion. In addition, temperature regulation is significantly more difficult to control in these patients without any compensatory vasoconstriction or dilatation, even if depressed by anesthesia. Forced air warming of these patients as well as using warmed IV fluids can help. The key is temperature monitoring as overenthusiastic warming can lead to hyperthermia [15].

Emergence

Because these patients are being kept "deep" to avoid blood pressure swings during the procedure, it is important to have a controlled emergence and loading of adequate amounts of narcotic to prevent a hypertensive crisis on emergence. The challenge remains to weigh the return of adequate respiratory function [15]. The ability to clear secretions, adequate tidal volume, and minute ventilation all contribute to the decision of when to extubate. The right balance between residual narcotic, inhalation anesthesia, and muscle relaxant all make the decision to extubate often a difficult one.

Spinal and Epidural Versus Regional Anesthesia

Spinal and epidural anesthesia have been used successfully in patients with SCI without any adverse effects on their injury [14]. There is no evidence that it worsens the neurological state of a chronic and stable spinal cord injury. Peripheral nerve blocks can be used as well in patients with nerve injuries, both of the lower and upper extremities. As we have already discussed, the greatest challenge with these patients is their autonomic hyperreflexia. One of the best ways to prevent this is to block the afferent pathways at the level of the spinal cord, so the reflex loop is cut. Both epidural and subarachnoid blocks can achieve this reliably, as opposed to topical or local anesthesia that does not impact the afferent loop at all. Spinal anesthesia is particularly useful in blocking stimulus at the sacral roots, commonly stimulated in urological procedures. Lumbar epidural anesthesia does not provide consistently reliable relief at the sacral levels but can be more effective at higher levels and is slowly titratable to the required level [19].

The respiratory and cardiac difficulties that are the hallmark of general anesthesia are often easier to manage under a regional block. These blocks also provide good muscle relaxation with the use of paralytics. For abdominal operations, an epidural needs to be used in conjunction with a general anesthetic for patient's comfort and safety. The use of epidural or spinal narcotics also helps to block opiate receptors that inhibit autonomic reflexes.

Regional anesthesia is not without its challenges. It's often difficult to determine the level of the block because of the sensory deficit so it is difficult to ascertain if block is at an appropriate level to sufficiently counteract autonomic reflexes until the procedure starts. A test dose through the epidural is difficult to evaluate for subarachnoid injection and intravascular injection putting the patient at risk for total spinal and hemodynamic instability.

Neuraxial anesthetics result in often complete sympathetic blockade, making them difficult to manage in patients with SCI who are often hypovolemic, anemic, brady- or tachycardic, and hemodynamically unstable. Patients will typically need fluid resuscitation and vasoactive agents immediately available. It is also often technically difficult to do neuraxial anesthesia in these patients. They often have integumentary issues like decubitus ulcers and excoriations on the lumbar spine area, muscle spasm, and distortion of the vertebral column. Osteoporosis and previous spinal fusion can also be a problem along with difficulty in positioning.

Spinal and epidural anesthesia can be very effective in preventing autonomic hyperreflexia but can be problematic. Assessment of anesthetic level can be difficult; in addition, a test dose during epidural anesthesia is not useful. Technical difficulties are common. Vertebral column deformities, surgery, and infection may make access to CSF difficult [14].

Regional anesthesia has little or no role in the care of spinal cord-injured patients. It neither blunts an autonomic hyperreflexive response nor provides analgesia to an already denervated area.

Treatment of Autonomic Hyperreflexia

Autonomic hyperreflexia needs to be treated immediately and aggressively as soon as it occurs. It can cause increased morbidity and mortality both intraoperatively and postoperatively (Box 3.2). Stroke remains the second most common cause of death in these patients [20]. Treatment starts with the removal of the precipitating stimulus. This may require deepening the level of general anesthesia, raising the level of an epidural, or placing a catheter to empty the bladder. The underlying cause must be identified and treated. Pharmacologic agents should be used simultaneously to lower the blood pressure until the inciting cause is

- Urological
  - Bladder distension, urinary tract infection, urological procedures (e.g., cystoscopy, urodynamics), and genital stimulation (including assisted ejaculation)
- Gastrointestinal
  - Rectal distension, anorectal conditions, anorectal procedures, and acute abdomen
- Musculoskeletal
  - Fractures, dislocation, and heterotopic ossification
- Others
  - Skin problems (e.g., ulceration, infection), pregnancy, and labor
    Reproduced from *Autonomic dysreflexia: a medical emergency*, J Bycroft, I S Shergill, E A L Choong, N Arya, P J R Shah, 81, p. 232–235, 2004

identified. The agents should be easily administered, rapid in onset, and short in duration of action as well as easily titratable.

- *Hydralazine* [21]
  - Very useful agent in this scenario
  - Pure arteriolar vasodilator, with quick onset and easily titratable
  - Often associated with reflex tachycardia that helps alleviate the bradycardia
  - Dosed in 5–20 mg IV
- *Enalapril*
  - ACE inhibitor that dilates blood vessels by inhibiting the conversion of angiotensin I to angiotensin II (vasoconstrictor)
  - Causes a gentle vasodilation generally without a reflex tachycardia
  - Dosed in increments of 1.25 mg, up to 5 mg IV
- *Nitroprusside*
  - Direct arteriolar and venous vasodilator, easily titratable and always effective
  - Requires an arterial line for titration
  - Prolonged administration can result in cyanide toxicity
- *Clevidipine*
  - Intravenous calcium channel blocking infusion
  - Arteriolar vasodilator
  - Start with doses of 1–2 mg/h and titrate up to 1 mg/h every 90 s until desired BP
- *Nifedipine*
  - Also calcium channel blocker that can be used sublingually as well as orally
  - Rapid onset and short duration of action
  - Can also be used prophylactically when given prior to a procedure
- *Labetalol*
  - Commonly used antihypertensive, but its role in this situation is limited because bradycardia from beta-blocker effect can make the reflex bradycardia from autonomic hyperreflexia worse

Special Cases: Peripheral Nerve Reconstruction

When performing surgery for peripheral nerve reconstruction, there are a few considerations from an anesthetic perspective. Frequently, the surgeons will use intraoperative nerve monitoring, and care must be taken not to interfere with the signal. This means limited use of neuromuscular blocking agents for intubation. Due to muscle spasm, rigidity, previous surgery, or injury, these patients often have a difficult airway, and succinylcholine is the muscle relaxant of choice. A limited dose of a non-depolarizing muscle relaxant can be used as long as it has worn off before nerve monitoring commences. Inhalation anesthetics provide amnesia, analgesia, and hypnosis but need to be kept to less than half-MAC, standard dosing measure of inhalation anesthetics, to avoid interference with neuromuscular monitoring. Total intravenous anesthesia (TIVA) can either be used alone or in conjunction with small doses of inhalation agents. Often the surgeon requests limited movement on emergence to prevent injuring a fresh nerve repair.

Suctioning the airway while the patient is still deep and ensuring adequate analgesia when awakening help reduce "bucking" and straining on the endotracheal tube.

Postoperative Considerations

Postanesthesia Care

In the postanesthesia care unit, the patient still remains at risk for autonomic hyperreflexia. Care must be taken to prevent bladder distention and distended rectum.

The biggest concern remains in the respiratory system. Inadequate respiration can cause atelectasis and hypoxia. Inability to handle secretions is common in this patient population who often require suctioning [14]. It is important to insure that all muscle relaxants are reversed and patients meet all criteria prior to extubation. Frequently these patients need prolonged ventilation after major surgery. Do not hesitate to leave the patient intubated if it is not clear that he or she can protect his or her airway, clear secretions, and adequately ventilate.

Long-Term Care

Frequent episodes of autonomic hyperreflexia can be managed with nifedipine as well as removing the causative stimulus [22]. Occasionally, cordectomy or neurectomy of pudendal or pelvic nerves is necessary. Selective dorsal rhizotomy can relieve spasticity in intractable cases [23]. Bilateral paravertebral blocks can also be used to block the response. Since bladder distention is the most common cause of autonomic hyperreflexia, efforts should be directed to relieving and preventing this.

Acute Pain Management

The postoperative pain management of these patients starts with a thorough history of pain management medications and muscle relaxants as well as all medications of which the patient does not tolerate the side effects. Some narcotics are better tolerated than others and this varies from patient to patient. This is particularly important in these patients who often have problems with ileus secondary to denervation or are on narcotics and other medicines preoperatively that slow bowel motility. A thorough history of the pain medicines, both narcotic medications and those used to treat neuropathic pain, that the patient is already on preoperatively is critical to knowing the patient's baseline need for pain medication and muscle relaxants. For example, it would be an error to put a patient on what appears to be an appropriate amount of pain medicine for the procedure and then realize the patient takes more than that dose at home prior to the procedure. It is important to understand the patient's chronic pain needs before treating acute pain.

When thinking about acute pain management in patients with SCI or nerve damage, it is important to think first about multimodal therapy [23]. This is the approach of using nonnarcotic analgesics, muscle relaxants, and anti-inflammatory medications to reduce the amount of narcotic that is required to keep a patient comfortable. Narcotics can commonly cause nausea, ileus, and dysphoria and often require larger doses when chronically used to release pain. The short-term addiction potential is small when used to relieve pain but can create dependency over time.

When thinking about multimodal therapy, we use different medications that work on different areas of the nociceptive pathways. Below is a list of some of the drugs that can be used and suggested doses. These drugs are meant to be used in combination, reflecting a larger goal in pain management.

- *Acetaminophen*
  - Mechanism thought to be inhibition of COX2 enzyme centrally
  - No local anti-inflammatory effects peripherally
  - Administered IV or orally
    - IV dose is more efficacious immediately post-op in the face of poor GI motility and absorption.

- IV can reduce narcotic requirements of 40–60 % in most patients when used on a regular basis as opposed to as needed.
- After 48–72 h, transition to oral doses.
  - Dosage and safety concerns
    - Up to 4 g/day in patients with normal liver function.
    - Dosage reduced in patients with impaired liver function demonstrated by elevated bilirubin or prolonged PT in the face of no anticoagulation.
    - Care needs to be taken to consider other combination agents (Percocet, Lortab, etc.) that contain acetaminophen when calculating the total dose.
    - We recommend not using combination agents and giving acetaminophen around the clock to a total of 4 g/day and supplement with narcotics as needed.
- *Nonsteroidal anti-inflammatory drugs (NSAIDs)*
  - Peripheral anti-inflammatory effect.
  - Analgesic effects both centrally and peripherally.
  - They work mainly by inhibiting cyclooxygenases (COX1 and COX2).
  - Side effects
    - Increase bleeding by inhibiting platelet aggregation
    - One of the leading causes of GI bleeding from ulcers and erosive gastritis
    - Cause acute renal failure if used in the face of impaired renal function or dehydration, particularly in the elderly
    - Important to follow the BUN and creatinine tests and keep the patients well hydrated
  - Despite these drawbacks, extremely efficacious in the treatment of acute pain in the perioperative setting
  - Multiple oral versions of these drugs with different strengths and duration of actions as well as different preferences for COX1 or COX2 receptors
  - IV formulations used in pain management
    - Ketorolac (Toradol).
      - Inexpensive agent
      - Duration of action of 4–6 h and dosed q6 h

  - Not recommended to be used for more than 5 days.
- Other IV NSAIDs are diclofenac and naproxen.
  - Similar concerns and varying degrees of COX1 vs. COX2 effects
- NSAIDs, in combination with acetaminophen, provide most of the narcotic dose reduction in multimodal therapy.
- *Corticosteroids*
  - Reduce inflammation at the site of injury
  - Reduce concentration of cytokines and other mediators of pain in the inflammatory reaction
  - Single dose at the time of the procedure or a short course after a procedure
- *GABA analogs*: *gabapentin and pregabalin*
  - Used to treat neuropathic or "burning" pain
    - All pain from injury, particularly nerve injury, has a component arising from the nerve itself.
    - Possibly works through an inhibitory effect on nerve transmission.
    - Evidence that using these agents in multimodal therapy reduces the incidence of chronic pain syndromes after acute pain episodes.
- Ketamine
  - Works through the NMDA receptor
  - Both dissociative and analgesic
  - Occasionally used in low doses intraoperatively to reduce narcotic requirements
  - Usually 0.5 mg/kg/h loading and 0.1 mg/kg/h infusion

Narcotic use in these patients is frequently required. A background level is obtained by using a long-acting agent, whether by the oral route or as a patch supplemented by as needed doses of IV or oral agents. A patient-controlled analgesia pump can be used with morphine or dilaudid to allow for pain control and determination of the patient's narcotic requirements. The dose of the long-acting agents can be adjusted to reflect additional requirements and converted to oral form or weaned as the patient improves. A background of multimodal therapy reduces the narcotic requirement significantly, making fewer complications and higher patient satisfaction.

Summary

Anesthesia for rehabilitative surgery requires taking into account the unique challenges of SCI. The loss of internal autonomic function can cause wide blood pressure swings as well as exaggerated response to a severed spinal cord reflex loop. These patients also present positioning problems secondary to contractures, previous surgeries, and muscle spasm. They are often dehydrated with both chronic and acute renal problems, including infection and calculi.

Chronic pain syndromes are common in these patients, who are frequently on narcotics preoperatively that need to be considered in determining their intra- and postoperative pain regimen. Temperature measurement and regulation while these patients are under anesthesia can be a challenge as they are poikilothermic.

References

1. National Spinal Cord Injury Statistical Center, Birmingham, AL. Annual report for the model spinal cord injury care system. Birm; 2005.
2. Frankel HL, Coll JR, Charlifue SW, et al. Long term survival in spinal cord injury: a fifty year investigation. Spinal Cord. 1998;36:266.
3. Hagen EM, Lie SA, Rekand T, et al. Mortality after traumatic spinal cord injury: 50 years of follow-up. J Neurol Neurosurg Psych. 2010;81:368–73.
4. Bycroft J, Shergill IS, Chung EA, et al. Autonomic dysreflexia: a medical emergency. Postgrad Med J. 2005;81:232–5.
5. Karlsson AK. Autonomic dysreflexia. Spinal Cord. 1999;37:383–91.
6. McKinley WO, Jackson AB, Cardenas DD, De Vivo MJ. Long term medical complications after traumatic spinal cord injury: a regional model system analysis. Arch Phys Med Rehab. 1999;80:1402–10.
7. Bellucci CH, Wollner J, Gregorini F, et al. Acute spinal cord injury- do ambulatory patients need urodynamic investigations? J Urol. 2013;189:1369–73.
8. Chiodo AE, Scelza WM, Kirshblum SC, et al. Spinal cord injury medicine. 5. Long-term Medical Issues and Health Maintenance. Arch Phys Med Rehabil. 2007;88:S76–83.
9. Lazo MG, Shirazi P, Sam M, et al. Osteoporosis and risk of fracture in men with spinal cord injury. Spinal Cord. 2001;39:208.
10. Desmond J. Paraplegia: problems confronting the anaesthesiologist. Can Anaesth Soc J. 1970;17:435–51.
11. Vandam LD, Rossier AB. Circulatory, respiratory and ancillary problems in acute and chronic spinal cord injury. In: Hershey SG, editor. Refresher courses in anesthesiology. Philadelphia: JB Lipincott; 1975. p. 171–82.
12. Rocco AG, Vandam LD. Problems in anesthesia for paraplegics. Anesthesiology. 1959;20:348–54.
13. Marz DG, Schreibman DL, Matjasko MJ. Neurologic diseases. In: Katz J, Benumof JL, Kadis BL, editors. Anesthesia and uncommon diseases. 3rd ed. Philadelphia: Saunders; 1990. p. 560–89.
14. Giffin JP, Grush K, Karlin AD, et al. Spinal cord injury. In: Newfield P, Cottrell JE, editors. Handbook of neuroanesthesia: clinical and physiologic essentials. Boston: Little Brown; 1991. p. 338.
15. Gronert GA, Theye RA. Pathophysiology of hyperkalemia induced by succinylcholine. Anesthesiology. 1975;43:89–99.
16. Welply NC, Mathias CJ, Frankel HL. Circulatory reflexes in tetraplegics during artificial ventilation and general anaesthesia. Paraplegia. 1975;13:172–82.
17. Schonwald G, Fish KJ, Perkash I. Cardiovascular complications during anesthesia in chronic spinal cord injured patients. Anesthesiology. 1981;55:550–8.
18. Fraser A, Edmonds-Seal J. Spinal cord injuries. Anesthesia. 1982;37:1084–98.
19. Raeder JC, Grisvold SE. Perioperative autonomic hyperreflexia in high spinal cord lesion: a case report. Acta Anesthesiol Scand. 1986;30:672–3.
20. Lindan R, Joiner E, Freehafer AA, Hazel C. Incidence and clinical features of autonomic dysreflexia in patients with spinal cord injuries. Paraplegia. 1980;18:285–92.
21. Steinberger RE, Ohl DA, Bennett CJ, et al. Nifedipine pretreatment for autonomic dysreflexia during electroejaculation. Urology. 1990;36:228–31.
22. Mulcahy JJ, Young AB. Long-term follow-up of percutaneous radiofrequency sacral rhizotomy. Urology. 1990;35:76–7.
23. Gordon DB, Dahl JL, et al. American pain society recommendations for improving the quality of acute and cancer pain management. Arch Intern Med. 2005;165:1574–80.
24. Randall B, editor. Physical medicine and rehabilitation. 2nd ed. Philadelphia: WB Saunders Company; 2000.

Deep Venous Thrombosis in the Operative Rehabilitation Patient

4

Jonathan Weiswasser

Venous thromboembolic disease remains a particularly common source of morbidity in hospitalized patients and is considered one of the most common preventable causes of hospital death, accounting for 50–75,000 of the 200,000 venous thromboembolic (VTE) deaths per year in the USA [1]. The principal determinant of VTE risk seems to be the patient's indication for hospitalization; hence, all studies of this risk have been based upon comparison of different groups based on a group risk assignment. Moreover, most thrombophylaxis trials have employed venous imaging and invasive venograms as a marker for DVT, rather than symptoms, duplex findings, pulmonary embolism (PE), or fatal PE. The goal of thrombophylaxis in patients undergoing any type of surgery must therefore be to accurately assess DVT risk, understand the types and benefit of therapy, and balance the benefit of prophylaxis with the associated risk of complications, namely, bleeding.

Special attention by the astute clinician should be given to the patient who is immobilized due to neurologic disease (e.g., para-/tetraplegia) or through orthopedic injury. The increase in risk for DVT in those with neurologic disease with extremity paresis increases threefold, and in those who have sustained orthopedic trauma, that risk may be as high as 12-fold [2]. D-dimer levels of greater than 16 ug/dL measured two weeks following injury can be predictive of the development of DVT with a 77% sensitivity, especially when added to careful physical exam and duplex ultrasound [3]. Indeed, the need for aggressive prophylaxis in this surgical group demands careful attention to the balance between DVT/VTE prophylaxis and the risk of bleeding which, in the trauma group, may be prohibitive. Unfortunately, there exists no steadfast algorithm for the use of prophylaxis in patients with spinal cord injury or in patients immobilized from multipoint trauma or surgery, which requires that the clinician base prophylaxis based on individual patient risk.

Many schema have been designed to characterize risk stratification among perioperative hospitalized patients (see Table 4.1). Procedure length, positioning, an orthopedic or neurosurgical component, a bariatric patient, malignancy, and other comorbidities should factor heavily in the estimate of DVT risk, as patients undergoing reconstructive surgery often may present several compounding factors which may be additive in terms of risk.

While there have been few randomized controlled trials of perioperative DVT prophylaxis in patients undergoing reconstructive surgery as a whole, the general consensus of recommendations is based upon a general surgical population. The degree of thrombophylaxis is commensurate with overall risk and includes external

J. Weiswasser, MD
The Plastic Surgery Center, Institute for Advanced Reconstruction, 535 Sycamore Ave, Shrewsbury, NJ 07702, USA
e-mail: jweiswassermd@theplasticsurgerycidernj.com

© Springer International Publishing Switzerland 2017
A.I. Elkwood et al. (eds.), *Rehabilitative Surgery*, DOI 10.1007/978-3-319-41406-5_4

compression stockings, intermittent pneumatic compression boots (IPC), low-dose ultrafractionated heparin (LDUH), low molecular weight heparinoids (LMWH), fondaparinux, and aspirin.

Table 4.1 Risk stratification in plastic and reconstructive surgery patients

AT9 VTE risk category/Caprini score	Estimated baseline risk without prophylaxis (%)	Risk of VTE with prophylaxis (%)
Very low/0–2	NA	<0.5
Low/3–4	0.6	1.5
Moderate/5–6	1.3	3
High/>6	2.7	6

Adapted from Gould et al. [1]

Table 4.2 lists the recommendations for perioperative thrombophylaxis based on risk.

Finally, with surgery there is always a risk of bleeding. Perioperative DVT prophylaxis in most cases only compounds the risk of significant bleeding as a complication, and it is up to the clinician to balance this risk with that of DVT and subsequent VTE. Table 4.3 lists the risk factors for major bleeding among patients generally. Other complications that arise from DVT prophylaxis include reactions to heparinoids, which in the case of certain types of heparin-induced thrombocytopenias can be severe and life threatening. It is incumbent upon the physician to monitor platelet counts following the administration of any type of heparinoid.

Table 4.2 Recommendations for thrombophylaxis

Risk of VTE	Risk of major bleeding complication	
	Average	High/severe
Very low (<0.5 %)	No prophylaxis	
Low (1.5 %)	Mechanical/IPC	
Moderate (3 %)	LDUH, LMWH, or IPC	IPC alone
High (6 %)	LDUH or LMWH plus ES or IPC	IPC with pharmacologic prophylaxis when bleeding risk subsides
High-risk cancer surgery	LDUH or LMWH plus IPC/ES and extended-duration prophylaxis with LMWH post discharge	IPC with pharmacologic prophylaxis when bleeding risk subsides
High-risk LDUH and LMWH contraindicated or not available	Fondaparinux or low-dose aspirin, IPC, or both	IPC with pharmacologic prophylaxis when bleeding risk subsides

Adapted from Gould et al. [1]
IPC intermittent pneumatic compression, *LDUH* low-dose ultrafractionated heparin, *LMWH* low molecular weight heparin, *ES* elastic stockings

Table 4.3 Risk factors for major bleeding complications

General risk factors

Active bleeding

Previous bleeding

Untreated bleeding disorder

Renal or hepatic failure

Thrombocytopenia

Acute stroke

Uncontrolled hypertension

Lumbar puncture, epidural, or spinal anesthesia within last 4 h or next 12 h

Use of anticoagulants

Procedure-specific risk factors

Abdominal surgery

Male sex

Pancreaticoduodenectomy

Sepsis

Hepatic resection

Cardiac surgery

Use of aspirin

Use of clopidogrel 3d before surgery

BMI >25 kg/m^2

Older age, renal insufficiency

Thoracic surgery

Procedures in which bleeding complications have especially severe consequences

Craniotomy

Spinal surgery

Spinal trauma

Reconstructive procedures involving free flap

Adapted from Gould et al. [1]

References

1. Gould MK, Garcia DA, Wren SM, et al. Prevention of VTE in nonorthopedic surgical patients. Chest. 2012;141(2 Suppl):e227S–77s.
2. Heit JA, Silverstein MD, Mohr DN, et al. Risk factors for deep vein thrombosis and pulmonary embolism. Arch Intern Med. 2000;160:809–15.
3. Masuda M, Ueta T, Shiba K, et al. D-dimer screening for deep venous thrombosis in traumatic cervical spinal injuries. Spine J. 2015;15:2338–44.

Part III

Pain Management

Evaluation and Management of Chronic Pain

5

Peter S. Staats and Sean Li

Introduction

Chronic pain is one of the greatest health-care crises affecting Americans today. It is a major cause of disability and a leading reason for physician office visits. Moreover, the indiscriminate treatment of chronic pain with systemic opiates has become a major cause of morbidity and mortality. There are close to 16,000 deaths each year attributed to the use of prescription opiates in the United States. It is crucially important for physicians to have an appropriate algorithm for managing patients with pain.

Any strategy begins with a comprehensive evaluation that leads to establishing an accurate diagnosis. To achieve an accurate diagnosis, it is important for caregivers to include a detailed history and physical examination, any necessary imaging, a psychosocial evaluation, understanding the options for patients with chronic pain, and implementing the most conservative options [1]. When the correct diagnosis is made, one can develop the safest and most effective care plan to managing pain.

What Is Pain?

The International Association for the Study of Pain (IASP) defines pain as "an unpleasant sensory and emotional experience associated with actual or potential tissue damage, or defined in such terms" [1]. As such, there is typically an emotional component as well as a biologic component of most human pain states [2]. The challenge for the treating physician is to assess the patient from a psychosocial as well as from a biologic perspective and come up with the most appropriate accurate diagnosis, from which a therapeutic plan can be developed.

Physicians need to recognize that pain syndromes are complex and have the ability to treat pain or organize care from a biological, psychological, and social perspective. For most physicians who are trained primarily in the biological approach, it can be challenging to evaluate a patient with severe chronic pain with comorbid psychiatric disorders. In the reverse, many psychiatrists and psychologists who are expert pain clinicians may lack the expertise to diagnose and manage the biological underpinnings. For example, specific nerve injuries can manifest with diffuse pain problems. A clinician needs to be able to recognize these problems and establish the underlying pain generator. Sometimes this will lead to a cure, while at other times the most appropriate management strategy can be achieved.

P.S. Staats, MD, MBA (✉) • S. Li, MD
Interventional Pain Physician, Premier Pain Centers, 170 Ave. at the Common, Suite 6, Shrewsbury, NJ 07702, USA
e-mail: sstaatsne@gmail.com; sli@premierpain.com

© Springer International Publishing Switzerland 2017
A.I. Elkwood et al. (eds.), *Rehabilitative Surgery*, DOI 10.1007/978-3-319-41406-5_5

Patients with similar injuries can present with dramatically different experiences of pain. This can occur for a variety of reasons that are not always evident. For example, some patients with psychological disorders like severe depression and anxiety will frequently present with increased pain beyond what would be expected based on the injury or objective findings. Discrete lesions can be missed, but psychological factors can amplify pain as well. Patients with negative thoughts will experience more pain compared with others with neutral and positive thoughts [3]. On the other extreme, individuals can have genetic disorders leading to lack of pain fibers and experience no pain following an otherwise traumatic injury. These patients with "congenital insensitivity to pain" truly feel no pain [4]. There are multiple gradations in between with sensitivity to nerve injuries.

Pain generally begins in the periphery at specific nociceptors and is conducted to the central nervous system via specific pathways. There is processing and neuromodulation that occurs at the dorsal root ganglion, the spinal cord, and further up the central nervous system [5]. The plasticity that occurs throughout the nervous system has been shown to modify and amplify pain in chronic pain conditions. We have recently learned that at each step along this pathway, the pain signal can be modulated. The pain physician is like a general contractor and should be facile with clinical diagnosis and with the general treatment strategies. If necessary, a pain physician will consult with "subcontractors" who are specialized in addressing focal nerve injury.

If one looks closely enough, most patients we see in clinical practice have an identifiable biologic basis for their pain. However, most patients also have an emotional component that leads to suffering. In some cases this suffering, especially if associated with some psychologic morbidities, can overwhelm the physician. A consultation with psychology should be strongly considered if there is any question of overlapping diagnoses. The job of the pain physician is not only to determine biological source of pain but also to apportion the component of pain that emanates from both the biological underpinnings and the emotional overlay. This evaluation can be quite complex and may involve a more comprehensive evaluation with psychology. In this setting a multidisciplinary evaluation of the patient with pain is recommended.

Diagnostic Workup

This chapter certainly does not attempt to make the reader an expert in all of the different disorders that can cause pain. There are entire treatises devoted to the diagnosis and management of chronic pain [6, 7]. There are no simple X-rays or laboratory tests that indicate if a patient has severe pain. Physicians should, on the other hand, do their best to establish a diagnosis and come up with the most appropriate therapeutic plan. This is achieved by taking a detailed history, performing a physical examination, and obtaining the appropriate workup.

The expectation is understanding that not all patients have a "chronic pain syndrome," and some present with pure psychological pathology. Rather, in most cases, specific biologic correlates or underpinnings can be identified that may explain a patient's pain. While most patients do have some component of emotional overlay, psychological morbidity is rarely the primary pathology. Once a diagnosis has been established, a care plan can be formulated. Whenever possible, the source of the pain should be identified, and the clinician-patient team should predetermine a treatment goal. Only with this framework can we expect to come up with an appropriate therapeutic plan.

The complete history and physical examination for all painful disorders is beyond the scope of this chapter. However, the concept of establishing a presumptive diagnosis before embarking on the therapy cannot be overstated. The visit begins with a comprehensive history and physical examination. Prior to considering implementation of a long-term strategy for chronic intractable pain, the physician should establish a diagnosis or at least a presumptive diagnosis. With a diagnosis in hand, one can come up with the most appropriate therapeutic plan [8].

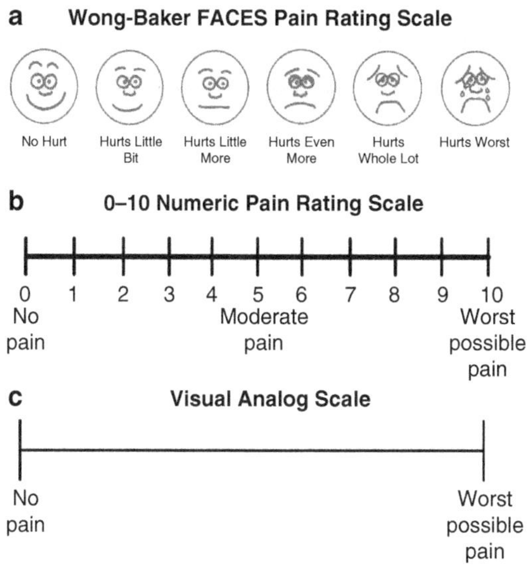

a   **Wong-Baker FACES Pain Rating Scale**

No Hurt | Hurts Little Bit | Hurts Little More | Hurts Even More | Hurts Whole Lot | Hurts Worst

b   **0–10 Numeric Pain Rating Scale**

0   1   2   3   4   5   6   7   8   9   10
No   Moderate   Worst
pain   pain   possible
                                            pain

c   **Visual Analog Scale**

No   Worst
pain   possible
                                            pain

Fig. 5.1 Pain severity scales. Various tools have been developed to help patients and clinicians quantify the severity of pain. The following are examples of common pain scales: (**a**) Wong-Baker FACES Foundation (2015). Wong-Baker FACES® Pain Rating Scale. Retrieved [Date] with permission from http://www.WongBakerFACES.org. (**b**) numerical pain rating scale, and (**c**) visual analog scale (Note: for permission please see Wong-Baker FACES pain rating scale: From Wong et al. [9]. Copyrighted by Mosby, Inc. Reprinted with permission, 0–10 numerical pain rating scale: From McCaffery and Pasero [10]. Copyrighted by Mosby, Inc. Reprinted by permission, Visual analog scale and verbal pain intensity scale: From *Pain Management: Theory and Practice*, edited by RK Portenoy & RM Tanner, copyright 1996 by Oxford University Press, Inc. Used by permission of Oxford University Press)

Begin with a chief complaint. Why is the patient here to see you? What is the primary pain problem? The secret to taking a good history is being a good listener. Figure 5.1 illustrates several common pain severity scales utilized to assess pain. During an initial intake, one needs to take a history and understand the inciting events, the time course and character, and the severity of the pain. What makes the pain better or worse? Verbal descriptors of pain, e.g., "burning sensation," can help determine if the pain is neuropathic or not. Confounding variables, such as work history and satisfaction with the job, will be important as well, and the end result should be a medical documentary of the patient's pain history. The pain history should include:

1. Anatomic location (body part)
2. Severity (0–10 scale; faces; mild, moderate, severe)
3. Verbal descriptors (shooting or burning, dull or achy)
4. Time course (When is it bad? Does it wax and wane throughout the day, week, or month?)
5. Alleviating factors (What makes it better?)
6. Aggravating factors (What makes it worse?)
7. Changes in functional status caused by pain
8. Review of diagnostic workup (previous EMG, MRI, laboratory tests)
9. Review of the previous treatment (previous surgery, medication, and rehabilitation strategies)

Obtaining a past medical history is part of the comprehensive evaluation for pain. Comorbid diseases can be central in defining a differential diagnosis. Patients with a history of many disorders, including diseases such as cancer or diabetes, can develop painful conditions as a result of the disease or its treatment. A complete understanding of the patient's history thus can be helpful when trying to establish a diagnosis. For example, patients with uncontrolled diabetes may develop peripheral neuropathies that can be quite painful. The practitioner should understand that part of the treatment of the pain is to work with the primary care physician/endocrinologist to get diabetes under control. As part of the comprehensive evaluation, one should understand what treatments have been tried to date and what the outcome has been of previous treatments. Has a patient previously tried medications, injections, physical medicine modalities, or surgical interventions?

The pain practitioner typically takes a history and follows with a focused physical examination that is determined by the history. This helps the physician narrow the differential, or presumptive, diagnosis. This typically involves inspection, palpation, provocative maneuvers, and a neurologic examination. Laboratory workup can be used to help make a diagnosis or determine if it is safe to proceed with a planned course of therapy. In addition, with the use of some pharmacologic agents, specific laboratory testing may help identify complications that can occur with treatment strategies. More commonly, laboratory workup may be used to determine if it is safe to proceed with interventional pain procedures.

The reason to obtain additional studies is to establish a diagnosis and to help guide the therapy. One should only perform the additional studies below as a guide to therapy. Plain X-rays use X-ray radiation to take a picture of the hard and soft tissue in the spine. These can be helpful in arthritic disorders and evaluating other connective tissues. Flexion-extension films of the spine are taken with patients in multiple positions to assess stability of the spine if a fracture (spondylosis) is suspected. This test also helps to determine spinal instability. In addition, by carefully orienting the patient in the correct plane, fractures and foraminal compromise can be identified and correlated with a patient's symptoms.

Computed tomography uses a series of X-ray-generated images formatted into two-dimensional and now three-dimensional images of both soft and hard tissues. Scans can help identify hard tissue abnormalities, cancer, and spinal pathology. Ultrasound images internal structures by measuring their capacity to transmit and reflect high-frequency sound waves, making them good for evaluating soft tissue abnormalities. Because of the refractive elements of bony structures, they cannot be used to visualize structures deep to the bony tissue. In the soft tissue, patterns of tears and can be seen in muscles, and abnormal activity can be seen in the soft tissue. This highly sensitivity modality is frequently used to evaluate muscle and ligamentous tears as well as soft tissue structures such as cysts.

Magnetic resonance imaging utilizes strong magnetic fields to assess soft tissues. The detailed images allow for detailed evaluation of the internal soft tissue, such as the nervous tissue or herniated disks in the spine. In the spine, there is clearer definition of the spinal cord, surrounding CSF, and extradural structures, such as disks. Moreover architecture of the disks and level of disk dehydration can be assessed by changes in signal intensity in the spine. MRI with and without contrast will help distinguish malignancy and inflammatory or scar tissues from a re-herniation.

EMG, or electromyography, measures electrical activity within muscles. Various patterns of altered activity can indicate both primary muscle pathology and denervation. Electromyography records voltage changes within a muscle by placing a needle into the muscle. Electrical activity is then recorded in the muscle and displayed on an oscilloscope. Various patterns correlate with diseases of the muscle and other pathologic processes. Nerve conduction velocity (NCV) tests help determine if there is damage along the path of specific nerves. Nerve conduction studies measure velocity and amplitude of electrical activity of the nervous tissue. Abnormalities in electrical activity and conduction can indicate pathology of the nervous tissue, and can be used to identify entrapment syndromes, lesions along the course of a nerve or intrinsic problems within a nerve. The pattern of abnormalities identified can help distinguish between radiculopathies, plexopathies, and primary nerve injuries. These patterns can be used to guide therapy.

Radionucleotide bone scanning is used to assess tissue that has high bone turnover, as seen in fractures, metastatic tumor, and infection. Because this technique is relatively sensitive, it can be used to identify subtle lesions that are missed with other techniques. Biopsy to obtain a tissue diagnosis can be helpful with some neurologic and rheumatologic pain states, visceral pain syndromes, as well as with cancer diagnosis.

In an interventional pain, physicians will also perform diagnostic blocks in order to determine if a structure is involved in pain. This involves placing low volumes of local anesthetic around a peripheral nerve. If pain relief follows a local anesthetic block, an ablative procedure is entertained [11]. For example, diagnostic blocks are frequently performed in the spine (medial branch blocks), viscera (celiac plexus block), or peripheral (specific neural structures, i.e., radial nerve) to determine if the structure innervated by that nerve or plexus is the source of the problem [12]. Table 5.1 illustrates the various types of pain and the associated characteristics. If the practitioner is not clear on the diagnosis, it is appropriate to obtain consultation with pain physicians or members of other specialties.

Treatment Strategies

All too often practitioners may have not established a diagnosis or have an inaccurate diagnosis before beginning treatment. The treatment strategy chosen should be determined after one has established a presumptive diagnosis and a treatment goal. Broadly speaking, there are several general approaches to treating patients with chronic pain. These include medical approaches, anatomic or surgical approaches, neuromodulatory approaches, psychological approaches, alternative approaches, and interventional approaches. Figure 5.2 illustrates a pain treatment ladder that was adapted from the World Health Organization's pain treatment.

Generally, the practitioner should consider conservative modalities prior to the more invasive options. One should generally have a clinical matrix in place, understanding the risks of the therapies being recommended, the likelihood of curing or managing the problem, the risks of the proposed therapy for any given patient, and the costs of the therapies over both the short and long term. If a patient presents with back pain, it is crucial to understand the pathology, as well as the patient's comorbid medical disorders, prior to making decisions on the appropriate treatment strategy. A young patient with new onset neurologic deficit, herniated disk, and classic radicular findings may benefit from a micro-diskectomy early in the treatment algorithm. Alternatively an elderly patient with comorbid medical disorders and back pain may benefit from early treatment with physical therapy, chiropractic care, or medication management. Each treatment strategy is based on the judgment of the practitioner and an understanding of the entire clinical picture for an individual patient.

Medication Management

There are several classes of medications frequently used in the treatment of pain. They can be used for a variety of indications (see Table 5.2). Within each class of medication, there are multiple medications that are commonly used as well as numerous side effects and risks that define the category. The class of medication chosen is determined by the patient's disorder and side effect profile of the agent(s) chosen. For example, neuropathic pain can be most effectively treated with

Table 5.1 Types of pain

Types of pain	Characteristics
Nociceptive pain	Transient, response to noxious stimuli
Neuropathic pain	Damage or dysfunction of the nervous system
Inflammatory pain	Response to tissue damage and inflammation
Postsurgical pain	Transient pain, nociceptive, and inflammatory
Cancer pain	Associated with malignancy

Benzon et al. [13]

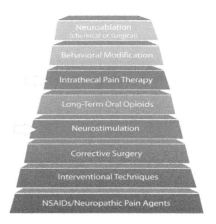

Fig. 5.2 World Health Organization pain treatment ladder. The WHO pain treatment ladder was originally devised to treat cancer pain (This is an adapted version for treating chronic nonmalignant pain (http://www.who.int/cancer/palliative/painladder/en/#, Krames [14], Stamatos et al. [15])

In contrast to earlier thinking on the order of treatments in the pain treatment continuum, it has been proposed that device therapies be considered at an earlier stage.

Neuroablation (chemical or surgical)

Behavioral Modification

Intrathecal Pain Therapy

Long-Term Oral Opioids

Neurostimulation

Corrective Surgery

Interventional Techniques

NSAIDs/Neuropathic Pain Agents

Table 5.2 Common pain medications and their routes of administration

Class of medication	Mechanism of action	Route	Concerns	Notes
Nonsteroidal anti-inflammatory	Inhibits prostaglandin synthesis	Oral and IV	GI Bleeding/platelet dysfunction Renal dysfunction Cardiovascular risk	Acute chronic and cancer
Acetaminophen	Central	Oral and IV	Hepatotoxicity in higher doses or chronic use	Hidden in many other combo medications and OTC formulations
Steroids	Potent anti-inflammatory	Oral IV topical	Bone Immune depression Hyperglycemia associated with GI bleeding Autologous steroid depression	Not a long-term option
Antiseizure medications	Multiple mechanisms	Oral	Gingivitis, aplastic anemia Drug-drug interactions	Neuropathic pain
Antidepressant medications	Can alter reuptake of serotonin and norepinephrine	Oral	Serotonin syndrome a rare side effect Anticholinergic effects	Neuropathic pain
Opiates	Bind opiate receptor	Oral IV, IM, intrathecal	Respiratory depression Endocrine Addiction Constipation Death	Neuropathic Nociceptive pain (Limited)
Cytokine modulators	Affects TNF-alpha	Oral intravenous	Immune suppression	Rheumatoid arthritis
Local anesthetics	Blocks Na channels	Topical Epidural and intrathecal	Seizures Tachyphylaxis	Less common oral or IV
NMDA receptor antagonists	Blocks N-methyl-D-aspartate receptor	Topical Intravenous	Hallucination Sialorrhea	May affect tolerance and
Alpha-2 agonists	Binds the alpha-2 receptor centrally and peripherally	Topical/intrathecal	Hypotension	Sympathetically maintained pain
Bisphosphonates	Inhibit pyrophosphate metabolism	Oral Intravenous	Jaw disease	Used in clinical trial for CRPS type 1 osteoporosis

Table 5.3 Antiseizure medications

Drug	Mechanism of action	Starting dose	Typical daily dose	Primary clinical use	Special considerations
Gabapentin	Binds to voltage-gated calcium channels	300 mg	1800–3600 mg	Postherpetic neuralgia (general neuropathic pain)	Start at low dose and slow titration upward
Pregabalin	Binds to voltage-gated calcium channels	50 mg	150–300 mg	Diabetic peripheral neuropathy, fibromyalgia, spinal cord injury	Start at low dose and slow titration upward
Topiramate	1. Blocks voltage-gated Na channels 2. Augments GABAA receptors 3. Antagonizes AMPA/kainate receptors 4. Inhibits carbonic anhydrase (isozyme II and IV)	50 mg per day	100–200 mg	Primary indication seizure disorder Effective in migraine prophylaxis	1. Side effect is weight loss 2. Used in bipolar disorder 3. Effective with headaches
Gabapentin enacarbil (Horizant)	Extended release gabapentin	600 mg	1200 mg	Restless leg syndrome and neuropathic pain	Different pharmacokinetic profile than gabapentin
Gabapentin (Gralise)	Extended release gabapentin	300 mg	1800 g once daily in the evening	Postherpetic peripheral neuropathy and neuropathic pain	Different pharmacokinetic profile than gabapentin
Phenytoin	Voltage-dependent block of voltage-gated sodium channels Class 1b antiarrhythmic	100 mg tid	200 mg tid	Treatment of trigeminal neuralgia (second choice to carbamazepine)	Narrow therapeutic index

antiepileptic medications and antidepressant medications. If a patient were to present with chronic burning pain and a comorbid depression, the physician may choose an antidepressant class of medication. Severe lancinating pain is more commonly treated with antiseizure medications (see Table 5.3).

Opiates require a specific discussion. Opiates can be used in chronic pain, but there is a paucity of data supporting their use in long-term administration. Lower doses should be considered at early phases as part of a rehabilitative strategy. However, not all patients with chronic pain should be placed on opiates. There arc significant risks of systemic opiates that include death. Clinical guidelines support the use of opiates in certain clinical settings [16].

Opioid therapy should be reserved for patients with moderate to severe persistent chronic pain refractory to non-opioid and intervention pain management modalities to improve functioning and quality of life. This should be only started after careful assessment of the risks and benefits

of opioid therapy for the individual patient. The initiation, titration, monitoring, and maintenance of opioid medications should only be carried out under the care of an adequately trained pain management specialist and mental health or addiction specialist [17]. Much of what is practiced in the prescribing of opioids for chronic pain has been adapted from experiences with treating cancer pain. The "analgesic ladder" (ref. to fig. or to other chapters) was first introduced by the World Health Organization (WHO) in the 1980s [18]. The short-term (less than 6 months) use of opioids for the treatment of non-cancer chronic pain has been shown to be effective in several systematic reviews. Furlan et al. reviewed 41 randomized trials in 6019 patients suffering from nociceptive, neuropathic, mixed, and fibromyalgia pain and concluded that opioid use over 5–16 weeks was more effective than placebo despite a 33 % dropout rate [19]. Chou and Huffman found opioids to be moderately effective in the treatment of chronic non-cancer pain compared to placebo based on study periods less than 12 weeks [20]. Interestingly, tramadol was the only pain medication to show fair evidence in the treatment of chronic osteoarthritis pain in the systematic review by Manchikanti et al. [21]. In this comprehensive systematic review of 111 trials, only four studies evaluated the effectiveness of opioid use beyond 6 months. Furthermore, Trescot et al. reviewed the efficacy of chronic opioid therapy in terms of functional improvement among chronic pain patients in addition to their pain relief. For treatment of chronic noncancer pain beyond 6 months, there is a weak evidence supporting morphine and transdermal fentanyl; there is limited evidence for other more commonly used opioids including hydrocodone and oxycodone [22].

Physical Medicine Modalities

Physical modalities include all modalities designed to modify the muscular or painful tendinous insertions. The key pillars in this treatment modality include identifying altered mechanics, promoting healing, and restoring proper mechanics and function. Complimentary treatments such as chiropractic care and acupuncture should be considered along with conventional therapies such as manipulation, physical therapy of the deep tissue including massage, exercise, heat, and cooling, and transcutaneous electric nerve stimulation (TENS) therapy. All of these approaches can be effective for various types of pain.

Psychological Approaches

Many patients with chronic pain can benefit from a comprehensive psychological evaluation. The degree of suffering and comorbid psychologic disorders can be reduced. Biofeedback can decrease arousal of pain and provide additional pain relief. Relaxation techniques such as biofeedback, guided visual imagery, and hypnosis are few of the coping mechanisms that contribute to the multimodal pain treatment strategy. The restoration of sleep in the activity-rest cycle is a key element in the psychosocial component of chronic pain. Treatment is often maintained through self-management interventions that may comprise of scheduled group sessions utilizing the social support and peer interactions.

Cognitive and Behavioral Approaches

An important aspect of treating chronic pain is bridging the gap between patient's expectations of the treatment plan and the reality of what is actually achieved. Utilizing cognitive behavioral therapy, the focus of pain relief is redirected from "the pain" itself to goal-oriented improvement of function. Negative mechanisms such as catastrophizing are replaced with adaptive and more constructive mechanisms such as self-reassurance. This cognitive restructuring focuses on the value of attitudes, beliefs, and emotional responses to pain and allows the sufferer to resume pleasurable activities and activities of daily living.

Interventional Pain Management

Interventional pain management is the discipline of medicine devoted to the diagnosis and treatment of pain-related disorders, principally with the application of interventional techniques in managing subacute, chronic, persistent, and intractable pain, independently or in conjunction with other modalities of treatment. Interventional pain management techniques are minimally invasive procedures, including percutaneous precision needle placement, with placement of drugs in targeted areas or ablation of targeted nerves, and some surgical techniques, such as laser or endoscopic diskectomy, intrathecal infusion pumps, and spinal cord stimulators, for the diagnosis and management of chronic, persistent, or intractable pain [23]. The lack of knowledge or fear of the risks of some of these techniques leads to over-prescribing of opiate analgesics. Some primary care physicians hesitate to refer out for these procedures, considering them risky or may not know of their efficacy. However, when used judiciously and in appropriate patients, it is possible to decrease the amount of opiates and the complications related

Epidural Steroid Injections

One of the classic interventional or minimally invasive approaches is epidural steroids, application of small amounts of steroids to specific sites within the epidural space [26]. Usually performed with the aid of fluoroscopic guidance, this technique involves placing a needle into the epidural space. The needle may be placed translaminarly, through the caudal canal, or transforaminally. Each technique can be performed with and without a catheter. Multiple types of steroids, local anesthetics, and contrast are used in the performance of the procedure. It is thought to decrease inflammation, improve pain scores, and function and decrease opiate consumption in patients with acute radiculopathies secondary to disk herniations. They are also infrequently performed in patients with cancer, PHN, and vascular insufficiency pain.

Epidural Infusions of Local Anesthetics

Less frequently, epidural catheters are placed to run an infusion of local anesthetics. The local anesthetic quality can be used to decrease pain and improve function in patients undergoing rehabilitation or in the immediate perioperative period following extremity, abdominal or thoracic surgery, or trauma. This technique has superior pain control over systemic opiates alone. Risks of this technique include epidural bleeding or trauma and should be considered carefully in patients who require anticoagulation.

Sympathetic Ganglion Blocks

Sympathetic blocks are used most frequently in the diagnosis and management of complex regional pain syndrome (formerly known as reflex sympathetic dystrophy or RSD), first reported by Weir Mitchell during the civil war in soldiers who suffered limb injuries. This was later named Sudeck's dystrophy with observed muscle atrophy and bone demineralization. In 1947, Evans refined the diagnosis with the term reflex sympathetic dystrophy (RSD) with assumed involvement of the sympathetic nervous system with observed abnormal activity in the periphery. It was recently in 2003, the International Association for the Study of Pain (IASP) formed a consensus group in Budapest who outlined the diagnosis criteria for complex regional pain syndrome or CRPS (see Fig. 5.3) [27]. Type I and II differ by the presence (type II) or absence (type I) of named nerve injury. Disproportionate pain is the hallmark of this syndrome that leads to peripheral sensitization and associated with sensory (allodynia), vasomotor (temperature asymmetry), sudomotor (abnormal sweating), motor (atrophy), and trophic (hair and nail growth abnormalities) changes. Variants of complex regional pain syndrome have been described to include sympathetically maintained pain and sympathetically independent pain. Sympathetic blocks are used to distinguish between the two types of the disorder. Table 5.4 describes various treatment options for CRPS including sympathetic nerve block.

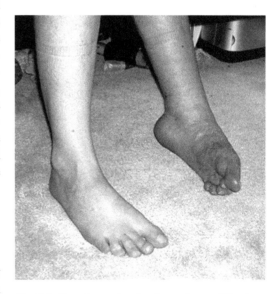

Fig. 5.3 Complex regional pain syndrome. This photo illustrates the typical syndrome of persistent disproportionate pain in the setting of sensory, vasomotor, sudomotor, motor, and trophic changes

Table 5.4 Complex regional pain syndrome (CRPS): treatment options

Psychological	Pharmacological	Physiological	Interventional
Cognitive behavioral therapy	Corticosteroids	Occupational	Sympathetic nerve block
Biofeedback	NSAIDs	Physical	Intravenous
Relaxation training	Anticonvulsants	Desensitization	Neuromodulation
Coping skills	Antidepressants		Intrathecal
	Opioids		

The use of multidisciplinary approach including diagnostic/therapeutic sympathetic nerve block strives to achieve overall goal of functional restoration in the treatment of CRPS

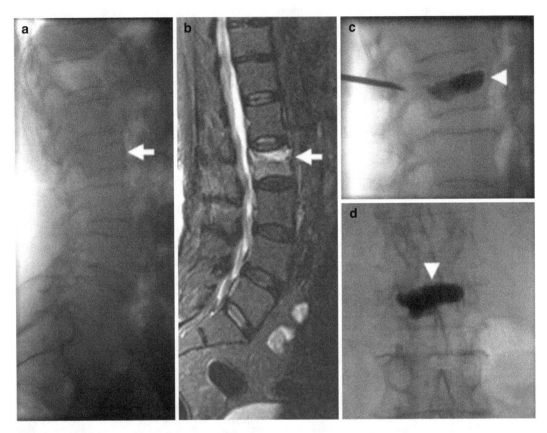

Fig. 5.4 Vertebral augmentation. Acute vertebral compression fractures can be stabilized with percutaneous vertebroplasty. The following is an example of an L2 vertebral compression fracture shown on X-ray (**a**), and MRI (**b**). There is evidence of bone marrow edema on the MRI suggesting acute inflammation. Panel (**c**) (lateral view) and (**d**) (AP view) illustrates the vertebral body after injection of bone cement via vertebroplasty. Kyphoplasty is a similar procedure that utilizes the addition of a pneumatic balloon (not shown) to create a cavity in the vertebral marrow prior to injection of bone cement

Vertebroplasty and Kyphoplasty

This therapy is indicated for patients with focal pain due to a spinal compression fracture. These are minimally invasive, fluoroscopically guided techniques to restore the structural instability of a fractured vertebral body by placing a small amount of bone cement either directly through a cannula. The compressed vertebral body height may be restored during a kyphoplasty by first placing a pneumatic balloon into the crushed vertebrae. This newly created cavity is then filled with bone cement to stabilize the augmented vertebral body. Both of these procedures have been demonstrated to improve pain and decrease opiate consumption in patients with semi-acute and acute vertebral compression fractures (Fig. 5.4) [28].

Minimally Invasive Lumbar Decompression

Minimally invasive lumbar decompression has been recently developed to treat lumbar spinal stenosis as a result of ligamentum flavum hypertrophy. Patients with spinal stenosis present with progressive neurogenic claudication where low back and/or lower extremity pain is exacerbated with standing or walking. This is a minimally invasive, fluoroscopically guided technique for decompressing the narrowed spinal canal by removing portions of the ligamentum flavum through 5 mm trocar sites. This procedure may help chronic pain patients obtain pain relief with less risk than open spinal surgery. Numerous well-controlled trials have been performed with the level one evidence pending [29].

Neuromodulation

Neuromodulation is the field of medicine where electrical energy or medications are targeted to the nervous system through which the conduction of pain signals is modulated and reduced. The use of electricity in the treatment of pain dates back to 46 A.D. where torpedo fish were used by Scribonius Largus to treat headaches. In 1967, Dr. Norman Sheely pioneered the use of electrical leads in the dorsal epidural space to treat intractable cancer pain. This concept has evolved into sophisticated electronic devices that can help patients manage chronic pain. Targeted drug delivery to the intrathecal space was first described by Dr. August Bier in 1898 when he described the first spinal anesthetic [30]. Similarly, the delivery of specific medications has also evolved into the application of implanted computer-controlled pumps capable of delivering precise amounts of analgesic medication(s) to the intrathecal space.

Spinal Cord Stimulation

Spinal cord stimulation involves implanting electrodes into the epidural space to modify pain or disease. The therapy has been demonstrated to be more effective than repeat back surgery and then medication management in the control of pain [31, 32]. Traditional, or tonic stimulation, has been used since the 1960s and is a widely accepted approach to managing neuropathic pain. Traditional stimulation would layer a sensation of "buzzing" over an area of pain, effectively masking the painful sensation with a gentle buzzing sensation. In order to experience pain relief with traditional stimulation parameters, there was a requirement of stimulating the area of pain. Both rechargeable and non-rechargeable power sources have been used to control pain. Figure 5.5 illustrates a typical implanted spinal cord stimulator system. These therapies have been traditionally most effective for neuropathic pain of the trunk and limbs.

New frequencies are also improving the efficacy of spinal cord stimulation. High-frequency spinal cord stimulation involves utilization of frequencies in the 10,000 Hz range and requires a larger energy requirement. It is typically set subthreshold, so the patient feels no paresthesia as they typically do with traditional or tonic stimulation. High-frequency spinal cord stimulation was recently compared to traditional or tonic stimulation in a FDA clinical trial. In a noninferiority study design, high-frequency stimulation demonstrated superior pain control for both the back and leg over traditional or tonic stimulation [33]. Burst stimulation involves utilizing novel frequencies that have bursts of electrical activity followed by a quiescent period. It is also widely used in Europe and Australia and is the subject of FDA-approved clinical trials in the United States [34].

Novel Targets and Frequencies

Newer stimulation targets or approaches may even improve on the success of traditional spinal cord stimulation. For example, DRG stimulation

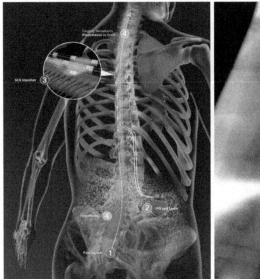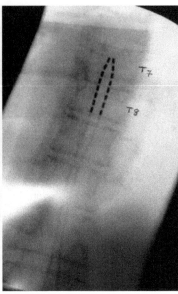

Fig. 5.5 Spinal Cord Stimulation. Chronic refractory neuropathic pain of the trunk and limb can be treated with electrical stimulation of the pain fibers within the dorsal horn of the spinal cord. Placement of electronic leads within the epidural space creates paresthesia based stimu- lation to the painful areas. Left panel illustrates the place- ment of spinal cord stimulator leads within the epidural space to modulate ascending pain signals (Image courtesy of Boston Scientific). The right panel is an example of multi-contact leads placed in the thoracic epidural space

involves placing the electrodes directly on the dorsal root ganglion (DRG) and stimulating the DRG that is presumed to be involved in the pro- cessing of painful stimuli. It appears to be supe- rior to traditional spinal cord stimulation in certain settings [35]. Electrodes are also placed on peripheral nerves in the head and neck to mod- ulate headaches. A novel approach approved in Europe and Australia stimulates the vagus nerve noninvasively as a prophylaxis and treatment for cluster headaches and migraines and has been approved in Europe for GI disorders, asthma anx- iety, and depression [36].

Intrathecal Drug Therapy

Intrathecal therapy has been relegated to a sal- vage approach for most patients with severe can- cer and non-cancer-related pain [37]. Intrathecal therapy involves placing a catheter into the intrathecal space and connecting it to an implant- able pump to deliver analgesics including opi- oids. It has been demonstrated to be effective in both cancer and non-cancer populations. In the cancer population, intrathecal opiates have been shown to improve pain with less side effects and possibly improve life expectancy when com- pared to medical management alone [38]. In addition, when compared to the costs of sys- temic opiates, intrathecal therapy becomes cost- effective after 28 months. The high upfront costs of the device are offset by the lower costs of maintenance of intrathecal opiates. Furthermore, with close to 16,000 deaths attributed each year to systemic opiates, the overall higher safety profile of controlled delivery is favorable on multiple fronts [39].

In addition, the use of non-narcotics in the intrathecal space to manage severe pain is quite common. Novel agents, including intrathecal ziconotide, have been demonstrated to be effec- tive in patients with severe pain related to cancer and AIDS and in non-cancer-related pain [40, 41]. Algorithms have been developed that guide physicians through various medications [42, 43]. The therapy is widely considered a safe therapy and is used for patients with chronic severe pain who have failed an adequate response to other conservative therapies including low-dose opiate therapy.

Summary

There are multiple treatment strategies that are effective in the management of cancer and non-cancer-related pain. While opiates remain an important tool for physicians, it should not be considered the only tool that physicians have in managing pain. In the treatment of chronic pain, pain should be regarded as the disease state rather than a symptom. Whichever treatment strategy the physician chooses, he/she should begin with a thorough history and physical examination. Based on this, a presumptive diagnosis should be established. This diagnosis thus should lead the physician down an individualized treatment algorithm. The risks of all therapies should be evaluated when developing the appropriate therapeutic plan. All strategies, from simply ignoring the pain to complex surgical procedures, involve some risk. Understanding the treatment options should facilitate treatment with safest and most conservative option, working up in a hierarchical fashion.

Portions of this manuscript have been published in Staats Li Silverman, *Alternative options in treating pain* (ed Staats PS, Silverman, Controlled Substance Management Springer 2015).

References

1. Merskey H, Bodguk N. Classification of chronic pain: descriptions of chronic pain syndromes and definition of pain terms. 2nd ed. IASP Press. Seattle. 1994.
2. Staats PS, Hekmat H, Staats AW. Psychological behaviorism theory of pain: a basis for unity. Pain Forum. 1996;5:194–207.
3. Staats PS, Staats A, Hekmat H. The additive impact of anxiety and a placebo on pain. Pain Med. 2001;2: 267–79.
4. Thrush D. Congenital insensitivity to pain. Brain. 1973;96:369–86.
5. Ashburn MA, Staats PS. The management of chronic pain. Lancet. 1999;353:1865–9.
6. Staats PS, Wallace MS. Pain medicine: just the facts. 2nd ed. McGraw Hill; New York. 2015.
7. Diwan S, Staats PS. The Diwan Staats atlas pain medicine procedures. McGraw Hill; New York. 2015.
8. Gupta R, Staats PS. Diagnostic tools in the management of pain. In: Expert pain management. Springhouse Corporation; North Wales. 1997.
9. Wong DL, Hackenberry-Eaton M, Wilson D, Winkelstein ML, Schwartz P. Wong's essentials of pediatric nursing. 6th ed. St. Louis; Missouri. 2001, p. 1301.
10. McCaffery M, Pasero C. Pain: clinical manual. St. Louis; Missouri. 1999, p. 16.
11. Guarino A, Staats PS. Diagnostic neural blockade in the management of pain. Pain Digest. 1997;7:194–9.
12. Boswell MV, Singh V, Staats PS, Hirsch JA. Accuracy of precision diagnostic blocks in the diagnosis of chronic spinal pain of facet or zygapophysial joint origin. Pain Physician. 2003;6:449–56.
13. Benzon HT, et al. Essentials of pain medicine. 3rd ed. Elsevier, Philadelphia. 2011
14. Krames ES. Intraspinal opioid therapy for nonmalignant pain: current practices and clinical guidelines. J Pain Symptom Manage. 1996;11:333–52.
15. Stamatos JM, et al. Live your life pain free. Based on the interventional pain management experience of Dr. John Stamatos. McKinney, TX. 2005.
16. Manchikanti L, Abdi S, Atluri S, Balog CC, Benyamin RM, Boswell MV, et al. American Society of Interventional Pain Physicians (ASIPP) guidelines for responsible opioid prescribing in chronic non-cancer pain: Part 2—guidance. Pain Physician. 2012;15(3 Suppl):S67–116.
17. Chou R, Fanciullo GJ, Fine PG, et al. Clinical guidelines for the use of chronic opioid therapy in chronic non-cancer pain. J Pain. 2009;10:113.
18. World Health Organization. Cancer pain relief. Geneva: World Health Organization; 1990.
19. Furlan AD, Sandoval JA, Mailis-Gagnon A, et al. Opioids for chronic non-cancer pain: a meta-analysis of effectiveness and side effects. Can Med Assoc J. 2006;174:1589–94.
20. Chou R, Huffman L. Use of chronic opioid therapy in chronic non-cancer pain: a systematic review. American Pain Society; 2009.
21. Manchikanti L, Koyyalagunta L, Datta S, et al. A systematic review of randomized trials of long-term opioid management for chronic non-cancer pain. Pain Physician. 2011;14:91–121.
22. Trescot AM, Helm S, Benyamin R, et al. Opioids in the management of chronic non-cancer pain: an update of the American Society of Interventional Pain Physicians (ASIPP) guidelines. Pain Physician. 2008; 11:S5–62.
23. MLA citation– Medicare Payment Advisory Commission (U.S.). Report to the Congress: Paying for Outpatient Services In Cancer Hospitals. Washington, DC: MedPac. 2001.
24. Staats PS. The effect of pain on survival. In: Interventional pain management Anesthesiology Clinics of North America. Guest Ed Staats PS. Philadelphia: Lippincott, Williams and Wilkins, 2003;

25. Staats PS. Pain, depression and survival. Am Fam Physician. 1999;60:42–4.

26. Manchikanti L, Staats PS, Nampiaparampil DE. What is the role of epidural injections in the treatment of lumbar discogenic pain: a system 4/2015. Korean J Pain. 2015;28:75–87.

27. Harden RN, Bruehl S, Stanton-Hicks M, Wilson PR. Proposed new diagnostic criteria for complex regional pain syndrome. Pain Med. 2007;6:326–31.

28. Anselmetti CG, et al. Percutaneous vertebroplasty in osteoporotic patients: an institutional experience of 1,634 patients with long-term follow-up. J Vasc Intervent Radiol. 2011;22:1714–20.

29. Benyamin R, Staats PS, Davis K, et al. Accepted for publication. Midas Encore, Pain Physician 2015.

30. Li S, Staats PS. Permanent implant (intrathecal drug delivery). The atlas of interventional pain care. New York: McGraw-Hill; 2015.

31. North RB, Kidd DH, Shipley J. Spinal cord stimulation versus reoperation for failed back surgery syndrome: a cost effectiveness and cost utility analysis based on a randomized controlled clinical trial. Neurosurgery. 2007;61:361.

32. Kumar K, et al. The effects of spinal cord stimulation in neuropathic pain are sustained: a 24 month follow up of the prospective randomized controlled multicenter trial of effectiveness of spinal cord stimulation. Neurosurgery. 2008;63:762–70.

33. Buyten V, et al. High-frequency spinal cord stimulation for the treatment of chronic back pain patients: results of a prospective multicenter European Clinical Study. Neuromodulation. 2013;16:59–66.

34. DeRidder D, et al. Burst stimulation for back and limb pain. World Neurosurg. 2013;80:642–9.

35. Kramer J, Draper CE, Deer TR, et al. Dorsal root ganglion stimulation: anatomy physiology and potential for therapeautic targeting in chronic pain. In: Diwan S, editor. The Diwan Staats Atlas of pain medicine procedures. McGraw Hill; New York. 2015. p. 626–31.

36. Deer TR, Mekhail N, Petersen E, Krames E, Staats P, Pope J, Saweris Y, Lad SP, Diwan S, Falowski S, Feler C, Slavin K, Narouze S, Merabet L, Buvanendran A, Fregni F, Wellington J, Levy RM. The appropriate use of neurostimulation: stimulation of the intracranial and extracranial space and head for chronic pain. Neuromodulation. 2014;17:551–70.

37. Pope J, Deer T, McRoberts WP. The Burden of being positioned as a salvage therapy. Pain Med. 2015; 16(10):2036–8.

38. Smith TJ, Coyne PJ, Staats PS, Deer T, Stearns LJ, Rauck RL, Boortz-Marx RL, Buchser E, Català E, Bryce DA, Cousins M, Pool GE. An implantable drug delivery system (IDDS) for refractory cancer pain provides sustained pain control, less drug-related toxicity, and possibly better survival compared with comprehensive medical management (CMM). Ann Oncol. 2005;16:825–33.

39. Kumar K, et al. Treatment of chronic pain by using a intrathecal drug delivery compared to conventional treatments. A cost effectiveness analysis. J Neurosurg. 2002;97:803–10.

40. Staats PS, et al. Intrathecal ziconotide in the treatment of refractory pain in patients with cancer or AIDS: a randomized controlled clinical trial. JAMA. 2004;1:291.

41. Wallace MS, Charapata S, Fisher R, Staats PS, et al. The Ziconotide Nonmalignant Pain Study Group. Intrathecal Ziconotide in the treatment of chronic nonmalignant pain: a randomized double blind placebo controlled trial. Neuromodulation. 2006;9:75–86.

42. Prager J, Deer T, Levy R, et al. Best practices for intrathecal drug delivery for pain. Neuromodulation. 2014;17(4):354–72.

43. Deer TR, Prager J, Levy R, Rathmell J, Buchser E, Burton A, Caraway D, Cousins M, De Andrés J, Diwan S, Erdek M, Grigsby E, Huntoon M, Jacobs MS, Kim P, Kumar K, Leong M, Liem L, McDowell II GC, Panchal S, Rauck R, Saulino M, Sitzman BT, Staats P, Stanton-Hicks M, Stearns L, Wallace M, Willis KD, Witt W, Yaksh T, Mekhail N. Polyanalgesic Consensus Conference 2012: recommendations for the management of pain by Intrathecal (Intraspinal) drug delivery: report of an interdisciplinary expert panel. Neuromodul Technol Neural Interface. 2012;15:436–66.

44. WHO's pain ladder for adults. World Health Organization Web site. http://www.who.int/cancer/palliative/painladder/en/#. Accessed May 5 2013.

Part IV

Nervous System and Spine

Jonathan Lustgarten, David Estin, Ty Olson,
Timothy Link, and Henry Moyle

Cerebrovascular Disease

Stroke Overview

Stroke refers to any new neurological symptoms with sudden onset. This commonly used term can refer to any cerebrovascular disease of the nervous system that interrupts neural tissue function abruptly. When patients present to the emergency room with an abrupt onset of new focal neurologic deficits, the etiology of 95 % will be vascular (i.e., stroke), and 5 % will be other disease processes such as seizures, tumor, or psychogenic. Stroke is most commonly used to describe an ischemic event involving an acute occlusion of an artery supplying neural tissue. However, stroke can also result from loss of neural tissue function secondary to sudden hemorrhage into

J. Lustgarten, MD (✉) • D. Estin, MD
T. Link, MD • H. Moyle, MD
Neurosurgeons of New Jersey, 121 Hwy 36 West,
Suite 330, West Long Branch, NJ 07764, USA
e-mail: jLustgarten1@gmail.com;
d.estin@verizon.net; timothy.link.md@gmail.com;
HMoyle@barnabashealth.org

T. Olson, MD, FACS
Monmouth Medical Center, Long Branch, NJ, USA

Columbia University Medical Center,
New York, NY, USA
e-mail: to103@columbia.edu

the neural tissue. Approximately 85 % of all strokes are ischemic in nature, while the remaining 15 % of strokes are hemorrhagic in nature [1].

Cerebral Ischemia or Cerebral Infarction

Cerebral ischemia is a decrease in blood flow to a part of the brain. If blood flow is too low or cutoff completely, the brain tissue begins to die. The result is cerebral infarction. This is by far the most common pathology, occurring much more frequently than the hemorrhagic causes of sudden neurological symptoms listed below.

Hemorrhagic Stroke

Spontaneous hemorrhage into the brain leads to the sudden onset of neurological symptoms. Aneurysmal subarachnoid hemorrhage results from the rupture of a cerebral aneurysm. This typically leads to the sudden onset of headache and/or other neurological symptoms and is one of the most common forms of brain hemorrhage. Other sources of sudden hemorrhage into the brain include arteriovenous malformation, arteriovenous fistulas, cavernous malformation, and venous sinus thrombosis. Intracerebral hemorrhage can result from blood vessel disease, such as amyloid angiopathy, vasculitis, and vasculopathy such as Moyamoya disease. Moyamoya involves gradual intimal thickening of the supraclinoid internal carotid arteries leading to eventual occlusion. The abnormal collateral vessels formed are prone to spontaneous hemorrhage.

Pathophysiology of Ischemic Stroke

Ischemic stroke is a stroke caused by inadequate blood flow to a part of the brain. Because the brain requires a continuous supply of oxygen and other nutrients from the blood, this interruption in blood flow leads to dysfunction of the brain and death of the cells in the affected area. With complete obstruction of blood flow, neuronal death will occur within 2–3 min. In most strokes, there is a salvageable *penumbra* (tissue at risk) that retains viability for a period of time through suboptimal perfusion by collateral vessels. Progression of local cerebral edema resulting from the ischemic injury results in compromise of these collaterals and progression of ischemic penumbra to infarction if flow is not restored and maintained. Treatments discussed below are aimed at revascularizing penumbra tissue by reopening the occluded vessel.

The most common interruption to cerebral blood flow is from a blood clot that forms in a more proximal artery and then lodges into a distal downstream artery that supplies the brain. Blood clots can form in many areas and have many causes. One of the most common causes of cerebral infarction is carotid stenosis. The carotid artery is prone to the development of atherosclerosis and the resultant narrowing or stenosis of the artery, particularly in patients with high blood pressure, high cholesterol levels, and diabetes mellitus. Smoking, obesity, and a sedentary lifestyle also contribute highly to the development of atherosclerosis. The narrowing of the carotid artery and the atherosclerotic plaque in the artery can lead to clot formation. Often, these clots break free and travel distally downstream, lodging into a smaller artery in the brain as an embolic event. Other causes of ischemic embolic stroke can include blood clots from aneurysms, heart condition such as atrial fibrillation, septal defects, or valve disease, although these sources of emboli are less common than carotid stenosis.

When blood flow is decreased at the periphery of adjacent vascular territories, e.g., the middle cerebral artery and anterior cerebral artery, due to a disturbance in the flow of one or both arteries, infarction can occur in the most distal portions of the adjacent territories leading to a watershed infarct. This pattern of ischemia is seen in proximal vessel occlusion such as interruption of flow in the internal carotid artery, affecting the watershed between the anterior and middle cerebral arteries. Low flow states such as cardiogenic shock can also result in watershed infarcts. Risk factors for these types of brain infarctions are identical to the risks for coronary artery disease and other blood vessel diseases. Patients most at risk for ischemic stroke are often the same patients who have heart disease or other peripheral vascular disease.

Occasionally, small blockages of an artery can be resolved quickly on their own. If the blockage is reversed soon enough, in these cases the new neurological symptoms may reverse completely. These temporary neurosymptoms are often referred to as transient ischemic attacks (TIAs). While they do not lead to permanent disability on their own, they usually occur in patients at high risk for stroke and often predict further ischemic injuries including full cerebral infarction [2].

Presenting Symptoms of Ischemic Stroke

The symptoms caused by an ischemic stroke are extremely variable and depend on which cerebral arteries are involved, the severity of ischemia, and ultimately the areas of brain that are damaged. Almost any neurological symptom can occur. However, one of the most common sites involved is the middle cerebral artery. Ischemic stroke in the region of the middle cerebral artery typically causes weakness of the opposite side of the body (hemiparesis). If the ischemia involves the dominant hemisphere (usually the left side), then language and speech can be affected. In the case of very large infarctions of the middle cerebral artery territory, the brain can swell significantly, leading to increased intracranial pressure that can lead to coma or death.

It is important to consider a differential diagnosis in patients with these symptoms. Other causes leading to sudden neurologic deficits include hemorrhage, tumor, seizure, complicated migraines, reversible cerebral vasoconstrictive syndrome (RCVS), and psychogenic causes. Typically, the acute interruption of cerebral blood flow results in the sudden onset of neurologic deficits that are characterized by the territory of the brain that is normally supplied by the interrupted vessel. The hallmark of stroke is that symptoms are acute in onset and generally result in the sudden loss of function.

Intracerebral hemorrhage (ICH) should be suspected with smooth onset of symptoms over minutes to hours, presence of severe headaches, frequent vomiting, and when depression of level of consciousness is prominent, in contrast to ischemic infarct which typically has significant motor or sensory deficits with little or no impairment consciousness except if massive or with brainstem involvement. Lobar hemorrhages resulting from amyloid angiopathy often are clinically not as severe as other causes of intracerebral hemorrhage and are more common in the elderly and are frequently associated with Alzheimer's dementia [3, 4].

Postictal states following seizures can involve weakness or aphasia and a history of seizure disorder, witnessed seizure activity, or the loss of bowel, and bladder control can help to make the diagnosis of seizure. The neurologic symptoms resulting from tumor are usually late in the course of tumor progression and preceded by other more chronic symptoms including headache and seizure. Complicated migraine with transient neurologic deficits can usually be differentiated from stroke by obtaining an accurate patient history of recurring intermittent symptoms; however, auras are the most recognizable symptom associated with migraines. Patients who present for the first time with complicated migraines require a full stroke evaluation. RCVS is characterized by a week-long course of thunderclap headaches, occasional focal neurologic signs, and seizures. The diagnosis is made by angiographic demonstration of diffuse reversible cerebral vasospasm [5].

Evaluation and Management of Ischemic Stroke

The key components to look for when taking the history of a suspected acute ischemic stroke are the last time when seem normal and any potential contraindications to the administration of intravenous tPA (tissue plasminogen activator). tPA administered within 4.5 h of symptom onset is the standard of care for ischemic stroke [6, 7]. tPA is a thrombolytic drug used to reopen occluded vessels by directly breaking up blood clots [8]. Contraindications to the use of tPA include intracerebral hemorrhage, clinical presentation of subarachnoid hemorrhage even in the setting of a negative head CT, known intracranial aneurysm or arteriovenous malformation (AVM), active internal bleeding, known bleeding diathesis, serious head trauma, stroke or internal surgery within the last 3 months, or blood pressure that cannot be controlled (SBP >185 or DBP >110) [8]. A noncontrast head CT is necessary to rule out hemorrhagic infarct prior to the administration of intravenous tPA.

Examination of the patient includes neurologic assessment utilizing the NIH Stroke Score (NIHSS). This examination helps to localize the lesion and quantitates the severity of the stroke. This is important because an NIHSS greater than eight is a strong predictor for large vessel occlusion. Large vessel occlusion refers to occlusion of the internal carotid artery, proximal segment of the middle cerebral artery, or basilar artery. Reopening of large vessel occlusion has been less effective with IV tPA treatment alone and is associated with poor clinical outcomes [9].

Recent prospective randomized trials have demonstrated improved outcomes in ischemic stroke due to large vessel occlusion when utilizing mechanical clot retrieval (thrombectomy) [10]. This technique uses aspiration micro catheters or retrievable stents placed directly into the occluded vessel to remove the clot. This technique requires neuroendovascular capability (neurointerventional trained physician and a neuroendovascular interventional angiography suite). These studies also required a noninvasive test confirming large vessel occlusion prior to thrombectomy. CT angiogram (CTA) has been the choice study to confirm large vessel occlusion. At our institution, we also utilize CT perfusion scans obtained simultaneously with the CTA to determine the amount of penumbra tissue that can be salvaged. Thrombectomy can be performed together with the administration of IV tPA or as a stand-alone procedure for patients who do not qualify for IV tPA. Thrombectomy has to be started within 6 h from the last time seen normal.

Patients who awaken with stroke symptoms are generally out of the time windows for IV tPA or thrombectomy treatments. These patients comprise 25 % of ischemic strokes. There is growing evidence for positive outcomes in the setting of wake up strokes, and these patients may still benefit from thrombectomy provided the CT perfusion scan demonstrates an infarct volume less than 70 cc and a reasonable volume of salvageable penumbra [11]. Other studies utilized in assessing ischemic stroke include brain MRI perfusion imaging and MRA studies of the cervical carotid arteries and intracranial circulation. These studies are generally not as useful in the setting of acute stroke management due to limited accessibility and time required to obtain the studies.

Management of a patient who has had a TIA or stroke following their acute management and treatment involves the evaluation for an underlying cause. Cervical carotid arteries are evaluated by duplex ultrasound, CTA, or MRA looking for atherosclerosis and any blockage that could have been the source of the clot. If this is not found, other sources including the heart may be studied to determine if the patient has a clot inside the heart that could be the source, as can occur with atrial fibrillation. A medical evaluation for an underlying hypercoagulable disorder is also appropriate, especially in the younger stroke patient. In about 41 % of ischemic stroke, no underlying cause will be identified [12].

Long-term management of ischemic stroke is aimed at modifying vascular risk factors through diet, lifestyle modification, exercise, medications, and surgery. This includes weight reduction, tobacco cessation and management of hypertension, hypercholesterolemia, and diabetes. Patients can also benefit from antiplatelet medications. Patients with atrial fibrillation can benefit from anticoagulation therapy. Carotid endarterectomy (CEA) is indicated for symptomatic carotid stenosis greater than 50 % and in asymptomatic male patients with carotid stenosis greater than 70 % [13].

Pathophysiology, Evaluation, and Management of Spontaneous Intracerebral Hemorrhagic Stroke

Hemorrhagic stroke is the result of damage to brain tissue resulting from hemorrhage directly into the brain tissue. Although it is thought that the primary etiology of hemorrhagic stroke is hypertension, this is still controversial. Hemorrhagic stroke is the second most common form of stroke accounting for 15–30 % of all strokes, but it is associated with a much higher mortality rate compared to ischemic stroke. The actual volume of the hematoma correlates with morbidity and mortality.

Risk factors associated with hemorrhagic stroke including increasing incidence after the age of 55 years and doubling with each decade until age greater than 80 years where the incidence is 25 times that of the previous decade. Hemorrhagic stroke is more common in males. History of previous CVA of any type increases the risk of hemorrhagic stroke 23:1. Acute and chronic alcohol consumption increases the risk of hemorrhagic stroke. Street drugs such as cocaine, amphetamines, and phencyclidine are associated with increased risk of hemorrhagic infarct.

Eighty to ninety percent of hemorrhagic infarcts are located in the basal ganglia, putamen, thalamus, cerebellum, or brainstem. Only 10–20 % of hemorrhagic infarcts are located in the cerebral white matter. Hemorrhagic infarction involving cerebral white matter is thought to be related to amyloid angiopathy, direct extension from deeper hemorrhage, hemorrhagic conversion of previous ischemic infarction, or an underlying vascular malformation such as an AVM, aneurysm, or cavernous malformation.

Patients presenting with hemorrhagic stroke typically have a history of smooth progressive onset of symptoms over minutes to hours often accompanied by severe headaches, vomiting, and alterations in level of consciousness. During the initial evaluation, it is important to gather information regarding a history of hypertension, drug use particularly amphetamines and cocaine, use of nasal decongestants or appetite suppressants and anticoagulants, antiplatelet medications, alcohol abuse, coagulopathies, previous stroke, history of vascular malformations, history of tumors, and history of recent childbirth particularly if eclampsia preeclampsia was involved. Although noncontrast head CT will make a definitive diagnosis of intracerebral hemorrhage for patients greater than 45 years of age with preexisting hypertension and hemorrhage in the thalamus putamen and posterior fossa, patients outside of these criteria should undergo a cerebral vascular study such as a CT angiogram, MRA, or catheter angiogram to rule out an underlying lesion such as an AVM.

Initial management of hemorrhagic stroke involves primarily medical treatment. The patient should be admitted to the intensive care unit and intubated if their level of consciousness compromises airway protection or if needed for intracranial pressure management. Both physiologic and drug-induced coagulopathies should be reversed if possible. Patients should have strict blood pressure control with the target systolic blood pressure less than 140 and a diastolic blood pressure less than 90. In our practice we also obtain a delayed noncontrast head CT 6–12 h after the initial scan to determine clot stability. It has been demonstrated that approximately one third of hemorrhagic strokes will increase in volume within the first 3 h of onset. If clot volume leads to increased intracranial pressures, critical care specialists should be involved for elevated intracranial pressure management.

To date there have been no randomized prospective trials that have demonstrated the advantage of surgical evacuation over the best medical management. It is however widely accepted that posterior fossa hemorrhagic infarcts require surgical evacuation in patients who are considered surgical candidates. This is almost always in the setting of mass effect on the brainstem or obstructive hydrocephalus. There is one large prospective randomized trial that trended toward better outcomes with surgical evacuation of hematomas that came within 1 cm of the cortical surface [14]. The decision to operate on hemorrhagic stroke must be individualized based on patient's neurologic condition, size and location of hematoma, patient's age, and the patient's and family's wishes concerning heroic measures in the face of catastrophic illness.

Cerebrovascular Lesions Causing Intracranial Hemorrhage

It is beyond our scope to describe in detail other less common causes of intracranial hemorrhage. Below, other known cerebrovascular etiologies of intracranial hemorrhage are summarized briefly.

Aneurysmal Subarachnoid Hemorrhage (SAH)

The most common cause of subarachnoid hemorrhage is trauma. The most common cause of spontaneous subarachnoid hemorrhage is a ruptured intracranial aneurysm accounting for 75–80 % of spontaneous subarachnoid hemorrhage. Patients presenting with acute subarachnoid hemorrhage from ruptured aneurysm will present with sudden onset of worst headache of life accompanied by meningismus and photophobia. Often patients will have associated nausea vomiting and decreased level of consciousness.

Initial evaluation of a patient with suspected aneurysmal subarachnoid hemorrhage involves a noncontrast head CT. If there is no evidence of acute hemorrhage, a lumbar puncture should be performed. The key result from the lumbar puncture is xanthochromia of the supernatant. Elevated red blood cell counts that do not decrease from the first to the last collection tubes may suggest subarachnoid hemorrhage but can also be seen in traumatic lumbar punctures. CT angiogram may also be useful in identifying an aneurysm. Once a subarachnoid hemorrhage is confirmed or suspicion is high enough, a catheter angiogram is required for definitive diagnosis. Because of the high mortality associated with rebleeding (15–20 % first 2 weeks) of a ruptured aneurysm, early treatment within the first 24 h of presentation is recommended. Treatment options include surgical clipping and no interventional embolization. Treatment of aneurysmal subcutaneous arachnoid hemorrhage should always involve neurosurgeons, neurointensivists, and neurointerventionalists. Subarachnoid hemorrhage from aneurysmal rupture carries a grave prognosis with 15 % of patients expiring before reaching medical care. Overall mortality is approximately 45 % with approximately 30 % of survivors having moderate to severe disabilities [15].

Arteriovenous Malformations (AVM)

An arteriovenous malformation is an abnormal tangle of blood vessels that can form in the brain or spinal cord during development. This form of cerebrovascular disease is considered congenital, meaning that they are present at birth. Most do not present clinically until childhood or early adulthood. An AVM is generally comprised of arteries that carry blood into a "nidus" of tangled, abnormal blood vessels that then drain directly to a vein. Because of the high flow of blood into the abnormal bed of vessels, many of them are prone to rupture and bleeding.

The symptoms associated with an AVM vary considerably from patient to patient depending on the location of the malformation, its size, and whether it bleeds or not. Some patients can present with seizures. Others present with focal neurological deficits such as weakness, for example, if it is located in the motor part of the brain. Not infrequently, an AVM can rupture and bleed. Frequency of arteriovenous malformation hemorrhage is thought to be 2–4 % per year [16]. Bleeding is typically into the brain tissue itself but can also bleed into the subarachnoid space around the brain or into the ventricles, the fluid-filled spaces within the brain. Depending on the severity of bleeding, symptoms can include sudden headache, seizures, or other neurological deficits that vary depending on the location of the

hemorrhage. Very severe bleeds or bleeding into the brainstem can lead to a depressed level of consciousness, coma, or death.

When a patient presents with symptoms suggestive of an arteriovenous malformation, following a neurological exam, an imaging study such as a CT scan or MRI scan is often performed. MRI can show the abnormal tangle of blood vessels in many cases. CT is good for demonstrating any bleeding that may have occurred. However, the best study to detect an AVM is a catheter cerebral angiogram.

Treatment for arteriovenous malformation varies depending on several factors. Generally, symptomatic patients with an AVM in a surgically accessible region of the brain will be recommended to have surgery. In some cases, endovascular techniques are used to occlude some of the AVM from within the vessels prior to surgery. This type of treatment is generally not curative and requires surgery for stereotactic radiosurgery. The goal of surgery is to completely remove the abnormal blood vessels while preserving the normal brain and normal blood vessels in the area.

Stereotactic radiation therapy is also used to treat surgically non-accessible arteriovenous malformations. This treatment option requires that the nidus of the AVM be less than 3 cm. Over the subsequent years, the malformation will slowly involute and become occluded; however, patients are still at risk of hemorrhage during this time until the arteriovenous malformation has occluded. The treatment plan for AVM cannot be generalized as there are several variables that may make one option or a combination of treatment options better for an individual patient.

Cavernous Malformation (Cavernoma)

A cavernous malformation, also known as a cavernous angioma or cavernoma, is an abnormal collection of blood vessels in the brain. It consists of multiple, small dilated sacs which resemble blood vessels but do not have a direct connection with other blood vessels. The appearance on MRI imaging has been described as resembling a mulberry. Cavernous malformations can rupture, leading to bleeding into the adjacent brain.

Generally, this bleeding tends to be small to moderate as compared to the large amount of bleeding that can be seen from an arteriovenous malformation. A cavernous malformation may increase in size over time, often with evidence of leakage of blood products at multiple times in the past at the time of presentation.

Bleeding or leakage of blood produced from a cavernoma can be silent or symptomatic. With bleeding, neurological symptoms related to the location of the cavernoma can occur. These vary considerably depending on what part of the brain the malformation effects. A cavernoma in the brainstem can be much more dangerous than a small peripheral lesion in less important parts of the brain. As the malformation enlarges and irritates the brain around it, particularly if there have been episodes of bleeding in the past, seizures or progressive neurological dysfunction can occur. Again, these vary depending on the location of the lesion. Headaches are nonspecific symptoms that can occur in some patients.

If a patient presents with neurological symptoms, they typically undergo some form of imaging study after a neurological examination. A CT scan or MRI scan can generally detect these lesions and show evidence of bleeding if any has occurred. Cavernous malformations have a quite characteristic appearance on MRI imaging, and thus the diagnosis can often be made with a high degree of accuracy. Occasionally, asymptomatic cavernomas can be discovered on a CT or MRI scan incidentally, if the patient gets these tests for another reason. Interestingly, cavernomas, despite being of blood vessel origin, are not visible on cerebral angiograms, unlike most other cerebrovascular malformations such as cerebral aneurysms or arteriovenous malformations.

Treatment varies depending on location, symptoms, and size of these malformations. For some patients, they are simply watched and only treated at a later date if symptoms become progressively severe. In those that decide on treatment, surgical removal of the malformation is generally curative. These are not tumors so if removed completely they do not generally recur.

Brain Tumors

Introduction

Neurosurgical treatment of brain tumors has been revolutionized over the past several decades. Advances in radiological diagnosis, surgical and neuroanesthetic management, perioperative pharmacology, and aggressive rehabilitation have rendered what in the past was a dreaded procedure associated with high morbidity into an often very smooth, uneventful intervention in many cases. Unfortunately, the overall prognosis for long-term survival remains poor for malignant primary brain tumors, despite significant advances in adjuvant treatment that are showing great promise. From the standpoint of a physiatrist caring for brain tumor patients, patients who recover uneventfully from routine brain tumor surgery may only require physical therapy assistance with their early mobilization. Many patients are able to be discharged safely to home as early as a day or two following some of these surgeries in the modern practice of neurosurgery. Other patients may have significant neurological deficits or functional impairment requiring prolonged multimodality inpatient rehabilitation.

Advances in Operative Technique and Treatment Options

The advent of the neurosurgical microscope, which came into widespread practical use in the 1960s, is one of the key technical advances leading to improved outcome from intracranial neurosurgery. In the last two decades, there has been an explosion in the field of "surgical navigation." Surgical navigation systems integrate digitized instruments with advanced imaging modalities and computers. This allows mapping of tumors preoperatively and accurate intraoperative localization. Real-time intraoperative CT and MRI also are utilized in some centers.

Advanced anesthetic and electrophysiological techniques, often in combination with surgical navigation, allow identification and protection of critical brain areas during surgery near eloquent areas of the brain, for example, those involving motor or language areas. For the mapping and protection of critical language areas in the brain, patients can be operated upon while awake without discomfort. Specialized endoscopes are also increasingly utilized in the resection of neoplasms involving the ventricular system and CSF pathways. In certain cases of tumor-associated obstructive hydrocephalus, these endoscopes can be used to bypass the site of obstruction, obviating the need for indwelling shunts that may be prone to infection or malfunction. In some cases, tumors can be resected endoscopically through a simple burr hole rather than requiring an open craniotomy. These technologies and others have dramatically enhanced the accuracy of brain tumor surgery, enabling surgeons to be at the same time more aggressive in pursuing complete resections while minimizing the invasiveness and improving the safety of such surgery.

The modern neurosurgical armamentarium allows accurate diagnosis and aggressive resection of many intracranial tumors, pursuing a surgical cure for certain tumors, and therapeutically beneficial debulking for others. While some tumors remain "inoperable," the definition of this term clearly has shifted in the last several decades as these technologies have been introduced and exploited to optimize multimodality management of intracranial neoplasms.

Treatment options have also expanded for tumors that are not primarily amenable to resection. The combined expertise of neurosurgeons, radiation oncologists, and radiation physicists has led to another explosion in the therapeutic options for brain tumors known as *stereotactic radiosurgery*. This term refers to several different technologies designed to deliver tumoricidal doses of radiation in very brief discrete treatments while minimizing radiation exposure to normal brain structures. These treatments are called "radiosurgery" to differentiate them from standard radiation therapy typically involving broader treatment fields, lower radiation doses, and longer courses of treatment.

Radiosurgery (e.g., the Gamma Knife or Cyberknife) is conceptually more like a surgical intervention and is generally done in a collaborative fashion involving neurosurgery and radiation oncology. These technologies are based on the concept of using multiple extremely focal beams of radiation delivered along varied pathways such that the radiation exposure to normal brain structures along any single pathway through the brain is quite small, but the beams coalesce in a tightly delineated highly "conformal" manner to deliver large radiation dosages to the target while sparing adjoining brain structures.

Stereotactic radiosurgery is a very important treatment especially for smaller or deep-seated tumors that are relatively inaccessible to open surgery. It is used extensively for small solitary or multiple brain metastases, meningiomas in surgically inaccessible locations, vestibular schwannomas (a.k.a acoustic neuromas), and a variety of other intracranial neoplasms. Its role is more limited for malignant gliomas. It may also be used as an adjuvant to open surgery for residual or recurrent disease. Since it is fully noninvasive and does not require anesthesia, it is an important treatment option for elderly patients or patients with significant medical comorbidities that increase the relative risks of open surgery.

The goal of the modern brain tumor surgeon is to utilize all of these tools in a rational manner that takes into account the nature and location of the tumor, as well as the underlying health and age of the patient, to optimize a treatment strategy to diagnose and treat the tumor *while avoiding any neurological complications or functional impairment*. Preoperative neurologic function is an important predictor of postoperative functional outcome. In essence, we try to ensure that the patient comes through surgery requiring the least amount of therapy and rehabilitation as is possible. Of course that goal is impossible to achieve in all cases.

Depending on the age, vigor, and underlying health of the patient, the location of the neoplasm and the aggressiveness of resection needed or pursued, and the skill and experience of the surgeon and his or her team, a range of neurologic and functional outcomes occur following intracranial tumor surgery. Expected neurological deficits or unanticipated complications may necessitate significant assistance from the various experts in the fields of physiatry, physical and occupational therapy, speech and cognitive/behavioral therapy, psychiatry, neuropsychology, and related fields. Prevention of delayed complications from intracranial tumor surgery can depend very importantly on the care rendered by treating physiatrists. A practical working knowledge of the postoperative management goals, strategies, and pitfalls of post-op care of these patients and of the issues specific to certain tumors and procedures is of importance.

Intracranial Tumor Types and Treatment Considerations

Any standard neurosurgical textbook lists the numerous types of tumors that occur intracranially. From a physiatry standpoint, it is helpful to understand different categories or types of tumors that affect the treatment goals and perioperative issues. Broadly speaking, intracranial tumors may be intrinsic or intraaxial, i.e., arising from within the brain parenchyma, or extraaxial. An important example of the extraaxial tumors is meningiomas, typically arising from the meningeal linings of the calvarium. Extraaxial lesions may invade the brain to varying degrees as they grow away from the relatively noncompliant cranium.

Common intraaxial tumors include gliomas which may be low grade and slow growing or high grade and rapidly progressive. Most gliomas cannot be cured surgically due to their infiltrative nature. Aggressive surgical resection of low grade gliomas has been shown to result in long-term remission in many cases and improved functional survival [17]. Aggressive surgical debulking of malignant gliomas and glioblastoma also improves quality of life and survival [18].

In recent years, the advent of multifaceted molecular and chromosomal analysis has allowed the development of more sophisticated and targeted adjuvant therapy. Surgical resection of tumors provides adequate pathological material to facilitate these more sophisticated therapeutic approaches. Stereotactic needle biopsy alone may not be sufficient for the tissue analysis

required to optimize adjuvant therapies. For intrinsic or glial neoplasms, tumor location and pattern of growth are the key factors that determine resectability. Factors that favor resection include younger age of the patient, large size, superficial or accessible location, a relatively well-circumscribed growth pattern, and edema or mass effect on surrounding structures. Counterintuitively, relatively benign tumors may be the brain tumors whose resection actually offers the most benefit relative to the more malignant gliomas. Tumors that are deep seated, are situated in eloquent brain areas, or demonstrate a diffuse, poorly circumscribed, or multilobar pattern of growth at presentation are less likely to be beneficially resected.

Accessible solitary or large symptomatic brain metastases from systemic cancers are often excised surgically as well. Stereotactic radiosurgery plays a very important role in the management of brain metastases, either as a primary treatment for single or multiple small or surgically inaccessible metastases or as adjuvant treatment to the bed of a surgically resected metastasis to lessen likelihood of local recurrence. Whole-brain radiation therapy (WBRT) historically was the primary treatment for brain metastases, prior to data showing that outcomes may be improved by aggressive surgical or "radiosurgical" management of solitary or relatively small numbers of brain metastases [19–21].

For appropriately selected patients, these strategies may help cancer patients avoid some of the long-term cognitive and memory impairment that may occur in some patients as a delayed complication of whole-brain radiation. Whole-brain RT continues to play an important role for patients with very numerous metastases and may help control recurrence from microscopic disease. It may also remain the treatment of choice for highly radio-sensitive tumors, for example, small cell lung carcinoma. The decision whether to use local therapies alone such as surgery or radiosurgery or to add adjuvant WBRT is a complex one factoring in the extent and aggressiveness of systemic disease, tumor biology, patient functional status, neurologic condition, and patient preferences.

Surgical treatment of extraaxial neoplasms involves generally similar surgical principles to the intrinsic brain neoplasms but varies in some of its achievable goals and technical considerations. Many meningiomas can be surgically cured, especially if it is technically feasible to excise not only the main bulk of the tumor but also a broad enough margin of dura mater surrounding the site of tumor origin and dural attachment. When possible, the dural site of origin is completely excised and replaced with an autograft, allograft, or synthetic patch with an attempt to achieve relatively watertight closure to avoid postoperative cerebrospinal fluid leakage.

Typically meningiomas are benign and slow growing. Incidentally noted or asymptomatic meningiomas may thus often be followed with periodic radiographic surveillance and only treated if they are observed to grow or become symptomatic. A small percentage of meningiomas may demonstrate atypical or even malignant phenotype, with an increased likelihood of invading adjoining structures, growing rapidly, and recurring following surgical resection. Some advocate empiric postsurgical treatment of resected meningiomas of aggressive subtype with radiation therapy or radiosurgery to the area of tumor resection.

It is worthwhile for allied medical specialists involved in the treatment of brain tumor patients to have a working knowledge of a few specific intracranial tumor types and locations that require special attention in the perioperative period. In general, both supratentorial and infratentorial tumors can be operated on with a good margin of safety, although there are some considerations specific to surgery in the posterior fossa. Due to the closed or contained nature of the intracranial compartment, intracranial masses such as tumors or hemorrhages tend to increase intracranial pressure.

The posterior fossa has a tendency to act as an even more critically enclosed space, containing vital brainstem structures within a smaller intracranial compartment constrained by the tentorium. Tumors and tumor-induced brain edema tend to become highly symptomatic in the posterior fossa, inducing nausea, vomiting, and gait ataxia that can progress quickly to life-threatening brainstem compression. Relative to supratentorial tumors, postradiation or radiosurgically induced edema may not be tolerated. It may be preferable to surgically excise tumors in this location if they have mass effect. Masses or postoperative edema can obstruct the fourth ventricle and cause acute hydrocephalus. All these factors may necessitate more aggressive management of these patients with antiemetic agents and steroids, with slower tapering of postoperative steroid dosages.

Neurosurgeons also draw an important distinction between tumors whose operative exposure is achieved via conventional exposures through the cranial vault and those involving the skull base, i.e., situated such that extensive or complex dissection or drilling of the skull base is required to access them. A host of varied pathologies may involve these areas, including meningiomas, pituitary adenomas, chordomas, dermoid and epidermoid cysts, vestibular and other cranial nerve schwannomas, glomus jugulare tumors, sarcomas, and metastases. Relative to many tumors arising near the skull base, pituitary adenomas are relatively accessible via open or endoscopic approaches via the nasal passages and sphenoid sinus, a.k.a. transsphenoidal approaches, and have been addressed via variations of that route for many years.

Skull-base surgery is a recognized discipline within the field of neurosurgery, sometimes involving allied specialties, e.g., otolaryngology, ophthalmology, or plastic surgery, with fellowships dedicated to developing expertise in this challenging area. These surgeries may be extremely prolonged and entail a higher risk of postoperative complications and morbidity. Potential special issues in this patient population are the risks of cranial neuropathies, including very problematic lower cranial dysfunction sometimes requiring PEG tubes or tracheostomies, risk of pituitary or hypothalamic dysfunction, as well as a higher likelihood of postoperative CSF leakage, which may present as rhinorrhea or otorrhea.

Technical advances in endoscopic neurosurgery are having a significant impact in this field, allowing some lesions that were previously accessible only via highly destructive or extensive approaches to be addressed with less invasiveness and morbidity. Even more revolutionary is the widespread and very successful application of stereotactic radiosurgery to the treatment of pathology of the skull base. Many patients who in the past would have required an extremely formidable skull-base surgery for fairly common problems such as vestibular schwannoma (acoustic neuroma) or meningioma of the cavernous sinus or parasellar region are now treated noninvasively with stereotactic radiosurgery and often achieve cure or at least long-term satisfactory "biological control" (arrest of tumor progression) with this treatment modality.

In the modern practice of neurosurgery, many patients requiring more routine craniotomy may need little assistance from physiatry as their recuperation from this surgery may often be very uneventful. However, patients requiring "skull-base approaches" still pose a formidable technical challenge for neurosurgery, and these patients may yet require more prolonged and intensive postoperative care and rehabilitation.

As in any surgical field, there are also special challenges that arise for the neurosurgeon in patients who require reoperation in the same area as the previous surgery. This situation often arises in patients with recurrence of a glioma, metastasis, or meningioma. In the case of the malignant gliomas, recurrence near the original treatment site usually occurs at some point in the course of the illness, and reoperation is frequently considered as an option. Frequently these patients may have received chemotherapy and/or radiation, and some may be systemically challenged by side effects of chemotherapy drugs or systemic illness in the case of brain metastasis patients. The scalp in these situations may be thin, atrophic, and avascular and heal poorly. Risk of wound healing problems and wound infection is higher in this situation. Meticulous wound care is of particular importance for these patients, and often sutures or staples may be left in place significantly longer than is customary for the primary surgery. Collaboration with plastic surgery colleagues can be helpful, and physiatrists and health-care professionals should coordinate wound care for these patients closely with the operating surgery team.

Postoperative Management of Brain Tumor Patients

As noted above, the postoperative management of many patients requiring neurosurgery for a brain tumor need not be complicated. Generally early mobilization of patients is advisable. We observe most patients one night in an ICU setting unless they have specific issues requiring a longer stay. Patients who awaken from surgery with unexpected neurologic deficits undergo urgent CT scan. Postoperative MRI scans with and without contrast are generally obtained routinely postoperative day one to assess extent of tumor resection and rule out residual tumor in patients harboring malignant pathology or intrinsic neoplasms. These images are an important baseline for guiding future treatment. Surgical staples are often used to close craniotomy incisions and *do not* contraindicate postoperative MRI, i.e., they are MRI compatible.

In patients who recover uneventfully, diet is advanced, catheters and lines are removed, and the patient is mobilized out of bed on the morning following surgery. Deep venous thrombosis prophylaxis is used intraoperatively (compression stockings) and mini-dose heparin or equivalent DVT prophylaxis begun in most patients on the first postoperative day. Careful blood pressure management is observed especially in the first 24 h following surgery. Normotensive blood pressure is typically the goal. Patients with hypertension may predispose to postoperative brain hemorrhage and those with hypotension to ischemic complications. Fluid management is typically directed at keeping the patient euvolemic with isotonic fluids. Hypotonic fluids are avoided so as not to exacerbate cerebral edema. Careful monitoring of electrolytes is important, with particular attention to derangements of sodium metabolism that can occur in craniotomy patients, for example, cerebral salt wasting or SIADH.

Most brain tumor patients will be on dexamethasone to control perioperative cerebral edema, which is typically tapered following surgery. The numerous side effects of steroids include hyperglycemia, hypertension, sodium and water retention, agitation including steroid psychosis, gastritis and peptic ulcers, and avascular necrosis of the hip. Prolonged usage induces iatrogenic Cushing's syndrome with symptoms including obesity and hirsutism. The guiding principle of steroid management is to taper the patient as quickly as possible to the lowest dose that keeps them free of symptoms of cerebral edema such as headache, nausea, and focal neurologic symptoms that reverse at higher doses. Patient requirements for steroids may fluctuate, and higher doses are often needed following radiation therapy or adjuvant radiosurgical treatment. More aggressive dosing of steroids and slower tapers are used in patients presenting preoperatively with more marked edema radiographically or more symptoms of elevated intracranial pressure. For extraaxial tumors such as meningiomas, steroids are fully tapered. Patients being treated for malignant intrinsic neoplasms may need to be maintained on steroids from the postoperative period through postoperative radiation therapy depending on the extent of edema present.

Seizures are present in about 20–40 % of patients by the time their tumor is diagnosed. Patients with a history of seizure should be maintained on anticonvulsants perioperatively. If surgical treatment ultimately results in resolution of perilesional edema, these patients may be considered for weaning off of anticonvulsants electively in a delayed fashion under neurological supervision. Prophylactic anticonvulsants are not currently used routinely for newly diagnosed brain tumors [22]. In patients undergoing craniotomy for supratentorial tumors, prophylactic anticonvulsants are typically used perioperatively but may be tapered starting a week after surgery. Seizures are rare after posterior fossa surgery.

Postoperative craniotomy wound management seems to vary based on the preferences and practices of various surgeons and may vary depending on the type of closure utilized, i.e.,

staples, sutures, or tissue glues or sealants. Typically head wraps or bandages are removed between 24 and 48 h postoperatively. While some surgeons and institutions prefer to maintain the incisions dry until removal of clips or sutures, many others prefer a head washing protocol with a mild shampoo starting 48–72 h postoperatively. In our institution, we prefer to maintain good scalp hygiene with the latter protocol, which is supported in the literature [23].

If caring for a craniotomy patient in a rehabilitation facility, the best practice is probably to ensure the facility is familiar with the preferences of the operating surgeon. If there is any concern regarding possible infection raised by erythema, swelling, drainage, or wound separation, it is imperative to alert the surgeon prior to instituting therapy, for example, with antibiotics. Empiric antibiotics prior to evaluation by their surgical team may ultimately limit the opportunity to obtain cultures permitting proper identification of causative organisms and thereby adversely affect the ability to target specific antimicrobial therapy. Prompt recognition and therapy for any infectious issue pertaining to a craniotomy wound is imperative. A minor stitch abscess dealt with promptly may minimally harm a patient's recovery and prognosis. However, if infection progresses to involve osteomyelitis of the bone flap requiring its surgical removal or a brain abscess, the consequences may be very significant and also may greatly delay the ability to offer needed adjuvant treatment such as chemotherapy or radiation.

Occasionally there may be significant accumulations of fluid postoperatively in the subgaleal compartment. These are often self-limited but may persist for weeks after surgery. In some cases surgeons may choose to aspirate these collections with or without the subsequent placement of a head wrap dressing to limit re-accumulation of the fluid. In general, it is very beneficial for physiatrists caring for post-craniotomy patients to coordinate wound care and evaluation closely and in a timely manner with the surgical team that has performed the initial surgery.

Evaluation of a post-craniotomy patient who deteriorates neurologically must proceed in a systematic and logical fashion. Often the cause may prove to be systemic or metabolic, such as a derangement of sodium metabolism, hypoxemia, or hypercarbia, for example, related to pulmonary embolism or intercurrent or postoperative pneumonia, or sepsis, for example, from a postoperative urinary tract infection. Primary infection of the craniotomy site or brain abscess is also a concern. Drug toxicity, e.g., anticonvulsant or pain medication overdose, is also possible. Patients with underlying CNS pathology such as brain tumor may be more sensitive to narcotics than might be expected otherwise.

Another common cause of worsening in a patient previously recuperating well may be a decrease in postoperative steroid dose that is too rapid for the degree of residual symptomatic edema. Delayed hemorrhage related to the craniotomy may occur, either intraparenchymal, subdural, or epidural. Obstructive or communicating hydrocephalus is also possible. Seizures, either observed or unobserved with subsequent lethargy or focal deficit (Todd's paralysis), may occur. Subclinical seizure or epilepsia partialis continua may be a cause of unexplained obtundation. Vascular complications such as ischemia, stroke, or venous thrombosis may occur in postoperative craniotomy patients.

Appropriate evaluation to elucidate the underlying cause should consist of careful clinical observation and documentation of the patient's neurologic exam, with careful consideration of the time course of symptom evolution. Blood work to evaluate for metabolic derangement, drug toxicity, and sepsis is important. Timely imaging with CT scan to assess for intraaxial or extraaxial hemorrhage, hydrocephalus, and pneumocephalus can be very helpful. MRI may be less practical as an initial evaluation but will more clearly show cerebral edema, ischemia, or stroke. Again, it is crucial for the physiatry team caring for a post-craniotomy patient who is worsening to have close communication with the surgical team who, having done the surgery, will best understand the specific risks and concerns for that particular patient.

The physiatric and rehabilitative component of a brain tumor patient's care is of great importance and underscores the critical nature of a team approach to the care of brain tumor patients. In the author's opinion, it is essential that, barring geographical obstacles, any patient currently diagnosed with a brain tumor must be treated in a center that offers a coordinated multispecialty approach to brain tumor treatment, whether in the community or academic setting. At a minimum, this requires collaborative input from specialists in neurosurgery, neurooncology, radiation oncology, neuroradiology, neuropathology, and physiatry. Physiatrists can play a crucial and important role not only in helping patients optimize recovery and community reintegration following surgical treatment for brain neoplasms but in helping to ensure that patients and their families have access to support services and especially to the key nonsurgical specialists, especially neurooncology and radiation oncology, in a timely fashion during their rehabilitation or after discharge from a rehabilitation facility.

Adult Cranial Neurosurgery: Developmental Disorders and Hydrocephalus

Many developmental syndromes and disorders exist in the realm of neurosurgery, ranging from craniofacial disorders to spina bifida. However, the following text is restricted to adult developmental issues and their presentation as well as treatments. Much of the following material can be found in Greenberg's *Handbook of Neurosurgery*, and if more information is desired on any of these topics, that text is an excellent source.

One of the most common neurosurgical developmental syndromes diagnosed in the adult age group is Chiari 1 malformation [24]. This must be distinguished from Chiari 2 (or Arnold-Chiari) malformation please see Table 6.1 [25]. Chiari 1 is a malformation of the hindbrain, resulting in cerebrospinal fluid circulation dysfunction, usually cerebellar tonsillar ectopia, and occasionally syringomyelia. A wide range of symptoms are

Table 6.1 Comparisons of Chiari type 1 and 2 anomalies

Finding	Chiari type 1	Chiari type 2
Caudal dislocation of the medulla	Unusual	Yes
Caudal dislocation into the cervical canal	Tonsils	Inferior vermis, medulla, fourth ventricle
Spina bifida (myelomeningocele)	May be present	Rarely absent
Hydrocephalus	May be absent	Rarely absent
Medullary "kink"	Absent	Present in 55 %
Course of upper cervical nerves	Usually normal	Usually cephalad
Usual age of presentation	Young adult	Infancy
Usual presentation	Cervical pain, suboccipital headache	Progressive hydrocephalus, respiratory distress

associated with Chiari 1, though many are controversial. These include, in order of commonality, headache, neck and suboccipital discomfort, weakness, numbness, loss of temperature sensation (often presenting with painless burns), unsteadiness, diplopia, dysphasia, tinnitus, vomiting, dysarthria, dizziness, deafness, and facial numbness [26]. Signs a practitioner may observe, also in order of commonality, include hyperreflexia of the lower extremities, nystagmus, gait disturbance, hand atrophy, upper extremity weakness, "cape-like" sensory loss, cerebellar signs, hyperreflexia of the upper extremities, lower cranial nerve dysfunction, Babinski sign, lower extremity weakness, dysesthesia, fasciculation, and Horner's sign [27]. It is important to distinguish between a simple radiographic diagnosis of Chiari 1, low-lying cerebellar tonsils, and the symptomatic clinical syndrome of Chiari 1. This distinction is often first made in the neurosurgeon's office.

Once the diagnosis of adult Chiari is made, treatment options include observation versus surgical intervention depending on the severity of symptoms and the presence or absence of syringomyelia. The goal of surgery is to normalize the flow of cerebrospinal fluid around the brainstem and cerebellum at the foramen magnum. This is usually accomplished by performing a midline suboccipital craniectomy and duraplasty. Posterior cervical laminectomies of C1, and occasionally C2 or lower, may be necessary to fully expose the descended cerebellar tonsils. Duraplasty may be performed with a dural substitute such as bovine pericardium or DuraGen or with autograft such as local pericranium or fascia lata. Surgical complications include leakage from the wound, shunt-requiring hydrocephalus, infection, aseptic meningitis, subdural hematoma, and respiratory depression. Complication rates range from 10 to 33 % depending on the series. Substantive and lasting improvement is generally in the 80–90 % range [28–30].

Clearly Chiari 1 malformation is a complex syndrome with still poorly understood pathophysiology. The multiplicity of presenting complaints, poor correlation with radiographic findings, and high surgical complication rates make it a formidable disease process. However, with careful patient selection and meticulous attention to surgical detail, Chiari 1 treatment can be extremely gratifying.

Normal pressure hydrocephalus (NPH) is an acquired diagnosis, usually seen in an older population. Similar to Chiari 1, it involves a disruption of cerebrospinal fluid flow dynamics. The classic triad of NPH includes dementia, gait disturbance, and urinary incontinence. NPH is an important diagnosis to evaluate in the setting of memory and cognitive impairment because it represents a remediable form of dementia. Many neurologic conditions, most commonly Alzheimer's dementia and Parkinson's disease, may present with symptoms similar to NPH. In addition, multiple other disease states can have similar findings please see Table 6.2 [31]. The gait disturbance of NPH is usually the first symptom to present and often manifests as short, shuffling, unsteady steps. Because of the perceived difficulty of lifting one's feet off the floor, this

Table 6.2 Conditions with similar presentations to NPH

Neurodegenerative disorders
Alzheimer's disease
Parkinson's disease
Lewy body disease
Huntington's disease
Frontotemporal dementia
Corticobasal degeneration
Progressive supranuclear palsy
Amytrophic lateral sclerosis
Multisystem atrophy
Spongiform encephalopathy
Vascular dementia
Cerebrovascular disease
Multi-infarct dementia
Binswanger's disease
CADASIL
Vertebrobasilar insufficiency
Other hydrocephalic disorders
Aqueductal stenosis
Arrested hydrocephalus
Long-standing overt ventriculomegaly syndrome
Non-communicating hydrocephalus
Infectious diease
Lyme disease
HIV
Syphilis
Urological disorders
Urinary tract infection
Bladder or prostate cancer
Benign prostatic hypertrophy
Miscellaneous
Vitamin B_{12} deficiency
Collagen vascular diseases
Epilepsy
Depression
Traumatic brain injury
Spinal stenosis
Chiari malformation
Wernicke's encephalopathy
Carcinomatous meningitis
Spinal cord tumor

gait is often described as "magnetic." Dementia presents with impaired memory with both bradyphrenia (slowness of thought) and bradykinesia (slowness of movement). Urinary incontinence is usually a later symptom and completely unwitting by the patient.

Because NPH shares signs and symptoms with so many disease states and has a poorly understood pathophysiology, it is difficult to diagnose. A good clinical history detailing the above symptoms presenting insidiously and progressively is important. Ventriculomegaly out of proportion to overall atrophy on CT or MR imaging is also useful but not a solely diagnostic criterion. A "tap test" or high-volume lumbar puncture is often performed. Opening pressures are generally in the upper range of normal (15 ± 4.5 cm H_2O) and 40–50 ml of CSF removed [31]. Many centers prefer a trial of ambulatory lumbar drainage in which a lumbar drain is inserted and CSF drained constantly for 3–5 days. Patients will often experience an improvement by day three and a slow relapse after the drain is removed. Radionuclide cisternography and cerebral blood flow measurement testing rarely yield helpful diagnostic information.

Once the diagnosis is established, CSF diversion is the treatment of choice. This can be performed with a lumbar-peritoneal shunt or more commonly with a ventriculoperitoneal shunt. Generally programmable shunt valves are employed in order to glean the most benefit from CSF diversion without exposing the patient to undue risk. A retrospective review of shunt insertion for NPH estimated a complication rate between 34 and 57 %, though this included long-term follow-up inclusive of delayed shunt malfunctions [32]. These complications included subdural hematoma, intracerebral hematoma, infection, seizure, and shunt malfunction. Estimated mortality directly associated with shunt insertion for NPH is 2 % [33].

Unlike most procedures where the risk is directly around the time of surgery, the risk of subdural hematoma is increased for the remaining lifetime of the patient, given the shunt is in good working order. As the usually enlarged ventricles are slowly drained and shrink, the mantle (tissue from the cortex or surface of the brain to the ventricular wall) may not proportionally expand. This makes the cortex more likely to sag away from the dural lining of the skull. The surface cortical veins are thus put on stretch and are more likely to rupture, resulting in a subdural hematoma. Moreover, as blood collects in the subdural space, placing pressure on the brain, the shunt will allow the ventricular system to further decompress, encouraging the hematoma to expand. Despite the relatively high reported morbidity and mortality rates associated with shunt insertion for NPH, most patients, and their families, opt for the procedure given the alternative bleak prognosis as well as the often near complete reversal of neurologic decline.

Chiari 1 and NPH represent two diagnoses relevant to the care of adults with neurologic deficits. They are both remediable disease processes, at least for a given amount of time, but if missed subject patients to a lifetime of progressive issues. However, with proper diagnosis and treatment, both Chiari 1 and NPH are extremely responsive to neurosurgical intervention instilling meaningful positive impact on lives of both patients and their families (Tables 6.1 and 6.2).

Neurosurgical Infections

Introduction

Infections may be encountered in the field of clinical neurosurgery under a number of circumstances. These include cerebral abscess, subdural empyema, parasitic infection, viral encephalitis, fungal infection, spinal epidural abscess, shunt infection, and neurosurgical postoperative infection. Each entity must be diagnosed and treated expediently to maximize the likelihood of a complete recovery. After treatment in the acute care setting, acute inpatient rehabilitation and subsequent outpatient rehabilitation services may be necessary and essential. What follows is a survey of some of the more common infections encountered in neurosurgery, along with their associated rehabilitation considerations.

Cerebral Abscess

A cerebral abscess is typically an encapsulated mass of purulent necrotic infected material within the brain parenchyma. An abscess may arise from hematogenous (through the blood) spread or contiguous spread. Hematogenous spread may originate in the lungs as a lung abscess, in the heart as endocarditis or in the gastrointestinal system such as a pelvic infection. These abscesses may be multiple in 10–50% of cases [34]. Contiguous spread may occur as a result of sinusitis, dental infection, penetrating trauma, or after a neurosurgical procedure. Streptococcus is the most common organism identified in brain abscess but the organism may be anaerobic or even multiple [35].

Clinically, cerebral abscess may present with a focal neurological deficit based on the location of the lesion (i.e., aphasia or hemiparesis), seizure, or symptoms due to increased intracranial pressure, such as headache, vomiting, or altered mental status. Fever may not be present, and white blood cell count may be normal. Blood cultures are often negative and the erythrocyte sedimentation rate can be normal as well. Diagnosis is made by neuroimaging, with computed tomography (CT) used as the initial screening test and magnetic resonance imaging (MRI) used for definitive diagnosis (Fig. 6.1).

Treatment consists of surgical drainage and intravenous antibiotics. Most abscesses can be drained by stereotactic needle aspiration. Surgical excision may be necessary in cases of traumatic abscess with retained foreign body. Initial antibiotic therapy is broad spectrum and then tailored by culture results and continued for 6–8 weeks. During acute rehabilitation, careful monitoring is needed to assess for signs of neurological worsening, infectious relapse, and poor wound healing. Seizure prophylaxis should continue in the setting of all supratentorial abscesses, and close follow-up with infectious disease and neurosurgery is critical. Prevention of deep venous thrombosis can be managed with subcutaneous heparin if immobility is an issue. Nutrition, bowel and bladder regimens, and prevention of skin breakdown also need to be addressed in debilitated patients. Subacute rehabilitation is important for treatment of neurological deficits, which may be present in up to 50% of patients.

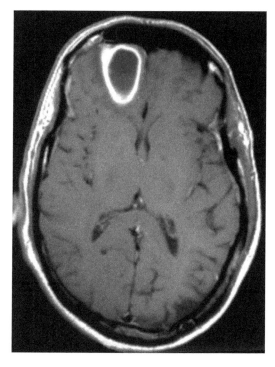

Fig. 6.1 Axial postcontrast T1 weighted MRI demonstrating brain abscess with typical hypotense center and ring enhancement

Subdural Empyema

Subdural empyema is a purulent infection within the subdural space, usually over the convexities of the brain. These mostly occur as a result of contiguous spread of infection of the paranasal sinuses. Much less likely are postsurgical, traumatic, and hematogenous origins. Clinically, they tend to present more acutely and fulminantly than cerebral abscesses might, with fever, headache, meningismus, weakness, and altered mental status [36]. Streptococci are the most common organisms. Once again, MRI allows for definitive diagnosis (Fig. 6.2).

Treatment is surgical and pharmaceutical. Burr hole drainage may be sufficient for an early fully liquefied empyema, but craniotomy is necessary in all other circumstances. Antibiotics are required for at least 4–6 weeks. The majority of patients have some degree of neurological deficit on discharge and therefore will require inpatient and outpatient rehabilitation.

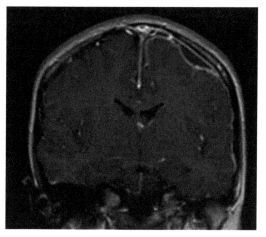

Fig. 6.2 Coronal postcontrast T1 weighted MRI showing subdural empyema along the left frontal convexity with marginal enhancement around a subdural hypodensity

Parasitic Infections

A number of parasitic infections may involve the central nervous system (CNS) and often occur in the setting of foreign travel or immunosuppression. Cysticercosis is the most common parasitic infection in the CNS and is caused by the pork tapeworm *Taenia solium*, endemic in Central and South America among other regions[37]. Cysts may develop in the brain parenchyma, subarachnoid space, or ventricles. Patients may present with seizures, signs of elevated intracranial pressure, and focal neurological deficits. The infection may be diagnosed by serum serology and CNS involvement by CT (which can identify a punctate high density scolex or head) and MRI (Fig. 6.3).

Treatment usually consists of antiparasitic agents, antiepileptic drugs, and steroids. Surgery is necessary only if diagnosis is in doubt, if a large cyst with mass effect is present, or if hydrocephalus is present due to ventricular location requiring shunting. Fifteen days of medical therapy may suffice.

The other parasitic infection seen with some frequency in neurosurgery is toxoplasmosis. This is a protozoan that is clinically significant only in an immunocompromised host. It is the most common mass lesion in patients with acquired immunodeficiency syndrome (AIDS). Toxoplasmosis

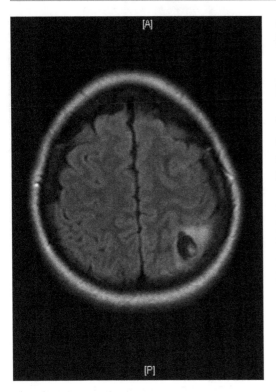

Fig. 6.3 Axial noncontrast proton density weighted MRI depicting a left parietal cysticercosis lesion with a bulls eye appearance of bright edema around a dark cyst around a bright scolex

presents as a mass lesion in the brain but must be distinguished from progressive multifocal leuko-encephalopathy (PML). This can usually be done with serologic testing, but occasionally the neurosurgeon is asked to perform a biopsy to make the diagnosis. Treatment is with antitoxoplasmosis agents.

Viral Encephalitis

Herpes simplex encephalitis is the viral entity that may be seen by a neurosurgeon and require biopsy for diagnosis. It is a fulminant disease that may rapidly progress to coma. Treatment with acyclovir should be initiated as soon as the diagnosis is even entertained. MRI imaging demonstrates edema in the temporal lobes, sometimes associated with hemorrhage [38]. Biopsy may be necessary in equivocal cases. Fourteen to twenty-one

days of treatment is indicated, and rehabilitation is critical to recovery of function.

Fungal Infection

These infections are typically seen in immuno-compromised patients. Aspergillus may occur as a cerebral abscess (Fig. 6.4) in organ transplant patients [39].

Cryptococcus can develop in normal or immunocompromised patients, as a cryptococcoma or pseudocyst or as meningitis. A neurosurgeon may be called to drain a large pseudocyst or manage intracranial hypertension if it exists. Some patients will develop hydrocephalus and require a shunt.

Spinal Epidural Abscess

Spinal epidural abscess is a purulent infection within the spinal canal that presents with a classic triad of symptoms consisting of fever, back pain, and spinal tenderness. Diagnosis may be delayed if fever is not present, leading to weakness and paralysis. Once again, the source may be hematogenous spread from another nidus of infection or direct extension. *Staphylococcus aureus* is the most common organism and it is often associated with vertebral osteomyelitis [40]. The diagnosis is typically made by MRI (Fig. 6.5), and the organism may or may not be identified by blood cultures.

Surgical treatment is necessary if there is a neurological deficit, if bacterial identification cannot be made, and if the spine is unstable. Postoperative intravenous antibiotics are continued for 6–8 weeks.

Rehabilitation will involve therapy to improve neurologic dysfunction of the involved limbs as well as truncal stability, activities of daily living, and other modalities used in the care of spinal cord injury patients. Care must be taken to assess patients for temperature, wound healing, and level of neurologic function to rule out treatment failure and relapse of disease. Pain level should also be monitored and instability considered if

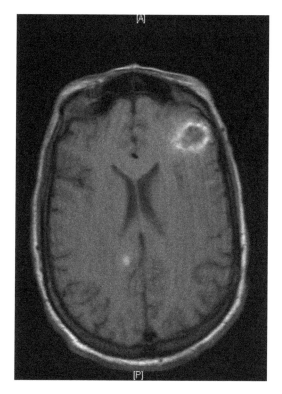

Fig. 6.4 Axial postcontrast T1 weighted MRI demonstrating a left frontal aspergillus abscess

discomfort increases over time rather than decreases. Any concerns should be communicated to the neurosurgeon in a timely manner.

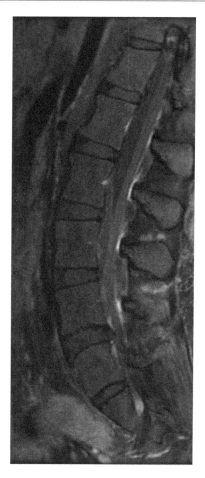

Fig. 6.5 Sagittal postcontrast T1 weighted lumbar MRI showing a spinal epidural abscess with diffuse enhancement within the spinal canal

Shunt Infection

The risk of infection after shunt surgery is relatively high, at about 7 % [41]. This may be partly related to the extensiveness of the foreign body inserted and its potential contact with the skin as it is inserted. The most common pathogen is *Staphylococcus epidermidis*. The clinical presentation is similar to that of a shunt malfunction or CNS infection or peritonitis. Headache, nausea and vomiting, fever, lethargy, and abdominal pain are common presenting symptoms.

The diagnostic workup includes routine blood work, a shunt tap to obtain CSF for culture, a CT to look for ventriculomegaly indicating shunt malfunction, and an abdominal CT that may show a pseudocyst around the peritoneal catheter tip. Treatment consists of antibiotics and removal of the shunt hardware. If the patient is shunt dependent, the shunt may be externalized by bringing the distal tubing out through a small incision at the clavicle and connecting it to a closed external drainage system until the infection is cleared. A completely new system can then be surgically placed. If a newly shunted patient is transferred from the hospital to a rehabilitation facility, the physiatrist and staff should monitor the patient for symptoms and signs of shunt infection, as discussed above. Any concerns should be relayed to the neurosurgeon and reevaluation in the acute care setting should be considered.

Postoperative Infection

Neurosurgical postoperative infection may take the form of a wound infection, meningitis, cranial osteomyelitis, brain abscess, or subdural empyema. Any postoperative fever should be evaluated for neurosurgical and non-neurosurgical causes. Non-neurosurgical causes may be noninfectious, such as atelectasis, drug fever, transfusion reaction, or deep venous thrombosis; or they may be infectious, such as pneumonia, urinary tract infection, or IV line infection. Neurosurgical causes that are not infectious include central fever and meningismus or chemical meningitis. This last entity is a sterile inflammatory reaction to blood spilled in the subarachnoid space. It causes fever and neck stiffness similar to bacterial meningitis. It should therefore be worked up as such, with a lumbar puncture, and treated as such with antibiotics, if bacterial meningitis is a significant possibility [42].

Central fevers are caused by intracranial pathology that affects the temperature regulatory centers in the hypothalamus. They are typically without peaks and troughs, are not affected by antipyretics, and are not associated with sweating. Wound infections are most commonly caused by *Staphylococcus* species. They present with classic signs of redness, warmth, and pain. These patients must be further evaluated with blood work, imaging, and possible lumbar puncture in order to exclude intracranial extension of the infection with associated meningitis, osteomyelitis, or brain abscess. Meningitis may cause nausea, vomiting, stiff neck, and altered mentation. It must be differentiated from chemical meningitis by CSF culture and treated with antibiotics.

Postoperative neurosurgical infection may extend intracranially as demonstrated on imaging and require surgical re-exploration. Abscess and empyema can then be evacuated, with irrigation and debridement of the involved structures. One controversial component is the craniotomy bone flap. This is a technically devitalized tissue and should be discarded as such, to prevent persistent or recurrent infection. However, this practice commits the patient to another future surgery: a cranioplasty to repair the cranial defect. To mitigate against this, some evidence has arisen in the literature suggesting that, if the bone flap is extensively soaked and scrubbed with antiseptic solution, it may be replaced and not discarded [43].

Traumatic Brain Injury (TBI)

TBI Overview

The spectrum of head trauma is broad, ranging from minor, negative imaging entities (i.e., CT and MRI of the brain reported as negative) such as concussion to more complex injuries involving obvious, severe intracranial injury. Depending on the type of rehabilitative facility, the percentage of patients with head injuries varies significantly. In general, these patients can be challenging. Frustration with an oscillating rehabilitative course is common. This chapter will help to introduce the reader to the different types of brain injuries and the usual post-injury course. A brief description of the inpatient experience for each is helpful to acquaint the reader with what might also present itself while in a rehabilitative facility, even weeks after discharge. To keep the information presented here brief, we will focus only on adult traumatic brain injury.

Concussion

Thanks to the growing popularity of American football, this "minor" type of head injury has received increasing attention. As a result, various grading scales have been used to develop return-to-work or play guidelines. These guidelines are now well published and readily available via government and neurology-/neurosurgery-supported websites. The reader is encouraged to further investigate these websites for further details. Of particular use is the AAN guidelines for sports-related concussion:

www.aan.com/go/practice/concussion
www.cdc.gov/headsup/providers/return_to_
activities.html

pediatrics.aappublications.org/content/
126/3/597.full
www.aans.org/Patient%20Information/
Conditions%20and%20Treatments/
Concussion.aspx

In general terms, concussion is when the brain is impacted and experiences sudden acceleration/deceleration forces. This temporary action results in disruption of the usual harmony of the various brain regions' communication with each other. This is thought to be secondary to different densities of brain regions moving at different velocities relative to one another. Additionally, cell injury results in the release of glutamate which further starts a chemical cascade of further local cell injury. The whole cellular milieu is deranged and as a result the normal well-tuned autoregulation of blood flow is disrupted [44]. The above processes result in desynchronization of the brain: the dynamic symphony of the brain is out now of tune. This is manifested in several ways including these typical symptoms:

Blank stare or befuddled expression
Delayed motor or verbal response
Easy distractibility, attention derangements
Speech alteration – slurred, incomprehensible, or perseverant
Incoordination
Emotional lability
Short-term memory deficits
Loss of consciousness

These symptoms may last for some time and reflect the degree of concussion. This also has a direct correlation to the duration of the post-concussive recovery. Generally, these patients are admitted, usually for observation and further evaluation of other injuries. Typically these patients do not proceed to rehabilitation but may be in inpatient facilities for concomitant injuries sustained elsewhere. It is important however to be familiar with the post-concussive syndrome that usually follows as this may also be present in the other types of traumatic brain injuries to be discussed [45–49].

Post-concussive symptoms may include the following involving somatic, cognitive, and psychological realms:

Headache
Dizziness
Light-headedness
Blurry visual or other visual disturbance
Anosmia
Tinnitus or other less common hearing difficulties including reduced acuity
Imbalance
Concentration difficulties
Judgment impairment
Emotional lability
Personality deviation
Loss of libido
Sleep/wake cycle disruption – insomnia or hypersomnolence
Fatigability
Photophobia or hyperacusis (increased sensitivity to sound)

Long-term sequelae include:

Dementia – though more common with multiple concussion within a short interval or multiple brain injuries during a single insult – now commonly referred to chronic traumatic encephalopathy (CTE). [50]
Increased rate of divorce or job loss due to the aforementioned sequelae.
Again much has been published on this topic and is readily available from trusted sources including the AAN, AANS, and the government-sponsored concussion websites including those endorsed by the NFL.

Contusion

In distinction to concussion, contusion is an actual pathological finding on imaging, such as CT or MRI [51]. Generally, it is considered an intraparenchymal hemorrhage of less than 1 cm. The mechanism of injury is usually high-velocity blunt trauma or penetrating (Fig. 6.6).

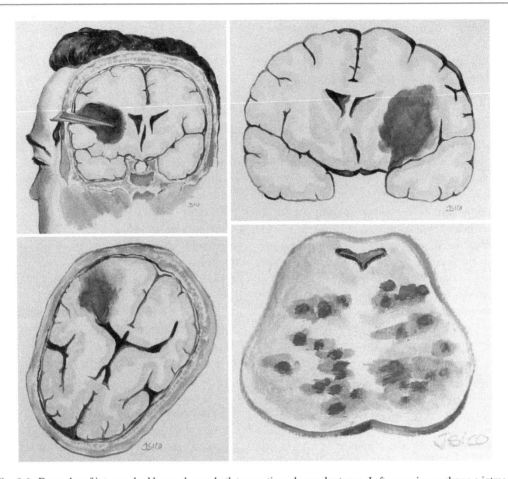

Fig. 6.6 Examples of intracerebral hemorrhages, both traumatic and vascular types. *Left upper image* shows a intracerebral hemorrhage as a result of penetrating trauma in which veins and arteries likely have been lacerated or disrupted. Right upper image illustrates a hypertensive hemorrhage which usually is non traumatic in etiology. *The left lower image* is representative of either a hemorrhagic stroke or a larger hemorrhage from a traumatic blunt head injury, though the former is the common appearance as represented. *The right lower image* illustrates multiple small hemorrhages in the brainstem (pons in this case) the after effects of brain herniation or after decompression via craniotomy, craniectomy, or removal of cerebrospinal fluid via a ventriculostomy

Similar derangements as discussed in concussion may be present. Typically patients are monitored for 24 h and released if imaging is stable and the hospital course uneventful. Here again, transition to a rehabilitative facility is unusual, although age may play a factor. Again, familiarity with aforementioned post-concussive syndrome is important. Things to be mindful of in this population include the possibility for delayed deterioration which will be discussed separately as there is significant overlap in the various types of traumatic brain injuries [52, 53].

Traumatic Subarachnoid Hemorrhage

There are two general types of subarachnoid hemorrhage: traumatic and aneurysmal. The etiology and source of these entities are very different. Aneurysmal subarachnoid hemorrhage results from the rupture of an intracranial aneurysm and usually nontraumatic in nature. The blood typically layers in the basal cisterns surrounding the brainstem and also involving the sylvian fissure. This entity is distinct from traumatic subarachnoid hemorrhage in which blood is within the subarachnoid space but within the sulci over the convexities of the cerebrum rather than along the larger diameter arteries in the basal cisterns and sylvian fissure. The etiology for this is thought to be secondary to tearing of small veins or arteries within the subarachnoid space. The typical hospital course is similar to contusion though with some potential ischemic variation to be discussed. Aneurysmal subarachnoid hemorrhage is further discussed elsewhere in this chapter but does share with traumatic subarachnoid the theoretical possibility of delayed ischemic events [54, 55]. This entity is well described and published in aneurysmal subarachnoid hemorrhage but only anecdotally mentioned in the literature for traumatic subarachnoid hemorrhage. My own research in rabbits suggests this is a physiologic possibility but does seem to correlate more with the arterial diameter within the foci of the subarachnoid blood and the presence of oxyhemoglobin from an arterial source [56]. Therefore, attention should be paid for neurological changes particularly 3–21 days after the ictus of injury. If this is suspected, a thorough neurological evaluation should be performed. CT imaging would be helpful to rule out new hemorrhage. Further workup, including transfer to a local medical center for neurological evaluation and MRI, might be warranted if a neurological deficit is present regardless of CT findings. Clearly any new CT findings would also warrant further evaluation as well regardless of neurological exam findings [57, 58]. Other types of delayed deterioration will again be discussed later.

Epidural Hematoma

Epidural hematomas are general secondary to laceration of the middle meningeal artery from a fracture calvarium typically as it courses under the normally thin temporal bone. This is the classical appearance (Fig. 6.7).

However, epidural hematomas can also result from inflow of venous blood from the venous lacunes within the diploic space of the calvarium (space between the inner and outer cortical tables of the skull) into the space between the dura and inner surface of the skull. Typically these venous variants tend to be small and infrequently require

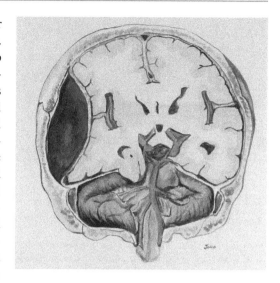

Fig. 6.7 Classic appearance of an epidural hematoma. The blood collects in the potential space between the inner table of the calvarium and the dura mater

evacuation. Arterial forms can continue to grow after initial recognition. A "lucid interval" is commonly described and accounts for the time in which this collection is enlarging. Patients have an initial concussive type of presentation then slowly decline as the hematoma creates increasing mass effect [59, 60]. Generally, these are evacuated via craniotomy if greater than 1 cm or producing a neurological deficit [61]. The goal of surgery is to remove the hematoma and stop the source of bleeding [62]. Patients may be monitored for several days and usually in an ICU setting. Age plays a role in which patients require further rehabilitative efforts after discharge. A post-concussive syndrome is typical. Delayed deterioration recognition and management will again be discussed later in this chapter.

Subdural Hematoma

Subdural hematomas form from tearing of the small bridging veins within the subdural space either from violent movement of the brain from trauma or from the fragility of these veins in the older population, often "encouraged" by anticoagulation or antiplatelet medications for other systemic disorders (Fig. 6.8).

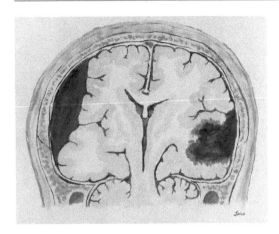

Fig. 6.8 *Left side of the image* (or the patient's right side by imaging orientation and presentation standards) illustrates the classic subdural hematoma in which the blood pools in the space between the dura mater and the subarachnoid layer. This typical appearance is usually from minor trauma or secondary to over-anticoagulation. *The right side of the image* (the patient's left) portrays a higher velocity injury in which the subdural hematoma spreads through the arachnoids layer which has been disrupted by the impact and into the subarachnoid space. This side of the images therefore shows both subdural hematoma and traumatic subarachnoid hemorrhage

Typically these torn veins will clot as this is a low pressure system. However, derangements of clotting will prevent proper clotting and bleeding may continue resulting in mass effect. Symptoms will vary from headache to focal neurological findings. A "lucid interval" has also been noted here though less robust as in epidural collections. Surgical indications and typical hospital management are similar to epidural hematomas, though chronic subdural collections which are more liquid in density may be relatively easily removed via a burr hole rather than a formal more time-intensive, morbid craniotomy [63–67].

Multicompartment Trauma

All the above types of hematomas can be found in a single patient if the degree of trauma is severe enough. The presence of an anticoagulated state will also increase the possibility of multiplicity

[68]. The GCS of these patients is important to trend. Prolonged hospital stays are common. Surgery in the form of craniotomy with hematoma removal may be required for a focal neurological deficit or for increasing intracranial pressure (ICP) [69]. Skull fracture elevation or calvarial vault reconstruction may be required for significant blunt trauma. Decompressive craniectomy in which a large piece of the skull is removed to provide space for a swollen brain may be required if intracranial pressure is difficult to control or the brain is noted to be severely swollen intraoperatively [70, 71]. Typically, intracranial pressure monitoring will be employed in those with a GCS < 8 with substantial CT findings. Removal of a part of the calvarium requires later reimplantation or placement of a prosthetic usually 2–3 months postoperatively. Obviously, care should be taken in these patients to avoid pressure on this portion of the brain as it lacks its usual protective boney covering.

Late Complications/Delayed Deterioration

Complications associated with TBI can be related to the surgery itself or the trauma suffered to the brain [72]. Those associated with surgery are well described previously in the section on brain tumors. Injury to the brain, whether traumatic or iatrogenic (yes, surgery), can put the brain at risk for seizure. Commonly, antiepileptics are recommended and have proven to reduce the frequency of TBI-related seizure when given for at least a week after injury [73, 74]. Those at high risk for posttraumatic (TBI) seizures include those with the following criteria/characteristics of injury:

Acute subdural, epidural, or intracerebral hematoma
Open-depressed skull fracture with contusion/parenchymal injury
Seizure during initial 24 h post-injury
Penetrating brain injury
History of significant alcohol abuse

Typically, antiepileptics are tapered after 1 week. Exceptions include those with history of seizure, those undergoing craniotomy, penetrating brain injury, and development of seizure after 7 days post-injury. Those remaining on antiepileptic medications for the above reasons should be maintained on the medications for at least 6 months and followed closely by a neurologist. Typically, an EEG will be required prior to removal of these medications. Driving is not allowed due to risk of harm to one's self or others should a seizure occur during operation of a motor vehicle.

Other potential late developments or complications for traumatic brain injury include:

Chronic headaches.

Otorrhea or rhinorrhea from basilar skull fractures – no role for antibiotics in this situation unless febrile or with leukocytosis [75].

Facial nerve dysfunction from mastoid or petrous bone fractures – generally treated with steroids by ENT – self-limited in most cases [76].

Delayed traumatic intracerebral hemorrhage – usually with 72 h of injury – thought to be secondary to early resumption of anticoagulants or coalescence of extravasated microhematomas [77].

Upper gastroduodenal ulceration and hemorrhage – proton pump inhibitors – are strongly recommended in the TBI patient to reduce this potential complication [78].

Infection – particularly in the postsurgical patient, whether an ICP monitor, ventriculostomy, or formal craniotomy.

Deep venous thrombosis – difficult to treat due to delayed traumatic intracerebral hemorrhage – anticoagulants, and antiplatelet agents are not recommended and this is best avoided with early mobilization and the use of sequential pneumatic devices and compression stockings [79, 80].

Communicating hydrocephalus – which may not present for several years or even decades and may present at idiopathic or normal pressure hydrocephalus (nicely described previously) [81, 82].

Post-concussive syndrome – as described above.

Hypogonadotropic hypogonadism (hypopituitarism that may require endocrine support, diabetes insipidus (DI) may be present in 40 % and usually is transient) [83, 84].

Alzheimer's disease [85, 86].

Chronic traumatic encephalopathy (CTE).

The last item has received a significant press in the era of the high-velocity, large mass collisions of the current NFL. CTE is a clinically distinct entity from Alzheimer's though pathologically they share the microscopic/histological characteristics of neurofibrillary tangles and β-amyloid plaques with the associated increased risk for intracerebral hemorrhage. The clinical features of CTE include:

Mental slowing or memory decline (usually short term > long term).

Personality changes:

Explosive behavior

Morbid jealousy

Pathological alcohol ingestion/intoxication

Paranoia

Motor changes:

Cerebellar dysfunction (intention tremor)

Pyramidal tract dysfunction (similar to Parkinson's)

Optimization of recovery from TBI clearly involves avoidance of the above potential complications but also includes:

Avoidance of hyperglycemia

Avoidance of the use of steroids [87]

Early parenteral feeding [88–92]

Early mobilization

Normalization of sleep/wake cycle – this may require stimulants in the morning to reset the patient's internal clock

The recovery from TBI is usually frustrating for all involved, including the caregivers, family, and patient. The process of rehabilitation from TBI is nicely described in *Living with Brain Injury* [93]. The reader is encouraged to delve further into this text for a well-organized approach to behavioral rehabilitation of the TBI patients. Briefly, a multistep process is suggested:

Evaluate a patient's specific needs and goals

Prevent complications

Educate on compensatory strategies for disabilities

Harness the brain's natural healing mechanisms (i.e., neural plasticity)

Maximize abilities that return early or remain unaffected

In general, it is a process of "mind over matter." In other words, it is cognitive reprogramming or remediation that is required to help patients adjust to their new deficits. Moreover, it is about developing appropriate problem solving and coping skills to maximize their abilities and develop or adapt new ones to overcome and improve their function limitations.

References

1. Go AS, Mozaffarian D, Roger VL, Benjamin EJ, Berry JD, Blaha MJ, Dai S, Ford ES, Fox CS, Franco S, Fullerton HJ, Gillespie C, Hailpern SM, Heit JA, Howard VJ, Huffman MD, Judd SE, Kissela BM, Kittner SJ, Lackland DT, Lichtman JH, Lisabeth LD, Mackey RH, Magid DJ, Marcus GM, Marelli A, Matchar DB, McGuire DK, Mohler 3rd ER, Moy CS, Mussolino ME, Neumar RW, Nichol G, Pandey DK, Paynter NP, Reeves MJ, Sorlie PD, Stein J, Towfighi A, Turan TN, Virani SS, Wong ND, Woo D, Turner MB, American Heart Association Statistics Committee and Stroke Statistics Subcommittee. Executive summary: heart disease and stroke statistics – 2014 update: a report from the American Heart Association. Circulation. 2014;129(3):399–410 12p.

2. Go AS, Mozaffarian D, Roger VL, Benjamin EJ, Berry JD, Blaha MJ, Dai S, Ford ES, Fox CS, Franco S, Fullerton HJ, Gillespie C, Hailpern SM, Heit JA, Howard VJ, Huffman MD, Judd SE, Kissela BM, Kittner SJ, Lackland DT, Lichtman JH, Lisabeth LD, Mackey RH, Magid DJ, Marcus GM, Marelli A, Matchar DB, McGuire DK, Mohler ER, Moy CS, Mussolino ME, Neumar RW, Nichol G, Pandey DK, Paynter NP, Reeves MJ, Sorlie PD, Stein J, Towfighi A, Turan TN, Virani SS, Wong ND, Woo D, Turner MB, American Heart Association Statistics Committee and Stroke Statistics Subcommittee. Heart disease and stroke statistics—2014 update: a report from the American Heart Association. Circulation. 2014;129:e28–292.

3. Chung YA, Hyun OJ, Kim JY, Kim KJ, Ahn KJ. Hypoperfusion and ischemia in cerebral amyloid angiopathy documented by 99mTc-ECD brain perfusion SPECT. J Nucl Med. 2009;50(12):1969–74.

4. Weller RO, Preston SD, Subash M, Carare RO. Cerebral amyloid angiopathy in the aetiology and immunotherapy of Alzheimer disease. Alzheimers Res Ther. 2009;1(2):6.

5. Mehdi A, Hajj-Ali RA. Reversible cerebral vasoconstriction syndrome: a comprehensive update. Curr Pain Headache Rep. 2014;18(9):1–10.

6. Adams Jr HP, del Zoppo G, Alberts MJ, Bhatt DL, Brass L, Furlan A, Grubb RL, Higashida RT, Jauch EC, Kidwell C, Lyden PD, Morgenstern LB, Qureshi AI, Rosenwasser RH, Scott PA, Wijdicks EF, American Heart Association; American Stroke Association Stroke Council; Clinical Cardiology Council; Cardiovascular Radiology and Intervention Council; Atherosclerotic Peripheral Vascular Disease and Quality of Care Outcomes in Research Interdisciplinary Working Groups. Guidelines for the early management of adults with ischemic stroke: a guideline from the American Heart Association/American Stroke Association Stroke Council, Clinical Cardiology Council, Cardiovascular Radiology and Intervention Council, and the Atherosclerotic Peripheral Vascular Disease and Quality of Care Outcomes in Research Interdisciplinary Working Groups: the American Academy of Neurology affirms the value of this guideline as an educational tool for neurologists. Stroke (00392499). 2007;38(5):1655–711 57p.

7. Albers GW, Amarenco P, Easton JD, Sacco RL, Teal P. Antithrombotic and thrombolytic therapy for ischemic stroke: American College of Chest Physicians Evidence-Based Clinical Practice Guidelines (8th edition). Chest. 2008;133(6 Suppl):630S–69S.

8. Hemphill 3rd JC, Greenberg SM, Anderson CS, Becker K, Bendok BR, Cushman M, Fung GL, Goldstein JN, Macdonald RL, Mitchell PH, Scott PA, Selim MH, Woo D, American Heart Association Stroke Council; Council on Cardiovascular and Stroke Nursing; Council on Clinical Cardiology. Guidelines for the management of spontaneous intracerebral hemorrhage: a guideline for healthcare professionals from the American Heart Association/American Stroke Association. Stroke J Cereb Circulation. 2015;46(7):2032–60.

9. Smith W, Tsao J, Billings M, Johnston S, Hemphill J, Bonovich D, Dillon W. Prognostic significance of angiographically confirmed large vessel intracranial occlusion in patients presenting with acute brain ischemia. Neurocrit Care. 2006;4(1):14–7.

10. Sarraj A, Gupta R. Endovascular treatment for ischemic strokes with large vessel occlusion: proven therapy and bright future. Stroke J Cereb Circulation. 2015;46(5):1431–2.

11. Feigin VL, Rinkel GJ, Lawes CM, et al. Risk factors for subarachnoid hemorrhage: an updated systematic review of epidemiological studies. Stroke. 2005;36(12):2773–80.

12. Adams Jr HP, Butler MJ, Biller J, Toffol GJ. Nonhemorrhagic cerebral infarction in young adults. Arch Neurol. 1986;43:793–6.

13. Ferguson GG, Eliasziw M, Barr HW, Clagett GP, Barnes RW, Wallace MC, Taylor DW, Haynes RB, Finan JW, Hachinski VC, Barnett HJ. The North American symptomatic carotid endarterectomy trial – surgical results in 1415 patients. Stroke. 1999;30(9):1751–8.

14. Morgenstern LB, Frankowski RF, Shedden P, Pasteur W, Grotta JC. Surgical treatment for intracerebral hemorrhage (STICH): a single-center, randomized clinical trial. Neurology. 1998;51:1359–63.

15. Rubin MN, Barrett KM. What to do with wake-up stroke. Neurohospitalist. 2015;5(3):161–72.

16. Yamane F, Takeshita M, Izawa M, Kagawa M, Sato K, Takakura K. Natural history of arteriovenous malformations: analysis of non-radically treated patients. J Clin Neurosci. 1998;5(suppl):26–9.

17. Berger MS, Rostomily RC. Low grade gliomas: functional mapping resection strategies, extent of resection, and outcome. J Neurooncol. 1997;34(1):85–101.

18. Eyüpoglu I, Hore N, Savaskan N, Grummich P, Roessler K, Buchfelder M, Ganslandt O. Improving the extent of malignant glioma resection by dual intraoperative visualization approach. Plos ONE. 2012;7(9):e44885.

19. Patchell RA, Tibbs PA, Walsh JW, et al. A randomized trial of surgery in the treatment of single metastases to the brain. New Eng J Med. 1990;322(8):494–500.

20. Patchell RA, Tibbs PA, Regine WF, et al. Postoperative radiotherapy in the treatment of single metastases to the brain: a randomized trial. J Am Med Assoc. 1998;280:1485–9.

21. Kondziolka D, Patel A, Lunsford LD, Kassam A, Flickinger JC. Clinical investigations: stereotactic radiosurgery plus whole brain radiotherapy versus radiotherapy alone for patients with multiple brain metastases. Int J Radiat Oncol Biol Phys. 1999;45:427–34.

22. Glantz MJ, Cole BF, Forsyth PA, Recht LD, Wen PY, Chamberlain MC, Grossman SA, Cairncross JG. Practice parameter: anticonvulsant prophylaxis in patients with newly diagnosed brain tumors: report of the quality standards subcommittee of the American Academy of Neurology. Neurology. 2000;54(10): 1886–93.

23. Ireland S, Carlino K, Gould L, Frazier F, Haycock P, Ilton S, Deptuck R, Bousfield B, Verge D, Antoni K, MacRae L, Renshaw H, Bialachowski A, Chagnon C, Reddy K. Shampoo after craniotomy: a pilot study. Can J Neurosci Nurs. 2007;29(1):14–9 6p.

24. Greenberg MS. Chiari malformation handbook of neurosurgery. 5th ed. New York: Thieme; 2001. p. 143–6.

25. Carmel PF. Management of the Chiari malformations in childhood. Clini Neurosurg. 1983;30:385–406.

26. Paul K, Lye R, Strang F, Dutton J. Arnold-Chiari malformation. Review of 71 cases. J Neurosurgery. 1983;58(2):183–7.

27. Levy W, Mason L, Hahn J. Chiari malformation presenting in adults: a surgical experience in 127 cases. Neurosurgery. 1983;12(4):377–90.

28. Alden TD, Ojemann JG, Park TS. Surgical treatment of Chiari I malformation: indications and approaches. Neurosurg Focus. 2001;11(1):E2.

29. Duddy JC, Allcutt D, Crimmins D, O'Brien D, O'Brien DF, Rawluk D, Sattar MT, Young S, Caird J. Foramen magnum decompression for Chiari I malformation: a procedure not to be underestimated. Br J Neurosurgery. 2014;28(3):330–4.

30. Vakharia V, Guilfoyle M, Laing R. Prospective study of outcome of foramen magnum decompressions in patients with syrinx and non-syrinx associated Chiari malformations. Br J Neurosurgery. 2012;26(1):7–11.

31. Greenberg MS. Handbook of neurosurgery. New York: Thieme; 2010.

32. Bergsneider M, Black P, Klinge P, Marmarou A, Relkin N. Surgical management of idiopathic normal-pressure hydrocephalus. Neurosurgery. 2005;57(3):29–39.

33. Malm J, Kristensen B, Stegmayr B, Fagerlund M, Koskinen LO. Three-year survival and functional outcome of patients with idiopathic adult hydrocephalus syndrome. Neurology. 2000;55:576–8.

34. Mamelak AN, Mampalam TJ, Obana WG, Rosenblum ML. Improved management of multiple brain abscesses: a combined surgical and medical approach. Neurosurgery. 1995;36:76–86.

35. Calfee DP, Wispelwey B. Brain abscess. Semin Neurol. 2000;20(3):353–60.

36. Dill S, Cobbs C, McDonald C. Subdural empyema: analysis of 32 cases and review. Clin Infect Dis. 1995;20(2):372–86.

37. Carpio A. Neurocysticercosis: an update. Lancet Infect Dis. 2002;20(12):751–62.

38. Tyler KL. Update on herpes simplex encephalitis. Rev Neurol Dis. 2004;1(4):169–78.

39. Minari A, et al. The incidence of invasive aspergillosis among solid organ transplant recipients and implications for prophylaxis in lung transplants. Transpl Infect Dis. 2002;4(4):195–200.

40. Darouiche RO. Spinal epidural abscess. N Engl J Med. 2006;355:2012–202.

41. Kanev PM, et al. Reflections on shunt infection. Pediatr Neurosurg. 2003;39(6):285–90.

42. Forgacs P, et al. Characterization of chemical meningitis after neurological surgery. Clin Infect Dis. 2001;32(2):179–85.

43. Bruce J, Bruce S. Preservation of bone flaps in patients with postcraniotomy infections. J Neurosurgery. 2003;98(6):1203–7.

44. Cold G. Cerebral blood flow in acute head injury. The regulation of cerebral blood flow and metabolism during the acute phase of head injury, and its significance for therapy. Acta Neurochir Suppl. 1990;49:1–64.

45. Parkinson D. Evaluating cerebral concussion. Surg Neurol. 1996;45(5):459–62.

46. Alves WM, Jane JA. Post-traumatic syndrome. In: Youmans JR, editor. Neurological surgery, vol. 3. 3rd ed. Philadelphia: WB Saunders; 1990. p. 2230–42.

47. Reilly P, Graham D, Hume Adams J, Jennett B. Patients with head injury who talk and die. Lancet. 1975;306(7931):375–7.

48. Duus B, Lind B, Christensen H, Nielsen O. The role of neuroimaging in the initial management of patients with minor head injury. Anna Emerg Med. 1994;23(6):1279–83.

49. Stein SC, Ross SE. Mild head injury: a plea for routine early ct scanning. J Trauma Injury Inf Critical Care. 1992;33(1):11–3.

50. Jordan BD, Kanik AB, Horwich MS, Sweeney D, Relkin NR, Petito CK, Gandy S. Apolipoprotein E epsilon 4 and fatal cerebral amyloid angiopathy associated with dementia pugilistica. Annals Neurol. 1995;38(4):698–9.

51. Wilberger JE, Deeb Z, Deeb W. Magnetic resonance imaging after closed head injury. Neurosurgery. 1987;20:571–6.

52. Cohen TI, Gudeman SK. Delayed traumatic intracranial hematoma. In: Narayan RK, Wilberger JE, Povlishock JT, editors. Neurotrauma. New York: McGraw-Hil; 1996. p. 689–701.

53. Cooper P, Maravilla K, Moody S, Kemp Clark W. Serial computerized tomographic scanning and the prognosis of severe head injury. Neurosurgery. 1979;5(5):566–9.

54. Taneda M, Kataoka K, Akai F, Asai T, Sakata I. Traumatic subarachnoid hemorrhage as a predictable indicator of delayed ischemic symptoms. J Neurosurgery. 1996;84(5):762–8.

55. Jaeger M, Schuhmann M, Soehle M, Nagel C, Meixensberger J. Continuous monitoring of cerebrovascular autoregulation after subarachnoid hemorrhage by brain tissue oxygen pressure reactivity and its relation to delayed cerebral infarction. Stroke (00392499). 2007;38(3):981–6 6p.

56. Link TE, Murakami K, Beem-Miller M, Tranmer BI, Wellman GC. Oxyhemoglobin-induced expression of R-Type Ca2+ channels in cerebral arteries. Stroke. 2008;39(7):2122–8.

57. Findlay J, Macdonald R, Weir B (n.d) Current concepts of pathophysiology and management of cerebral vasospasm following aneurysmal subarachnoid hemorrhage. Cerebrovascular Brain Metab Rev. . 1991 Winter;3(4):336–61.

58. Tian H, Xu T, Hu J, Cui Y, Chen H, Zhou L. Risk factors related to hydrocephalus after traumatic subarachnoid hemorrhage. Surg Neurol. 2008;69(3):241–6.

59. Rivas J, Lobato R, Sarabia R, Cordobes F, Cabrera A, Gomez P. Extradural hematoma: analysis of factors influencing the courses of 161 patients. Neurosurgery. 1988;23(1):44–51.

60. Mckissock W, Taylor J, Bloom W, Till K. Extradural hæmatoma. Observations on 125 cases. Lancet. 1960;276(7143):167–72.

61. Bullock R, Chesnut RM, Clifton G, Ghajar J, Marion DW, Narayan RK, Newell DW, Pitts LH, Rosner MJ, Wilberger JW. Guidelines for the management of severe head injury. Brain Trauma Foundation. Eur J Emerg Med Off J Euro Soc Emerg Med. 1996;3(2):109–27.

62. Bullock MR, Chesnut R, Ghajar J, Gordon D, Hartl R, Newell DW, Servadei F, Walters BC, Wilberger J, Surgical Management of Traumatic Brain Injury. Surgical management of traumatic parenchymal lesions. Neurosurgery. 2006;58(3 Suppl):S25.

63. Bullock MR, Chesnut R, Ghajar J, Gordon D, Hartl R, Newell DW, Servadei F, Walters BC, Wilberger JE, Surgical Management of Traumatic Brain Injury. Surgical management of acute subdural hematomas. Neurosurgery. 2006;58(3 Suppl):S16.

64. Robinson R. Chronic subdural hematoma: surgical management in 133 patients. J Neurosurgery. 1984;61(2):263–8.

65. Abouzari M, Armin R, Rezaii J, Esfandiari K, Asadollahi M, Aleali H, Abdollahzadeh M. The role of postoperative patient posture in the recurrence of traumatic chronic subdural hematoma after burr-hole surgery. Neurosurgery. 2007;61(4):794–7.

66. Sambasivan M. An overview of chronic subdural hematoma: experience with 2300 cases. Surg Neurol. 1997;47(5):418–22.

67. Sahuquillo-Barris J, Lamarca-Ciuro J, Vilalta-Castan J, Rubio-Garcia E, Rodriquez-Pazos M. Acute subdural hematoma and diffuse axonal injury after severe head trauma. J Neurosurgery. 1988;68(6):894–900.

68. Bouma G, Muizelaar J, Choi S, Newlon P, Young H. Cerebral circulation and metabolism after severe traumatic brain injury: the elusive role of ischemia. J Neurosurg. 1991;75(5):685–93.

69. Alberico A, Ward J, Choi S, Marmarou A, Young H. Outcome after severe head injury. Relationship to mass lesions, diffuse injury, and ICP course in pediatric and adult patients. J Neurosurgery. 1987;67(5):648–56.

70. Polin R, Shaffrey M, Bogaev C, Tisdale N, Germanson T, Bocchicchio B, Jane J. Decompressive bifrontal craniectomy in the treatment of severe refractory post-traumatic cerebral edema. Neurosurgery. 1997;41(1):84–94.

71. Aarabi B, Hesdorffer D, Ahn E, Aresco C, Scalea T, Eisenberg H. Outcome following decompressive craniectomy for malignant swelling due to severe head injury. J Neurosurgery. 2006;104(4):469–79.

72. Dacey Jr R, Alves W, Rimel R, Winn H, Jane J. Neurosurgical complications after apparently minor head injury: assessment of risk in a series of 610 patients. J Neurosurgery. 1986;65(2):203–10.

73. Chang B, Lowenstein D. Practice parameter: antiepileptic drug prophylaxis in severe traumatic brain

injury: report of the Quality Standards Subcommittee of the American Academy of Neurology. Neurology. 2003;60(1):10–6.

74. Bratton SL, Chestnut RM, Ghajar J, Hammond FFM, Harris OA, Hartl R, et al. Brain Trauma Foundation: anti-seizure prophylaxis. J Neurotrauma. 2007;24: S83–6.

75. Lewin W. Cerebrospinal fluid rhinorrhœa in closed head injuries. Br J Surg. 1954;42(171):1.

76. Esslen E. Electrodiagnosis of facial palsy. In: Miehlke A, editor. Surgery of the facial nerve. 2nd ed. Philadelphia: W B Saunders; 1973. p. 45–51.

77. Gudeman S, Kishore P, Miller J, Girevendulis A, Lipper M, Becker D. The genesis and significance of delayed traumatic intracerebral hematoma. Neurosurgery. 1979;5(3):309–13.

78. Chan KH, Lai EC, Tuen H, Ngan JH, Mok F, Fan YW, Fung CF, Yu WC. Prospective double-blind placebo-controlled randomized trial on the use of ranitidine in preventing postoperative gastroduodenal complications in high- risk neurosurgical patients. J Neurosurgery. 1995;82(3):413–7.

79. Kaufman HH, Satterwhite T, McConnell BJ, Costin B, Borit A, Gould L, Pruessner J, Bernstein D, Gildenberg PL. Deep vein thrombosis and pulmonary embolism in head injured patients. Angiology. 1983;34(10):627.

80. Bratton SL, Chestnut RM, Ghajar J, Hammond FFM, Harris OA, Hartl R, et al. Brain Trauma Foundation: deep vein thrombosis prophylaxis. J Neurotrauma. 2007;24:S32–6.

81. Poca M, Sahuquillo J, Arikan F, Mataró M, Benejam B, Báguena M. Ventricular enlargement after moderate or severe head injury: a frequent and neglected problem. J Neurotrauma. 2005;22(11): 1303–10.

82. Marmarou A, Foda MA, Bandoh K, Yoshihara M, Yamamoto T, Tsuji O, et al. Posttraumatic ventriculo-megaly: hydrocephalus or atrophy? A new approach for diagnosis using CSF dynamics. J Neurosurgery. 1996;85(6):1026–35.

83. Clark J, Raggatt P, Edwards O. Hypothalamic hypo-gonadism following major head injury. Clini Endocrinol (Oxf). 1988;29(2):153–65.

84. Edwards O, Clark J. Post-traumatic hypopituitarism: six cases and a review of the literature. Med (US). 1986;65(5):281–90.

85. Mayeux R, Ottman R, Tang M, Marder K, Stern Y, Gurland B, Noboa-Bauza L. Genetic susceptibility and head injury as risk factors for Alzheimer's disease among community-dwelling elderly persons and their first-degree relatives. Anna Neurol. 1993;33(5): 494–501.

86. Roberts G, Gentleman S, Lynch A, Murray L, Graham D, Landon M. β3 Amyloid protein deposition in the brain after severe head injury: Implications for the pathogenesis of Alzheimer's disease. J Neurol Neurosurgery Psychiatry. 1994;57(4):419–25.

87. Bratton SL, Chestnut RM, Ghajar J, Hammond FFM, Harris OA, Hartl R, et al. Brain Trauma Foundation: steroids. J Neurotrauma. 2007;24:S 91–5.

88. Deutschman C, Konstantinides F, Raup S, Thienprasit P, Cerra F. Physiological and metabolic response to isolated closed-head injury. Part 1: Basal metabolic state: correlations of metabolic and physiological parameters with fasting and stressed controls. J Neurosurgery. 1986;64(1):89–98.

89. Rapp R, Young D, Twyman D, Bivins B, Haack D, Tibbs P, Bean J. The favorable effect of early paren-teral feeding on survival in head-injured patients. J Neurosurgery. 1983;58(6):906–12.

90. Hadley M, Grahm T, Harrington T, Schiller W, McDermott M, Posillico D. Nutritional support and neurotrauma: a critical review of early nutrition in forty-five acute head injury patients. Neurosurgery. 1986;19(3):367–73.

91. Vespa PM, McArthur D, O'Phelan K, Glenn T, Etchepare M, Kelly D, Bergsneider M, Martin NA, Hovda DA. Persistently low extracellular glucose cor-relates with poor outcome 6 months after human trau-matic brain injury despite a lack of increased lactate: a microdialysis study. J Cereb Blood Flow Met. 2003;23(7):865–77.

92. Kaufman H, Bretaudiere J, Rowlands B, Stein D, Bernstein D, Wagner K, Gildenberg P. General metabo-lism in head injury. Neurosurgery. 1987;20(2):254–65.

93. Senelick R, Dougherty K. Living with Brain Injury. 2nd ed. Birmingham: HealthSouth Press; 2001.

Neil R. Holland

Introduction to the Motor System

There are two main sets of motor pathways that run between the brain and individual muscles to facilitate movement. The pyramidal system is a direct pathway from the motor cortex to spinal cord segments controlling individual muscle groups. It facilitates conscious volitional movements such as writing, typing, picking up a cup, or kicking a ball. The extrapyramidal system consists of multiple discrete indirect pathways connecting the brainstem nuclei and the cerebellum to larger groups of muscles. It facilitates subconscious motor tasks such as maintenance of stance and posture. Both motor pathways are referred to as upper motor neurons as they descend through the spinal cord.

These pathways converge into the anterior horn cells in the gray matter of the spinal cord, whose axons, the lower motor neurons, are the final common connection to muscle fibers (Fig. 7.1). Anterior horn cells are also affected by local reflex circuits within the spinal cord designed continuously and automatically to adjust muscle tone based on sensory receptors

within muscles and tendons. This myotactic or stretch reflex is the basis for the knee or ankle jerk. Other spinal reflexes facilitate reciprocal inhibition: when a muscle is voluntarily activated, its antagonistic muscles must be simultaneously relaxed to allow movement (Fig. 7.2). Some descending upper motor neurons directly activate the lower motor neuron anterior horn cells causing movement, while others modulate local reflex circuits in the spinal cord to make reflexive movements more adaptive [1].

Lower Versus Upper Motor Neuron Injury

Injuries to peripheral nerves and spinal segments result in partial or complete weakness of innervated muscle and interruption of associated spinal reflex arcs. Such lower motor neuron lesions are easy to recognize and localize based on the pattern of weakness and interruption of the appropriate local reflex arc. For example, both radial nerve and C7 nerve root lesions will cause weakness of wrist and elbow extension and an absent triceps reflex, but the C7 nerve root lesion will also cause wrist flexion weakness through its contribution to the median nerve.

Upper motor neuron lesions are more complicated. First, many such lesions selectively affect the pyramidal pathway with loss of fine motor skills in the affected limb in the absence of complete paralysis. Affected patients will

N.R. Holland, MBBS, MBA, FAAN
Neurology, Geisinger Health System,
Danville, PA, USA

Medicine (Neurology), Commonwealth Medical College, Scanton, PA, USA
e-mail: nholland1@geisinger.edu

© Springer International Publishing Switzerland 2017
A.I. Elkwood et al. (eds.), *Rehabilitative Surgery*, DOI 10.1007/978-3-319-41406-5_7

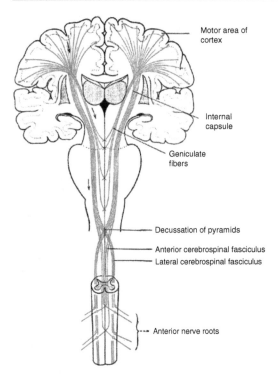

Fig. 7.1 Motor pathways, upper motor neuron pathway (the brain and spinal cord), and lower motor neuron pathway in nerve root and peripheral nerve (Source: Henry Gray (1918) Anatomy of the Human Body, a public domain image – http://en.wikipedia.org/wiki/Upper_motor_neuron#/media/File:Gray764.png)

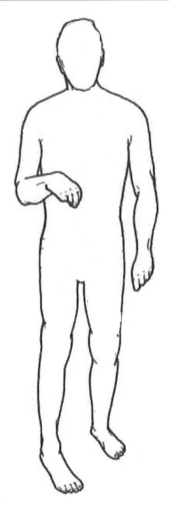

Fig. 7.3 "Pyramidal" distribution weakness. This stroke patient has a spastic right hemiparesis from selective involvement of the pyramidal tract. Unopposed descending input from the extrapyramidal pathways results in disproportionate flexion in the upper extremity and extension in the lower extremity

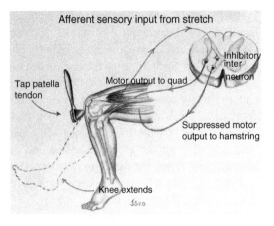

Fig. 7.2 The spinal reflex arc, tendon stretch, is transmitted via a sensory neuron into the spinal cord, where it activates the motor fibers to quadriceps and at the same time inhibits the motor fibers to hamstrings, in order to extend the knee (knee jerk). This reflex can be facilitated or inhibited by descending central influences

subconsciously keep the upper limb flexed and lower limb extended based on unopposed activity via the unaffected descending extrapyramidal pathways (Fig. 7.3). Second, in addition to loss of motor function, upper motor neuron lesions will also lead to loss of modulation (inhibition) of the local spinal reflexes. Uninhibited, these myotactic reflexes become overactive leading to exaggerated resistance to passive stretching (spasticity) and loss of reciprocal inhibition. In other words, muscle weakness from an upper motor lesion can stem from both loss of volitional

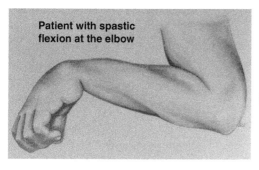

Patient with spastic flexion at the elbow

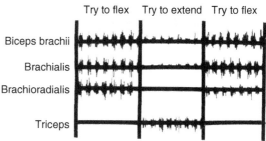

Try to flex   Try to extend   Try to flex

Biceps brachii

Brachialis

Brachioradialis

Triceps

Fig. 7.4 Spasticity with loss of central inhibition. This patient has a spastic arm with weakness of extension and flexion at the wrist and elbow. Multichannel EMG record-ing shows that biceps is activated during attempted elbow extension; the "weakness" is from persistent activity in the flexor muscles (i.e., a failure to relax antagonistic groups)

activation and also failed relaxation or resistance to passive stretching of the antagonistic muscles, somewhat akin to driving with the hand brake on. Multichannel dynamic EMG recordings can be helpful in sorting this out (Fig. 7.4). Treating the spasticity – or releasing the hand brake – can be enough to improve function in some patients. Other patients require more complicated proce-dures to improve function. In extreme cases, this can involve lesioning and neurotization. In other words, this converts an upper motor neuron lesion into a simpler lower motor neuron lesion and then fixes the lower motor neuron lesion.

Spasticity

Clinical Features

Spasticity is an involuntary increase in muscle tone that can cause pain and deformity in addition to exacerbating upper motor neuron pattern weak-ness. This increased tone results from interruption of descending inhibition of myotactic stretch reflexes. Spasticity is velocity-dependent: the resistance will build up as the muscle is stretched faster until it suddenly gives away, known as the "clasp knife phenomenon." This velocity-depen-dent change in tone is what distinguishes spastic-ity from other positive motor phenomena like the rigidity seen in Parkinson's disease, the sustained dystonic movement seen in Wilson's disease, or the neuropsychiatric phenomenon of catatonia. Spasticity can also cause reflexive painful grouped

muscle spasms in response to a somatic or vis-ceral trigger or change in posture. The increased tone from spasticity can be so severe as to appear as a fixed contracture. This distinction is impor-tant, since the latter will not respond to medical therapy. An examination under anesthesia may be necessary to differentiate the two.

Treatment

Treating spasticity not only improves motor function but also can relieve pain, improve pos-ture and positioning (and hence prevent pressure sores), and facilitate hygiene. Treatment modali-ties can include physical therapy, splinting, and medical and surgical interventions, depending on the extent and severity of the symptoms (Fig. 7.5). This necessitates a multidisciplinary approach to spasticity management, beginning with the iden-tification of reasonable outcome goals.

Physical Therapy
Spastic limbs can be passively stretched using bands, splints, or pressure garments (dynamic fabricated orthoses) to reduce tone and prevent fixed contracture [2]. Fixed contractures can be slowly stretched out using progressive splinting (Fig. 7.6). Standing frames allow paraplegic patients to remain upright for prolonged periods, using gravity to reduce spasticity and prevent contractures. Strengthening exercise regimens for weak muscles can make it easier to overcome spasticity and improve function; in particular,

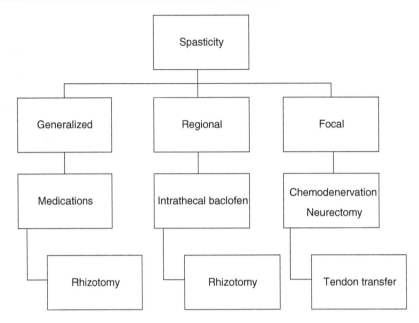

Fig. 7.5 Algorithm for treating spasticity based on extent and severity of symptoms

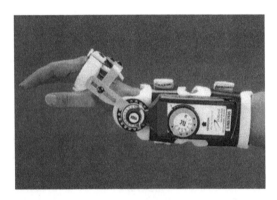

Fig. 7.6 An adjustable wrist splint can be adjusted to provide gradual correction of spastic tone and soft tissue contracture from progressive splinting

forced use of a hemiparetic limb by constraining the unaffected side in stroke patients can reduce spasticity [3].

Oral Medications

Oral drugs used to treat spasticity work by increasing GABA-mediated inhibition of spinal reflexes (baclofen and benzodiazepines), suppressing the release of the excitatory neurotransmitter glutamate (tizanidine via activation of alpha-2 adrenergic receptors) or blocking calcium

release in muscle cells to reduce contractility (dantrolene) (Table 7.1). Drug regimens can be very helpful in specific situations. For example, a dose of clonazepam at bedtime can reduce nocturnal spasms and improve sleep. However, although widely prescribed to spastic patients, for the most part, these drugs have limited efficacy and cause such significant side effects including drowsiness and worsening weakness that most patients are noncompliant with prescribed doses [4–6].

Chemodenervation

Botulinum neurotoxin prevents the release of acetylcholine from presynaptic nerve terminals at the neuromuscular junction. When injected intramuscularly, its effects are maximal at the injected muscle, causing a temporary dose-dependent blockage of neuromuscular transmission that reduces muscle contraction within 7–10 days and lasts for 3–4 months [7]. The resultant partial paralysis can alleviate spasticity and improve function. Adverse effects can include excessive weakness (temporary) and transient ptosis and/or difficulty in swallowing if the drug is administered to head and neck muscles.

Table 7.1 Oral drugs commonly prescribed for spasticity

Drug	Mechanism of action	Dose	Side effects
Baclofen	GABA agonist	5 mg three times daily, increased by 5–10 mg weekly up to a max dose of 90–120 mg in 3 divided doses	Increased weakness, drowsiness, and dizziness. Sudden withdrawal may cause rebound spasticity, seizures, and hallucinations
Tizanidine	Alpha-2 adrenergic receptor agonist inhibits glutamate release	2 mg at bedtime, increased by 2 mg weekly up to a max dose of 36 mg in 3–4 divided doses	Dry mouth, GI upset, low blood pressure, abnormal liver tests
Benzodiazepines Clonazepam Diazepam	Increased GABA	Clonazepam 0.5–1.0 mg at bedtime Diazepam 2.5 mg once a day, increased by 2.5 mg every 2–3 days up to a max dose of 30–40 mg in 3–4 divided doses	Sedation, lethargy, incoordination Dependency
Dantrolene	Blocks calcium release from the sarcoplasmic reticulum in skeletal muscle	300 mg once daily, increase by 300 mg every 2–3 days up to a max dose of 3600 mg in 3 divided doses	Weight gain, GI upset, confusion, hepatotoxicity, prolonged QT interval

Intrathecal Baclofen

As mentioned earlier, oral baclofen alleviates spasticity but has a high incidence of side effects, limiting compliance and outcome. However, much smaller doses of baclofen administered intrathecally can achieve a relatively high concentration of drug within the spinal cord, alleviating spasticity with fewer systemic side effects. Potential patients can be screened with a test dose of medication administered via lumbar puncture. Patients responding to the test dose can then undergo surgical implantation of a programmable pump that continuously delivers medication directly into the spinal subarachnoid space via a catheter (Fig. 7.7). Intrathecal baclofen therapy has been shown to be effective for spasticity resulting from spinal cord injury, stroke, and multiple sclerosis [8]. However, instances of life-threatening drug withdrawal can occur from failure to refill the pump regularly, catheter failure, and/or programming error, so these patients need close and frequent follow-up.

Surgical Treatment

Spastic contracture can be treated by surgical lengthening or transfer of tendons. For example, spastic elbow flexion can be alleviated by

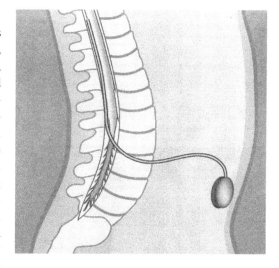

Fig. 7.7 Schematic representation of an intrathecal baclofen pump implanted in an abdominal pocket, connected to the spine via an implanted catheter

release and lengthening of the biceps brachii, brachialis, and/or brachioradialis tendons [9] (Fig. 7.4). Spastic talipes equinovarus ankle deformity can be reversed by tendon lengthening, then transferring the tibialis posterior tendon onto the tibialis anterior tendon so that the unopposed action of tibialis posterior now everts and dorsiflexes the foot, reversing the deformity [10]. Multichannel EMG recordings made during active movement can demonstrate which muscles are under volitional control, working in or out of phase, and the presence or absence of antagonistic muscle co-contracture. This can be critical for planning surgical management such as which nerves or tendons to sacrifice and/or transfer in order to restore function (Figs. 7.8 and 7.9).

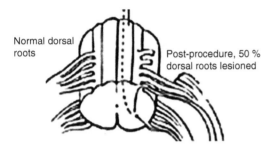

Fig. 7.8 During selective dorsal rhizotomy, exposed dorsal nerve root is identified, and a portion (around 50 %) is lesioned to reduce afferent input into the spinal reflexes which mediate spasticity

Spasticity is caused by exaggerated myotactic stretch reflexes (Fig. 7.2) and can be treated by surgically interrupting these pathways. Dorsal rhizotomy is a surgical procedure used for spastic paraparesis, which involves a lumbar laminectomy followed by identification and surgical lesioning of the dorsal (sensory) roots, interrupting the afferent arc of this reflex while sparing the motor (efferent) arc to avoid exacerbating weakness (Fig. 7.6). The rootlets selected for lesioning may be identified by intraoperative electrodiagnostic testing [11]. This technique has been most used in children and adolescents with cerebral palsy leading to improved ambulation and range of motion [12, 13].

Neurolysis or neurotomy is the destruction of specific peripheral nerves either by intraneural injection of phenol or alcohol or direct surgical lesioning to alleviate regional spasticity [14]. Unlike selective dorsal rhizotomy, this process will destroy both motor and sensory fibers, so on its own cannot improve motor function. Selective tibial neurotomy has been used to alleviate ankle spasticity in nonambulatory

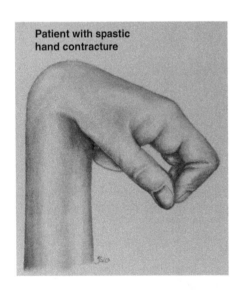

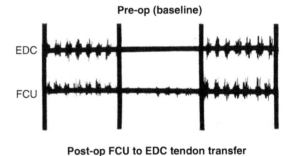

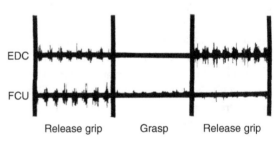

Fig. 7.9 Selective tendon transfer for contracted wrist and hand. (*Top right*) Baseline multichannel EMG showing abnormal co-contraction of flexor carpi ulnaris (FCU) with extensor digitorum communis (EDC) muscles when a patient tries to release a grip. FCU is not only antagonizing extension but activating out of phase. The patient undergoes FCU to EDC tendon transfer. Postoperatively (*bottom right*) the FCU muscle is still active during grip release but now facilitates finger extension instead of inhibiting it

patients with spastic diplegic equinovarus deformity [15]. However, neurotomy followed by tendon transfer or neurotization can be effective for both alleviating spasticity and restoring function. This of course is essentially converting a central nervous system injury into a peripheral nervous system injury and then surgically repairing it. Obviously, performing the tendon transfer or neurotization without the neurotomy first might not be effective, since active movement cannot be restored without first removing passive resistance. For example,

cross-chest C7 nerve root transfer had been used to neurotize avulsed nerves from brachial plexus injuries with successful outcomes [16]. This technique has been recently also applied to spastic hemiplegic upper limbs. The C7 nerve root on the spastic side is first transected and then neurotized from the C7 nerve root on the normal side using intervening cross-chest sural nerve grafts. Treated patients were less spastic and developed functionally significant improvements of hand, wrist, and elbow strength over a 2-year observation period [17].

Summary of Key Points
- Upper motor neuron injuries are more complicated than lower motor neuron injuries, because of more primitive motor pathways that are spared, exaggerated myotactic reflexes (spasticity), and loss of reciprocal inhibition.
- Simply restoring power without accounting for these other issues may not improve function.
- Management of spasticity can include any combination of physical therapy, oral medications, chemodenervation,

intrathecal baclofen, tendon transfer, neurectomy, and/or rhizotomy. Realistic goals and a multidisciplinary approach are paramount.
- Surgical functional restoration may include neurectomy followed by neurotization and/or tendon transfer – i.e., converting the upper motor neuron lesion into a simpler lower motor neuron lesion then fixing it.
- Multichannel dynamic EMG recordings can be critical in planning these procedures.

References

1. Knierim J. Spinal reflexes and descending motor pathways. Neuroscience online, an electronic textbook for the neurosciences. 1997. http://neuroscience.uth.tmc.edu/s3/chapter02.html. Accessed May 2015.
2. Jo HM, Song JC, Jang SH. Improvements in spasticity and motor function using a static stretching device for people with chronic hemiparesis following stroke. NeuroRehabilitation. 2013;32:369–75.
3. Kagawa S, Koyama T, Hosomi M, Takebayashi T, Hanada K, Hashimoto F, et al. Effects of constraint-induced movement therapy on spasticity in patients with hemiparesis after stroke. J Stroke Cerebrovasc Dis. 2013;22:364–70.
4. Taricco M, Pagliacci MC, Telaro E, Adone R. Pharmacological interventions for spasticity following spinal cord injury: results of a Cochrane systematic review. Eura Medicophys. 2006;42:5–15.
5. Montane E, Vallano A, Laporte JR. Oral antispastic drugs in nonprogressive neurologic diseases: a systematic review. Neurology. 2004;63:1357–63.
6. Halpern R, Gillard P, Graham GD, Varon SF, Zorowitz RD. Adherence associated with oral medications in the treatment of spasticity. PM R. 2013;5:747–56.
7. Wissel J, Ward AB, Erztgaard P, Bensmail D, Hecht MJ, Lejune TM, et al. European consensus table on the use of botulinum toxin type A in adult spasticity. J Rehabil Med. 2009;41:13–25.
8. Zahavi A, Geertzen JH, Middel B, Staal M, Rietman JS. Long term effect of intrathecal baclofen on impairment, disability and quality of life in patients with severe spasticity of spinal origin. J Neurol Neurosurg Psychiatry. 2004;75:1553–7.
9. Kolessar DJ, Keenan MA. Surgical management of upper extremity deformities following traumatic brain injury. Phys Med Rehabil. 1993;7:623–35.
10. Roper BA, Williams A, King JB. The surgical treatment of equinovarus deformity in adults with spasticity. J Bone Joint Surg Br. 1978;60:533–5.

11. Holland NR. Intraoperative EMG. In: Elkwood AI, Kaufman M, Schneider LF, editors. Rehabilitative surgery: an interdisciplinary approach to restoring functionality. New York: Springer; 2016.

12. Steinbook P. Selective dorsal rhizotomy for spastic cerebral palsy; a review. Childs Nerv Syst. 2007;23:981–90.

13. Hurvitz EA, Marciniak CM, Daunter AK, Haapala HJ, Stibb SM, McCormick SF, Muraszko KN, Gaebler-Spira D. Functional outcomes of childhood dorsal rhizotomy in adults and adolescents with cerebral palsy. J Neurosurg Pediatr. 2013;11:380–8.

14. Kocabas H, Salli A, Demir AH, Ozerbil OM. Comparison of phenol and alcohol neurolysis of tibial nerve motor branches to the gastrocnemius muscle for treatment of spastic foot after stroke: a randomized controlled pilot study. Eur J Phys Rehabil Med. 2010;46:5–10.

15. Abdennebi B, Boutagene B. Selective neurectomies for relief spasticity focalized to the foot and to the knee flexors. Results in a series of 58 patients. Acta Neurochir (Wien). 1996;138:912–20.

16. Gu YD, Zhang GM, Chen DS, Yan YG, Cheng XM, Chen L. Seventh cervical nerve root transfer from contralateral healthy side for treatment of brachial plexus root avulsion. J Hand Surg Br. 1992;17:518–21.

17. Hua XY, Qiu YQ, Li T, Zheng MX, Shen YD, Jiang S, Xu JG, Gu YD, Xu WD. Contralateral peripheral neurotization for hemiplegic upper extremity after central neurologic injury. Neurosurgery. 2015;76:187–95.

Electrodiagnostic Testing for Nerve Injuries and Repairs

Neil R. Holland

Introduction

The evaluation and management of patients affected by peripheral nerve injuries necessitates a thorough knowledge of peripheral neuroanatomy, neurophysiology, and electrodiagnostic medicine. In general, every nerve injury can be classified according to its completeness and predominant pathophysiology. Complete injuries disrupt all the neurons traversing the injured segment, causing total loss of distal motor or sensory function. Incomplete lesions disrupt some neurons but leave others unaffected, with some sparing of distal motor or sensory function. An incomplete nerve injury implies that at least part of the nerve remains in continuity and this usually indicates a more favorable prognosis for spontaneous recovery. Although peripheral nerves may be injured in various ways, there are only two possible pathophysiologic responses to trauma at the neuronal level – demyelination and axonal loss (Table 8.1). It is important to recognize that axonal nerve injuries evolve with time. Although axonal function is disrupted immediately, the disconnected distal segment will continue to conduct externally applied stimuli, until

N.R. Holland, MBBS, MBA, FAAN
Neurology, Geisinger Health System,
Danville, PA, USA

Medicine (Neurology), Commonwealth Medical
College, Scanton, PA, USA
e-mail: nholland1@geisinger.edu

it slowly degenerates in a centrifugal fashion over the course of the next 7–10 days by a process known as Wallerian degeneration. Furthermore, most nerve injuries consist of some combinations of these two processes, which one predominates will determine prognosis.

Electrodiagnostic medicine physicians may be called upon to assist in any one of three distinct roles. First, electrodiagnostic evaluations are needed to localize injuries, determine if they are complete or incomplete, and characterize the pathophysiology. Second, preoperative evaluation for planning tendon transfer repair may also necessitate multichannel electromyography during complex volitional activities as discussed in this book in Chap. 7 [1]. Finally, electromyographers may be asked to come to the operating room to provide additional information during the actual surgical exploration and repair.

Part I: Preoperative Electrodiagnostic Testing

A carefully planned electrodiagnostic study is critical for determining the localization, completeness, and pathophysiology of nerve injuries. Both nerve conduction studies and the needle electromyography (EMG) portion of the test contribute. However, the utility of nerve conduction studies to assess nerve injuries can be limited by the availability of conventional studies and stimulation sites. In general, sensory

Table 8.1 Pathophysiology of peripheral nerve injury with implications for prognosis

Neurapraxia (segmental demyelination)	Caused by a mild stretch or compression injury that disrupts the myelin sheath at the injury site, resulting in focal demyelination and leaving the axons intact. This causes a transient state of disrupted conduction along the injured segment	The axons remain intact, function can be restored by focal remyelination, usually within a matter of days to weeks
Axonotmesis	A more severe injury that disrupts axons but spares the supporting perineural connective tissue sheaths The axonal segment distal to the injury degenerates in a centrifugal pattern (Wallerian degeneration)	The axon may recover by axonal regeneration through the intact perineural sheath from the intact cell body, which is a slow process occurring at a rate of about 1 mm/day
Neurotmesis	The most severe injuries which disrupt the whole nerve, affecting both the axon and supporting connective tissue	These injuries are less likely to recover by axonal regeneration and more often require surgical repair
Mixed	Most nerve injuries will actually include a mixed pattern of both segmental demyelination and axonal loss. The prognosis is determined by which process predominates	Recovery from mixed lesions is usually biphasic. The neurapraxic component of the injury recovers quickly by remyelination and the axonal component of the injury recovers slowly by axonal regeneration

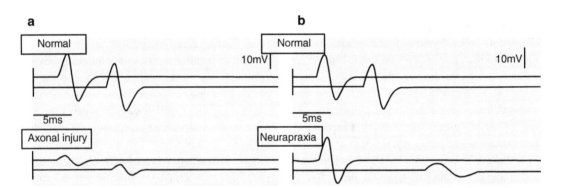

Fig. 8.1 Nerve conduction studies in nerve injury. (**a**) Axonal injury, once Wallerian degeneration has occurred, evoked responses are low amplitude or absent proximal and distal to the injury site. (**b**) Neurapraxia, the distal segment conducts normally, but proximal stimulation will result in conduction slowing and block across the injury site

conduction studies are affected earlier and more severely than motor studies in nerve injuries, and a low-amplitude or absent sensory response from an affected nerve is the most sensitive indication of peripheral nerve injury. Normal sensory responses are seen with nerve root injuries, even from clinically anesthetic regions, because the injured nerve segment is proximal to the dorsal root ganglion. In neurapraxic injuries, the compound muscle action potential elicited from stimulation of a motor nerve distal to the lesion is normal, with partial or complete conduction block from proximal stimulation. Late responses (F-waves) are occasionally useful with extremely proximal lesions where it is not possible to directly stimulate proximal to the injured segment. Once an axonal injury has fully evolved, nerve conduction studies will show low-amplitude responses from both proximal and distal stimulation (Fig. 8.1 and Table 8.2). Nerve injuries will cause reduced or absent motor unit potential recruitment in denervated muscles on needle electromyography (EMG) examination. The mere presence of any

Table 8.2 Electrodiagnostic findings in neurapraxia and axonal injury

	Motor nerve response from distal stimulation	Motor evoked response from proximal stimulation (or F-wave response)	Needle EMG examination
Neurapraxia	Normal	Low amplitude or absent	Reduced or absent motor unit recruitment
Axonotmesis	Low amplitude or absent	Low amplitude or absent	Abnormal spontaneous activity and reduced or absent motor unit recruitment
Neurotmesis	Low amplitude or absent	Low amplitude or absent	Abnormal spontaneous activity and reduced or absent motor unit recruitment

voluntary motor unit potentials in a clinically paralyzed muscle always indicates that the nerve injury, at least the branch or fascicle supplying that individual muscle, is partial and not complete. Abnormal spontaneous activity on needle EMG examination in the form of fibrillation potentials appears in muscles denervated by axonal nerve injury over 2–3 weeks.

In sum, although electrodiagnostic studies can be performed at any time after nerve injuries, maximal information can be obtained after 2–3 weeks, when the presence of conduction block on nerve conduction studies indicated neurapraxia, and the presence of low-amplitude motor and sensory responses and abnormal spontaneous activity on needle EMG examination indicate the degree of axonal loss (Table 8.2). Obviously every electrodiagnostic evaluation is tailored to the particular clinical situation. However, in general the study should include motor and sensory nerve conduction studies and proximal (F-wave) responses from affected nerves and from the contralateral limbs to compare amplitudes as well as a needle EMG examination of affected muscles to distinguish complete from incomplete injuries and neurapraxia from axonotmesis. In the case of axonal injuries, a repeat study may be indicated in 2–3 months to look for increased evoked amplitudes on nerve conduction studies as well as nascent or reinnervating motor unit potentials on needle EMG examination, both of which indicate ongoing recovery [2]. Planning for surgical repair should be considered for the case of complete

injury or where there is significant injury with the lack of ongoing reinnervation after 2–3 months. Even after nerve graft repair, recovery must occur by axonal regrowth from the proximal stump which occurs at a rate of 1 mm/day. Reinnervation must occur before the muscle undergoes irreversible muscle atrophy (within 12 months). In other words, nerve graft repair must be accomplished within 6 months, 3 months for proximal injuries, in order to obtain meaningful results.

Part II Intraoperative Electromyography

The value of having a preoperative clinical and electrodiagnostic evaluation as discussed in the first part of this chapter cannot be overemphasized. Before surgery, it will have already been determined if the nerve injury is axonal or demyelinating (neurapraxic), if axonal whether complete or incomplete, and if axonal and complete in the arm if a true plexus injury or root avulsion. Unfortunately, it is not possible to differentiate axonotmesis from neurotmesis in cases of complete axonal injury using a preoperative study. If the injury was axonometric, the patient will likely improve without surgery. However, if the injury was neurotmetric and the patient does not improve, the 3–6 month window for successful nerve repair will have been missed, limiting their chances of a meaningful surgical recovery [3].

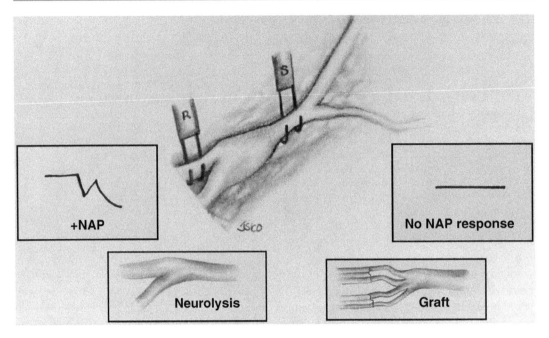

Fig. 8.2 Nerve action potential testing across an injury site (scar). An evoked response (*left*) indicates a regenerating nerve (axonotmesis), and surgery is limited to a neurolysis. No response (*right*) is more consistent with neurotmesis, which will require a nerve graft repair

Nerve Action Potentials

In some instances, even surgical exploration and direct visualization of the injured nerve segment will not differentiate these two processes since it may be impossible to determine how much internal derangement to nerve architecture has occurred from external inspection. Intraoperative nerve action potentials (NAPs) have been used in this situation to determine the extent of injury [4]. The nerve segment containing the injury is dissected free and lifted up on two pairs of bipolar electrodes separated by at least 3–4 cm. An attempt is made to conduct across this nerve segment using stimulus intensities of 10–200 V [5]. Identification of a nerve action potential response indicates the presence of at least several thousand moderate-diameter regenerating fibers. This number of fibers correlates with clinical recovery of injured nerves in experimental animal models [6]. Thus, the presence of a recordable nerve action potential across the injured segment 2–3 months after the nerve injury indicates the presence of ongoing renervation, indicating axonotmesis and not neurotmesis and

obviating the need for nerve graft repair. In these situations, surgical exploration, identification of the injury, and then intraoperative testing to determine whether the injury is axonometric (in which case surgery is limited to neurolysis) or neurotmetric (in which case nerve graft repair is needed) (Fig. 8.2). This approach has been shown to improve outcome from surgical exploration of the brachial plexus [7].

It is important to recognize that large-amplitude, fast-conducting nerve action potential responses can still be recorded from sensory nerve fibers in the brachial plexus even in the presence of complete nerve root avulsions proximal to both the stimulation site and the dorsal root ganglion. Any suspicion that this may be the case can usually be resolved by attempting to record cortical somatosensory responses from direct stimulation of proximal nerve segments. Responses will be absent in the case of root avulsions [8]. Tourniquets may cause false-negative nerve action potential responses because of peripheral nerve ischemia. The tourniquet should be deflated for at least 30 min before performing the test [9].

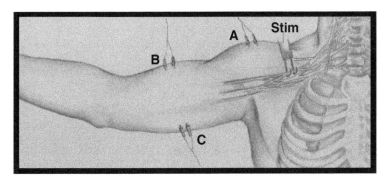
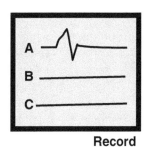

Fig. 8.3 Using stimulus-triggered EMG to identify nerves in brachial plexus. The exposed nerve is stimulated, with recordings made from multiple appropriate muscles. Identification of a compound muscle action potential in one muscle (*trace A, right*), but not the others, can identify the nerve and confirm that it is uninjured

Stimulus-Triggered EMG

Most peripheral nerve surgeons use a battery-powered handheld monopolar stimulator to help identify nerves during surgery by watching the limb for an evoked visible twitch. However, it can be hard to attribute a visible proximal arm twitch to the action of a particular nerve and muscle. Specific localization can be improved by using the EMG machine to provide current to a hand held stimulator in the field with simultaneous recordings made from multiple muscles using intramuscular needles. Identifying a time-locked evoked compound muscle action potential in only one of the recording channels will identify the individual nerve (Fig. 8.3). Obviously, this only works for uninjured normally conducting nerves in the absence of neuromuscular blocking drugs. This technique is particularly important for identifying the spinal accessory nerve during brachial plexus exploration, which is spared in plexus injury, and can be used both for orientation and as a potential donor for neurotization.

The concept of cross chest C7 nerve root transfer for repair of peripheral and central nervous injuries was discussed in another chapter [1]. Obviously, this necessitates the sacrifice of a nerve root from the healthy limb in a compromised patient with a potential for causing further neurologic deficit. Although reported cases have experienced only minor sensory loss or transient weakness because of relative redundancy of the C7 nerve root and co-innervation by adjacent nerve roots, cases of aberrant innervation are always possible [10]. Sequential stimulation of the exposed C6, C7, and C8 nerve roots with triggered responses recorded from major muscle groups can be used to rule out muscles with exclusive C7 innervation prior to transection [11].

Stimulus-triggered EMG can be also used during dorsal rhizotomy for surgical treatment of spasticity. The premise is that lesioning some of the dorsal roots can lessen spasticity without exacerbating weakness by partially interrupting segmental reflex arcs [1]. Triggered EMG responses are used by some surgeons to identify the dorsal rootlets which are contributing most to spasticity based upon "abnormal" evoked responses, either responses generated at abnormally low stimulus thresholds or abnormally sustained evoked EMG responses [12]. However, it is unclear if this type of testing has any merit compared to simply lesioning randomly chosen rootlets [13].

Summary/Key Points
- Preoperative diagnostic EMG evaluations are critical for evaluating and following nerve injury patients.
- A diagnostic EMG done 2–3 weeks after injury can localize nerve injuries, distinguish complete from incomplete injuries, and distinguish neurapraxia from axonal degeneration.
- Further intraoperative testing is usually needed to fully elucidate these injuries and plan surgical repair.

- A nerve action potential conducted across a visualized injured nerve segment can indicate axonotmesis, with ongoing renervation, obviating the need for nerve graft repair.
- Stimulus-triggered EMG can be used for orientation, localization, and exclusion of aberrant innervation prior to sacrificing a donor site.

References

1. Holland NR. Neurologic injury and spasticity. In: Elkwood AI, Kaufman MR, Schneider LF, editors. Rehabilitative surgery: an interdisciplinary approach to restoring functionality. New York: Springer; 2016.
2. Robinson LR. How electrodiagnosis predicts clinical outcome of focal peripheral nerve lesions. Muscle Nerve. 2015;52:321–33.
3. Jonsson S, Wiberg R, McGrath AM, Novikov LN, Wiberg M, Novikova LN, Kingham PJ. Effect of delayed peripheral nerve repair on nerve regeneration, Schwann cell function and target muscle recovery. PLoS One. 2013;8:e56484.
4. Oberle JW, Antoniadis G, Rath SA, Richter HP. Value of nerve action potentials in the surgical management of traumatic nerve lesions. Neurosurgery. 1997;41:1337–44.
5. Robert EG, Happel LT, Kline DG. Intraoperative nerve action potential recording: technical considerations, problems, and pitfalls. Neurosurgery. 2009;65(4 Suppl):A97–104.
6. Kline DG, DeJonge BR. Evoked potentials to evaluate peripheral nerve injuries. Surg Gynecol Obstet. 1968;127:1239–50.
7. Kandenwein JA, Kretschmer T, Engelhardt M, Richter HP, Antoniadis G. Surgical interventions for traumatic lesions of the brachial plexus: a retrospective study of 134 cases. J Neurosurg. 2005;103:614–21.
8. Landi A, Copeland SA, Wynn–Parry CD, Jones SJ. The role of somatosensory evoked potentials and nerve conduction studies in the surgical management of brachial plexus injuries. J Bone Joint Surg Br. 1980;62B:492–6.
9. Kline DG, Happel LT. A quarter century's experience with intraoperative nerve action potential recording. Can J Neurol Sci. 1993;20:3–10.
10. Chuang DCC, Wei FC, Noordhoff MS. Cross-chest C7 nerve root grafting followed by free muscle transplantations for the treatment of total avulsed brachial plexus injuries: a preliminary report. Plast Reconst Surg. 1993;92:717–27.
11. Holland NR, Belzberg AJ. Intraoperative electrodiagnostic testing during cross-chest C7 nerve root transfer. Muscle Nerve. 1997;20:903–5.
12. Fasano VA, Broggi G, Zeme S. Intraoperative electrical stimulation for functional posterior rhizotomy. Scand J Rhabil Med Suppl. 1988;17:149–54.
13. Steinbok P, Tidermann AJ, Miller S, Morteson P, Bowen-Roberts T. Electrophysiologically guided versus non-electrophysiologically guided selective dorsal rhizotomy for spastic cerebral palsy: a comparison of outcomes. Childs Nerv Syst. 2009;25:1091–6.

Spine Trauma

9

I. David Kaye and Peter G. Passias

Introduction

Spinal trauma, including spine fractures, dislocations, and spinal cord and/or nerve root injuries,
is a frequent musculoskeletal injury. Vertebral
column injuries occur in approximately 6 % of
trauma patients, with about half of these patients
sustaining a spinal cord or nerve root injury [1].
The incidence of spine fractures is about 64 per
100,000 people, with the overwhelming majority
occurring at the junctional regions of the spine,
such as the craniocervical, cervicothoracic, and
thoracolumbar areas [2]. Failure to properly diagnose and manage these injuries can result in neurologic deficits that may permanently impair a
patient's function and quality of life and may
even lead to death in some cases.

With increasing safety protocols, specifically
regarding automobiles, patients are now surviving initial traumas that previously would have
been lethal. These patients are now being tri-
aged with increasingly severe spinal injuries
that require urgent management. The advent of
advanced imaging has also aided detection and
guided management of spinal injuries, and
newer instrumentation has afforded better prognosis for some patients with spine trauma. The
goal of this chapter is to provide an overview of
cervical, thoracic, and lumbar trauma with a
focus on epidemiology, diagnosis, radiographic
evaluation, acute management, and rehab
strategies.

Anatomy

The spine is composed of 7 cervical, 12 thoracic, and 5 lumbar vertebrae. Five fused vertebrae form the inflexible sacrum that provides
relatively rigid fixation to the rest of the pelvis. Below the sacrum, four or five ossicles
comprise the coccyx. These bones constitute
97 diarthroses. An even greater number of
amphiarthroses with numerous processes on
each bone for ligamentous attachments provide stability for these articulations. The purpose of the spine is to provide neuroprotective
support to the trunk. Although some levels
have unique anatomical modifications, for
example, the axis and the atlas, an in-depth
description of these variances is beyond the
scope of this text.

Each vertebral unit is composed of an anterior
body, made of mostly trabecular bone, and a posterior structure, the dorsal vertebral arch, which
is attached to the dorsolateral aspect of the body

I.D. Kaye, MD (✉)
Division of Spine Surgery, The Rothman Institute at
Thomas Jefferson University Hospital, 925 Chestnut
Street, Philadelphia, PA 19107, USA
e-mail: iandavid.kaye@gmail.com

P.G. Passias, MD
Division of Spinal Surgery, NYU School of Medicine,
New York, NY, USA

© Springer International Publishing Switzerland 2017
A.I. Elkwood et al. (eds.), *Rehabilitative Surgery*, DOI 10.1007/978-3-319-41406-5_9

Fig. 9.1 Spinal anatomy.
(**a**) *Top image*: lumbar spine
anatomy. (**b**) *Lower image*:
upper cervical spine
anatomy

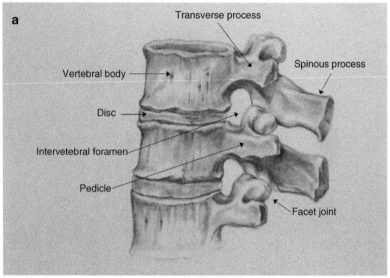

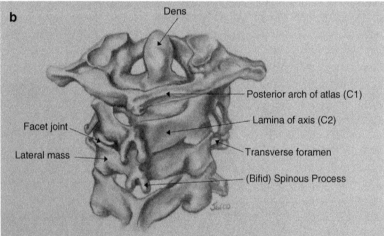

by stout pillars called pedicles. The pedicles are united posteriorly by the laminae and then give off a dorsal projection, the spinous process. Transverse processes project off the junction of the pedicles and lamina.

The spinal column houses the spinal cord, which in turn gives off dorsal and ventral nerve roots that pass through the subarachnoid space to form the spinal nerve (commonly referred to as root). This occurs approximately at the level of the intervertebral foramen. In the cervical spine, the spinal nerves exit the column one level above the numbered pedicle (e.g., C6 nerve root exits at the C5–C6 interspace). However, the thoracic and lumbar nerve roots exit below the numbered

pedicle (e.g., L4 nerve root exits at the L4–L5 interspace) (Figs. 9.1 and 9.2).

Spine Trauma Overview

Epidemiology

Injuries to the spine are most commonly secondary to high-energy trauma in the young but secondary to low energy forces, with minimal or even no trauma, in the elderly. In the cervical spine, injuries occur in 2–3 % of all patients who sustain blunt trauma [3]. Injuries are more common at the upper cervical region compared to the

Fig. 9.2 Spinal nerve. (**a**) *Top image*: lumbar spine roots exiting below the pedicle of their respective vertebral body. (**b**) *Lower image*: cervical spine nerve roots exiting above the pedicle of their respective vertebral body

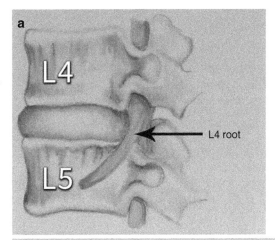

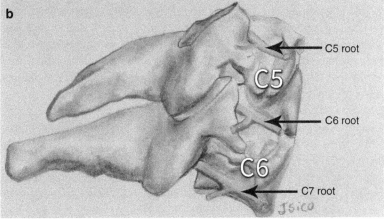

subaxial cervical spine with injuries most commonly secondary to high-energy trauma such as motor vehicle accidents or falls from height in the young as opposed to low-velocity falls in the elderly [4–7]. At the thoracic and lumbar spine, most isolated fractures are related to osteoporosis and involve minimal trauma. Osteoporosis leads to approximately 750,000 vertebral fractures each year in the United States [8]. Conversely, only about 15,000 thoracic or lumbar fractures related to trauma are reported annually [9].

Most spine fractures occur at the thoracic and lumbar regions, accounting for more than half of all spinal injuries in trauma victims with 60 % of those fractures occurring between the T11 and L2 vertebral levels [10–12]. Although spinal cord injury is exceptionally rare with osteoporotic fractures, neurologic injury occurs in one-fourth

of traumatic thoracic and lumbar fractures [12]. Overall, neurologic injury following thoracic or lumbar trauma is 3 % [12]. This rate is significantly lower than the rate of spinal cord injury after cervical spine fractures as spinal cord injury after cervical trauma accounts for 65 % of all traumatic spinal cord injuries [13].

The presence of a spinal cord injury dramatically affects a patient's mortality risk and his ultimate function and quality of life. For patients with a spinal cord injury, the overall mortality during the initial hospitalization was 17 % based on a study in the early 1980s, but more recently, the National Spinal Cord Injury Statistical Center estimates the mortality of traumatic spinal cord injury to be 2.6 % [1, 14]. However, some have suggested that the number is actually closer to 5–10 % [15].

Initial Care

The goal of any intervention following spine trauma is to achieve spinal stability. White and Panjabi describe clinical spinal stability as the "ability of the spine under physiologic loads to limit patterns of displacement so as not to damage or irritate the spinal cord or nerve roots and, in addition, to prevent incapacitating deformity or pain caused by structural changes" [16].

Any patient who has sustained a high-energy trauma should be assumed to have a spine injury until proven otherwise. In fact, at least 6 % of all trauma patients sustain a spine injury [1]. As a general rule, all trauma patients need to be fully investigated for spinal injury. Before proceeding with any intervention in the trauma setting, establishing the ABCs (airway, breathing, circulation) and applying the Advanced Trauma Life Support protocols are paramount. Field management of trauma victims requires vigilance for the possibility of an unstable spinal injury until spinal injury is definitively excluded or treated. Proper extrication of the patient and immobilization of the cervical spine at the accident scene are critical to avoid further neurologic injury [17]. The head and the neck need to be aligned with the long axis of the trunk and immobilized in this position with the use of a cervical collar, sandbags, tape, and spine board. Cervical extension should be avoided because it narrows the spinal canal more than flexion [18]. Logrolling precautions must be maintained, although logrolling has been shown to allow some degree of motion at the spinal injury site [19].

As part of the initial evaluation of ABCs, assessment of vital signs including blood pressure and heart rate may reveal abnormalities that must be accurately diagnosed to prevent potential catastrophe. Unlike other trauma patients who are more likely to suffer from hemorrhagic shock, patients with spine trauma may instead be in a state of neurogenic shock, which must be distinguished for safe resuscitation (Table 9.1) [20, 21]. Neurogenic shock results from a loss of sympathetic outflow leading to hypotension with simultaneous bradycardia in the face of warm

Table 9.1 Comparison of neurogenic and hypovolemic shock

	Neurogenic shock	Hypovolemic shock
Etiology	Loss of sympathetic outflow	Loss of circulating blood volume
Blood pressure	Hypotension	Hypotension
Heart rate	Bradycardia	Tachycardia
Urine output	Normal	Low
Skin	Warm extremities	Cool extremities

extremities and a normal urine output. It is generally treated with administration of vasopressors (e.g., dopamine), whereas treatment with fluid resuscitation, if confused with hemorrhagic shock, can actually precipitate pulmonary edema. A more favorable neurologic recovery has been found in those whose mean arterial pressure is maintained above 85 mmHg, allowing for adequate perfusion of the cord [22].

After acute stabilization, other injuries must be assessed. While a primary lesion may be suspected at a particular spinal level, injuries at noncontiguous levels have been reported to occur in as many as 15–20 % of patients [23]. Although cervical spine fractures are unlikely to be associated with an abdominal injury, with a reported rate of 2.6 % of cases, chest and abdominal injuries are commonly identified in patients with thoracic and lumbar fractures [24].

Physical Examination

A thorough physical examination, identifying any potential neurologic deficits, is critical for guiding management. A methodical evaluation of motor and sensory groups for each spine level must be performed (Table 9.2). Based on this examination, an American Spinal Injury Association (ASIA) score may be assigned. The ASIA classification is graded from A, complete motor and sensory deficit, to E, completely intact neurologic exam. Distal motor function and sacral sparing are important for prognosis [25].

Table 9.2 Myotome and dermatome spine exam

	Motor	Sensory	Reflex
C5	Deltoid	Lateral shoulder/arm	Biceps
C6	Biceps/wrist extensors	Lateral forearm/thumb and index finger	Brachioradialis
C7	Triceps/wrist flexors	Middle finger	Triceps
C8	Hand intrinsics/finger flexors	Ring and little finger/medial forearm	
T1	Hand intrinsics/finger abductors	Medial arm/axilla	
L2	Iliopsoas	Upper thigh proximal lateral/distal medial	
L3	Quadriceps/hip adductors	Middle thigh proximal lateral/distal medial	
L4	Tibialis anterior	Upper thigh laterally crossing knee/medial leg	Patella tendon
L5	Extensor hallucis longus/gluteus medius	Lateral thigh and leg	
S1	Gastrocnemius/soleus	Posterior thigh/leg	Achilles tendon

In fact, even in those who are initially found to have a motor complete lesion, the return of sacral pinprick sensation by 4 weeks post-injury carries an improved prognosis of regaining ambulatory potential [26, 27]. Similarly, pinprick preservation in more than 50 % of the lower extremity dermatomes L2–S1 in the first 72 h of injury is associated with improved prognosis for ambulation [28].

Although an ASIA score is given on admission, it is reassessed and rescored with each successive exam. The score may also be lower secondary to spinal shock [28]. Spinal shock occurs when the physical energy of the inciting trauma causes immediate depolarization of axonal membranes in the neural tissue, resulting in a functional neurologic deficit that exceeds the actual tissue disruption. Spinal shock may be related to depolarization of the entire cord. Spinal reflexes caudal to the injury are depressed. Typically, the effects of spinal shock resolve within 24 h, but some effects, such as return of deep tendon reflexes, may take weeks or even months [28]. Unfortunately, the delayed plantar reflex, the first sign of emergence from spinal shock, is present only transiently and can easily be missed. The return of other reflexes, such as the bulbocavernosus, cremasteric, or anal wink, may take several more days to return.

Neurologic Injury

Spinal cord injuries may be either complete or incomplete. Complete injuries affect motor and sensation below the level of the injury such that no function exists. Incomplete injuries are more varied (Table 9.3). The most common site of spinal cord injury is the cervical region, accounting for 50–64 % of traumatic spinal cord injuries, with incomplete injuries outnumbering complete ones by nearly a 2:1 ratio [13, 14]. Approximately 41 % of the patients with an acute spinal cord injury have a complete injury on initial evaluation [13].

Acute management of spinal cord injury is controversial. The results of the third National Acute Spinal Cord Injury Randomized Controlled Trial (NASCIS III) showed that steroid administration begun within 8 h of injury is beneficial. From that trial, the guidelines established are as follows: for injuries within three hours, an initial bolus of 30 mg/kg of methylprednisolone is given followed by 5.4 mg/kg/h infusion over the next 24 h, and if steroids are begun 3–8 h after the injury, the infusion is continued for 48 h [29–31]. Some have abandoned steroid administration claiming no benefit and increased pulmonary complications and infections. The decision to administer steroids has largely become a medicolegal one.

Table 9.3 Incomplete spinal cord injuries

Syndrome	Lesion	Characteristics
Central cord	Incomplete cervical white matter injury	Cervical injury with sacral sparing and greater weakness in arms > legs; usually from hyperextension injury
Anterior cord	Anterior gray matter, descending corticospinal motor tract, and spinothalamic tract injury with preservation of dorsal columns	Causes loss of pain and temperature sensation with preserved proprioception; usually from vascular insult to cord
Posterior cord	Posterior white matter and ascending gracile and cuneate fascicule	Causes loss of proprioception with preserved pain and temperature sensation
Brown-Sequard	Injury to one lateral half of cord and preservation of contralateral half	Causes ipsilateral weakness and loss of proprioception and contralateral loss of pain and temperature sensibility; most commonly from penetrating trauma
Cauda equina	Injury to the lumbosacral nerve roots within the neural canal	Characterized by saddle anesthesia, bowel/bladder dysfunction, diminished reflexes, weakness, and pain
Conus medullaris	Injury to the sacral conus and lumbar nerve roots	Similar presentation to cauda equina syndrome but weakness and sensory disturbances are rare

Radiographic Evaluation

White and Panjabi state that "the major practical consideration in the determination of clinical instability is the evaluation of the patient's radiographs" [16]. While determination of spinal stability is more nuanced, accurate and meaningful interpretation of radiographic imaging is still central to diagnosis and helps guide management.

Plain Films

Cervical Spine

Systematic and reproducible evaluations of plain film radiographs are crucial to preventing missed injuries. In the subacute trauma setting, a complete radiographic series of the cervical spine should include a minimum of AP, lateral, and open-mouth odontoid views, with oblique images obtained as necessary. Flexion–extension views in the acute setting are generally deferred as they are often nondiagnostic and may even be dangerous. When in pain, patients may have limited mobility related to muscle spasm, limiting cervical spine motion on dynamic views, leading to false negatives. More concerningly, unsupervised

or forceful flexion in a patient with an occult ligamentous injury may precipitate a neurologic injury.

Radiographic assessment should proceed in a proximal to distal fashion beginning with the occipitocervical junction and proceeding distally to the cervicothoracic junction. Plain radiographs may reveal fractures or dislocations at the occipitocervical junction, upper cervical spine or subaxial spine. Fracture characteristics such as displacement and angulation can be measured from plain films and may help dictate management.

Spinal stability may generally be assessed by evaluating for segmental kyphosis or vertebral translation, both of which may indicate compromise of the posterior ligamentous complex (PLC) and instability [16].

In the subaxial cervical spine, plain radiographs or CT scans can be used to screen for injuries, but it is absolutely necessary to fully visualize the cervicothoracic junction. Failure to evaluate this area radiographically represents an incomplete evaluation. When regular lateral films do not reveal the junction, a swimmer's view, performed by placing one of the patient's arms above their head and one below, may provide better resolution (Fig. 9.3).

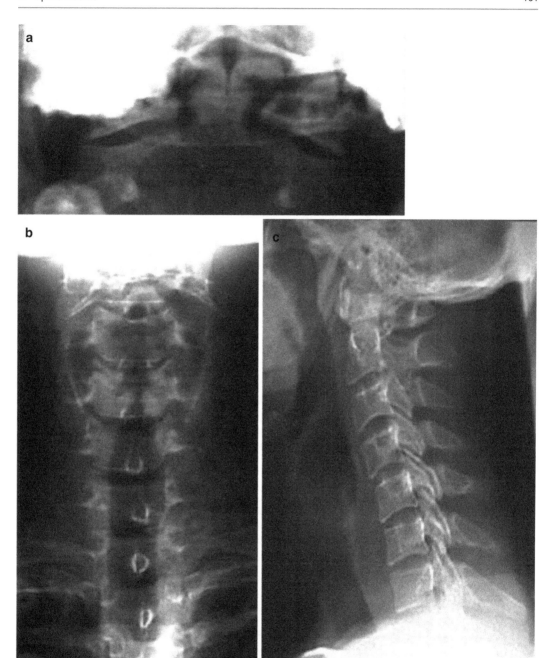

Fig. 9.3 Standard cervical spine radiographs. (**a**) Open-mouth odontoid view, (**b**) AP view, (**c**) lateral view

Thoracic and Lumbar Spine

Standard thoracic and lumbar evaluation includes AP and lateral projection. An AP view may reveal coronal malalignment or interpedicular widening characteristic of lateral displacement of burst fracture fragments, while lateral radiographs may be used to quantify sagittal deformity through measurement of Cobb angles.

As in the cervical spine, instability and posterior ligamentous disruption should be suspected with increased vertebral translation, angulation, or collapse.

In addition to the acute setting, plain imaging is also frequently used to monitor posttreatment follow-up. For example, for stable burst fractures managed with bracing, standing radiographs in the orthosis are obtained to ensure stability and that there is no progression of deformity once the patient is mobilized [32] (Fig. 9.4).

Computed Tomography

Plain radiographs may be limited by soft tissue shadows and preexisting spondylosis, while computed tomography (CT) displays high-resolution imaging of the spinal column that provides more information about the extent of a thoracolumbar injury than radiographs alone. One study found that for thoracolumbar trauma, plain radiographs alone may yield an incorrect diagnosis in as many as 25% of individuals with burst fractures and underestimate their amount of canal compromise by 20% [33, 34]. CT allows for more accurate assessment of comminution and perhaps, more importantly, the ability to detect retropulsed bony fragments which may influence treatment options. Because of its greater sensitivity and efficiency, a single helical CT scan has been

shown to be preferable to a series of plain radiographs for screening polytrauma patients who may have spinal injuries [35].

MRI

Cervical Spine

If there are no contraindications, an MRI scan is obtained in cases of cervical spine trauma when any of the following criteria are met: (1) the patient presents with a neurologic deficit; (2) the integrity of the PLC is unclear, and injury to this structure would have a direct influence on treatment, such as determining the need for surgery; and (3) the patient presents with a facet dislocation where there is concern regarding disk herniation into the spinal canal that may prevent safe reduction and cause difficulty in deciding on the correct approach for surgical intervention. T2-weighted images provide the best initial MRI review of cervical trauma. These studies have a so-called myelography effect, in that the cerebrospinal fluid (CSF) is bright and the discoligamentous structures are relatively dark or isointense. T2-weighted images may demonstrate increased signal within the disk, facet capsules, or posterior

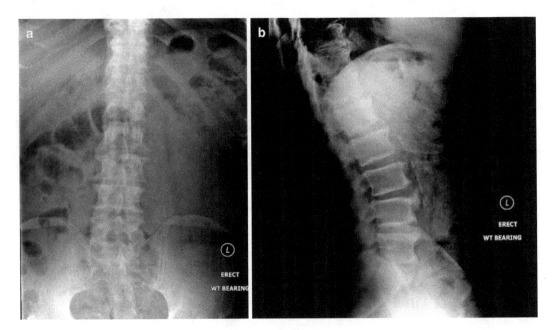

Fig. 9.4 Standard radiographs of lumbar spine. (**a**) AP view, (**b**) lateral view

interspinous process region, indicative of edema or frank disruption.

Thoracic and Lumbar Spine

Magnetic resonance imaging (MRI) is the "gold standard" technique for visualizing soft tissue injuries associated with thoracolumbar fractures including disk herniation, epidural hematoma, ligamentous injury, or intrasubstance injury to the spinal cord itself. In the thoracolumbar region, integrity of the PLC is crucial for determining stability, and MRI is the optimal modality for discernment [36]. On sagittal views of the spine, any edema involving the posterior supporting structures may be interpreted as a sign of a traumatic insult to the PLC, and the presence of a discrete stripe of fluid extending through these tissues on fat-suppressed T2-weighted images is indicative of a frank disruption of the posterior tension band (Fig. 9.5).

C-Spine Clearance

To reduce routine cervical spine imaging in trauma patients, two competing prediction rules have been developed and validated: the National Emergency X-ray Utilization Study (NEXUS) criteria (Fig. 9.6b) and the Canadian C-spine Rule (Fig. 9.6a) [37, 38]. The Canadian C-spine injury prediction rules have better sensitivity and specificity and reduce unnecessary imaging to a greater extent, but they are more complex to apply routinely [37–39]. Applying the Canadian C-spine Rules in the field may prevent 38 % of out-of-hospital spine immobilizations [40]. Many centers use these guidelines to help clear the cervical spine, and if the patient meets the NEXUS criteria or Canadian rules, then the cervical collar is removed.

Cervical Spine Injuries

The cervical spine is injured in about 2–3 % of all patients sustaining blunt trauma, and about two-thirds of those patients sustain injuries to the subaxial spine, with fracture of C7 or dislocation at

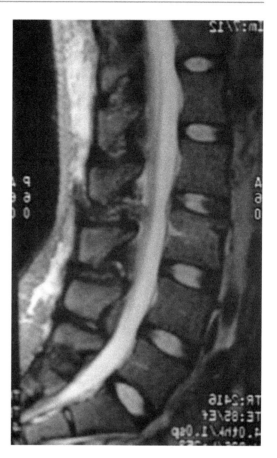

Fig. 9.5 MRI of lumbar spine. L3 Chance fracture with edema between L2 and L3 spinous processes suggestive of a PLC injury

C7–T1 accounting for almost 17 % of all injuries [41, 42]. In addition to the usual anatomy shared with the rest of the spine (i.e., anterior and posterior bony elements, intervertebral disks, joint capsules, ligaments), the cervical spine also houses the vertebral arteries in the transverse foramen (usually from C1 to C6).

The unique anatomy of the upper cervical spine, i.e., the atlas and the axis, lends it to unique fracture patterns (Table 9.4).

Regarding the subaxial cervical spine, several classifications have been proposed including Allen et al.'s, Harris et al.'s, and White and Panjabi's [16, 43, 44]. In 2008, the Spine Trauma Study Group devised a new classification scheme called the Subaxial Injury Classification system (SLIC) which identifies three major injury char-

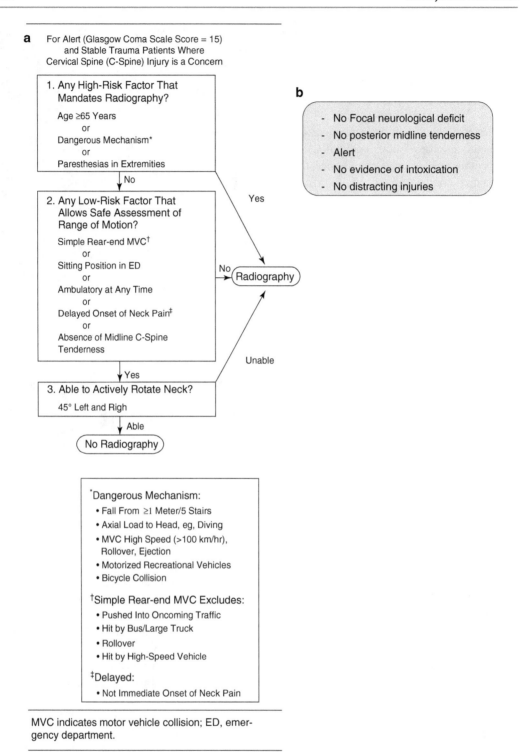

a For Alert (Glasgow Coma Scale Score = 15)
and Stable Trauma Patients Where
Cervical Spine (C-Spine) Injury is a Concern

1. Any High-Risk Factor That
   Mandates Radiography?

   Age ≥65 Years
   or
   Dangerous Mechanism*
   or
   Paresthesias in Extremities

2. Any Low-Risk Factor That
   Allows Safe Assessment of
   Range of Motion?

   Simple Rear-end MVC†
   or
   Sitting Position in ED
   or
   Ambulatory at Any Time
   or
   Delayed Onset of Neck Pain‡
   or
   Absence of Midline C-Spine
   Tenderness

3. Able to Actively Rotate Neck?

   45° Left and Righ

No → Radiography

Yes

No

Unable

Yes

Able

No Radiography

b

- No Focal neurological deficit
- No posterior midline tenderness
- Alert
- No evidence of intoxication
- No distracting injuries

*Dangerous Mechanism:
- Fall From ≥1 Meter/5 Stairs
- Axial Load to Head, eg, Diving
- MVC High Speed (>100 km/hr),
  Rollover, Ejection
- Motorized Recreational Vehicles
- Bicycle Collision

†Simple Rear-end MVC Excludes:
- Pushed Into Oncoming Traffic
- Hit by Bus/Large Truck
- Rollover
- Hit by High-Speed Vehicle

‡Delayed:
- Not Immediate Onset of Neck Pain

MVC indicates motor vehicle collision; ED, emergency department.

Fig. 9.6 (**a**) Canadian and (**b**) NEXUS criteria for traumatic cervical spine imaging and cervical collar clearance (From Stiell et al. [38] and Hoffman et al. [37], respectively)

Table 9.4 Summary of upper cervical injury characteristics and treatments

Injury	Characteristics	Treatment
Occipital condyle fracture	Types I–III depending on stability	Cervical collar vs. halo vest
Craniocervical dissociation	MRI evidence of dissociation vs. static film with dissociation	<2 mm displacement: no intervention >2 mm displacement: PSF occiput to C2
Atlas fracture	Stable (<7 mm of lateral mass displacement or isolated posterior arch) Unstable (>7 mm lateral mass displacement or unilateral sagittal split of lateral mass)	Stable: rigid collar vs. halo Unstable: posterior C1-C2 arthrodesis (possible halo vest for unstable lateral mass fractures)
Atlantoaxial dissociation	Subtypes based on stability of transverse atlantal ligament (increasing severity of rotation—>translation—>distraction)	TAL intact: closed reduction and immobilization TAL disrupted: C1–C2 arthrodesis
Dens fracture	Types I–III depending on location of fracture line	Avulsion: external immobilization Waist fracture: high risk of nonunion surgery Body fracture: halo vs. brace
Traumatic spondylolisthesis	C2 arch fracture with worsening severity depending on involvement of C2–C3 disk or facet dislocation	Usually halo vest unless significant risk to cord or in cases of dislocation when surgery indicated

acteristics (injury morphology, discoligamentous complex (DLC), and neurologic status) with additional subgroups based on minor characteristics (including spinal level, anatomical osseous injury descriptors, and injury confounders such as ankylosing spondylitis, diffuse idiopathic skeletal hyperostosis (DISH), prior surgery, ongoing cord compression, etc.) and grades the injuries accordingly (Table 9.5) [45].

Within this framework, injury morphology must be assessed radiographically. The alignment of the vertebral bodies, facet relationships, and soft tissue structures must be examined. The *compression*-type injury is defined by a loss of height of the vertebral body or disruption through the vertebral end plate. The *burst* modifier accounts for those compression fractures that extend into the middle column. The *distraction* injury pattern is identified by vertical dissociation of the spine, including hyperextension-type injuries causing disruption of the anterior longitudinal ligament and subsequent widening of the anterior disk space.

While fractures of the posterior elements (facets, laminae, and spinous processes) may be present, more typically, there may be perched or subluxated facets through a tensile failure of the ligamentous restraints. Lastly, the *rotation/translation* injury is defined by horizontal displacement of one vertebral body with respect to another and usually including unilateral and bilateral facet dislocations or fracture–dislocations. They may also include fracture separation of the lateral mass with vertebral subluxation and bilateral pedicle fractures with vertebral subluxation ("traumatic spondylolisthesis").

The SLIC also includes assessment of the DLC, which includes the intervertebral disk, anterior and posterior longitudinal ligaments, interspinous ligaments, facet capsules, and ligamentum flavum. Its integrity is classified as one of the three categories: disrupted, indeterminate, and intact. *Disruption* of the DLC may be represented by abnormal facet alignment (articular apposition < 50 % or diastasis > 2 mm through the facet joint), widening of the anterior disk space, translation or rotation of the vertebral bodies, or kyphotic alignment of the cervical spine. MRI may reveal high signal intensity on T2-weighted fat-suppressed sagittal sequences at the disk or posterior elements. The DLC may be noted to have an *indeterminate* injury when plain films and CT appear normal, but a hyperintense signal is found through either the disk or the posterior ligamentous regions on T2-weighted MR imaging images, suggesting edema and injury. The DLC is *intact* when there is normal spinal alignment in

Table 9.5 The subaxial injury classification (SLIC) system

Characteristic	Subtype	Points
Morphology		
	No abnormality	0
	Compression	1
	Burst	+1 (added to compression for a total of 2)
	Distraction	3
	Rotation/translation	4
Discoligamentous complex		
	Intact	0
	Indeterminate	1
	Disrupted	2
Neurologic status		
	Intact	0
	Root injury	1
	Complete cord injury	2
	Incomplete cord injury	3
	Ongoing cord compression in setting of a neurologic deficit	+1

Modified from Patel et al. [45]
If score is < or = 3, nonoperative management
If score is > or = 5, operative management
If score = 4, operative management is decided by individual surgeon

addition to normal disk space and ligamentous appearance. The last element, the neurologic status, may be the most important and may itself indicate the integrity of the spinal column. The status is categorized as follows: intact, root injury, complete cord injury, or incomplete cord injury. With translation or rotation injuries, the assessment of cord compression should be made after attempted reduction of the injury.

Surgical versus nonsurgical treatment is determined by a threshold value of the SLIC severity score. If the total score is < 4, nonoperative treatment is recommended. If the total is ≥ 5, operative treatment, including potential realignment, decompression, and stabilization, is recommended. Cases with a total score of 4 may be treated operatively or nonoperatively.

While the SLIC was generated to help standardize cervical spine trauma management, intervention may need to be individualized. In general, mechanical stability, neurologic compromise, and patient factors must be considered. According to White and Panjabi, mechanical instability may be assumed if there is > 3.5 mm of displacement or relative angulation of > 11°.

Patient factors to be considered include concomitant injuries, noncontiguous spinal injuries, smoking, comorbidities, and the ability to realistically treat an injury nonsurgically (e.g., the morbidly obese patient who cannot be fitted adequately for a halo brace).

Outcomes

Unfortunately, there is a paucity of quality data regarding management and outcomes for cervical spine surgery. Many of the purported advantages of spine trauma surgery, including the recommendation for intervention within 24 h, while well accepted, remain unsupported by high-quality evidence.

The sparse evidence available generally does support surgical intervention and good outcomes when indicated. Lee et al. reported a 100 % fusion rate when treating cervical spine flexion-type injuries with posterior interspinous wiring; however, they noted that the maintenance of sagittal alignment can be challenging [46]. Roy-Camille et al. used posterolateral mass screws and plates to treat lower cervical spine injuries and found

Table 9.6 The thoracolumbar injury classification and severity score (TLICS)

Characteristic	Subtype	Points
Morphology		
	No abnormality	0
	Compression	1
	Burst	+1 (added to compression for a total of 2)
	Rotation/translation	3
	Distraction	4
Posterior ligamentous complex		
	Intact	0
	Indeterminate	2
	Disrupted	3
Neurologic status		
	Intact	0
	Root injury	2
	Complete cord injury	2
	Incomplete cord injury	3
	Cauda equina	3

From Vaccaro et al. [54]
If score is < or = 3, nonoperative management
If score is > or = 5, operative management
If score = 4, operative management is decided by individual surgeon

that initial reduction and alignment was maintained in 85 % of cases [47].

As part of a prospective, randomized, controlled trial for unilateral facet injuries, Kwon and colleagues reported no difference in patient-based outcome measures between anterior and posterior fixation [48].

Postoperative Care

After internal fixation for cervical spine injuries, the need for postoperative external immobilization is diminished. The decision whether to use additional external fixation is determined individually and is generally dictated by the type of fixation and bone quality. Whereas a polyaxial screw–rod construct in normal bone may not necessitate external immobilization, osteoporotic bone fixed with wiring may.

Generally, a rigid cervical collar is prescribed for 6 weeks in awake and alert patients who will be ambulatory following surgery. When ventilator dependent, an orthosis is avoided to facilitate nursing and respiratory care. With rigid internal fixation, the patient can be seated to facilitate

pulmonary toilet and clearance of secretions. If indicated, postoperative thromboembolic chemoprophylaxis can be started on postoperative day 4 or 5, attempting to avoid an epidural hematoma with earlier administration.

Unfortunately, we do not, as yet, know which are the best outcome measures, which factors influence survival in the acute period, and how we can best maximize neurologic recovery (Table 9.6).

Thoracic and Lumbar Spine Injuries

Thoracolumbar injuries comprise 65–80 % of all spine injuries among polytrauma patients, the majority of these located at the thoracolumbar junction [10–12]. The annual incidence of fracture in patients younger than 60 years is 13 per 100,000 which rises to more than 50 fractures/100,000 in patients above 70 years of age and to above 100 fractures/100,000 for individuals older than 80 years [49]. This increase is largely secondary to osteoporotic fractures and is likely even higher given the number of undiagnosed fractures [49, 50]. Most of these fractures in the elderly are compression type and may be treated nonoperatively accounting for the relatively low rate of surgical intervention in elderly patients with thoracolumbar fractures compared to younger populations (2 % in ≥60 years old vs. 15 % in <60 years old) [49].

Approximately 20 % of patients with thoracolumbar fractures will develop some type of neurologic deficit [51]. In addition to the extensive morbidity sustained by these patients, the 1-year mortality rate of patients with paraplegia or other catastrophic thoracic or lumbar spinal cord injuries (SCIs) is approximately 4 % [52]. Although treatment algorithms are identical for elderly patients with thoracolumbar injuries provided the patient is healthy enough to undergo surgery, elderly patients with SCI and their families should be counseled regarding the relatively poor prognosis associated with their injury.

Classification

Early classification schemes for thoracolumbar fractures were aimed at defining stability at this part of the spine and intended to help guide management. Denis formulated a classification system dividing the spinal structures into three columns: anterior (anterior half of vertebra/disk and anterior longitudinal ligament), middle (posterior half of vertebra/disk and posterior longitudinal ligament), and posterior (posterior elements including the pedicles, facet joints, and remaining ligaments) [51]. From this system, four main fracture types exist—compression, burst, Chance, and fracture–dislocations—with an additional 16 subgroups. Any fracture that extends through the middle column is generally considered unstable.

While other classifications, including the AO (Magerl) classification, have been proposed, poor interobserver reliability has been documented [53].

In an effort to overcome the deficiencies of prior classification schemes, Vaccaro et al. developed the Thoracolumbar Injury Classification and Severity Score (TLICS) (TABLE) [54]. This scheme focuses on three parameters which influence spinal stability: (1) fracture morphology, (2) integrity of the PLC, and (3) neurologic status. Point values are

assigned based on these factors, and a total score is calculated that guides surgical decision-making. Regarding fracture morphology, three subtypes exist, increasing in severity: compression, rotation/translation, and distraction. *Compression* injuries are defined by a loss of height of the vertebral body or disruption through the vertebral end plate. The burst subtype is a compression variant which violates the middle column as well. *Rotation/translation* injury is identified by horizontal displacement of one vertebral body with respect to another. Other findings may include unilateral and bilateral dislocations, facet fracture–dislocations, and bilateral pedicle or pars fractures. *Distraction* is defined by vertical displacement, such as a hyperextension injury that causes disruption of the anterior longitudinal ligament, with subsequent widening of the anterior disk space. Fractures of the posterior elements (i.e., facet, lamina, spinous process) may exist.

As noted previously with cervical spine injuries, the patient's neurologic status is critical for surgical decision-making and often indicated the degree of spinal column injury. Neurologic status is described in increasing order of urgency: neurologically intact, nerve root injury, complete spinal cord or cauda equina injury, and incomplete spinal cord or cauda equina injury. Incomplete injuries are most urgent as they stand to potentially gain the most from surgical intervention.

The TLICS incorporates the integrity of the posterior ligamentous complex, including the supraspinous and interspinous ligaments, the ligamentous flavum, and the facet joint capsules, in determination of spinal stability. The PLC limits excessive flexion, rotation, translation, and distraction protecting the cord from damage. Once disrupted, the ligamentous structures demonstrate poor healing ability and generally require surgical stabilization. The PLC is graded as intact, indeterminate, or disrupted, determined radiographically. *Disruption* may be indicated by widening of the interspinous space or of the facet joints, empty facet joints, facet perch or subluxation, and dislocation of the spine. If frank disruption is more questionable, for example, with only edema on MRI, the integrity of the PLC may be defined as *indeterminate*.

Based on these factors, an aggregate score is calculated, and when > 4, surgical intervention is warranted, while < 4 suggests nonsurgical treatment. A patient with a score of 4 may be treated either surgically or nonsurgically. In the setting of multiple fractures, management is determined based on the injury with the greatest TLICS severity score.

Outcomes

As is the case with cervical spine fractures, outcome data and prospective studies comparing operative versus nonoperative management of thoracolumbar fractures are limited. Dai et al. reviewed 147 thoracolumbar fractures in polytrauma patients and found that the nonsurgical group, managed with immobilization, had increased rates of pneumonia and required longer hospital stays ($p < 0.05$) than the those managed operatively [55]. Siebenga et al. performed a multicenter, randomized prospective evaluation comparing short-segment posterior stabilization for stable burst fractures with immobilization in a Jewett brace and found that the operative cohort had improved kyphosis, better functional scores, and faster return to work ($p < 0.05$) [56]. However, Shen et al. found that while surgery allowed for greater initial correction of kyphosis and earlier pain relief than immobilization, at 2-year follow-up, there were no significant differences between the two groups [57].

Wood et al. performed a randomized, prospective study comparing surgical and conservative treatments for stable burst fractures without any neurologic deficits and at an average of 18 years follow-up could not identify meaningful improvements for the operative versus nonoperative group [58]. Those managed with orthoses reported less disability, greater pain relief, and fewer complications ($P < 0.001$).

Postoperative Care

There is currently little evidence to suggest that postoperative bracing regimens give rise to superior fusion rates or improved outcomes, especially if the fracture has been stabilized with internal fixation. Nevertheless, many immobilize these patients with a corset or thoracolumbosacral orthosis (TLSO) for up to 3 months depending upon the nature of the injury and healing response of the patient. Patients are encouraged to ambulate as soon as possible to reduce the risk of complications that commonly occur with prolonged recumbency. Standing radiographs should also be reviewed at regular intervals to evaluate for any radiographic signs indicative of pseudarthrosis such as worsening kyphosis or collapse of the fractured vertebra.

Conclusion

Patients sustaining spine trauma have suffered a potentially life-changing injury. Accurate and swift diagnosis is essential for dictating operative or nonoperative management, but a high index of suspicion and immediate triage in the form of immobilization and transportation to an equipped facility is paramount in the effort at achieving spinal stability. Injury prevention offers the best option for interventions aimed at decreasing the medical and social burden of these injuries. Strategies must aim to prevent or minimize functional loss by changing modifiable risk factors, altering the mechanics of the injury event, interrupting dangerous biological responses, and optimizing the initial and ultimate care through surgical or nonsurgical care.

References

1. Burney RE, Maio RF, Maynard F, et al. Incidence, characteristics, and outcome of spinal cord injury at trauma centers in North America. Arch Surg. 1993;128:596–9.
2. Hu R, Mustard CA, Burns C. Epidemiology of incident spinal fracture in a complete population. Spine. 1996;21:492–9.
3. Kwon BK, Vaccaro AR, Grauer JN, et al. Subaxial cervical spine trauma. J Am Acad Orthop Surg. 2006;14:78–89.
4. Harris MB, Reichmann WM, Bono CM, et al. Mortality in elderly patients after cervical spine fractures. J Bone Joint Surg Am. 2010;92:567–74.
5. Harris MB, Sethi RK. The initial assessment and management of the multiple-trauma patient with an

associated spine injury. Spine. 2006;31 suppl 11:S9–15.

6. Bono CM, Heary RF. Gunshot wounds to the spine. Spine J. 2004;4:230–40.

7. Farmer J, Vaccaro A, Balderston R, et al. The changing nature of admission to a spinal cord injury center: violence on the rise. J Spinal Disord. 1998;11:400–3.

8. Melton LJ. Epidemiology of spinal osteoporosis. Spine. 1997;22(24 suppl):2S–11.

9. Grazier H, Praemer A. Musculoskeletal conditions in the United States. Rosemont: American Academy of Orthopaedic Surgeons; 1999.

10. Wang H, Zhang Y, Xiang Q, et al. Epidemiology of traumatic spinal fractures: experience from medical university-affiliated hospitals in Chongqing, china, 2001–2010. J Neurosurg Spine. 2012;17:459–68.

11. Gertzbein SD. Scoliosis research society. Multicenter spine fracture study. Spine. 1992;17:528–40.

12. Hasler RM, Exadaktylos AK, Bouamra O, et al. Epidemiology and predictors of spinal injury in adult major trauma patients: European cohort study. Eur Spine J. 2011;20:2174–80.

13. Tator CH, Duncan EG, Edmonds VE, et al. Neurological recovery, mortality and length of stay after acute spinal cord injury associated with changes in management. Paraplegia. 1995;33:254–62.

14. Anon. Facts & Figures Sheet 5/01. Arch Phys Med Rehabil. 2008.

15. Ward WG, Nunley JA. Occult orthopaedic trauma in the multiply injured patient. J Orthop Trauma. 1991;5:308–12.

16. White AA, Panjabi MM. Clinical biomechanics of the spine. 2nd ed. Philadelphia: JB Lippincott Co; 1990.

17. Podolsky S, Baraff LJ, Simon RR, et al. Efficacy of cervical spine immobilization methods. J Trauma. 1983;23:461–5.

18. Ching RP, Watson NA, Carter JW, et al. The effect of post-injury spinal position on canal occlusion in a cervical spine burst fracture model. Spine. 1997;22:1710–5.

19. McGuire RA, Neville S, Green BA, et al. Spinal instability and the log-rolling maneuver. J Trauma. 1987;27:525–31.

20. American College of Surgeons Committee on Trauma. Advanced trauma life support for doctors-student course manual. Chicago: American College of Surgeons; 2008.

21. Levi L, Wolf A, Belzberg H. Hemodynamic parameters in patients with acute cervical cord trauma: description, intervention, and prediction of outcome. Neurosurgery. 1993;33:1007–16.

22. Vale FL, Burns J, Jackson AB, et al. Combined medical and surgical treatment after acute spinal cord injury: results of a prospective pilot study to assess the merits of aggressive medical resuscitation and blood pressure management. J Neurosurg. 1997;87:239–46.

23. Vaccaro AR, An HS, Lin S, et al. Noncontiguous injuries of the spine. J Spinal Disord. 1992;5:320–9.

24. Soderstrom CA, McArdle DQ, Ducker TB, et al. The diagnosis of intra-abdominal injury in patients with cervical cord trauma. J Trauma. 1983;23:1061–5.

25. Stauffer ES. Neurologic recovery following injuries to the cervical spinal cord and nerve roots. Spine. 1984;9:532–4.

26. Crozier KS, Graziani V, Ditunno JF, et al. Spinal cord injury: prognosis for ambulation based on sensory examination in patients who are initially motor complete. Arch Phys Med Rehabil. 1991;72:119–21.

27. Oleson CV, Burns AS, Ditunno JF, et al. Prognostic value of pinprick preservation in motor complete, sensory incomplete spinal cord injury. Arch Phy Med Rehabil. 2005;86:988–92.

28. Kakulas BA. Pathology of spinal injuries. Cent Nerv Syst Trauma. 1984;1:117–29.

29. Bracken MB, Collins WF, Freeman DF, et al. Efficacy of methylprednisolone in acute spinal cord injury. JAMA. 1984;251:45–52.

30. Bracken MB, Shepard MJ, Collins WF, et al. A randomized, controlled trial of methylprednisolone or naloxone in the treatment of acute spinal-cord injury. Results of the second national acute spinal cord injury study. N Engl J Med. 1990;322:1405–11.

31. Bracken MB, Shepard MJ, Holford TR, et al. Administration of methylprednisolone for 24 or 48 hours or tirilazad mesylate for 48 hours in the treatment of acute spinal cord injury. Results of the third national acute spinal cord injury randomized controlled trial. National acute spinal cord injury. JAMA. 1997;277:1597–604.

32. Mehta JS, Reed MR, McVie JL, et al. Weight-bearing radiographs in thoracolumbar fractures: Do they influence management? Spine. 2004;29:564–7.

33. Ballock RT, Mackersie R, Abitbol JJ, et al. Can burst fractures be predicted from plain radiographs? J Bone Joint Surg Br. 1992;74:147–50.

34. Keene JS, Fischer SP, Vanderby Jr R, et al. Significance of acute posttraumatic bony encroachment of the neural canal. Spine. 1989;14:799–802.

35. Hauser CJ, Visvikis G, Hinrichs C, et al. Prospective validation of computed tomographic screening of the thoracolumbar spine in trauma. J Trauma. 2003;55:228–34.

36. Lee JY, Vaccaro AR, Schweitzer Jr KM, et al. Assessment of injury to the thoracolumbar posterior ligamentous complex in the setting of normal-appearing plain radiography. Spine J. 2007;7:422–7.

37. Hoffman JR, Mower WR, Wolfson AB, et al. Validity of a set of clinical criteria to rule out injury to the cervical spine in patients with blunt trauma. National emergency X-radiography utilization study group. N Engl J Med. 2000;343:94–9.

38. Stiell IG, Wells GA, Vandemheen KL, et al. The Canadian C-spine rule for radiography in alert and stable trauma patients. JAMA. 2001;286:1841–8.

39. Stiell IG, Clement CM, McKnight RD, et al. The Canadian C-spine rule versus the NEXUS low-risk

criteria in patients with trauma. N Engl J Med. 2003;349:2510–8.

40. Blackmore CC, Emerson SS, Mann FA, et al. Cervical spine imaging in patients with trauma: determination of fracture risk to optimize use. Radiology. 1999;211:759–65.

41. Lowery DW, Wald MM, Browne BJ, Tigges S, Hoffman JR, Mower WR. Epidemiology of cervical spine injury victims. Ann Emerg Med. 2001;38:12–6.

42. Goldberg W, Mueller C, Panacek E, Tigges S, Hoffman JR, Mower WR. Distribution and patterns of blunt traumatic cervical spine injury. Ann Emerg Med. 2001;38:17–21.

43. Allen Jr BL, Ferguson RL, Lehmann T. A mechanistic classification of closed, indirect fractures and dislocations of the lower cervical spine. Spine. 1982;7:1–27.

44. Harris JH, Edeiken-Monroe B, Kopansiky DR. A practical classification of acute cervical spine injuries. Orthop Clin North Am. 1986;17:15–30.

45. Patel AA, Dailey A, Brodke DS, et al. Subaxial cervical spine trauma classification: the subaxial injury classification system and case examples. Neurosurg Focus. 2008;25:E8, 1–6.

46. Lee AS, Wainwright AM, Newton DA. Rogers' posterior cervical fusion: a 3-month radiological review. Injury. 1996;27:169–73.

47. Roy-Camille R, Saillant G, Laville C, et al. Treatment of lower cervical spinal injuries: C3 to C7. Spine. 1992;17:S442–6.

48. Kwon BK, Fisher CG, Boyd MC, et al. A prospective randomized controlled trial of anterior compared with posterior stabilization for unilateral facet injuries of the cervical spine. J Neurosurg Spine. 2007;7:1–12.

49. Jansson KA, Blomqvist P, Svedmark P, et al. Thoracolumbar vertebral fractures in Sweden: an analysis of 13,496 patients admitted to hospital. Eur J Epidemiol. 2010;25:431–7.

50. Cooper C, Atkinson EJ, O'Fallon WM, et al. Incidence of clinically diagnosed vertebral fractures: a population-based study in Rochester, Minnesota, 1985–1989. J Bone Miner Res. 1992;7:221–7.

51. Denis F. The three column spine and its significance in the classification of acute thoracolumbar spinal injuries. Spine. 1983;8:817–31.

52. Nicoll EA. Fractures of the dorso-lumbar spine. J Bone Joint Surg Br. 1949;31B:376–94.

53. Blauth M, Bastian L, Knop C, et al. Inter-observer reliability in the classification of thoraco-lumbar spinal injuries. Orthopade. 1999;28:662–81.

54. Vaccaro AR, Lehman Jr RA, Hurlbert RJ, et al. A new classification of thoracolumbar injuries: the importance of injury morphology, the integrity of the posterior ligamentous complex, and neurologic status. Spine. 2005;30:2325–33.

55. Dai LY, Yao WF, Cui YM, et al. Thoracolumbar fractures in patients with multiple injuries: diagnosis and treatment-a review of 147 cases. J Trauma. 2004;56:348–55.

56. Siebenga J, Leferink VJ, Segers MJ, et al. Treatment of traumatic thoracolumbar spine fractures: a multicenter prospective randomized study of operative versus nonsurgical treatment. Spine. 2006;31:2881–90.

57. Shen WJ, Liu TJ, Shen YS. Nonoperative treatment versus posterior fixation for thoracolumbar junction burst fractures without neurologic deficit. Spine. 2001;26:1038–45.

58. Wood KB, Buttermann GR, Phukan R, Harrod CC, Mehbod A, Shannon B, Bono CM, Harris MB. Operative compared with nonoperative treatment of a thoracolumbar burst fracture without neurological deficit: a prospective randomized study with follow-up at sixteen to twenty-two years. J Bone Joint Surg Am. 2015;97:3–9.

Matthew Kaufman, Thomas Bauer, Mary Massery, and John Cece

Introduction

The integration of advanced surgical methods aimed at restoring form and function in the human body into the paradigm of rehabilitation medicine has, until recently, lagged in the area of neuromuscular respiratory disorders. For several decades, reconstructive surgeons have been reporting on various procedures to improve function to a paralyzed arm or leg, including reconstructive nerve surgery, muscle or tendon transfers, and joint fusions. A natural synergy has occurred over time, where clinicians caring for patients with paralysis and spinal cord injury have an understanding of the surgical options and communicate with their surgical colleagues regarding proper patient selection for operative intervention.

M. Kaufman, MD, FACS (✉) • J. Cece, BAS
The Plastic Surgery Center, Institute for Advanced Reconstruction, 535 Sycamore Ave, Shrewsbury, NJ 07702, USA
e-mail: matthewrkmd@gmail.com; mkaufmanmd@theplasticsurgerycenternj.com; john.cece@gmail.com

T. Bauer, MD
Jersey Shore University Medical Center, 1945 NJ 33, Neptune, NJ 07753, USA
e-mail: TBauer@meridianhealth.com

M. Massery, PT, DPT, DSc (✉)
Massery Physical Therapy, 3820 Timbers Edge Lane, Glenview, IL 60025, USA
e-mail: mmassery@aol.com

However, neuromuscular dysfunction within the respiratory system has generally been the sole responsibility of the clinician, other than referral for tracheostomy or, more recently, diaphragm pacemakers. This lack of communication limits successful reversal of the disorder when noninvasive methods fail. It is the fault of neither the clinician nor surgeon in developing, recognizing, or promoting similar surgical options for patients with neuromuscular respiratory disorders. Rather, it has been a lack of focus or basic training of any surgical specialty to pursue functional restoration of the neuromuscular pathways in the respiratory system and a misconception that most central and/or peripheral nerve lesions within this system cannot be overcome.

An anatomical basis for pursuing surgical techniques to reverse respiratory paralysis exists just as it does for any other peripheral motor system in the human body. For direct insults to the primary peripheral respiratory nerve, i.e., the phrenic nerve, microsurgical methods of nerve reconstruction can be applied to restore or supplement axonal continuity and overcome diaphragmatic paralysis.

Successful surgical intervention to restore neuromuscular recovery following injury can occur provided the following basic principles apply. First, there must be inherent maintenance of the ability for peripheral nerve regeneration within the individual's nervous system. The capacity for nerve regeneration is maintained in peripheral nerves, even in patients with spinal cord injury. Second, surgical methods must be meticulous and precise. Surgical precision provides the scaffold upon which the regenerative process can occur. Finally, there must be adequate rehabilitation of the muscle once reinnervation has been confirmed. Restoration of normal or near-normal nerve conduction to a muscle, especially a rather large muscle like the diaphragm, will only result in muscle recovery and regrowth if intensive rehabilitation is instituted.

Insults to the central nervous system, including spinal cord injury, stroke, or tumor, may result in ventilator dependency when the neural pathways are interrupted between the brainstem respiratory centers and the peripheral circuitry. Diaphragm pacemakers, a topic discussed in detail in the following chapter 11, may offer a tremendous therapeutic benefit to reduce or eliminate the need for mechanical ventilation and minimize the associated morbidity and mortality associated with long-term ventilatory support. Unfortunately, there are a subset of patients for whom pacemakers will provide little or no benefit.

A requirement for successful application of a diaphragm pacemaker is phrenic nerve integrity. When individuals have insults to their central nervous system in locations that also results in loss of the anterior horn cells, there is resultant peripheral Wallerian degeneration in the phrenic nerves. It has been estimated that 18 % of all spinal cord injured patients have generalized peripheral axonal neuropathy, with tetraplegics having an even higher incidence [1]. These patients are often told to expect a life-long dependency on the ventilator. Recently, we have been able to demonstrate the restoration of phrenic nerve integrity using reconstructive nerve surgery, permitting successful use of a diaphragm pacemaker, a report that supplements an earlier, primary description of these methods [2, 3]. For these unfortunate patients, there may be an option to overcome the debilitating and life-shortening impact of chronic ventilator dependency.

In our quest to have a range of reconstructive surgical options to remedy the neuromuscular dysfunction regardless of severity, we are developing methods for diaphragm muscle replacement. Just as facial or upper extremity muscles can be

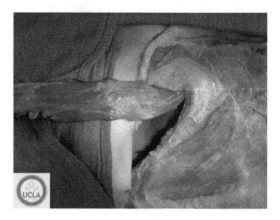

Fig. 10.1 Exposure of diaphragm through transthoracic approach and mobilization of pedicled rectus abdominis muscle flap in a cadaver (Courtesy and with gratitude to donors of UCLA Donated Body Program)

"replaced" by transferring vascularized, innervated muscle from somewhere else in the body, and expect it to function in a similar manner to that which it is replacing, the same may be true for the diaphragm. When these capabilities are realized through ongoing clinical evaluation, the surgical options would be comprehensive in nature in terms of replacing most major components of the neuromuscular pathways within the respiratory system. Specifically, the absence of a derived impulse due to the CNS (central nervous system) disorder could be overcome by the transmitted impulse from the diaphragm pacemaker, a nerve transfer to restore axonal circuitry to the degenerated phrenic nerve, and a muscle that has not undergone denervation atrophy (in a high cervical tetraplegic), such as the rectus abdominis, may be transferred to replace or enhance what may be an irreversibly atrophic diaphragm (Fig. 10.1).

Neuromuscular Anatomy and Physiology of the Respiratory System

Central Pathways

The anatomy and physiology of the respiratory system is somewhat unique. There is a baseline level of involuntary activity necessary to sustain breathing during sleep as well as a conscious "override" that may be invoked. Brainstem nuclei transmit impulses through the anterior horn cells to initiate an inspiratory effort. Alternatively, respiratory centers in the cerebral cortex may stimulate a respiratory event through a conscious effort. There are established connections between both sides of the brainstem, including a described "cross phrenic phenomenon," whereby a cord hemisection disrupting ipsilateral respiratory activity will be restored through a rerouting of impulses from the contralateral, uninjured side [4–6].

The Muscles of Respiration

After descending to the upper cervical region (C3-5), the conduction proceeds extradural through the cervical roots and phrenic nerves, downward toward each hemidiaphragm (Fig. 10.2). The

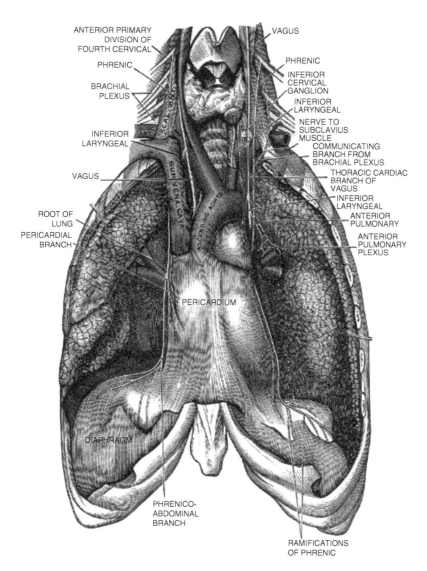

Fig. 10.2 Neuromuscular pathway of the respiratory system, including the phrenic nerves arising from the third through fifth cervical roots; the descent of the phrenic nerves through the cervical region, mediastinum, and chest cavities; and the intramuscular branching pattern of the phrenic nerve within the diaphragm to innervate all muscular segments

diaphragm is the primary inspiratory muscle, working in conjunction with several accessory respiratory muscles to expand the thoracic cavity in a vertical dimension, while intercostal muscles are primarily responsible for horizontal expansion of the ribcage. The entire process is a coordinated ensemble of contraction in the trunk musculature, including the trapezius, sternocleidomastoid, pectoralis major/minor, small strap muscles of the neck (hyoid musculature), intercostals, and abdominal muscles. The lung expands passively as a result of the facilitated increased thoracic domain, and an exchange of inspired gases occurs. The diaphragm maintains a critical role in this process through its action of increasing thoracic volume and opposing abdominal forces acting against it. The expiratory phase of breathing involves a different subset of muscles aimed at reversing the dimensions of the thoracic cavity back to its resting state.

The Phrenic Nerve

The phrenic nerve is a peripheral nerve arising from C3-5 and contains primarily motor fibers, although there are a small group of sensory fibers innervating primarily the pericardium. The course of the nerve is deep in the neck, subjacent to the prevertebral fascia, and just above the anterior scalene muscle (Fig. 10.3). A majority of

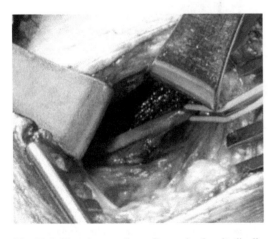

Fig. 10.3 Phrenic nerve (looped) coursing longitudinally along anterior scalene muscle (overlying prevertebral fascia has been cleared)

humans also have a smaller branch, called the accessory phrenic nerve, which runs a parallel but often variable course in the neck, typically joining the more dominant phrenic nerve proper at the base of the neck or in the mediastinum [7]. After entering the mediastinum, the phrenic nerve increases in caliber and travels between the lung and midline structures. In the region of the heart, the phrenic nerves on both sides are located close to or within the pericardial fat and descend within these tissues to reach their terminal insertions in the medial portions of each diaphragm. The nerves branch rather extensively within each hemidiaphragm in order to innervate all portions of these broad and wide muscles.

The Diaphragm

The primary respiratory muscle is skeletal in nature and is divided into two hemidiaphragms by its midline central tendon. The lateral attachments to each chest wall and its position in the center of the trunk account for its importance in body posture and stability. An excellent reference for the diaphragm's role as a postural stabilizer [8]. The structural makeup of the diaphragm consists of approximately 50 % slow-twitch (type I) and fast-twitch (type II) muscle fibers according to postmortem human research [9, 10]. The resting thickness of the diaphragm muscle when measured at its so-called zone of apposition is estimated to be roughly 1.5 mm, expanding by 2 mm with functional activation [11].

Diaphragmatic Paralysis

Incidence and Etiology

The true incidence of diaphragmatic paralysis is currently unknown, in part because of the variety of etiologies. The most common peripheral etiologies are iatrogenic or traumatic events impacting the neck, mediastinum, or chest (Table 10.1). Cardiac surgery procedures such as coronary artery bypass or valve replacement have been associated with phrenic nerve injury or abnormal diaphragm findings in anywhere from 1 to 80 % of cases [12–14].

Table 10.1 Suspected etiology of diaphragmatic paralysis in published series

Suspected etiology	No. (%)
Nerve block (interscalene/epidural)	18 (27)
Neck/spine trauma	16 (24)
Cardiac operation	11 (16)
Neck operation (thyroid, lymphadenectomy)	5 (7)
Chiropractic	5 (7)
Thymectomy	3 (4)
Radiofrequency ablation (cardiac)	3 (4)
Thoracic outlet operation	3 (4)
Carotid-subclavian bypass	2 (3)
Pulmonary lobectomy	2 (3)
Total	68 (100)

Reprinted with permission, Kaufman et al., *Annals of Thoracic Surgery*

Interscalene nerve blocks performed for shoulder surgery previously resulted in a 100 % incidence of temporary diaphragmatic paralysis as a result of anesthetic effect on the phrenic nerve. However, altered dosing regimens and use of ultrasound guidance have reduced the risk [15, 16]. Permanent diaphragmatic paralysis after interscalene block has been reported, though the incidence has not been determined [17, 18]. Chiropractic neck manipulation also has been associated with phrenic nerve injury in the neck, likely a result of either a traction-type nerve injury from the sudden jolting or perhaps a post-inflammatory effect on the nerve, especially if recurrent treatments prevent complete internal healing to occur [19, 20]. Other surgical procedures in the neck that have been reported to have an association with diaphragmatic paralysis include: carotid-subclavian bypass, thoracic outlet surgery, and cervical lymphadenopathy [21].

Mediastinal procedures such as thymectomy, especially for malignancy, have an association with phrenic nerve injury with a reported rate of 1–2 % [22, 23]. Aortic or mitral valve repairs/replacements may lead to phrenic nerve injury in the upper thoracic cavity. It is not yet known whether recently developed, minimally invasive methods of valve surgery will alter incidences of nerve injury. Phrenic nerve injury resulting from cardiac bypass surgery is most often due to either hypothermic damage from the use of heart cooling or direct injury during isolation and transfer of the internal mammary artery pedicle. Procedures performed to alleviate atrial fibrillation, such as the MAZE procedure and cardiac ablation, have both been reported to result in diaphragm paralysis. Patients with this etiology of phrenic nerve dysfunction have been evaluated, and their conditions are successfully reversed by the senior author (M.R.K) using techniques discussed below [3, 24].

Carcinoma of the lung requiring partial or complete resection may require intentional sacrifice of the phrenic nerve or, alternatively, result in diaphragmatic paralysis as an unintended consequence [25]. Patients undergoing lung transplantation may also suffer the effects of phrenic nerve injury due to the extensive restructuring of the thoracic cavity [26]. Trauma to the neck and chest may also lead to isolated phrenic nerve injuries or in combination with other neural structures, such as the brachial plexus or cranial nerves. A severe traction injury, when the shoulder is jolted forcefully in an opposite direction from the neck, puts substantial tension on the nerves coursing through the lower lateral cervical region [27]. Furthermore, there is often a resulting inflammatory process creating edema within the soft tissues of the neck. If this process does not resolve rather rapidly, the result is post-inflammatory fibrosis and adhesions.

Similar to other compression neuropathies in the upper and lower extremities, the phrenic nerve may easily be entrapped within the confines of its intra-fascial pathway, leading to conduction disturbances. A chronic, severe compression of any peripheral nerve may lead to segmental anoxia and axonal loss, a process that cannot be reversed spontaneously despite our inherent ability for nerve regeneration [28].

There may be certain patients who may be more susceptible to iatrogenic and traumatic phrenic nerve injury. The *double-crush* phenomenon, originally described by Upton and McKomas in 1973, describes the susceptibility of a second site of nerve injury along a neural pathway when one already exists [29]. For example, patients with cervical spine radiculopathy are more susceptible to carpal tunnel syndrome [30]. Similarly, patients with unilateral or bilateral phrenic nerve injuries resulting from trauma or surgery commonly present with degenerative cervical disease impacting the third through fifth cervical roots. We have also evaluated and treated numerous patients for diaphragmatic paralysis who have known, or subclinical cervical disease, but do not provide a clear traumatic or iatrogenic etiology. While the C-spine MRI often demonstrates foraminal narrowing or mild spinal stenosis in these patients, the only presenting clinical symptom is chronic dyspnea with exertion from a paralyzed diaphragm.

Idiopathic paralysis and viral neuritis (i.e., Parsonage-Turner syndrome) are other etiologies for diaphragmatic paralysis reported in the literature [31, 32]. Parsonage-Turner syndrome was originally described in 1948 as a condition that only affected the brachial plexus but is now used interchangeably, in addition to neuralgic amyotrophy, to describe isolated or combined insults to the brachial plexus and phrenic nerve(s) as a result of an inflammatory neuropathy. Although viral neuritis has very specific presenting sign and symptoms (e.g., fever, malaise, arm weakness, nausea/vomiting) that may be correctly diagnosed when exhibited in close temporal relation to the onset of dyspnea, idiopathic paralysis is truly a diagnosis of exclusion.

Central nervous system disorders may also cause diaphragmatic paralysis, often with bilateral muscle dysfunction, resulting in the need for oxygen supplementation or dependency on mechanical ventilation. Rates of ventilator dependence in high cervical spinal cord injury can reach as high as 71 % [33]. It is estimated that 20 % of these injuries will also result in Wallerian degeneration within the phrenic nerves as a result of the loss of anterior horn cells.

Amyotrophic lateral sclerosis (ALS) and other bulbospinal neuropathies lead to demyelination and axonal loss within the phrenic nerves. Diaphragmatic paralysis in ALS almost universally results in complete ventilator dependency in later stages of the disease and, ultimately, is one of the leading causes of mortality [34]. Other CNS conditions that are associated with diaphragmatic paralysis include: central hypoventilation syndrome, brainstem tumor, stroke, and cervical cord compression [35, 36].

Signs and Symptoms

Unilateral diaphragmatic paralysis will rarely result in a need for mechanical ventilation. However, in this clinical scenario, there is often a co-diagnosis of sleep-disordered breathing for which nocturnal positive pressure oxygen may be necessary [37]. Individuals with this disorder typically report dyspnea with exertion, orthopnea, and easy fatigability [38]. Quality of life assessments reveal disturbances on measures of physical functioning and indicate that traditional perceptions suggesting *one can live unaffected by a paralyzed diaphragm* have underestimated the significance of the problem [3]. Other presenting symptoms of unilateral paralysis include: gastroesophageal reflux for left-sided diaphragmatic paralysis, chest wall discomfort, abdominal bloating, chronic cough, breathlessness, depression, and postural asymmetries/pain.

On examination, the most obvious finding is diminished breath sounds at the base on the involved side when auscultating the lung fields. Occasionally, there will be a Tinel's sign in the supraclavicular region of the neck, supporting the diagnosis of a phrenic neuropathy in the cervical region. Unless the diagnosis is due to a major insult to the cervical roots and/or brachial plexus, examination of the upper extremities will be unremarkable. Alternatively, traumatic injury to the brachial plexus has a reported association with diaphragmatic paralysis due to phrenic nerve injury in 10–20 % of cases [39].

Evaluation

Diaphragmatic paralysis is most reliably diagnosed on a *sniff test* – chest fluoroscopy performed with a deep nasal inspiratory effort – and is revealed by either absence of movement or paradoxical (upward) movement, indicating a flail, atonic diaphragm muscle. Paretic muscle dysfunction, or partial paralysis, may also be diagnosed by observing reduced descent of the muscle upon inspiration, when compared to the contralateral, normally functioning side. For most patients, performing the diagnostic study in supine and upright positions can reveal differences that may assist in qualifying the severity of the dysfunction. The sniff maneuver may also be performed while observing with ultrasonography, thus permitting more accurate measurements of diaphragm thickness.

Spirometry evaluation in patients with diaphragmatic paralysis will typically reveal a restrictive ventilatory deficit, though well-conditioned individuals with unilateral paralysis may often have the percent predicted values within a normal range for their age. Alternatively, there are other patients with diaphragmatic paralysis who develop secondary pulmonary disorders, such as asthma or sleep-disordered breathing, and demonstrate mixed restrictive-obstructive deficits on spirometry testing. When bilateral diaphragmatic dysfunction is present, for example, in patients with cervical stenosis, the results of spirometry testing will usually indicate much more severe restrictive ventilatory deficiencies.

Radiographic imaging using CT or MRI modalities is almost always appropriate to rule out organic pathology, such as degenerative cervical disease or tumor, and should be recommended based on the particulars of patient history. For example, individuals with a history of neck or back pain, especially with concomitant upper extremity weakness or paresthesias, require cervical MRI to look for cord compression. Alternatively, patients with diaphragmatic paralysis, whose history is significant for benign or malignant tumors of the thyroid, thymus, breast, or lung, require imaging to eliminate tumor pathology causing neural injury.

Electrodiagnostic evaluation is important for quantifying the extent of phrenic nerve injury and severity of muscle atrophy and is discussed more thoroughly in its own chapter. The phrenic nerve conduction study is often performed in conjunction with an upper extremity evaluation to assess conduction velocity and latency. Normative values have been described. In cases of unilateral paralysis, the normally functioning side is often used as the baseline for comparison [40]. Diaphragm electromyography is included in a comprehensive evaluation to assess motor amplitude deficits and assists in stratifying those patients that may be candidates for phrenic nerve reconstruction. The technical difficulty of this assessment supersedes that of most other electrodiagnostic testing due to the muscle not being readily accessible transcutaneously and the inherent risk of pneumothorax.

Neuromuscular Pathology

The pathological processes responsible for diaphragmatic paralysis typically involve one or more sites of insult to the neuromuscular pathway. This pathway originates in the brain and cervical spine, emerges through the cervical roots 3–5, extends down the phrenic nerve, and terminates beyond the neuromuscular junction in the diaphragm itself. Aside from the central nervous system disorders previously described, e.g., stroke, spinal cord injury, and ALS, direct injury to the cervical roots and/or phrenic nerve may occur in any number of ways.

Peripheral nerve injury can result from complete transection or alternatively can be the consequence of traction, (hypo-)thermal, compression, or pharmacological injury. Regardless of the manner in which the injury is sustained, in all non-transection processes, the end result is usually segmental nerve anoxia leading to demyelination and, ultimately, axonal loss. This description follows the nerve injury classification system of Seddon and Sunderland that has gained universal acceptance and forms the basis for current surgical treatment algorithms [41].

Treatment Options for Diaphragmatic Paralysis

Positive Airway Pressure Supplementation (CPAP/BiPAP)

Continuous positive airway pressure (CPAP) and bi-level positive airway pressure (BiPAP) are two treatment modalities for respiratory sleep disorders that effectively maintain airway patency and reduce or prevent apneic events. The reduction in inspiratory muscle force that occurs with diaphragmatic paralysis commonly leads to sleep abnormalities detectable on polysomnography. Positive airway pressure supplementation using either CPAP or BiPAP is a recommended treatment, although the ability to maintain higher pressures during inspiration and then provide a lower level during the expiratory phase would seem to favor BiPAP for an inspiratory muscle disorder. This may distinguish sleep disorders due to isolated diaphragmatic paralysis from obstructive sleep apnea patients with upper airway obstruction that could benefit from higher pressures during both phases of breathing. Khan et al. (2014) retrospectively reviewed 66 patients with unilateral or bilateral diaphragmatic paralysis, all of whom exhibited abnormal sleep studies consistent with sleep-disordered breathing [42]. Patients exhibited demonstrable improvements using positive airway pressure supplementation. Unsurprisingly, less than 40% tolerated CPAP with the rest requiring BiPAP.

Plication of the Diaphragm

This section will focus on mechanics, method, timing, and results of diaphragmatic plication. The surgical restructuring of the diaphragm attempts to expand the thoracic volume and eliminate paradoxical motion in order to improve ventilation mechanics and pulmonary function and decrease symptomatic dyspnea. Diaphragmatic plication is indicated when symptomatic dyspnea occurs secondary to permanent phrenic nerve paralysis, and other methods of reinnervation or pacing are not available. Contraindications are relative and depend on the severity of the comorbidity and the significance of the dyspnea.

The vital role of the diaphragm in respiration is obvious, though its contribution varies based on position and sleep. The diaphragm is responsible for 56% of the tidal volume in the awake, supine patient and up to 81% during periods of deep sleep [43]. The aim of plication is to minimize the loss of thoracic space and prevent paradoxical motion. Plication decreases atelectasis of the involved lung and improves ventilation perfusion mismatch [44, 45]. Wright et al. demonstrated this diaphragmatic correction results in a signifi-

cant increase in total lung capacity, vital capacity, expiratory reserve volume, functional residual capacity, and arterial PaO_2. Diaphragm plication has also been found to improve spirometry results when testing is performed in both sitting and supine positions [46].

The traditional approach is through standard posterolateral thoracotomy [46–49]. With the advent of modern, minimally invasive surgery, a video-assisted thoracic surgical (VATS) approach has slowly replaced open thoracotomies [49, 50]. Gazala and colleagues examined 126 studies on diaphragmatic paralysis, reviewing 13 representing the best evidence of repair, and compared VATS approach with thoracotomy. They found that a VATS approach achieves similar results based on pulmonary function tests (PFTs), dyspnea scores and functional assessment with shorter length of stay, lower complications rates, and mortality rate [51]. Several authors have supported a laparoscopic approach [52–54]. Both VATS and laparoscopic approaches are minimally invasive and offer unique benefits. There is no clear benefit of either, and the approach should be dictated by the surgeon's preference and experience [54]. The technique involves a suture line running parallel to the thoracotomy that is repeated until appropriate tension is created [46, 47]. Others have described a series of horizontal mattress sutures with or without pledgets in varying directions [44, 50, 52, 54].

The timing of the repair is based on the likely mechanism of injury. Cold ice slurry cardioplegia is probably the most thoroughly studied etiology of phrenic nerve injury. Several studies have demonstrated that cold injury to the phrenic occurs in 52–69% of patients, though it may resolve up to 2 years after the initial insult [14, 38, 48, 55, 56]. Although no conclusive studies exist on the perfect timing of repair in permanent injury, a 6-month waiting period typically allows for sufficient recovery from the time of injury in order to determine permanent damage. Plication should be reserved for those patients with documented diaphragmatic paralysis and a significant dyspnea score. Morbidly obese patients and those with long-standing paralysis seem to be less likely to benefit from this repair [49]. Although only one of four vent-dependent patients was weaned from the ventilator after plication, 17 of 19 patients who were unable to work secondary to dyspnea were able to return to work by 6 months following plication [44].

Phrenic Nerve Reconstruction

Background

Scattered case reports in the 1980s and 1990s have described typically the acute repair of the phrenic nerve following trauma or after tumor resection [57, 58]. Until recently, it was not widely accepted to pursue delayed nerve repair in patients with unilateral or bilateral diaphragmatic paralysis. While brachial plexus injuries have been treated for decades in an acute or delayed manner using well-established nerve reconstruction methods, there has not been the same focus for phrenic nerve injuries, leaving diaphragm plication as the only interventional therapy. In 2011, the primary author published the first small series on successful phrenic nerve reconstruction, demonstrating partial or complete diaphragmatic recovery in 89 % of the treatment group [24].

Surgical Treatment

The successful surgical treatment of phrenic nerve injuries occurs in a clinical scenario of a segmental nerve injury in the neck, mediastinum, and/or chest cavity. These injuries are amenable to a combination of nerve decompression and interposition grafting or neurotization. For example, patients with phrenic nerve injury occurring from interscalene nerve blocks performed during rotator cuff surgery are often found intraoperatively to have dense fibrous and vascular adhesions in the region of the C5 root contribution to the phrenic nerve and proximal phrenic nerve proper. Appropriate therapy consists of meticulous nerve decompression and interpositional grafting to "bypass" the site of lesion. Both techniques are believed crucial to maximizing success since it is not possible to confirm during

surgery whether decompression has sufficiently reversed the pathological process.

We have described pathological findings from various causative etiologies of phrenic nerve injury, including "Red Cross syndrome." In this syndrome, the phrenic nerve is subject to compression neuropathy from an adherent and torturous transverse cervical artery and/or vein, likely the result of a post-inflammatory process (Table 10.1) [59]. Similar to other peripheral nerve surgical procedures, a successful outcome is based upon various factors, most notably superb technical methods and intensive rehabilitation to strengthen the atrophic muscle once reinnervation has been confirmed. Accordingly, the recovery process can be prolonged, often requiring 2–3 years for optimal recovery.

Outcomes

Comparing results of phrenic nerve reconstruction to both historical cohorts from a meta-analysis of diaphragm plication outcomes, and a control group of nonsurgical observation, we have demonstrated at least a functional equivalency to plication at 1-year follow-up and results that are far superior to no treatment [3]. Furthermore, electrodiagnostic recovery, including both a 69 % improvement in conduction latency and a motor amplitude increase of 37 %, was significant in the phrenic nerve surgery group. This improvement did not occur with plication surgery or the nonsurgical group. Based upon the likelihood of slow, progressive improvement expected with aggressive rehabilitation protocols, we believe that successful outcomes of phrenic nerve surgery would likely supersede those of plication with longer follow-up.

Treatment Algorithm

In developing successful nerve reconstruction methods to restore function to a paralyzed diaphragm, it is now possible to create a comprehensive treatment algorithm for this condition that includes both phrenic nerve surgery and diaphragm plication for cases of unilateral

paralysis. An important concept in this algorithmic approach is that failure to reinnervate the
paralyzed diaphragm after phrenic nerve surgery
does not preclude a subsequent attempt at plication, whereas the failed plication would not be
favorable for nerve surgery due to the likelihood
of dense scarring in the muscle itself. Therefore, if
electrodiagnostic testing reveals intact voluntary
motor units, phrenic nerve surgery should be
offered as the first-line treatment. Alternatively, if
progressive deterioration in the muscle is evident
on electromyography or the patient is a poor candidate (i.e., elderly, diabetic neuropathy, immuno-
suppressed), the likelihood of reinnervation is
vastly reduced, and the patient is better served
with a plication procedure (Figs. 10.4 and 10.5).

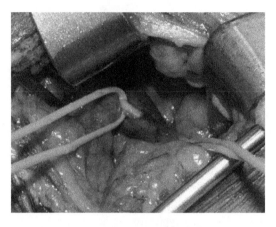

Fig. 10.4 Intraoperative example of "Red Cross syndrome," a vascular compression of the phrenic nerve
(looped proximal and distal to the crossing blood vessel)
caused by the transverse cervical artery

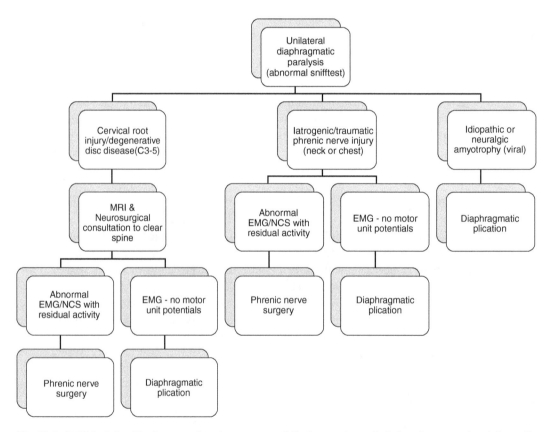

Fig. 10.5 Published algorithmic approach to the treatment of diaphragmatic paralysis based upon results of electrodiagnostic evaluation (Reprinted with permission, Kaufman et al. CHEST)

Ventilator Dependency

Demographics

Spinal cord injury in the cervical region leads to complete or incomplete tetraplegia, with a 38 % incidence of ventilator dependency at the time of hospital discharge [60]. Based on an estimated 12,500 new spinal cord injuries annually in the United States, roughly 60 % of which are partial or complete tetraplegia, there are approximately 1600 new cases per year of ventilator dependency associated with this debilitating condition. The premature morbidity and mortality associated with ventilator dependency in these patients have been clearly documented as well as the increased healthcare costs accrued despite a reduction in longevity.

Amyotrophic lateral sclerosis (ALS) is another neurological disorder leading almost universally to ventilator dependency. There are an estimated 5600 new cases of ALS annually in the United States or an incidence of 2 per 100,000 per year [61]. Similar to spinal cord injury statistics, the impact of ventilator dependency is profound, with respiratory causes of mortality as the primary source of early mortality in this disease. There are several other central nervous system disorders frequently leading to partial or complete ventilator dependency, including central hypoventilation syndrome, stroke, Pompeii's disease, and brainstem tumors.

Consequences of Positive Pressure Ventilation on the Diaphragm

A landmark study by Levine et al. (2008) clearly demonstrated rapid disuse atrophy occurring in the diaphragm muscles of patients requiring positive pressure ventilation [62]. After only 18 h of mechanical ventilation, there was a 57 % decrease in the more functional type I slow-twitch fibers compared to controls. Oxidative stress and proteolysis were seen even with limited periods of inactivity. Although it is unclear whether the early and rapid deterioration is reversible, the implications are likely profound

pertaining to the impact on the diaphragm in patients requiring anything more than a few days of mechanical ventilation.

In ventilator-dependent cervical tetraplegics, it is necessary to evaluate carefully the effectiveness of noninvasive weaning methods and consider the negative consequence of prolonging inevitable weaning failure. Although, in many cases, the implementation of well-established weaning methods leads to independent respiratory activity over a period of weeks to months following injury, it must be remembered that interventional treatment options, such as diaphragm pacemakers, require an intact phrenic nerve and at least some functional muscle to be effective. Long-term ventilator dependency undoubtedly leads to the transgression of a threshold beyond which there is profound irreversible diaphragmatic atrophy. Especially in patients who have cervical spinal cord injury and concomitant phrenic nerve degeneration, that timeframe is likely to be 18–24 months, after which time there may be complete loss of the motor end plates and a dramatic reduction in the success of any surgical intervention [63].

Treatment Options

Diaphragm pacemakers can be extremely effective at partially or completely reversing ventilator dependency in high cervical tetraplegia [64]. The history of diaphragm pacing and an explanation of the technique will be detailed in another chapter. However, it is critical to also focus on those patients that are deemed unsuitable for this therapeutic option. As mentioned previously, when there is loss of phrenic nerve integrity, diaphragm pacemakers will be ineffective. These unfortunate patients are often told there is no chance at ventilator weaning, and they must accept a life on mechanical ventilation with the associated morbidity and early mortality.

In 2000, Krieger and Krieger published the first report of simultaneous nerve transfers and pacemaker implantation to overcome ventilator dependency in patients with combined spinal cord injury and phrenic nerve degeneration [2].

The rationale for the dual approach was to first restore phrenic nerve integrity by transferring an intact nerve source that could subsequently permit pacemaker activation of the diaphragm. More recently, the primary author (M.R.K.) demonstrated a 93 % reinnervation rate in 14 patients undergoing nerve transfers and pacemaker implantation [65]. Partial or complete ventilator weaning was achieved in 62 %, and it was believed that due to an average interval of 34 months between injury and treatment, many patients had suffered significant and irreversible diaphragm atrophy preventing clinical success.

Increasingly, rehabilitation efforts for spinal cord injury patients have focused on functional electrical stimulation of peripheral nerves to prevent irreversible muscle atrophy [66]. Although this has been applied primarily for the upper and lower extremities, conceptually this could also prevent diaphragmatic atrophy in patients that may eventually be weaned or in more severe injuries when noninvasive methods are more likely to be unsuccessful, thus necessitating surgical intervention. The application of electrical stimulation in this latter setting would most certainly increase the likelihood of achieving independent respiratory activity with or without a pacemaker. Unfortunately, the technical difficulty of placing transcutaneous electrodes near the phrenic nerve or nerve-muscle interface makes noninvasive stimulation therapy more challenging than it is for the extremities.

In spinal cord injury patients who have suffered irreversible and severe diaphragmatic atrophy, it is possible to consider the most sophisticated reconstructive techniques for restoring the neuromuscular components of the respiratory system. In addition to the use of nerve reconstruction and implantation of a diaphragm pacemaker, an atrophic diaphragm may be "replaced" or "enhanced" by transferring an intact muscle with its own neurovascular connection. This application would not be unique to the respiratory system but is considered standard practice for the most severe injuries in the facial muscles and extremities [67]. Replacing or restoring diaphragm neuromuscular activity has also been reported in young children with congenital diaphragmatic hernia [68]. As of this writing, we have begun clinical application of this comprehensive procedure and have demonstrated immediate, intraoperative activity of the neo-diaphragm using an implanted pacemaker.

References

1. Nogajski J, Engel S, Kiernan M. Focal and generalized peripheral nerve dysfunction in spinal cord-injured patients. J Clin Neurophysiol. 2006;23:273–9.
2. Krieger LM, Krieger AJ. The intercostal to phrenic nerve transfer: an effective means of reanimating the diaphragm in patients with high cervical spine injury. Plast Reconstr Surg. 2000;105:1255–61.
3. Kaufman MR, Elkwood AI, et al. Functional restoration of diaphragmatic paralysis: an evaluation of phrenic nerve reconstruction. Ann Thorac Surg. 2014;97:260–6.
4. Fuller DD, Sandhu MS, Doperalski NJ, et al. Graded unilateral cervical spinal cord injury and respiratory motor recovery. Respir Physiol Neurobiol. 2009;165:245–53.
5. Golder FJ, Fuller DD, Davenport PW, et al. Respiratory motor recovery after unilateral spinal cord injury: eliminating crossed phrenic activity decreases tidal volume and increases contralateral respiratory motor output. J Neurosci. 2003;23:2492–501.
6. Vinit S, Gauthier P, Stamegna JC, Kastner A. High cervical lateral spinal cord injury results in long-term ipsilateral hemidiaphragm paralysis. J Neurotrauma. 2006;23:1137–46.
7. Loukas M, Kinsella Jr CR, Louis Jr RG, et al. Surgical anatomy of the accessory phrenic nerve. Ann Thorac Surg. 2006;82:1870–5.
8. Hodges PW, SC Gandevia. Activation of the human diaphragm during a repetitive postural task. J Physiol. 2000;522 Pt 1:165–175.
9. Mizuno M, Secher NH. Histochemical characteristics of human expiratory and inspiratory intercostal muscles. J Appl Physiol. 1985;67:592–8.
10. Mckenzie DK, Gandevia SC, Shorey CD. A histochemical study of human inspiratory muscles. Proc Int In Physiolol. 1983;40:351–4.
11. Bruin P, Ueki J, Bush A, et al. Diaphragm thickness and inspiratory strength in patients with Duchenne muscular dystrophy. Thorax. 1997;52:472–5.
12. Mehta Y, Vats M, Singh A, et al. Incidence and management of diaphragmatic palsy in patients after cardiac surgery. Indian J Crit Care Med. 2008;12:91–5.
13. Efthimiou J, Butler J, Woodham C, et al. Diaphragm paralysis following cardiac surgery: role of phrenic nerve cold injury. Ann Thorac Surg. 1991;52:1005–8.
14. Devita M, Robinson LR, Rehder J, et al. Incidence and natural history of phrenic neuropathy occurring during open heart surgery. Chest. 1993;103:850–6.

15. Mak P, Irwin M, Ooi C, et al. Incidence of diaphragmatic paralysis following supraclavicular brachial plexus block and its effect on pulmonary function. Anaesthesia. 2001;56:352–6.

16. Guirguis M, Karroum R, Abd-Elsayed AA, Mounir-Soliman L. Acute respiratory distress following ultrasound-guided supraclavicular block. Ochsner J. 2012;12:159–62.

17. Saint Raymond C, Borel JC, Wuyam B, et al. Persistent phrenic palsy following interscalene block, leading to chronic respiratory insufficiency and requiring long-term non-invasive ventilation. Respir Med. 2008;1:253–5.

18. Robaux S, Bouaziz H, Boisseau N. Persistent phrenic nerve paralysis following interscalene brachial plexus block. Anesthesiology. 2001;95:1519–21.

19. Tolge C, Iyer V, McConnell J. Phrenic nerve palsy accompanying chiropractic manipulation of the neck. South Med J. 1993;86:688–90.

20. Schram DJ, Vosik W, Cantral D. Diaphragmatic paralysis following cervical chiropractic manipulation: case report and review. Chest. 2001;119:638–40.

21. Coleman J. Complications in head and neck surgery. Surg Clin N Amer. 1986;66:149–67.

22. Bulkley GB, Bass KN, Sephenson GR, et al. Extended cervicomediastinal thymectomy in the integrated management of myasthenia gravis. Ann Surg. 1997;226:324–34.

23. Salati M, Cardillo G, Carbone L, et al. Iatrogenic phrenic nerve injury during thymectomy: the extent of the problem. J Thorac Cardiocasc Surg. 2010;139:e77–8.

24. Kaufman M, Elkwood A, Rose M, et al. Reinnervation of the paralyzed diaphragm: application of nerve surgery techniques following unilateral phrenic nerve injury. Chest. 2011;140:191–7.

25. Willaert W, Kessler R, Deneffe G. Surgical options for complete resectable lung cancer invading the phrenic nerve. Acta Chir Belj. 2004;104:451–3.

26. Sano Y, Oto T, Toyooka S, et al. Phrenic nerve paralysis following lung transplantation. Kyobu Geka. 2007;60:993–7.

27. Coene LN. Mechanisms of brachial plexus lesions. Clin Neurol Neurosurg. 1993;95(Suppl):S24–9.

28. Burnett M, Zager E. Pathophysiology of peripheral nerve injury: a brief review. Neurosurg Focus. 2004;16:E1.

29. Upton AR, McComas AJ. The double crush in nerve entrapment syndromes. Lancet. 1973;2:359–62.

30. Richardson JK, Forman GM, Riley B. An electrophysiological exploration of the double crush hypothesis. Muscle Nerve. 1999;22:71–7.

31. Valls-Sole J, Solans M. Idiopathic bilateral diaphragmatic paralysis. Muscle Nerve. 2002;25:619–23.

32. Marvisi M, Balzarini L, Mancini C, et al. A rare case of dyspnoea the parsonage-turner syndrome. J Med Cases. 2012;3:169–71.

33. Como J, Sutton E, McCunn M, et al. Characterizing the need for mechanical ventilation following cervical spinal cord injury with neurologic deficit. J Trauma. 2005;59:912–6.

34. Shoesmith C, Findlater K, Rowe A, et al. Prognosis of amyotrophic lateral sclerosis with respiratory onset. J Neurol Neurosurg Psychiatry. 2006;78:629–31.

35. Moris G, Arias M, Terrero J, et al. Ipsilateral reversible diaphragmatic paralysis after pons stroke. J Neurol. 2011;259:966–8.

36. Parke WW, Whalen JL. Phrenic paresis--a possible additional spinal cord dysfunction induced by neck manipulation in cervical spondylotic myelopathy (CSM): a report of two cases with anatomical and clinical considerations. Clin Anat. 2001;14:173–8.

37. Steier J, Jollet CJ, Seymour J, et al. Sleep-disordered breathing in unilateral diaphragm paralysis or severe weakness. Eur Respir J. 2008;32:1479–87.

38. Summerhill EM, El-Sameed YA, Glidden TJ, et al. Monitoring recovery from diaphragm paralysis with ultrasound. Chest. 2008;133:737–43.

39. Karaoğlu P, Yiş U, Öztura I, et al. Phrenic nerve palsy associated with brachial plexus avulsion in a pediatric patient with multitrauma. Pediatr Emerg Care. 2013;28:922–3.

40. Chen R, Collins S, Remtulla H, et al. Phrenic nerve conduction study in normal subjects. Muscle Nerve. 1995;18:330–5.

41. Sunderland S. Nerves and nerve injuries. 2nd ed. New York: Churchill Livingstone; 1978.

42. Khan A, Morgenthaler T, Ramar K. Sleep disordered breathing in isolated unilateral and bilateral diaphragmatic dysfunction. J Clin Sleep Med. 2014;10:509–15.

43. Tusiewicz K, Moldofsky H, Bryan AC, et al. Mechanics of the rib cage and diaphragm during sleep. J Appl Physiol Respirat Environ Exerc Physiol. 1977;43:600–2.

44. Freeman R, Wozniak T, Fitzgerald E. Functional and physiologic results of video-assisted thoracoscopic diaphragm plication in adult patients with unilateral diaphragm paralysis. Ann Thorac Surg. 2006;81:1853–7.

45. Tsakiridis K, Visouli A, Zarogoulidis P, et al. Early hemi-diaphragmatic plication through a video assisted minithoracotomy in post cardiotomy phrenic nerve paresis. J Thorac Dis. 2012;4:56 68.

46. Wright D, Williams J, Ogilvie C, et al. Results of diaphragmatic plication for unilateral diaphragmatic paralysis. J Thorac Cardiovasc Surg. 1985;90:195–8.

47. Graham D, Kaplan D, Hind CR, et al. Diaphragmatic plication for unilateral diaphragmatic paralysis: a 10-year experience. Ann Thorac Surg. 1990;49:248–52.

48. van Onna I, Metz R, Jekel L, et al. Post cardiac surgery phrenic nerve palsy: value of plication and potential for recovery. Euro J Card Thorac Surg. 1998;14:179–84.

49. Freeman R, Van Woerkom J, Vyverberg A, et al. Long term follow-up of the functional and physiologic results of diaphragm plication in adults with unilateral diaphragm paralysis. Ann Thorac Surg. 2009;88:1112–7.

50. Gharagozloo F, McReynolds SD, Snyder L. Thoracoscopic plication of the diaphragm. Surg Endosc. 1995;9:1204–6.

51. Gazalaa S, Hunt I, Bédard E. Diaphragmatic plication offers functional improvement in dyspnea and better pulmonary function with low morbidity. Interact Cardio Vasc Thorac Surg. 2012;15:505–8.

52. Huttl TP, Wichmann MW, Reichart B, et al. Laparoscopic diaphragmatic plication. Long-term results of a novel surgical technique for postoperative phrenic nerve palsy. Surg Endosc. 2004;18:547–51.

53. Hu J, Wu Y, Wang J, et al. Thoracoscopic and laparoscopic plication of the hemidiaphragm is effective in the management of diaphragmatic eventration. Pediatr Surg Int. 2014;30:19–24.

54. Groth SS, Rueth NM, Kast T, et al. Laparoscopic diaphragmatic plication for diaphragmatic paralysis and eventration: an objective evaluation of short-term and midterm results. J Thorac Cardiovasc Surg. 2010;139:1452–6.

55. Cohen A, Katz M, Katz R, et al. Phrenic nerve injury after coronary artery grafting- is it always benign? Ann Thorac Surg. 1997;64:148–53.

56. Gayan-Ramirez G, Gosselin N, Troosters T, et al. Functional recovery of diaphragm paralysis: a long term follow up study. Respir Med. 2008;102:690–8.

57. Brouillette RT, Hahn YS, Noah ZL, et al. Successful reinnervation of the diaphragm after phrenic nerve transection. J Pediatr Surg. 1986;21:63–5.

58. Schoeller T, Ohlbauer M, Wechselberger G, et al. Successful immediate phrenic nerve reconstruction during mediastinal tumor resection. J Thorac Cardiovasc Surg. 2001;122:1235–7.

59. Kaufman M, Willekes L, Elkwood A, et al. Diaphragm paralysis caused by transverse cervical artery compression of the phrenic nerve: the Red Cross syndrome. Clin Neurol Neurosurg. 2012;114:502–5.

60. Kornblith LZ, Kutcher ME, Ra C, et al. Mechanical ventilation weaning and extubation after spinal cord injury: a western trauma association multicenter study. J Trauma Acute Care Surg. 2013;75(6):1060–9.

61. The ALS Association. http://www.alsa.org/about-als/facts-you-should-know.html. 2015. Accessed 2 Sept 2015.

62. Levine S, Nguyen T, Taylor N, et al. Rapid disuse atrophy of diaphragm fibers in mechanically ventilated humans. N Engl J Med. 2008;358:1327–35.

63. Wiertz-Hoessels EL, Krediet P. Degeneration of the motor End-plates after neurectomy in the Rat and the rabbit. Acta Morphol Neerl Scand. 1965;6:179–93.

64. Tedde M, Vasconcelos F, Hajjar L, et al. Diaphragmatic pacing stimulation in spinal cord injury: anesthetic and perioperative management. Clinics. 2012;67:1265–9.

65. Kaufman M, Elkwood A, Aboharb F, et al. Diaphragmatic reinnervation in ventilator-dependent patients with cervical spinal cord injury and concomitant phrenic nerve lesions using simultaneous nerve transfers and implantable neurostimulators. J Reconstr Microsurg. 2015;31: 391–5.

66. Leem M, Kiernan M, Macefield V, et al. Short-term peripheral nerve stimulation ameliorates axonal dysfunction after spinal cord injury. J Neurophysiol. 2015;113:3209–18.

67. Magden O, Tayfur V, Edizer M, et al. Anatomy of gracilis muscle flap. J Craniofac Surg. 2010;21:1948–5.

68. Horta R, Henriques-Coelho T, Costa J, et al. Fascicular phrenic nerve neurotization for restoring physiological motion in a congenital diaphragmatic hernia reconstruction with a reverse innervated latissimus dorsi muscle flap. Ann Plast Surg. 2015;75:193–6.

Mary Massery

Introduction

Decreased endurance and dyspnea may be the primary presenting symptoms of unilateral or bilateral diaphragm paralysis, but further evaluation may expose a host of other adverse physical consequences. In order to understand the wide array of physical symptoms reported with unilateral or bilateral diaphragm paralysis, it is critical to understand the diaphragm's role as the body's major pressure regulator.

The diaphragm plays a major role in dynamic stabilization of the trunk and spine [1, 2]. The diaphragm is situated in the middle of the trunk, completely separating the thoracic and abdominal cavities, with external valves at the top (vocal folds) and at the bottom (pelvic floor). Hence, the diaphragm's movements cause a constant fluctuation in intra-abdominal and intrathoracic pressures, allowing the diaphragm to simultaneously manage respiration and spinal stabilization needs [3, 4]. This can be easily visualized as a soda pop can which uses internal pressure to stabilize the flimsy aluminum walls (dynamic spinal stability) (see Fig. 11.1) [5]. The ability of the trunk to control multiple functions, such as respiration, spinal stability, balance, limb force production, voicing, and continence, is dependent on finely regulated pressure changes, with the diaphragm as the prime contributor [6–8]. Thus, with diaphragm paralysis, besides the obvious breathing impairment, a whole range of unintended consequences need to be assessed.

When disease or trauma, such as a phrenic nerve injury, prevents or limits the diaphragm from significantly contributing to inspiration, there is a substantial risk of secondary problems with balance and spinal control [9, 10]. The altered motor control of the trunk can lead to musculoskeletal consequences including chronic pain (most often low back, neck, shoulder, or hip pain), shoulder range of motion restrictions, and/or pelvic floor dysfunction [8, 11]. The relationship of the diaphragm to upright postural control goes far beyond inspiration. The critical relationship of the diaphragm to respiratory and postural control function means that all patients with phrenic nerve paralysis should be screened for impairments of both functions.

Physical Therapy (PT) Preoperative Assessment

A physical therapist should assess the patient's breathing and postural presentation with this broader understanding of the diaphragm's multiple roles. Recommended assessments are listed in Table 11.1.

M. Massery, PT, DPT, DSc
Massery Physical Therapy, 3820 Timbers Edge Lane,
Glenview, IL 60025, USA
e-mail: mmassery@aol.com

© Springer International Publishing Switzerland 2017
A.I. Elkwood et al. (eds.), *Rehabilitative Surgery*, DOI 10.1007/978-3-319-41406-5_11

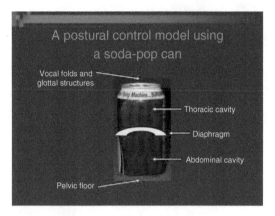

Fig. 11.1 Soda pop can model of postural control. The diaphragm is the body's major pressure regulator, completely separating the thoracic and abdominal chambers. Together with the superior valve (vocal folds) and inferior valve (pelvic floor), the diaphragm simultaneously controls trunk pressure for breathing and postural stability, which functionally links the *top* and the *bottom* of the can

Table 11.1 Preoperative PT assessment should ideally address the following potential impairments

Respiration	Pulmonary function tests
	Compensatory breathing patterns, assessed in multiple postures and activities
	Chest wall excursion (CWE)
	Sleep-disordered breathing
Endurance	Mobility tests (i.e., 6-min walk test)
	Perceived exertion during activities
Postural alignment in upright, especially	Spine and neck
	Rib cage
	Shoulders
	Pelvis/hips
	Pediatric vs. adults
Postural stability	Balance
	Gait deviations
	Pain
	Continence

Respiration

Pulmonary Function Tests (PFT) The combination of forced vital capacity (FVC) and the ratio of forced expiratory volume in one second to FVC (FEV1/FVC) are commonly used to clarify the severity of the lung restriction [12].

Compensatory Breathing Patterns Analysis of the patient's breathing pattern should be screened to identify which substitution patterns are used to achieve inspiratory lung volumes at rest (tidal volume) and with effort (vital capacity). Did the patient compensate in a functional manner or did the adaptive strategy add a burden to their pulmonary efficiency or postural control? PTs should assess the patient's breathing strategy in multiple postures and activities presurgically for post-nerve regeneration comparison. Specific manual palpation exam of both hemidiaphragms during inhalation should be done to determine the contributing function of each hemidiaphragm for postsurgical comparison. Where available, a videofluoroscopy or an ultrasound test can confirm or refute the therapist's manual palpation findings, which will be helpful for postoperative comparison [13, 14].

Chest Wall Excursion (CWE) CWE measurements can quantify the chest movements and have been shown to have good inter-/intra-tester reliability after minimal training [15, 16]. Suggested measurement sites that capture the common variations of breathing patterns are (1) level of the third rib (axilla), (2) xiphoid process, and (3) half the distance from xiphoid to umbilicus [17] (Fig. 11.2). CWE should be tracked through rehabilitation, hopefully showing a shift downward (increased diaphragm excursion and decreased upper chest accessory muscle recruitment), and a more symmetrical response.

Sleep Breathing assessment should encompass the entire day, thus including sleep. Bilateral diaphragm paralysis will require nocturnal support such as CPAP (continuous positive airway pressure), BPAP (bi-level positive airway pressure), or mechanical ventilation, but mounting evidence suggests that unilateral diaphragm paralysis results in sleep-disordered breathing, cespecially during REM sleep, that often goes undetected [18–21]. Sleep studies should be a routine. PTs' expertise in positioning may help patients and their physicians determine optimal sleep postures for oxygenation.

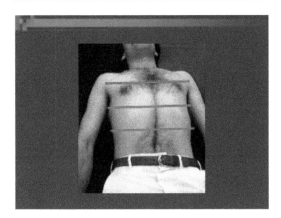

Fig. 11.2 Chest wall excursion (CWE) circumferential measurement sites: *Top line*: level of the third rib (axilla). *Middle line*: xiphoid process. *Bottom line*: half the distance between the xiphoid process and the umbilicus

Endurance

Endurance tests must be individually chosen to ensure that the measure will be sensitive enough to capture a change postsurgically. A 6- or 12-min walk test is easy to administer clinically. The length of the test is determined by the patient's level of impairment. A patient who is very weak may not be able to walk even 6 full minutes, whereas a patient with lesser impairment won't show an endurance limitation until pushed a greater distance, like the full 12-min test [22]. There are many tests to choose from that are appropriate to the patient's activity level [23].

Endurance could also be measured in terms of perceived exertion [24]. These subjective tests are particularly sensitive measures for patients who are very weak and may not show an increase in functional endurance such as walking further, but who may report less perceived effort for the same breathing and/or ADL skills recorded preoperatively.

Postural Alignment

Compensatory breathing patterns and the secondary impairments in balance may cause postural abnormalities [9]. This is particularly true for long-standing phrenic nerve paralysis where dis-

use has caused decreased chest wall and spinal mobility. Postural compensations may have developed slowly, and the patient may not even be aware of how much his posture has changed. Manual assessment of the entire rib cage and spine is necessary as restrictions are common in long-standing phrenic nerve paralysis. Shoulder range of motion (ROM) is often restricted secondary to diaphragm dysfunction. The weakness/paralysis disrupts the normal coupling effect between the shoulder and rib cage, especially when reaching above 90° of shoulder flexion [25, 26]. Limitations may also be noted at the hip/pelvis or neck due to compensatory breathing and/or postural control strategies. PTs should anticipate the need to mobilize noted musculoskeletal restrictions in order to regain maximal breathing and postural control function.

Postural impairments secondary to unilateral diaphragm paralysis are unique. These patients should be specifically screened for asymmetrical presentations. The development of chronic pain from asymmetric muscle use is a common complaint in this population but not yet researched (Fig. 11.3). Recent research suggests that patients with unilateral diaphragm paralysis have increased balance impairments because their center of mass is disturbed with every breath on a coronal plane, rather than just a sagittal plane [9]. Compensations to correct for this added postural burden could lead to repetitive muscle stress resulting in pain.

Pediatrics Special consideration must be made in pediatrics as their chest wall and spine have not yet matured. Chronic phrenic nerve paralysis may lead to hypoplasia of the rib cage on the side of the paralysis which in turn will contribute to scoliosis forces and increased likelihood of more pronounced asymmetric postural alignment throughout the trunk (Fig. 11.4). Balance compensations will increase the risk of repetitive stress injuries as the child matures, which could lead to pain. Recent research shows that patients with chronic low back pain have weaker diaphragms than controls [27]. Long-term research has not yet been done with children with pediatric

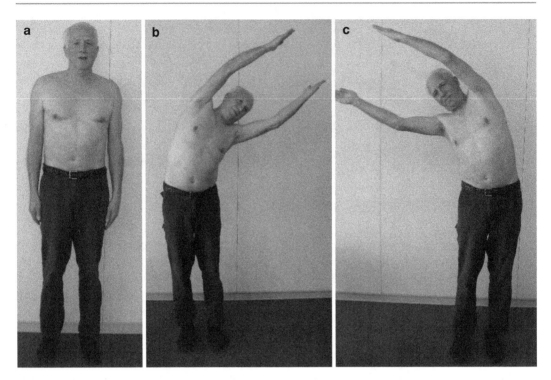

Fig. 11.3 Common postural compensations/abnormalities with unilateral phrenic nerve injury. Previously healthy, fit 67-year-old man with left paralyzed phrenic nerve of >12-month duration. Phrenic nerve graft surgery ~4 months prior to these pictures. One PT visit thus far. (**a**) Subject's trunk is shortened on the left. He reported no postural asymmetry problems before phrenic nerve injury. (**b**) Lateral side bending to left shows normal range of motion for the right rib cage and lower trunk (intact phrenic nerve). Patient shows normal weight shift of hips to the right when side bending to left. (**c**) Lateral side bending to the right shows moderate restrictions in left lower rib cage and lower trunk (left paralyzed phrenic nerve). Note: (1) increased effort in his face, (2) decreased elbow extension, (3) decreased shoulder flexion, and (4) decreased weight shift onto left lower extremity. These restrictions limit more than inspiratory lung volumes, such as limitations in balance, gait, and reach, and may lead to chronic pain from long-standing altered mechanics

phrenic nerve injuries but would suggest that maturing with a chronically weak or paralyzed diaphragm would predispose these children to an increased risk of developing low back pain.

Postural Stability

There are numerous functional presentations of postural instability. Four specific impairments are detailed below.

Balance The contributions of the diaphragm to postural stability are well established; thus, the assessment of balance (postural instability) should be a routine screening module of the PT evaluation. There are numerous balance tests from simple sitting perturbation tests, to timed single-limb stance tests, to sophisticated computerized limits of stability tests. Balance tests should be chosen for their sensitivity to change, availability of resources, and specificity to each individual patient's capabilities [28].

Gait Postural control impairments may be reflected as abnormal gait patterns and are highly variable with this population. Patients with mild postural instability are likely to stiffen their trunks in an attempt to improve postural stability. Common gait deviations associated with rigid trunks include decreased arm swing, decreased trunk rotation, slower cadence, and shorter steps. This pattern is very similar to other physical impairments such as chronic low back pain, neuromuscular weakness (Parkinson's, multiple sclerosis, stroke, etc.), incontinence, and lower

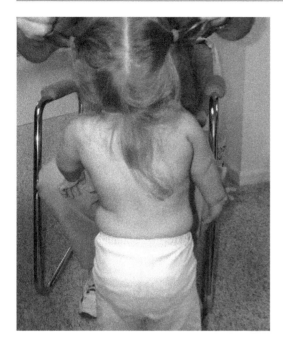

Fig. 11.4 Pediatric postural impairments 1–1/2-year-old girl surviving a traumatic vaginal birth with resultant bilateral phrenic nerve injury (left more impaired than right). Note postural shift of her trunk to left side (increased weight bearing on left leg) and increased lateral trunk flexion to left (increased skin fold), both likely balance compensations. Long term, this posturing will lead to greater scoliotic forces on her developing spine and greater risk of repetitive stress injuries (pain)

gastrointestinal dysfunctions (constipation, irritability, etc.) [29–31]. Careful screening is needed to ascertain gait deviations due to phrenic nerve paralysis vs. other underlying problems.

Patients with severe postural instability can't stiffen their trunk because of extreme weakness or motor control issues. Their trunk is too floppy, and their gait pattern typically shows deviations such as excessive arm swing and excessive trunk movements, especially in the coronal plane. If the trunk is markedly unbalanced, the patient may require an assistive device or may no longer be ambulatory.

Pain

A possible long-term consequence of altered motor plans is pain due to malalignment or overuse syndromes [32, 33]. Pain conditions may reflect overuse of the accessory muscles due to the diaphragm

weakness (neck or chest pain) or due to postural instability (pain anywhere from neck to hips) [34]. Patients with unilateral diaphragm paralysis may have pain related to rotational (torsion) forces due to asymmetric and rotary forces across their spine. Compensatory trunk postural strategies could result in pain down in the knee or ankle joints. All patients should be screened for secondary pain conditions.

Continence

The deep abdominal muscle shell that controls intra-abdominal pressure is comprised of the diaphragm as the top dome, the transversus abdominis and multifidus as the long cylinder, and the pelvic floor as the bottom sling. When one of those four muscles is impaired, it impairs the function of the whole abdominal complex. Thus, diaphragm dysfunction is highly associated with pelvic floor consequences, such as incontinence, and should be screened in this population [6, 8].

Summary

Diaphragm paralysis has marked implications for motor dysfunction beyond breathing and endurance impairments and should be carefully assessed and documented preoperatively in order to accurately assess the long-term outcomes of the phrenic nerve graft surgery. However, because this surgery is so specialized, requiring many patients to travel a great distance, there is little likelihood that the same PT will do the pre- and post-surgery which may limit the reliability of the measures. Research is needed to determine the optimal pre-/posttests that could be performed reliably on a nationwide basis.

Physical Therapy Rehabilitation

PT Reassessment

Following phrenic nerve graft surgery and after the confirmation from the surgeon that it is safe to start rehabilitation, the patient should be reassessed by PT. If the patient was not seen by PT preoperatively, the PT evaluation described earlier in the chapter should be done. Two specific tests should be included in the postsurgical rehabilitation phase of PT: (1) integument restrictions and (2) diaphragm responsiveness.

Integument Surgical scars on the calf and chest, as well as surrounding tissue, should be evaluated for fascial restrictions or scar adhesions which can limit mobility [35]. If restricted, the PT should include myofascial releases and scar massage to affected areas to maximize range of motion and ease of movement.

Diaphragm Each hemidiaphragm should be reassessed with manual facilitation to determine if the diaphragm is now contracting. This is a clinical examination. Where possible, the results should be compared with a videofluoroscopy or an ultrasound of the diaphragm for confirmation [13, 14].

PT Rehabilitation Treatment

PTs are very familiar with designing treatments to address issues such as impaired endurance, poor posture, poor core stability, impaired balance, fascial/scar restrictions, gait deviations, pain, and stress incontinence. PT treatments uniquely related to phrenic nerve rehabilitation will be specifically addressed below: (1) thoracic spine and rib cage musculoskeletal restrictions, as well as (2) breathing neuromotor retraining.

Thoracic Spine and Rib Cage Musculoskeletal Restrictions Restrictions of the spine and rib cage are very common in this population due to disuse and atrophy over a prolonged period of time. Rehabilitation often includes (1) spinal mobilization techniques in the sagittal and transverse planes, sometimes in the coronal plane, and (2) rib mobilizations. The PT will need to determine if the entire rib cage or only one side (unilateral phrenic nerve injuries) needs musculoskeletal interventions. Typically, treating these trunk restrictions includes a combination of joint mobilizations, soft tissue releases, and fas-

cial releases in order to maximize functional gains following the regeneration of the phrenic nerve [36]. Compensatory breathing and/or postural control strategies may lead to additional musculoskeletal problems which should be addressed on an individual basis.

Breathing Neuromotor Retraining Significant neuromotor retraining is necessary to stimulate and strengthen the diaphragm's response both unilaterally and bilaterally. The diaphragm also needs to be coupled with the intercostals to optimize inspiratory lung volumes [37, 38]. Adequate intra-abdominal pressure to optimize the diaphragm's length-tension relationship is imperative, so focusing on core strength is a hallmark of a diaphragm rehab program [39]. If the patient is too weak to generate adequate intra-abdominal pressures on their own, then an abdominal binder should be trialed [40].

Reduce Postural Demands on the Diaphragm Reducing the postural demand on the diaphragm will allow the diaphragm to focus on its respiratory role rather than its postural role. Thus, early in rehabilitation, facilitation of the diaphragm in recumbent postures (less postural demand) is usually more successful than upright postures. Manual facilitation techniques based on the neurophysiologic response of the diaphragm as well as the physiologic need to breathe (survival response) will bolster the clinician's efforts to elicit a response from the recovering diaphragm [41] (Fig. 11.5). Long term, the goal is to restore the diaphragm's ability to function simultaneously as a breathing and a postural control muscle; thus, recruitment of the diaphragm in higher-level postures, such as sitting, standing, walking, and running, is an important progression of treatment. Combining diaphragm breathing with complex movements including upper extremity reaching (coupling the diaphragm and intercostals) and/or gait (coupling the diaphragm with the abdominals and pelvic floor) will promote restoration of the diaphragm to its previous complex motor functions (Fig. 11.6). Resisted movements, such as with proprioceptive neuromuscular facilitation (PNF) exercises, will drive a greater motor response

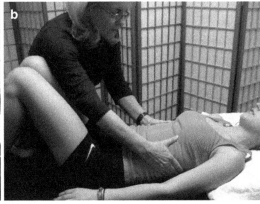

Fig. 11.5 Neuromotor retraining: handling techniques to maximize the response of a weak diaphragm contraction. (**a**) "Diaphragm scoop" neuromotor facilitation technique can be used as a diagnostic screening tool to assess bilateral or unilateral diaphragm contraction and used to stimulate the diaphragm's contraction. Resistance is added once the diaphragm is consistently activating. Rehabilitation starts with isolated diaphragm facilitation techniques but quickly moves to integrated complex neuromotor retraining that includes coordinating simultaneous postural control responses of the diaphragm with the breathing responses of the diaphragm (ventilatory strategies). (**b**) "Lateral costal" neuromotor facilitation technique progresses from a focus on facilitation of a central response of the diaphragm (hemidiaphragm or bilateral) to a coupled response with the intercostals (progression toward normal multipurpose reaction)

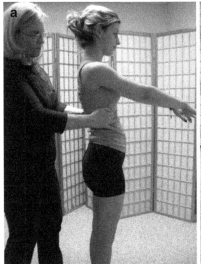
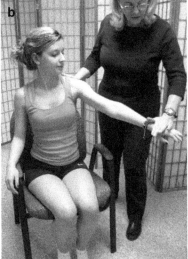
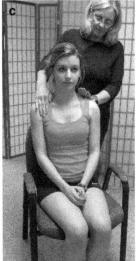

Fig. 11.6 Sample of techniques that promote integration of diaphragm with higher-level postural stability such as standing, reaching, and axial trunk rotation. (**a**) Mid-trunk dynamic stabilization resistance training in standing requires the diaphragm to move dynamically for breathing as well as postural stability (balance). The therapist applies resistance at the mid-trunk to actively engage the diaphragm in balance response. Submaximal resistance allows breathing and postural control responses. Avoid maximal resistance as it will elicit a static breath-hold response and is not a desired outcome. (**b**) Distal resistance shown here on the arm, but can also be done on the leg, demands that the diaphragm respond as a postural muscle. Be careful to use submaximal resistance so that the diaphragm can relearn how to breathe and "hold" at the same time (dynamic stability). (**c**) Rotary resistance of the trunk, shown here in sitting but can be done in any upright posture, focuses on the role of the diaphragm for balance responses (maintenance of axial control of the trunk in upright)

from the diaphragm and trunk muscles which will aid in strengthening the reemerging complex neuromotor plans [42–44].

Unilateral Paralysis Diaphragm Neuromotor Retraining Specific neuromotor retraining techniques that bolster the response of the weak side of the diaphragm are particularly helpful. This author highly recommends using proprioceptive neuromuscular facilitation (PNF) "timing for emphasis" technique to use the strength of the strong diaphragm to get an overflow response to the weak hemidiaphragm [41, 45]. Immediately after eliciting the motor response, the diaphragm's efforts should be reinforced by pairing inspiration with activities that naturally couple the diaphragm with the intercostals and abdominals such as reaching or trunk rotation. This will aid in reinforcing the diaphragm's inspiratory response and promote the diaphragm's role as a postural stabilizer as well.

Endurance Training for the Diaphragm Once the diaphragm responds consistently, ventilatory muscle training programs (inspiratory and expiratory muscle trainers) can be initiated to increase endurance and reinforce neuroplasticity [46]. Don't start these programs until the diaphragm has adequate strength or the other inspiratory muscles may overpower the diaphragm's response, which would have the unintended outcome of reinforcing the compensatory pattern instead of strengthening the diaphragm.

Airway Clearance If the patient has a history of decreased ability to clear lung secretions secondary to diaphragm weakness or paralysis, then a comprehensive airway clearance program should be developed, including assistive cough techniques [47].

Summary

Rehabilitation of the diaphragm following a phrenic nerve graft involves a detailed multisystem evaluation by the PT to determine the extent of the impairment (primary and secondary) as a result of the long-standing unilateral or bilateral phrenic nerve paralysis. A bilateral paralysis has a devastating impact on the patient's survival, often requiring mechanical ventilation, but unilateral paralysis is also devastating due to balance impairments, endurance impairments, sleep disruptions, musculoskeletal restrictions/pain, and an ongoing risk of respiratory complications. If the consequences of phrenic nerve paralysis are not fully understood, assessed, and treated, the patient's long-term quality of life outcomes may be impaired.

Dr. Kaufman's surgical approach to phrenic nerve paralysis is an innovative procedure. Research with spinal cord injury gives PT's guidance for the development of an appropriate treatment approach to this population, but research specific to phrenic nerve restoration is needed.

References

1. Hodges PW, et al. Coexistence of stability and mobility in postural control: evidence from postural compensation for respiration. Exp Brain Res. 2002; 144:293–302.
2. Hodges PW, et al. Intra-abdominal pressure increases stiffness of the lumbar spine. J Biomech. 2005;38: 1873–80.
3. Gandevia SC, et al. Balancing acts: respiratory sensations, motor control and human posture. Clin Exp Pharmacol Physiol. 2002;29:118–21.
4. Hodges PW, Gandevia SC. Activation of the human diaphragm during a repetitive postural task. J Physiol. 2000;522:165–75.
5. Massery M. Multisystem consequences of impaired breathing mechanics and/or postural control. In: Frownfelter D, Dean E, editors. Cardiovascular and pulmonary physical therapy evidence and practice. 4th ed. St. Louis: Elsevier Health Sciences;2006. p. 695–717.
6. Hirayama F, et al. Association of impaired respiratory function with urinary incontinence. Respirology. 2009;14:753–6.
7. Massery M, et al. Effect of airway control by glottal structures on postural stability. J Appl Physiol. 2013;115:483–90.
8. Smith MD, Russell A, Hodges PW. The relationship between incontinence, breathing disorders, gastrointestinal symptoms, and back pain in women: a longitudinal cohort study. Clin J Pain. 2014;30:162–7.
9. Hamaoui A, et al. Postural disturbances resulting from unilateral and bilateral diaphragm contractions: a phrenic nerve stimulation study. J Appl Physiol (1985). 2014;117:825–32.
10. Hamaoui A, Gonneau E, Le Bozec S. Respiratory disturbance to posture varies according to the respiratory mode. Neurosci Lett. 2010;475:141–4.

11. Smith MD, et al. Balance is impaired in people with chronic obstructive pulmonary disease. Gait Posture. 2010;31:456–60.

12. Aaron SD, Dales RE, Cardinal P. How accurate is spirometry at predicting restrictive pulmonary impairment? Chest. 1999;115:869–73.

13. Yi LC, Nascimento OA, Jardim JR. Reliability of an analysis method for measuring diaphragm excursion by means of direct visualization with videofluoroscopy. Arch Bronconeumol. 2011;47:310–4.

14. Summerhill EM, et al. Monitoring recovery from diaphragm paralysis with ultrasound. Chest. 2008;133:737–43.

15. Massery M. Asthma: multi-system implications. In: Campbell S, Palisano R, Orlin M, editors. Physical therapy for children. St. Louis: Elsevier;2012. p. 815–44.

16. LaPier TK, et al. Intertester and intratester reliability of chest excursion measurement in subjects without impairment. Cardiopulm Phys Ther. 2000;11:94–8.

17. Massery MP, et al. Chest wall excursion and tidal volume change during passive positioning in cervical spinal cord injury. (Abstract). Cardiopulm Phys Ther. 1997;8:27.

18. Steier J, et al. Sleep-disordered breathing in unilateral diaphragm paralysis or severe weakness. Eur Respir J. 2008;32:1479–87.

19. Khan A, Morgenthaler TI, Ramar K. Sleep disordered breathing in isolated unilateral and bilateral diaphragmatic dysfunction. J Clin Sleep Med. 2014;10:509–15.

20. Baltzan MA, Scott AS, Wolkove N. Unilateral hemidiaphragm weakness is associated with positional hypoxemia in REM sleep. J Clin Sleep Med. 2012;8:51–8.

21. Wolkove N. Sleep-related desaturation in patients with unilateral diaphragmatic dysfunction. In: Chest 2005 annual conference. Montreal; 2005.

22. American-Thoracic-Society. ATS Statement: Guidelines for the six-minute walk test. Am J Respir Crit Care Med. 2002;166:111–7.

23. Scherer SA, Noteboom JT, Flynn TW. Cardiovascular assessment in the orthopaedic practice setting. J Orthop Sports Phys Ther. 2005;35:730–7.

24. Scherer S, Cassady SL. Rating of perceived exertion: development and clinical applications for physical therapy exercise testing and prescription. Cardiopulm PhysTher J. 1999;10:143–7.

25. Flynn TW. The thoracic spine and rib cage: musculoskeletal evaluation and treatment. Newton: Butterworth-Heinemann; 1996.

26. De Troyer A, Wilson TA. Effect of acute inflation on the mechanics of the inspiratory muscles. J Appl Physiol. 2009;107:315–23.

27. Janssens L, et al. Greater diaphragm fatigability in individuals with recurrent low back pain. Respir Physiol Neurobiol. 2013;188:119–23.

28. Glave AP, et al. Testing postural stability: are the star excursion balance test and biodex balance system limits of stability tests consistent? Gait Posture. 2016;43:225–7.

29. Brumagne S, et al. Persons with recurrent low back pain exhibit a rigid postural control strategy. Eur Spine J. 2008;17:1177–84.

30. Grenier SG, McGill SM. When exposed to challenged ventilation, those with a history of LBP increase spine stability relatively more than healthy individuals. Clin Biomech. 2008;23:1105–11.

31. Smith MD, Coppieters MW, Hodges PW. Is balance different in women with and without stress urinary incontinence? Neurourol Urodyn. 2008;27:71–8.

32. Lunardi AC, et al. Musculoskeletal dysfunction and pain in adults with asthma. J Asthma. 2011;48:105–10.

33. Koh JL, et al. Assessment of acute and chronic pain symptoms in children with cystic fibrosis. Pediatr Pulmonol. 2005;40:330–5.

34. Kolar P, et al. Postural function of the diaphragm in persons with and without chronic low back pain. J Orthop Sports Phys Ther. 2012;42:352–62.

35. Stecco C, et al. The fascia: the forgotten structure. Ital J Anat Embryol. 2011;116(3):127–38.

36. Massery M. Musculoskeletal and neuromuscular interventions: a physical approach to cystic fibrosis. J R Soc Med. 2005;98(Supplement 45):55–66.

37. De Troyer A, Kirkwood PA, Wilson TA. Respiratory action of the intercostal muscles. Physiol Rev. 2005;85:717–56.

38. De Troyer A, Leduc D. Role of pleural pressure in the coupling between the intercostal muscles and the ribs. J Appl Physiol. 2007;102:2332–7.

39. Hodges PW, Gandevia SC. Changes in intra-abdominal pressure during postural and respiratory activation of the human diaphragm. J Appl Physiol. 2000;89:967–76.

40. Wadsworth BM, et al. Abdominal binder improves lung volumes and voice in people with tetraplegic spinal cord injury. Arch Phys Med Rehabil. 2012;93:2189–97.

41. Frownfelter D, Massery M. Facilitating ventilation patterns and breathing strategies In: Frownfelter D, Dean E, editors. Cardiovascular and pulmonary physical therapy evidence and practice. 4th ed. St. Louis: Elsevier Health Sciences; 2006. p. Chapter 23.

42. Hindle KB, et al. Proprioceptive neuromuscular facilitation (PNF): its mechanisms and effects on range of motion and muscular function. J Hum Kinet. 2012;31:105–13.

43. Mitchell UH, et al. Neurophysiological reflex mechanisms' lack of contribution to the success of PNF stretches. J Sport Rehabil. 2009;18:343–57.

44. Gong W. The effects of dynamic exercise utilizing PNF patterns on abdominal muscle thickness in healthy adults. J Phys Ther Sci. 2015;27:1933–6.

45. Sullivan PE, Markos PD. Clinical procedures in therapeutic exercise. 2nd ed. Stamford: Simon and Schuster Co.; 1996.

46. Sprague SS, Hopkins PD. Use of inspiratory strength training to wean six patients who were ventilator-dependent. Phys Ther. 2003;83:171–81.

47. Frownfelter D, Massery M. Facilitating airway clearance with coughing techniques. In: Frownfelter D,Dean E, editors. Cardiovascular and pulmonary physical therapy evidence and practice. 4th ed. St. Louis: Elsevier Health Sciences; 2006. p. Chapter 22.

Recovery of Diaphragm Function Through Functional Electrical Stimulation: Diaphragm Pacing

Raymond P. Onders

Introduction

Mechanical ventilation (MV) has saved countless lives. Since MV was introduced, it is the primary therapy for respiratory failure and a fundamental treatment in intensive care units. Whether MV is used during a surgical procedure or to treat respiratory failure, it is generally a time-limited therapy that, when withdrawn, has no untoward sequelae. However, there are a number of patients who become dependent on MV. These patients, often referred to as "failure to wean" (FTW), present a significant physiologic and economic burden to the healthcare system.

FTW patients arise from those who required "prolonged" MV (PMV), defined as greater than 96 h of MV. Patients on PMV or FTW have longer hospital days (median 17 days vs. 6), higher comorbidities, poor functional outcomes, and increase cost [1]. Damuth reviewed worldwide data of PMV patients with 124 studies ultimately included in results. This report showed a 1-year mortality of 58 % in ICU patients. Only 50 % of patients were ever liberated from mechanical ventilation [2]. Additional reports have mortality ranging from 20 to 50 %. The 1-year functional outcomes in PMV patients demonstrate only 9 % being able to perform activities of daily living independently. Conversely, 65 % were completely dependent on others. PMV incur substantially greater hospital costs than patients who are able to wean, with 1-year survival costs averaging $306,000.00 US dollars. The number of patients requiring PMV is growing 5.5 % annually, 4.4 % higher than the total hospital admission growth rate. It is estimated that by the year 2020, there will be 605,000 patients requiring PMV with hospital costs of $64 billion.

Multiple medical conditions, such as heart failure, severe respiratory disease, critical illness neuropathy, and respiratory muscle weakness, can lead to PMV. In addition to medical etiologies, MV has its own deleterious effects. Positive pressure MV leads to inactivity of the diaphragm muscle, causing atrophy and weakness. Because the diaphragm is the primary inspiratory muscle, ventilator-induced diaphragm dysfunction (VIDD) is widely recognized as a major contributing factor to FTW [3]. For this chapter, it will be important to remember the diaphragm is innervated by the phrenic nerve, composed of nerve roots from cervical level 3 to 5.

High level spinal cord injury (SCI) is another condition that lends itself to PMV. Approximately 4 % of the 12,000 SCI patients per year in the USA require chronic long-term MV. Respiratory complications are the leading cause of death in SCI, with pneumonia being the leading cause of death in those on MV. Patients with the same

R.P. Onders, MD
Department of Surgery, University Hospitals
Case Medical Center, Case Western Reserve
University School of Medicine,
11100 Euclid Avenue, Cleveland, OH, USA
e-mail: Raymond.onders@uhhospitals.org

© Springer International Publishing Switzerland 2017
A.I. Elkwood et al. (eds.), *Rehabilitative Surgery*, DOI 10.1007/978-3-319-41406-5_12

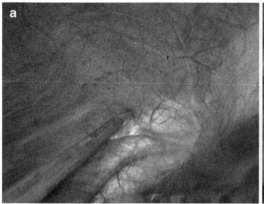
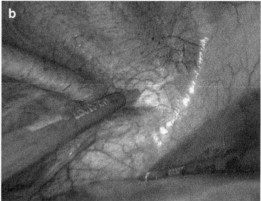

Fig. 12.1 (a) The laparoscopic dissector is placed against the right diaphragm, an electrical burst from the clinical station externally will allow contraction if the phrenic nerve is intact, and subsequent mapping will show ideal location for implantation; (b) the diaphragm has a diffuse but weak contraction which will improve with diaphragm conditioning

level of injury who require MV have significantly shorter life spans. Chronic long-term MV is associated with increased anxiety for both patient and caregiver. It alters speech patterns, decreases sense of smell, adds bulk and weight to wheelchairs, and impedes mobility, and noise and tubing attract unwanted attention [3]. The presence of a tracheostomy increases secretions and may cause tracheal malacia and tracheal erosion.

Surgical Intervention with Diaphragm Pacing

Diaphragm pacing (DP) was developed to provide natural negative pressure ventilation in SCI patients on PMV. DP involves laparoscopically placed electrodes at the motor point of each hemidiaphragm where stimulation provides maximal contraction of the diaphragm. Essentially, DP electrically stimulates intact lower motor units in the spinal column replacing the upper motor neuron signal. It has been shown to decrease, delay, or replace MV.

Surgical implantation of DP begins with patients receiving deep vein thrombosis prophylaxis through sequential compression devices and appropriate warming apparatuses. General anesthesia is administered without neuromuscular blocking agents. Short-acting agents such as propofol for amnesia and remifentanil for pain along with inhalation agents are the preferred anesthetic management for patients undergoing DP [4]. Standard four-port laparoscopy begins with generous amounts of preemptive local anesthetic being placed into the incisions to decrease pain and intraoperative spasms. The abdomen is insufflated, and the falciform ligament is divided allowing easier access of the implant instruments to the diaphragm. Then a 12-mm epigastric port is placed for the implant instrument and to provide an unimpeded exit for the pacing electrodes.

The next step of DP surgery is mapping of the diaphragm. This process identifies the motor point. The tip of a laparoscopic dissector is touched against the diaphragm muscle (Fig. 12.1 a, b). A twitch stimulus is delivered from a clinical station to the instrument, and both qualitative and quantitative data are obtained. Quantitatively, changes in abdominal pressure are measured through tubing that is attached to one of the surgical ports and connected to the clinical station. A greater change in pressure indicates closer proximity to the motor point of the phrenic nerve and a larger diaphragm muscle contraction. Qualitatively, visual observation of the diaphragm is made during stimulation.

The area of electrode placement is chosen based on location of larger contraction with strong preference for the posterior diaphragm to facilitate posterior lung lobe ventilation that will

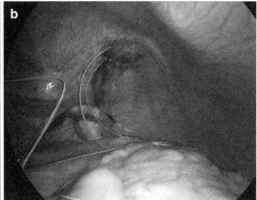

Fig. 12.2 (a) The implant instrument houses the diaphragm pacing electrode which is a double helix of 14 stainless steel wires that are Teflon coated. The needle of the implant instrument enters the diaphragm muscle and a polypropylene barb allows the electrode to be fixated. (b) Two electrodes in the left diaphragm

decrease atelectasis. Two electrodes are then implanted into the right and left diaphragm muscle. Placement of two electrodes in each diaphragm provides redundancy and synergy for maximal muscle recruitment. The electrodes are implanted using an implant instrument (Fig. 12.2 a, b). The electrode is threaded through the instrument to the tip of the needle. The needle at the end of the instrument is skived into the muscle, and the polypropylene barb on the end of the electrode releases upon withdrawal of the needle. The four electrodes and an anode are then tunneled subcutaneously to an appropriate exit site. A chest x-ray is taken at the end of the case to assess for the presence of a capnothorax that may result from carbon dioxide tracking from the abdominal cavity into the pleural space from the diaphragm. Small capnothoraxes resolve spontaneously where a larger one may need to be aspirated [5].

The implanted intramuscular electrodes are connected to a four-channel external pulse generator (EPG) (Fig. 12.3). This stimulator provides capacitively coupled charge-balanced biphasic stimulation to each subcutaneous electrode. The EPG is programmed with patient-specific parameters of pulse amplitude, pulse duration, inspiratory time, pulse rate, and respiratory rate by a clinician. DP users simply connect and turn the device on and/or off. The maximal settings for patient safety are 25 mA for amplitude, 200 for pulse width, and 20 for Hz. Patients should never exceed these parameters [5]. The goal for patient settings is to use the highest settings within the safety parameters that do not cause any patient discomfort.

Once implanted, the device can be utilized immediately to begin diaphragm conditioning. Each patient should have a customized conditioning program that entails initiation of DP use which gradually increases over time. Patients often begin with 30 min of DP use several times daily and increase usage every 3–5 days [3, 5]. DP conditioning will convert the atrophied muscle fibers from fast-fatigable type 2B muscle fibers to slow-twitch type 1.

Results of Diaphragm Pacing

The initial FDA multicenter clinical trial of DP in SCI dependent on tracheostomy MV showed 100 % of implanted patients were able to breathe for four consecutive hours with DP alone. Over 50 % of patients utilized DP for over 24 h of continuous use. The patients ranged in age from 18 years to 74 years (36 years old average). There were 37 males with the majority of injuries resulting from motor vehicle accidents followed by sports injuries. Patients were on PMV from 3 months to 27 years prior to DP implant with the average time of injury to implant being 5.6 years. This trial reports no pneumonia deaths.

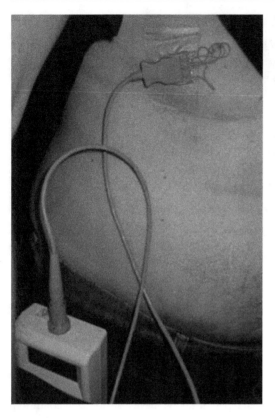

Fig. 12.3 The four implanted electrodes along with a subcutaneously placed ground electrode are placed in a block that connects to the external pulse generator that is programmed to provide diaphragm conditioning and subsequent ventilation

Another study done with DP in SCI but focused on SCI patients who had a permanent internal cardiac pacemaker was completed in 2010. The study included 20 SCI patients who had both cardiac pacemaker and DP. This study also showed all patients were able to achieve tidal volumes to meet their basic metabolic needs with 71 % able to replace MV with DP full time. The internal cardiac pacemakers were interrogated at the time of DP implant with DP being set at maximal stimulation settings and the cardiac pacemakers being set at their most sensitive. No device interactions were noted [6].

DP has been implanted successfully in pediatric patients. A report of six pediatric SCI patients ranging in age 3–17 years (average age 9 years old) with an average weight of 32.6 kg was successfully implanted with no technical difficulties.

Unique to the pediatric population is growth that may require DP reprogramming and scoliosis, which may need to be addressed prior to implantation and/or may affect ventilator weaning. Pediatric patients experienced the same success with being liberated from MV as their adult counterparts [7].

More recent and exciting data on DP in the SCI population was published in 2014 [8]. This study focused on early implantation of DP. Their analysis included 29 patients, 22 of whom were implanted and 7 patients had denervated "dead diaphragms" at surgery. The average time frame of injury to implant was 3–112 days with a median of 33 days. Seventeen percent of patients were weaned completely off MV in an average of 13.1 days. A subset of patients implanted within 11 days of injury weaned off MV in 5.7 days. Some patients (36 %) implanted early after injury had recovery of respiration and were able to wean off of DP. This study highlighted the potential of electrical stimulation from DP and neuroplasticity of the spinal cord allowing recovery of phrenic nerve function. Also noteworthy was the fact that early identification of those patients with "dead diaphragms" will save significant amounts of time, frustration, and money on futile ventilator weaning and also allow early consideration of the growing use of nerve transfer techniques to allow recovery.

Recent uses of DP expanded from SCI to diaphragm dysfunction. DD can be either unilateral or bilateral with varying degrees of symptomatology ranging from asymptomatic to respiratory failure requiring mechanical ventilation. Onders reported the use of DP in a group of 21 patients. The study identified six patients with non-stimulable diaphragms at surgery. Of note, preoperative testing, which included radiographic exams, phrenic nerve conduction studies, and pulmonary testing, showed no statistical difference between the two groups. Ten of the implanted patients had false-negative phrenic nerve conduction studies with no measurable muscle action potentials. The average duration of symptoms for those implanted was 41 months compared to 22 months in the non-stimulable group. Four patients were on tracheostomy mechanical ventilation. Diaphragm dysfunction was a result of phrenic nerve injury from thoracic surgery, shoulder surgery, idiopathic and one spinal muscle atrophy (SMA), one Charcot-Marie-Tooth disease, and one diaphragm flutter (belly dancer syndrome). Sixty-two percent had clinically relevant improvements in respiration. All four mechanically ventilated patients were weaned off tracheostomy mechanical ventilation and ultimately decannulated and weaned off DP with electrodes removed. Two people decreased noninvasive ventilation use; two were weaned off oxygen therapy and two had resolution of paradoxical motion of the diaphragms and three additional patients having improved diaphragms on chest x-ray. Using an adapted cable, the implanted DP electrodes were used to assess diaphragm electromyographic activity that not only allowed for identification of abnormalities such as central apneas but also provided an avenue for monitoring of diaphragm recovery [9].

Conclusion

Prolonged mechanical ventilation is a significant and growing healthcare predicament. DP has been successfully used in SCI to replace or decrease mechanical ventilation. Early implantation of DP has substantial benefits and no known drawbacks. The more recent utilization of DP in DD is a foundation for DP to be used in critical care units. Duplication of the success of DP in weaning patients from tracheostomy mechanical ventilation would change the paradigm of therapy in intensive care units.

Conflict of Interest Disclosure Dr. Raymond Onders, University Hospitals of Cleveland, and Case Western Reserve University School of Medicine have intellectual property rights involved with the diaphragm pacing system and equity in Synapse Biomedical who manufactures the device.

References

1. Criner G. Long-term ventilator dependent patients: new facilities and new models of care. The American perspective. Port Rev Pneumol. 2012;18:214–6.
2. Damuth E, Mitchell J, Bartock B, Roberts B, Treciak S. Long-term survival of critically ill patients treated with prolonged mechanical ventilation: a systematic review and met-analysis. Lancet Resp Med. 2015;3:544–53.
3. Elmo M, Kaplan C, Onders R. Diaphragm pacing: helping patients breathe. AANLCP J Nurse Life Care Plann. 2012;12:600–11.
4. Onders RP, Carlin AM, Elmo MJ, Sivashankaran S, Katirji B, Schilz R. Amyotrophic lateral sclerosis: the Midwestern surgical experience with diaphragm pacing stimulation system shows that general anesthesia can be safely performed. Am J Surg. 2009;197:386–90.
5. Onders RP, Elmo M, Khansarinia S, Bowman B, Yee J, Road J, Bass B, Dunkin B, Ingvarsson PE, Oddsdottir M. Complete worldwide experience in laparoscopic diaphragm pacing: results and differences in spinal cord injured patients and amyotrophic lateral sclerosis patients. Surg Endosc. 2009;23:1433–40.
6. Onders RP, Khansarinia S, Weiser T, Chin C, Hungness E, Soper N, DeHoyos A, Cole T, Ducko C. Multi-center analysis of diaphragm pacing in tetraplegic with cardiac pacemakers: positive implications for ventilator weaning in intensive care units. Surgery. 2010;148:893–7.
7. Onders RP, Ponsky TA, Elmo MJ, Lidsky K, Barksdale E. First reported experience with intramuscular diaphragm pacing in replacing positive pressure mechanical ventilators in children. J Pediatr Surg. 2011;46:72–6.
8. Posluszny JA, Onders R, Kerwin AJ, Weinstein MS, Stein DM, Knight J, Lottenberg L, Cheatham ML, Khansarinia S, Dayal S, Byeno PM. Multicenter review of diaphragm pacing in spinal cord injury: successful not only in weaning from ventilators but also in bridging to independent respiration. J Trauma Acute Care Surg. 2014;76:303–10.
9. Onders R, Elmo MJ, Kaplan C, Katirji B, Schilz R. Extended use of diaphragm pacing in patients with unilateral of bilateral diaphragm dysfunction: a New therapeutic option. Surgery. 2014;156:772–86.

Acute and Long-Term Surgical Management of the Spinal Cord Injury Patient

Melissa Baldwin, Patricia Ayoung-Chee, and H. Leon Pachter

Introduction

One quarter of the 2.5 million injured Americans who required hospitalization in 2013 required post-acute care rehabilitation services [1]. Many injured patients have ongoing medical needs that require prolonged hospital stays even when stable enough to progress to the recovery phase of care. Though this experienced functional decline is due primarily to traumatic injury, prolonged immobilization in the hospital, inadequate nutrition, and procedural and infectious complications increase patient debility and lengthen recovery time. The importance of early mobilization is being recognized and instituted not just in the acute care areas but in the intensive care units as well. Therefore, a better understanding and increased familiarity with early procedures and associated appliances are important for the safe treatment of the injured patient.

M. Baldwin, MD (✉)
General Surgery, NYU School of Medicine,
New York, NY, USA
e-mail: Melissa.Baldwin@nyumc.org

P. Ayoung-Chee, MD
Division of Trauma, Emergency Surgery and Surgical Critical Care, Department of Surgery, NYU School of Medicine, New York, NY, USA
e-mail: patricia.ayoungchee@gmail.com

H.L. Pachter, MD
Department of Surgery, NYU School of Medicine,
New York, NY, USA
e-mail: Leon.Pachter@nyumc.org

Damage Control Surgery

Damage control surgery describes initial non-definitive treatment of traumatic injuries in unstable patients who may only tolerate an abbreviated operation [2]. This type of intervention has been shown to increase survival by decreasing initial stressors, avoiding worsening coagulopathy and allowing time to adequately resuscitate the patient before definitive treatment [3]. Damage control surgery generally applies to control of hemorrhage and contamination of intra-abdominal injuries, but the same principles can apply to intrathoracic and extremity injuries.

Some indications for damage control laparotomy include abdominal compartment syndrome, perforation, or intra-abdominal or pelvic vascular injuries. After the initial procedure, the abdominal cavity is left open with a negative-pressure vacuum dressing to prevent abdominal compartment syndrome during the resuscitation period. Definitive repair of injuries is performed once the patient is stabilized. The abdomen is either closed primarily within a week of the initial operation, or a delayed closure with split-thickness skin graft over exposed viscera can be performed in a few weeks with formal repair of the ventral hernia performed in 6 months to 1 year [3].

With the use of commercially available portable vacuum dressings, there is less concern for evisceration. This allows for earlier extubation and quicker mobilization with participation in physical therapy. It is important to make sure the vacuum dressing has little or no leak so that the dressing remains intact. These temporary abdominal closure methods are associated with long-term risks, such as enterocutaneous (EC) fistula, although this is more likely to occur with graft material than a vacuum dressing or silo bag alone [3].

Enterocutaneous and Enteroatmospheric Fistulas

A fistula is an abnormal connection between two epithelialized surfaces. In an enterocutaneous (EC) fistula, the bowel is connected to the epidermis, and stool contents drain from the skin surface (Fig. 13.1 – enteroatmospheric fistula (EAF)). The majority of EC fistulas occur postoperatively, while a small portion present after radiation therapy or from inflammatory changes [4]. In a patient with an EC fistula, some important considerations are control of ostomy output, maintenance of patient nutrition, and proper wound care.

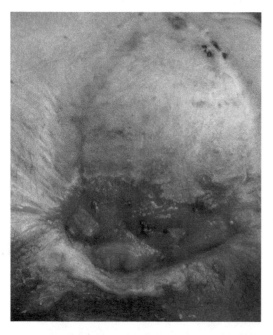

Fig. 13.1 Enteroatmospheric fistula – a section of small bowel is visible protruding through the lower pole of the abdominal wound

Once an EC fistula is diagnosed, usually within the first week postoperatively, drainage should be recorded to allow for proper resuscitation. A high-output fistula, draining >500 cc/day, puts the patient at greater risk of malnutrition and electrolyte imbalances, eventually requiring nutritional support [5]. Parenteral nutrition (PN) has been shown to result in increased rates of fistula closure compared to enteral nutrition (EN), although enteral nutrition (EN) is the preferred route as long as fistula output does not significantly increase once EN is begun [6]. Local wound care is important to protect the skin in preparation for surgical closure. The bowel effluent contains bacteria, digestive enzymes, and bile, which can cause skin breakdown around the fistula. Stoma barriers and creams are very helpful in protecting the skin around the fistula site, and the use of negative-pressure wound dressings has allowed for contained control of the drainage.

Although spontaneous fistula closure may occur, a fistula arising from the proximal gut, with a short tract of < 2 cm or a large skin defect of > 1 cm, is less likely to close spontaneously and may require operative closure. Patients with abscesses, inflammatory bowel disease, foreign body, or malnutrition are also more likely to require operative closure. Generally, colonic EC fistulas will close within a month, and small bowel EC fistulas may take up to 2 months to close [5]. If closure does not occur within this time, the patient should be optimized for surgical closure of the fistula with a procedure similar to an ostomy reversal. Continued optimal nutrition is important to allow for healing of the new wounds and preventing fistula recurrence.

Ileostomy and Colostomy

Stomas of the colon (colostomy) or small bowel (ileostomy) are created for fecal diversion or as a permanent orifice for the passage of stool. In the setting of trauma, a stoma may be used for temporary diversion if the bowel is perforated with intra-abdominal fecal contamination. This is performed as an end colostomy, where the rectum is stapled off and the segment of colon is brought to the skin surface (Hartmann's procedure), or as a loop ileostomy/colostomy, where a loop of bowel is brought up through the incision in the abdomen. An end ostomy has one lumen, whereas a loop ostomy has two lumens within the same stoma site (Fig. 13.2a, b). A red rubber catheter is initially placed between the lumens to maintain external positioning. With a loop ostomy, the afferent limb stoma is maintained for stool output, while the efferent limb stoma is connected to the distal bowel without expected output. After dissection of the abdominal wall is performed and the segment of bowel is everted, the enterocutaneous anastomosis is performed. The bowel should appear pink and viable extruding a few centimeters above the skin edge once the ostomy is completed [7].

The ostomy should begin to produce gas and stool within a few days after the operation. Early stoma-related complications include high output, obstruction, and ischemia. A high-output stoma, producing greater than two liters per day, is more common with an ileostomy than a colostomy [8]. Patients should be evaluated for signs of dehydra-

tion, and electrolytes should be regularly monitored during the first few weeks postoperatively. Patients may be started on antimotility agents such as loperamide or opiates such as a tincture of opium to slow gut transit. In addition, medications to reduce stomach acid production or bile acid-binding resins may be helpful in decreasing output [9]. Early obstruction can occur when the fascial incision for the stoma is too small, causing the rectus muscle to contract around the bowel. This is diagnosed clinically by inability to digitalize the ostomy and usually requires reoperation.

Other late complications include peristomal skin irritation due to a poor fitting appliance, peristomal hernia, prolapse, stenosis, and complications related to small bowel obstruction after surgery. Parastomal hernias may be managed conservatively with a belt appliance or repaired surgically with or without mesh, although recurrence rates are high. A prolapsed stoma will be evident by protruding mucosa beyond the usual stoma site and should be easily and gently reduced. If there is edema of the mucosa and a prolapsed stoma appears incarcerated, the use of

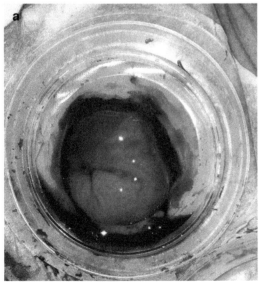 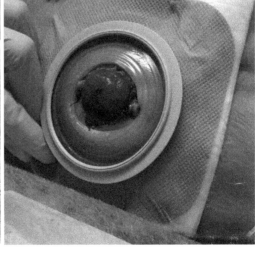

Fig. 13.2 (**a**) Colostomy – sigmoid colon anchored to the abdominal wall, pictured postoperative day one with mild edema and a small hematoma. (**b**) Loop ileostomy – a loop of small bowel has been brought out through an abdominal incision with a red rubber catheter in place; the catheter helps keep the ostomy elevated in the early postoperative course. The larger afferent limb and smaller efferent limb are in the superior and inferior positions, respectively

sugar on the mucosa to draw out excess fluids and allow for reduction has been shown to be effective [10, 11]. Bleeding from the stoma site may occur with minor trauma to the tissue, but bleeding may also be related to parastomal varices. Minor bleeding may be managed with light pressure, although significant bleeding may indicate erosion into a larger vessel and a surgical emergency. Bleeding or mucous discharge from the rectum associated with abdominal or perianal pain after a colostomy may be a sign of diversion colitis. This is treated with short-chain fatty acid enemas and earlier reversal if possible. Bowel obstruction should be suspected if a patient stops producing gas and stool from the ostomy and begins to complain of abdominal pain and bloating. In this case, a CT scan with oral and intravenous contrast should be obtained, and the patient should be prepared for inpatient admission if obstruction is evident. In general, ostomies are reversed no earlier than 3 months after creation or last intra-abdominal surgery.

Nutrition

Because the body is in a hypercatabolic state after trauma, it is important to maintain optimal nutritional support for wound healing and immune function. Non-oral nutrition is recommended if the patient is in a malnourished state at baseline or is expected to be without nutrition for longer than 1 week. Nutritional needs will be determined based on pre-injury nutritional state and stress level. When the gastrointestinal tract is functional and safe to use, enteral nutrition (EN) is preferred over parenteral nutrition (PN). EN is more efficiently utilized by the body due to first-pass metabolism in the liver and helps support the functional integrity of the gut. However, parenteral nutrition may be used when enteral feeding is not tolerated, as with a mechanical bowel obstruction, severe gastrointestinal bleeding, short gut syndrome, or a proximal enterocutaneous or enteroatmospheric fistula [12].

When the patient is unable to tolerate oral feeding, enteral nutrition may be administered through a nasogastric, nasojejunal, gastrostomy, or jejunostomy tube. Generally, nasogastric or nasojejunal tubes are used as a temporary measure until the patient is able to take in oral nutrition, e.g., patients with altered mental status or dysphagia. For patients who are expected to take no oral nutrition for 4 weeks or more, placement of a gastrostomy or jejunostomy tube is recommended [13]. This may include patients with neurological disorders such as stroke or traumatic brain injury, patients presenting after significant trauma, with cancer or recent surgery of the upper gastrointestinal tract [7]. A gastrostomy tube is sufficient for most patients, but a jejunostomy tube is preferred in patients requiring post-pyloric feeding due to injury or gastroparesis (Fig.13.6, Fig 13.7).

Enteral access procedures can be performed in a variety of settings, including at the bedside, in the endoscopy or interventional radiology suite, or in the operating room. The options for long-term feeding tube placement include laparoscopic or open gastrostomy or jejunostomy tube placement, percutaneous endoscopic gastrostomy (PEG) tube placement, and laparoscopic-assisted PEG tube placement (Fig. 13.3a, b). Open or laparoscopic gastrostomy and jejunostomy feeding tubes allow for fixation of the bowel wall to the anterior abdominal wall (see Box for procedure details). While a PEG tube is the preferred method, anatomic considerations may require open or laparoscopic techniques. After the procedure, the tubing is left to drain, and feedings are gradually begun the next day. The tubing should not be changed for 4–8 weeks to allow time for an epithelialized tract to form. When the patient recovers and feeding assistance is no longer needed, the tube can be removed, leaving the tract to granulate and heal.

Nutrition and electrolytes should be assessed while the patient is receiving enteral or parenteral nutrition. Early complications include surgical site bleeding and tube dislodgement, both of which require urgent surgical consultation. If tube dislodgement occurs after the 4 weeks, it can be carefully replaced with a Foley or red rubber catheter and intraluminal placement confirmed with radiologic contrast study.

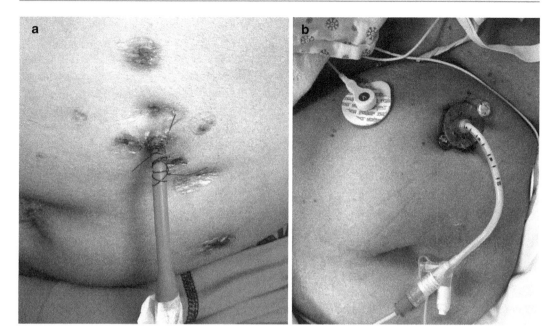

Fig. 13.3 (**a**) Jejunostomy tube – external tubing after a laparoscopic jejunostomy tube placement. (**b**) PEG tube – external tubing from a percutaneous endoscopic gastrostomy tube

Procedure in Details

1. Gastrostomy tube placement – Two concentric purse-string sutures are placed near the greater curvature of the stomach, and a gastrostomy is made in the center. The gastrostomy tubing is advanced through a small skin incision into the gastrostomy site, and the balloon is inflated. The purse-string sutures are tightened, cinching gastric mucosa around the tubing. The stomach is then anchored to the anterior abdominal wall at four points. The gastrostomy tubing is then secured to the skin.

2. Jejunostomy tube placement – The purse-string sutures are placed in an area 30–45 cm distal to the ligament of Treitz. The enterotomy is made on the antimesenteric side of jejunum, and a red rubber tubing is inserted through a small skin incision into the enterotomy.

The purse strings are tightened, and a serosal tunnel of a few centimeters is created around the tube to secure it in place, and the site is then sutured to the abdominal wall with nonabsorbable sutures.

3. PEG tube placement – Endoscopic gastrostomy is performed, and the stomach is insufflated to appose the anterior abdominal wall. A small skin incision is made, and the Seldinger technique is used to percutaneously introduce a needle and wire into the gastric lumen. The wire is grasped with the endoscope and extracted through the patient's oral cavity as the endoscope is removed. The gastrostomy tubing is tied to the wire, which is pulled through the skin incision until the bumper sits just abutting the gastric mucosa. An anchor is placed around the gastric tubing and secured to the skin [3].

Other complications after gastrostomy tube placement include infection or bleeding around the tubing site, "buried bumper" syndrome, ulceration or peristomal leakage, and gastric outlet obstruction [14]. A relatively common feeding tube problem is blockage of the tubing, which occurs more often with jejunostomy tubes. The first step in management is flushing the tube with warm water, carbonated beverages, juices, or an enzymatic solution. If this fails to unclog the tube, mechanical unclogging may be performed at the bedside with an approved device. To prevent blockage, the tubing should be flushed with 15–30 cc of water prior to and after each use, and all medications should be given as liquids or crushed thoroughly prior to administration.

Gastric outlet obstruction may be suspected when a patient complains of abdominal pain and nausea with emesis. In this case, the gastrostomy tube should be placed to gravity to allow stomach contents to drain. There are commercially available gastrostomy–jejunostomy (G–J) tubes so that the jejunostomy tube can be used for feeding, while the gastrostomy tube is used for gastric decompression. "Buried bumper" syndrome occurs when the inner bumper becomes impacted between the gastric wall mucosa and the skin. This may lead to infection or necrosis and can be managed endoscopically or surgically. To help prevent buried bumper syndrome, ulceration, or peristomal leakage, the distance markers along the tubing should be used to ensure that there is not undue tension or too much slack in the appliance. In general, these markings are at 2–3 cm at the skin, but this length can vary depending on the depth of a patient's abdominal wall thickness. Marker placement should be confirmed with the physician performing the tube placement.

Wound Complications

Wound complications after surgery range from a benign seroma to a life-threatening necrotizing fasciitis. A seroma is a clear, yellow fluid composed of liquefied fat, lymphatic drainage, or serous fluid. Procedures with large skin flaps and deep soft tissue pockets, such as axillary or groin dissection, mastectomy, or mesh repair, may be prone to developing seromas. Clinically, this appears as a small, localized swelling near the incision site. A seroma may be left alone, and the body will resorb the fluid, or the collection may be sterilely drained. A pressure dressing and the use of drains can prevent a seroma from recurring [6].

A hematoma is a collection composed of blood rather than serous fluid. Hematomas are more prone to infection and may be caused by inadequate hemostasis, coagulopathy, or trauma to the wound. After a trauma, wounds may be more prone to developing hematomas due to coagulopathy from cellular dysfunction, inflammation, or factor consumption. Unlike seromas, hematomas can expand rapidly in a small compartment leading serious complications, such as airway compromise or abdominal compartment syndrome. In patients with suspected hematomas, a complete blood count, prothrombin time/international normalized ratio, partial thromboplastin time, and type and screen should be assessed. Patients may need to go back to the operating room for exploration and washout of the wound and control of hemostasis [6].

Wound dehiscence is a serious complication following large abdominal procedures with fascial repairs. Abdominal musculoaponeurotic layers separate with concern for impending evisceration of abdominal contents. A patient is most prone to develop wound dehiscence 7–10 days after an operation, and dehiscence may be more likely to occur after an emergent operation in the setting of trauma (Fig. 13.4). Other risk factors include hematoma, infection, technical error, steroid use, obesity, and malnutrition. The classic sign of dehiscence is drainage of clear, salmon-colored fluid from the wound. If wound dehiscence is suspected, the wound should be covered with gauze and the operating team called to the bedside. It is possible to treat a small area of dehiscence with local wound packing. However, if eviscerated intestines are noted, a sterile saline-moistened gauze should be placed over the contents, and the patient should be taken immediately to the operating room for further management [6].

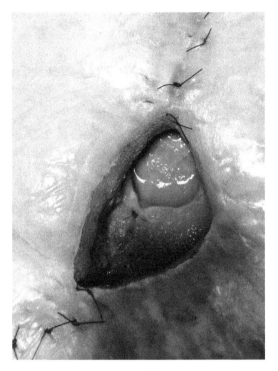

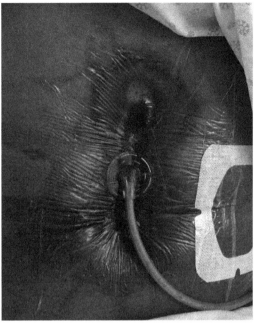

Fig. 13.5 Vacuum-assisted dressing – midline abdominal wound with vacuum dressing to suction

Fig. 13.4 Wound dehiscence – fascial separation with exposed bowel is seen in this midline incision after an open colon resection

Despite efforts by operating room staff and surgeons to reduce the incidence of surgical site infection (SSI), there is a risk for infection after any procedure. In trauma operations, this risk may be higher due to emergent procedures performed in a non-sterile setting. In addition, operations in a trauma setting may already be classified as dirty and more prone to developing SSI. With a scheduled operation, smoking cessation, corticosteroid weaning, proper blood glucose control, and adequate nutrition can help with wound healing, immunity, and prevention of SSI.

Surgical site infections usually present within a week of the operation with erythema, edema, pain, or purulent drainage from the wound. If an SSI is suspected, skin staples or sutures may be removed at the bedside with careful probing of the wound. If cellulitis or systemic signs of infection are present, empiric antibiotics are started. Crepitus, gray dishwater-looking fluid, or rapidly expanding necrosis of the fascial layer indicates necrotizing fasciitis, and emergent surgical debridement should be performed. Any infected wound should be left to heal by secondary intention or delayed primary closure.

Treatment of SSIs requires local wound care after removal of skin staples/sutures. With a small wound, wet-to-dry dressings are applied to assist in debridement of the wound with each dressing change. Gauze dressing is lightly moistened with saline and packed loosely into the wound. Dry gauze dressing is then placed over this to help absorb any excess drainage and prevent the skin from breakdown. When the wound is larger or deeper without signs of active infection, a vacuum-assisted dressing may be beneficial, e.g., KCI V.A.C.® dressing. With this dressing, a sponge is cut to fit the wound cavity and covered by a watertight dressing, allowing continuous negative pressure on the wound (Fig. 13.5). This keeps the outer skin dry with constant evacuation of drainage while promoting angiogenesis and granulation of the wound. Dressing changes occur every 3–5 days, and devices are portable allowing for mobilization and active participation in rehabilitation therapy. In a superficial wound with little drainage, nonstick dressings, like Adaptic® or

Xeroform, may be used to prevent debridement and painful dressing changes while also having antibacterial properties.

Surgical Drains

Surgical drains are used to remove or prevent fluid collections after surgery. Most drains used in surgery are closed drains with tubing connected to a suction device or bag. Active drains are connected to self-suction or wall suction. Passive drains work by means of gravity or pressure differentials. Either type of drain should be stitched in place and the output closely monitored. Drains are very effective but may also be linked to postoperative issues such as infection or inefficient drainage. A sudden increase in amount or character of drainage could be concerning for infection, and a sudden decrease in output could indicate the tubing is clogged. Dressings around drains should be changed daily to prevent surrounding infection.

There are many types of surgical drains. The most commonly used systems are Jackson-Pratt (JP), Blake®, Penrose, and pigtail drains. JP drains are under continuous self-suction with a low-negative-pressure system. They are most commonly used because they contain small fenestrations, preventing intra-abdominal contents from being sucked into the tubing. Uncapping the plug, squeezing the air out of the bulb, and recapping it create suction. When output is sufficiently decreased, removal of the drain requires uncapping the plug to release suction, cutting the suture at the skin level, and slowly withdrawing the tubing.

Blake® drains are connected to a similar suction bulb, but they have a large-diameter single-hole suction at the end of the drain. Penrose drains are a soft rubber tubing which is sutured in a wound to allow passive drainage [15]. These can be slowly withdrawn over time or pulled when the drainage is significantly decreased. Pigtail drains are long thin catheters with locking fenestrated tips, which curl once inserted. Pigtail drains are always placed, usually by interventional radiologists, in order to reach small cavities or lumens. In order to remove the pigtail catheter, the string on the outside must be cut to release the curl of the inner catheter and allow for a smooth withdrawal. If at any time a drain is unintentionally removed, the managing surgeon should be notified.

Fig. 13.6 Gastrostomy feeding tube

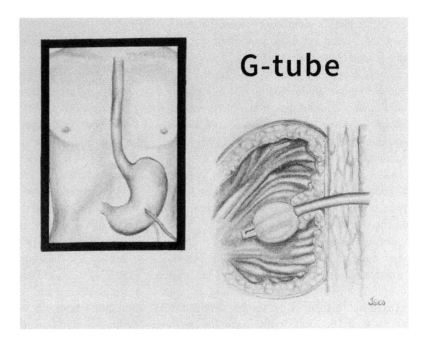

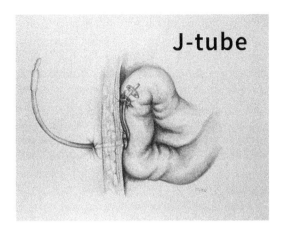

J-tube

Fig. 13.7 Jejunostomy feeding tube

Compartment Syndrome

Compartment syndrome is a consequence of increased pressure in a confined space, limiting blood flow and leading to ischemia of vital tissue. The sequelae can be devastating if not diagnosed in a timely manner. Compartment syndrome most commonly presents after fracture of an extremity, but it may present after blunt trauma, arterial injury, reperfusion injury, prolonged malpositioning, and crush or burn injury. It can also present very late after a patient's injury if a cast is ill-fitting.

The symptoms of compartment syndrome are pain, pallor, paresthesias, pulselessness, paralysis, and poikilothermia (coolness on palpation). If the extremity or compartment feels tense or the patient complains of tenderness upon palpation or with passive movement, there should be concern for impending compartment syndrome. Sensory deficits may be present early on, while pulselessness and pallor are very late findings. Generally, compartment pressures greater than 30 mmHg are considered concerning for compartment syndrome and require fasciotomy to prevent permanent muscle and nerve damage. There are many needle and catheter devices to measure compartment pressures, but these may not be necessary once a clinical diagnosis is made.

The treatment for compartment syndrome is fasciotomy, and the techniques vary based on the extremity involved. The goal of fasciotomy is to open up the fascial layer in all compartments to relieve the underlying built-up pressure. In the lower extremity, a four-compartment fasciotomy usually involves a single- or double-incision technique to release the anterior, lateral, deep posterior, and superficial posterior compartments [16]. The incisions are left open, and viability of the muscles and tissues are determined in the coming days. Wet-to-dry dressings are applied during this time, and the patient is brought back to the operating room for debridement after a couple of days. Delayed primary closure, split-thickness skin grafting, and healing by secondary intension are all options for closure of the fasciotomy wounds. Rotational flaps may also be necessary to cover vital structures prior to skin closure. When the wound is left to heal by secondary intention, wound vacuum devices may be used to assist in wound healing. If compartment syndrome is diagnosed and treated in a timely manner, usually within the first six hours, the extremity should heal and regain full function.

Tracheostomy

Many studies have looked at benefits of early tracheostomy within 4 days of admission compared to late tracheostomy in critically ill patients. Data has not shown a significant difference in 30-day mortality or secondary outcomes, including length of sedation, antibiotic use, or time in the intensive care unit [17]. However, many practitioners believe early tracheostomy in patients requiring long-term mechanical ventilation does have clinical benefits.

Indications for tracheostomy placement include ventilator dependence, airway obstruction from angioedema, burns, traumatic obstruction, neoplasm, laryngeal dysfunction, neck irradiation, or neurologic injury inhibiting a patient from protecting his/her airway [18]. The expected length of time a patient will require intubation is often the determining factor for performing tracheostomy. Frequently, a tracheostomy is performed within 7 days of intubation if the expected time of intubation is greater than 2 weeks. Some advantages to a tracheostomy are increased patient comfort, decreased need for ventilator dependence, and decreased risk of subglottic or laryngeal stenosis compared to intubation. There are few contraindications to performing a tracheostomy, but surrounding infection or distorted anatomy may increase the risk of the procedure [19].

A tracheostomy can be performed via open or percutaneous technique. A 2–3-cm incision is made about 2 cm above the sternal notch while the patient's neck is extended. When performed percutaneously, the Seldinger technique is applied. In this technique, a needle is used to access the trachea, a guidewire is then passed through the needle, and serial dilations are performed until a tracheostomy tube can be advanced over the wire. In an open technique, the platysma and strap muscles are dissected and divided to directly visualize the trachea, an incision is made between the second and fourth tracheal rings, and a tracheostomy appliance is inserted [19].

One of the most concerning complications after tracheostomy is accidental decannulation of the tracheostomy tube within the first week, before the tract has epithelialized. If this occurs, the patient should be placed in a recumbent position with a bump under the neck to keep the airway open, while supplies for re-cannulation are obtained. For this reason, spare supplies should always be kept at the patient's bedside. Other early complications include surgical site bleeding and obstruction of the inner cannula. For surgical site bleeding, the primary surgical team should be notified, while suctioning is performed and pressure applied. If the inner cannula is obstructed, it should be removed, while the patient is oxygenated and ventilated through the tracheostomy.

Other complications of tracheostomy include stoma site infection or stricture from ischemic necrosis at the cuff site, due to high cuff pressures or an oversized tube. Stridor, wheezing, or signs of airway obstruction may indicate tracheomalacia, where the airway collapses on expiration leading to air trapping, retained secretions, recurrent infection, or respiratory failure. Tracheoesophageal fistula is a rare complication of tracheostomy associated with high cuff pressures or simultaneous nasogastric tube placement, which can be diagnosed by CT scan or barium swallow. An even rarer complication, tracheo-innominate fistula, may occur within the first few weeks of placement after a low tracheostomy incision. It should be suspected if a pulsating tube or small bleed is evident, and the cuff should be inflated or a finger placed into the stoma to occlude the bleeding site against the sternum [20, 21].

When a patient without upper airway obstruction no longer requires mechanical ventilation or frequent pulmonary toilet, the patient is likely ready for decannulation. A capping trial may be performed for 24 h prior to decannulation, while oxygen saturation and breathing are monitored. After decannulation, the patient should be monitored for another 24 h, while the stoma site is covered with an occlusive dressing and left to heal.

Acute Abdomen in Spinal Cord Injury Patients

Diagnosis of an acute surgical abdomen relies on clinical exam, which is difficult in patients with spinal cord injury (SCI), especially those with high-level injury or complete transection. Severe pain, tenderness, rebound, and fever may all be absent in these patients, delaying diagnosis and management. Some signs of an acute abdominal injury in SCI patients include autonomic dysreflexia and referred shoulder pain due to irritation of the diaphragm. Abdominal distention is still very important to monitor, and increased distension with or without rigidity, nausea, or vomiting may be the only sign of a concerning intraabdominal process in these patients. While autonomic dysreflexia is a common response to noxious stimuli in SCI patients, it should be a warning sign in those patients with concern for abdominal injury after trauma or bowel perforation from chronic constipation or stress ulcers after a long, immobile hospitalization [22].

In a study looking at paraplegic or quadriplegic patients, it was determined that the correct diagnosis was made 77 % of the time by radiologic studies rather than history and physical exam. The most common presenting signs or symptoms were abdominal pain in the low-cord lesion patients, abdominal distension, shoulder pain, fever, and less commonly autonomic dysreflexia with hypertension, headaches, diaphoresis, and arrhythmias. The most common diagnoses were biliary-associated infections (e.g., acute cholecystitis), perforated ulcers, renal diseases, and other gastrointestinal pathology. It is recommended that an abdominal plain film is obtained as an initial diagnostic test, followed by an ultrasound to evaluate the hepatobiliary system or any obvious abscesses, and a CT scan if necessary thereafter. A low threshold to obtain imaging or take the patient for a diagnostic laparoscopy should be maintained in SCI patients [23].

Although spinal cord injury patients may suffer from constipation, impaction was noted to be a less common cause of acute abdomen in these patients. In any patient with a history of constipation presenting with an acute abdomen, the diagnosis of stercoral colitis should not be overlooked. In general, these patients present with severe constipation and an inflammatory process, often progressing to septic shock. The diagnosis is made on CT scan with evidence of a large fecaloma and proximal colonic dilatation. Wall thickening and fat stranding are often present with this diagnosis, and mortality rates are high even with prompt diagnosis. A low threshold to obtain a CT scan should be maintained if stercoral colitis is suspected [24].

Summary

After traumatic injury or surgery, patients may require continued care and rehabilitation despite completion of acute medical care. Postoperative nutrition, wound care, and prevention of infection and procedural complications need to be monitored during this transition of care where patients are working to regain function and mobility. It is important for practitioners to have an understanding of the needs of these patients and potential complications that may arise under their care.

- In an unstable patient, initial damage control laparotomy may be necessary, where the abdomen is left open with a vacuum dressing and closed at the next operation or weeks later with the use of split-thickness skin grafts. Despite having a large ventral hernia, patients can maintain a functional lifestyle.
- Enterocutaneous or enteroatmospheric fistulas may arise after surgery or from an inflammatory process. It is important to maintain adequate nutrition and decrease fistula output while awaiting spontaneous or operative closure.
- Patients with ostomies should be monitored for adequate fluid intake and nutrition, in addition to signs of possible complications including obstruction, hernia, high output, or prolapse.
- Maintaining adequate nutrition is very important in any injured or postoperative patient. Enteral nutrition is generally preferred and can be given through nasogastric, gastrostomy, or jejunostomy tubes, when oral intake is inadequate.
- Wound infection, dehiscence, or evisceration can be a devastating complication after surgery. Other wound complications such as a hematoma or seroma may require operative drainage if infection or compression of surrounding structures occurs.
- Surgical drains are used to prevent fluid collections, which may be prone to infection. Jackson-Pratt and Blake drains are most commonly used to allow for continuous suction, although Penrose drains may be placed for passive drainage from superficial spaces.
- Compartment syndrome most commonly occurs in the extremities after trauma or ischemia or in the abdomen with significant edema. A high index of suspicion is key to diagnosis, and prompt operative treatment is required.
- In patients requiring prolonged respiratory support, there are many advantages to a tracheostomy. Patients with a tracheostomy should be monitored for accidental decannula-

tion and respiratory compromise, bleeding, obstruction, or airway stenosis.

- In the patient with spinal cord injury, an acute abdomen may present with findings other than abdominal pain, such as shoulder pain or autonomic dysreflexia. A low threshold for imaging and diagnostic laparoscopy should be maintained in these patients.

References

1. Centers for Disease Control and Prevention, National Center for Injury Prevention and Control. Web-based Injury Statistics Query and Reporting System (WISQARS) [online]. (2016) [cited Year Month (abbreviated) Day]. Available from URL: www.cdc.gov/injury/wisqars
2. Pape H. Damage control management in the polytrauma patient. New York: Springer; 2010.
3. Godat L, Kobayashi L, Costantini T, Coimbra R. Abdominal damage control surgery and reconstruction: world society of emergency surgery position paper. World J Emerg Surg. 2013;8:53.
4. Galie KL, Whitlow CB. Postoperative enterocutaneous fistula: when to reoperate and how to succeed. Clin Colon Rectal Surg. 2006;19:237–46.
5. Pritts TA, Fischer DR, Fischer JE. Postoperative enterocutaneous fistula. In: Holzheimer RG, Mannick JA, editors. Surgical Treatment: evidence-based and problem-oriented. Munich: Zuckschwerdt; 2001.
6. Sabiston D, Townsend C. Sabiston textbook of surgery. Philadelphia: Elsevier Saunders; 2012.
7. Fischer JE, Jones DB, Pomposelli FB, Upchurch Jr GR. Fischer's mastery of surgery. 6th ed. Philadelphia: Lippincott Williams & Wilkins; 2011.
8. Bafford AC, Irani JL. Management and complications of stomas. Surg Clin North Am. 2013;93:145–66.
9. Steele SR. Complications, considerations and consequences of colorectal surgery. Surg Clin North Am. 2013;93:xv–xvi.
10. Husain SG, Cataldo TE. Late stomal complications. Clin Colon Rectal Surg. 2008;21:31–40.
11. Kwiatt M, Kawata M. Avoidance and management of stomal complications. Clin Colon Rectal Surg. 2013;26:112–21.
12. Wilson WGC, Hoyt D. Trauma. Hoboken: Taylor and Francis; 2013.
13. Cresci G. Nutrition support for the critically ill patient: a guide to practice. Francis T, editor. Boca Raton: Taylor & Francis; 2005.
14. Lynch C, Fang J. Nutrition issues in gastroenterology: prevention and management of complications of Percutaneous Endoscopic Gastrostomy (PEG) tubes. Pract Gastroenterol. 2004;22:66–76.
15. Beattie S. Surgical drains: modern medicine network. 2006 [cited 2015].
16. Granchi TS. Chapter 66 – Compartment syndromes. In: Trunkey JAAD, editor. Current therapy of trauma and surgical critical care. Philadelphia: Mosby; 2008. p. 489–96.
17. Young D, Harrison DA, Cuthbertson BH, Rowan K, TracMan C. Effect of early vs late tracheostomy placement on survival in patients receiving mechanical ventilation the TracMan randomized trial. JAMA-J Am Med Assoc. 2013;309:2121–9.
18. Freeman B. In: Vincent JL, editor. Indications for and management of tracheostomy by Freeman, BD. Elsevier. Philadelphia, PA. Textbook of critical care. 6th ed. 2011. p. 369–72.
19. Cameron JL, Cameron AM. Current surgical therapy. 11th ed. Philadelphia: Elsevier Saunders; 2011.
20. Morris LL, Whitmer A, McIntosh E. Tracheostomy care and complications in the intensive care unit. Crit Care Nurse. 2013;33:18–31.
21. Epstein SK. Late complications of tracheostomy. Respir Care. 2005;50:542–9.
22. Bar-On Z, Ohry A. The acute abdomen in spinal cord injury individuals. Paraplegia. 1995;33:704–6.
23. Neumayer LA, Bull DA, Mohr JD, Putnam CW. The acutely affected abdomen in paraplegic spinal cord injury patients. Ann Surg. 1990;212:561–6.
24. Saksonov M, Bachar GN, Morgenstern S, Zeina AR, Vasserman M, Protnoy O, et al. Stercoral colitis: a lethal disease-computed tomographic findings and clinical characteristic. J Comput Assist Tomogr. 2014;38:721–6.

Surgical Reconstruction of Pressure Ulcers

14

Tushar Patel, Eric G. Wimmers, Matthew Pontell, and Adam Saad

Introduction

Terminology

In its most basic terms, pressure sores are injuries to the skin and underlying tissue resulting from prolonged pressure on the skin. Pressure sores result from pressure breakdown in areas that bear seated weight, such as ischial tuberosities of spinal injury patients, and in areas with pressure due to devices, such as splints, ear probes, or rectal tubes. Decubitus ulcers occur over areas that have underlying bony prominences when the individual is recumbent, e.g., the sacrum, trochanter, heel, and occiput. Pressure is the most likely cause among many other factors that contribute to the development of pressure sores and hence is the most important etiologic factor.

Pressure sores do not only occur in the elderly or in people who are getting poor care. A pressure ulcer can happen to anyone who is in some sort of debilitated state. Unfortunately, healthcare providers may not aggressively evaluate patients routinely for pressure ulcers, which may be found incidentally while treating something else. Physical therapists tend to spend a lot of time with their patients. In a rehab or skilled nursing setting, a therapist may be with the patient for 1–2 h a day. A therapist might catch a glimpse of a pressure sore on a patient's sacrum while walking them to the bathroom. A pressure sore on the heel may be noticed while a therapist puts socks on their patient for ambulation. It is important to remember, even if you are not treating the wound or the pressure ulcer yourself, you might be the one to find it.

Epidemiology

A broad inquiry reviewing over 400,000 records from a survey between 1989 and 2005 found overall rates between 9.2 % in 1989 and 15.5 % in 2004 [1]. Rates were higher in long-term acute care facilities, at 27.3 % [2–4]. Overall, pressure ulcer prevalence appears relatively stable despite significant advances in treatment and prevention. Particular populations have been identified at higher risks. Hip fracture patients are at particularly higher risk for pressure sores ranging from 8.8 to 55 % [5–9]. Spinal cord injury (SCI) patients are also at particular risk for pressure sores due to the combination of immobility and insensitivity with reported rates between 33 and 60 % leading to the second leading cause of rehospitalization in these patients [10–15].

T. Patel, MD (✉) • E.G. Wimmers, MD • A. Saad, MD
The Plastic Surgery Center, Institute for Advanced Reconstruction, 535 Sycamore Ave, Shrewsbury, NJ 07702, USA
e-mail: tpatelmd@theplasticsurgerycenternj.com; ewimmersmd@theplasticsurgerycenternj.com; asaadmd@theplasticsurgerycenternj.com

M. Pontell, MD
Department of Surgery, Drexel University College of Medicine, Philadelphia, PA 19102, USA

© Springer International Publishing Switzerland 2017
A.I. Elkwood et al. (eds.), *Rehabilitative Surgery*, DOI 10.1007/978-3-319-41406-5_14

Economic Burden

Pressure sores are a costly problem for the health-care system. Direct cost calculations are difficult to perform due to inflation and the variability in admitted patients with pressure sores with ulcer-related problems. It is often difficult to separate out costs associated with the ulcer itself from other related expenses from concomitant mor-bidities. The Institute for Healthcare Improvement estimated the costs of managing pressure sores at nursing homes and healthcare facilities at 11 bil-lion dollars in 2006. The National Pressure Ulcer Advisory Panel (NPUAP) [16] has estimated the cost to treat hospital-acquired pressure sores to be $100,000 per patient.

Patients with pressure sores are generally inpatients three times longer than patients with-out a pressure sore. Patients with pressure sores as a primary diagnosis cost an average of $1200/day, while patients with pressure sores as a sec-ondary diagnosis cost an average of $1600/day. Mean cost per hospitalization are $16,800 and $20,400 for stays with a principal and secondary diagnosis of pressure sore, versus only $9900 for all other conditions [17].

Pathophysiology

Anatomic Distribution

In Meehan's 1994 review of 3487 patients with 6047 pressure sores, the most common site of occurrence was the sacrum (36 %), followed by the heel (30 %) [18]. In the acute phase of SCI, the sacral area seems to be the most common site of pressure sores [19]. In the chronic phase after SCI, the ischial area becomes the most predomi-nant site of pressure sores as patients begin to sit up in wheelchairs during their rehabilitation. In those individuals who use a wheelchair, pressure sores often occur on the skin over many sites. The tailbone/buttocks, shoulder blades/spine, and backs of arms/legs are all common areas as the patient rests against the chair. In individuals who are confined to a bed, common sites include the back/sides of the head, rim of the ears, shoulders/ shoulder blades, hip/lower back and the heels, and the ankles and skin behind the knees.

Basic Science

Pressure

Pressure ulcers are thought to result from pres-sure applied to soft tissue at a level higher than that found in the blood vessels supplying that area for an extended period of time [20]. Simply applying pressure in excess to an area will not always create an ulcer. Autoregulation of local blood flow will tend to increase blood pressure in response to increased applied pressure [21–23]. Dinsdale quantified the degree of pressure neces-sary to cause tissue damage as roughly double capillary closing pressure, applied for 2 h, to cause irreversible tissue damage [24]. Various tis-sues also have different susceptibilities to pres-sure. Pressure on the skin over a bone is more susceptible to injury than the skin over muscle [25–29] (Table 14.1).

Friction

Friction is the force resisting relative motion between two surfaces, which leads to shear. Friction develops between the patient's skin and contact surfaces, such as clothes, bedding, trans-port equipment, orthotics, wheelchairs, and other appliances. When friction is excessive, superficial skin injuries such as blisters and abrasions develop [30, 31]. Skin breakdown leads to transepidermal water losses and ultimately allows moisture to accumulate. Moisture promotes skin adherence to sheets and other contact surfaces [32].

Shear

Subcutaneous tissue lacks tensile strength and is easily susceptible to shear stress [33, 34]. Patient

Table 14.1 Changes at pressure > 32 mmHg

Time	Changes
30 min	Hyperemia
2–6 h	Ischemia
6 h	Necrosis
2 weeks	Ulceration

transfers, sliding, dragging, and the boosting of patients in bed all cause significant shear. Positions such as the semi-Fowler's or beach chair position as well as an individual sliding down a wheelchair create significant shear over the lower back and buttocks [35, 36].

Moisture

Excessive moisture leads to skin maceration and excoriation and is a risk factor for pressure sore development [37–39]. Incontinence is of particular concern in developing sores [40–42]. Urinary and fecal incontinence are common in the elderly, with even higher rates in institutionalized patients [43, 44].

Malnutrition

There is a strong correlation between malnutrition and pressure sores without any clear direct link [45]. Chronically ill patients with protein malnutrition typically have weight loss, poor wound healing, and immunosuppression, which correlate to increased susceptibility and definitive delayed healing of pressure sores [46–54].

Neurological Injury

Pressure sores are the most common complication and the second most common cause of hospitalization in spinal cord injury (SCI) patients [55–57]. Immobility in the bed or wheelchair causes increased pressure, friction, and shear with eventual pressure sore development. The lack of protective sensation in SCI patients leads to pressure sore development. Patients are unable to maneuver their bodies to off-load prolonged areas of direct pressure. Other causes frequent in this population for pressure sore development include incontinence, spasticity, and psychosocial issues [58, 59].

Prevention

As healthcare moves toward non-reimbursement for hospital-acquired pressure ulcers, there is increasing incentive to prevent these lesions. Although there have been numerous recommendations and studies, the overall incidence of pres-

sure ulcers is unchanged [3, 60]. Although there is no strategy that reduces the incidence to zero, there are several interventions that are now part of standard care, which contribute to the prevention of pressure ulcers [44].

Skin Care

Optimal skin care includes cleaning, hydrating, and protecting. Both nurses and physicians tend to neglect this time and labor-intensive care modality [61]. Most recommendations involve utilizing soap and water followed by rubbing or drying. The surfactants found in soaps, while effective in removing debris, can have a negative effect due to the chemical irritants [62]. The skin has a natural protective acidity that is counteracted by the alkaline nature of most soaps; this can result in a disturbance of the skin flora balance. Multiple alternate cleansers have been marketed to address the problems with soap and water; however, little data exist at this time to recommend any particular product [63].

The benefits of proper skin hydration are established, yet few data recommend any one hydrating product over another [43, 64–66]. The typical method in obtaining skin hydration is through the use of emollients, which occlude the skin surface with a hydrophobic layer. In addition, humectants can be instituted, which act by attracting water from the surrounding environment.

Barrier products protect the skin in the setting of fistulas, stomas, wounds, or incontinence. Traditional products create a protective film over the skin due to the liquid emulsion component. There are recent advances in barrier preparations utilizing a polymer which forms a thin semipermeable membrane over the skin [67]. Despite the widespread use and the proliferation of products, there is scant data on their effectiveness [68]. Although the data on individual agents is lacking, there is evidence that a clear skin care protocol can benefit patients. Cole and Nesbitt found a reduction from 17.8 to 2 % over a 3-year period, whereas Lyder et al. noted an 87 % reduction in a nursing home setting [69, 70].

Incontinence

The relationship between urinary incontinence and pressure sore incidence is not clear, with limited evidence to demonstrate a causal relationship. The use of diapers and sanitary pads in conjunction with skin care is a better option when compared to the risks associated with extended use of a urinary catheter [71].

On the other hand, fecal incontinence is shown to be a risk factor for pressure sores. The etiology of fecal incontinence is sometimes difficult to correct, such as cognitive impairment, radiation injury, inflammatory bowel disease, or sphincter dysfunction. Conservative measures include diet modification and a wide variety of antimotility agents. Diarrhea may be due to infection, which should be ruled out and treated prior to using antidiarrheal agents. If medical management is unsuccessful, surgery may be considered, ranging from attempts at sphincteroplasty to elective colostomy [72, 73]. Although most patients are reluctant to consider an elective diverting colostomy, there is evidence of improved quality of life in patients with severe fecal incontinence [73].

Spasticity

The impact of spasticity on quality of life is not straightforward. Spasticity has been shown to increase the risk of pressure sores and impair the ability to perform activities of daily living (ADL) [74]. In contrast, some cases of spasticity may increase stability in positioning and even facilitate transfers and ADLs and prevent osteopenia [75, 76].

Physical therapy is the first intervention in treating spasticity. Pharmacologic modulation is the next step. The various agents (diazepam, baclofen, clonidine, gabapentin) each have potential for adverse effects [77]. The side effects include sedation, nausea, diarrhea, muscle weakness, and cognitive impairment. Baclofen may also be delivered directly into the central nervous system (intrathecal administration). This route reduces the systemic side effects but introduces possible complications such as pump malfunction [78]. Another method to control spasticity is injection with chemodenervation agents such as ethanol or botulinum. Although the effects are temporary, long-term use of chemodenervation agents will result in denervation atrophy [79, 80].

Surgical intervention may be considered in refractory cases. Local tenotomy or tendon transfer has had mixed results in the treatment of spasticity [81]. Rhizotomy has been complicated by both inadequate treatment of spasticity and severe atrophy, depending on the technique employed [82]. These neurosurgical techniques may be of benefit but usually don't have prevention of pressure sores as their primary indication.

Pressure Relief

Extensive efforts have been made in pressure modulation, as this is the primary etiology of pressure ulcer pathogenesis. There are various surfaces and products, as well as protocols that direct patient positioning. The support surfaces and devices can be categorized as either constant low-pressure (CLP) devices or alternating-pressure (AP) devices. CLP devices distribute pressure over a large area to reduce the focal impact pressure in any specific area. They include static air, water, gel, bead, silicone, foam, and sheepskin supports. AP devices vary the pressure under the patient to avoid prolonged pressure at a specific anatomic point [83].

The two types of CLP devices that are most commonly used are low air loss (LAL) beds and air-fluidized (AF) beds. The LAL beds float the patient on air-filled cells that circulated warm air, which equalized the pressure and keeps the skin dry. These devices, when used properly, exert a maximum of 25 mmHg on any body part [84, 85]. AF devices work by circulating warm air through fine ceramic beads, creating a drying effect similar to LAL beds. The AF devices boast less than 20 mmHg pressure exerted on the patients; however, they are heavy and expensive [86].

Considerable evidence exists that the use of constant low-pressure overlays or sheepskin significantly decreases the incidence of pressure-related sores, when compared to standard hospital foam mattress [87–91]. Though several studies have compared CLP and AP devices, no clear advantage has been identified, despite attempts at pooled analysis [92].

Cushions for wheelchairs present a unique problem in that the typical wheelchair sling seat exerts a "hammocking" effect that can produce abnormal posture, leading to asymmetric pressure on the trochanter and ischium. Rigid-base cushions provide lumbar support and decrease ischial pressure by allowing wider weight distribution on the posterior thighs [93].

The development of pressure consciousness by the patient is essential in preventing pressure ulcers [94]. Release maneuvers should be performed every 15 min while the patient is seated.

Nutrition

Although limited evidence-based research is available, general consensus indicates that nutrition is an important aspect of a comprehensive care plan for prevention and treatment of pressure ulcers, and it is essential to address nutrition in every individual with pressure ulcers [95]. The body requires adequate calories, protein, fluids, vitamins, and minerals to maintain tissue integrity and prevent tissue breakdown. Little specific evidence exists related to medical nutrition therapy for preventing pressure ulcers [96, 97]. However, early nutrition screening and assessment are essential to identify risk of undernutrition and unintentional weight loss, which may precipitate pressure ulcer development and delay healing.

Diagnosis and Evaluation

Classification

The most commonly used system used for pressure sore classification is the NPUAP staging system [98]. Two recent additions to the staging classification are suspected deep tissue injury and unstageable [98, 99]. Pressure sores fall into one of the four stages based on their severity. The National Pressure Ulcer Advisory Panel (NPUAP), a professional organization that promotes the prevention and treatment of pressure ulcers, defines each stage as follows:

- Stage I: The beginning stage of a pressure sore where the skin is not broken but appears discolored (non-blanching erythema of the skin).
- Stage II: The outer layer of the skin (epidermis) and part of the underlying layer of the skin (dermis) are damaged or lost.
- Stage III: The sore is a deep wound where the skin is lost with exposed fat and appears crater-like.
- Stage IV: The sore shows large-scale loss of tissue with possible exposed muscle, bone, or tendons often with dead tissue at the bottom.

Patient Evaluation

A wide variety of factors must be considered when evaluating a new patient with a pressure sore. A thorough history and physical are imperative with meticulous examination of the wound and the patient. The wound history should include wound onset, duration, prior treatments, and current wound care regimens being used. The physical examination requires measurement in three dimensions, along with evaluating for tunneling or undermining [100]. The characteristics of the wound edges for eschar, slough, or necrotic tissue should be examined as well. If necrotic tissue is present, especially at the base, it should be debrided so accurate assessment of the base depth with exposed muscle, tendon, or bone can be determined.

In addition to a thorough history and physical, patient risk factors should also be assessed. The patient's local environment can provide substantial insight into sources of friction, moisture, shear, and pressure. Spasticity if present, especially in the SCI patient, may need to be controlled medically or surgically. Nutrition should also be assessed with evaluation of serum albumin and prealbumin along with having a good understanding of the patient comorbidities such as diabetes, hypertension, or cardiac disease [101].

Osteomyelitis

Unrecognized osteomyelitis is a major source of morbidity and increased cost due to lengthier hospital stays [102, 103]. Erythrocyte sedimentation rate (ESR) and C-reactive protein levels along with a surgical bone biopsy can help in diagnosing and following progression of wound osteomyelitis [104–110]. MRI appears to be most accurate and is noninvasive while providing detailed anatomic information in regard to the ulcer [111, 112]. Bone biopsy also has consistent accuracy and assists in determining length of antibiotic therapy [113–115].

Surgical Management of Pressure Ulcers

The management of pressure ulcers is largely focused on preventative measures. Early identification and elimination of risk factors are paramount in arresting ulcer progression. Failure of nonoperative intervention is often associated with the development of large, advanced stage, recalcitrant ulcers [116]. It is at this stage that the plastic surgeon is often consulted to evaluate the patient for wound reconstruction.

The basic rules of pressure sore reconstruction are as follows. The ulcer, surrounding scar tissue, and encompassing bursa should be completely excised along with any associated calcified tissue. Underlying necrotic bone and associated heterotopic ossification should also be excised. During the reconstructive process, remaining bony appendages should be padded, and dead space should be resurfaced. The donor site should also be addressed, and occasionally additional grafts are required to ensure flap donor site healing. In general, the flaps should be comprised of a generous amount of tissue, and suture lines should be placed away from areas that are subject to high pressures. Some authors advocate for muscle-sparing flaps to preserve functionality in

patients who remain ambulatory [116]. If possible, the initial flap harvest should not encroach on other potential donor sites, as recurrence rates are high despite even the most meticulous reconstruction [117].

Reconstructive Concepts

Surgical debridement is a quintessential step in the reconstructive process and, as such, deserves special recognition. Debridement begins with identifying the extent of the connective tissue bursa that encompasses the wound. This can be done simply by dissection and observation or with the assistance of methylene blue application. The wound appearance is often misleading as these connective tissue shells are frequently much larger than they appear on primary examination. Appropriate excision must include the entire bursa along with any other scar tissue or heterotopic ossification. Tissue should be excised down to a healthy, pliable bed, and when bony involvement is present, debridement should be carried down to healthy, hard, bleeding bone. The importance of adequate debridement cannot be stressed enough. It is the first step in creating a suitable recipient site for tissue transfer, and inadequate debridement is a common cause of flap failure [116].

After adequate debridement to healthy tissue, an appropriate operative approach must be selected. The analysis begins by exploring the different types of tissue transfer available. Isolated muscle flaps offer several theoretical advantages including increased bulk, rich vascular network, and the opportunity for a single-stage reconstructive procedure [117–119]. Animal model studies have also shown that the interposition of muscle between the skin and bone may disperse pressure and decrease the ulceration incidence [28]. However, other studies suggest that muscle flaps carry an increased risk of ischemic necrosis that may not be evident due to intact overlying skin [25, 120]. Despite these theoretical advantages, the success of muscle flaps is not largely proven in the scientific literature, and their indications remain poorly defined [121]. Musculocutaneous flaps, on the other hand, have shown promising results in preventing the vertical spread of underlying osteomyelitis when compared with random skin flaps and are commonly performed [122].

Perforator flaps are also commonly used for pressure sore reconstruction. These flaps generally involve isolating a fasciocutaneous segment and its associated vascular pedicle for transposition. These flaps maintain a rich vascular supply and also spare the underlying muscle, potentially preserving functionality in some patients while also preserving another possible donor site [123, 124]. Free flaps involve transposing a tissue unit and its associated vascular supply to a site distant from the initial harvest. They are not commonly used in pressure ulcer reconstruction [125–128]. The tensor fasciae latae flap (TFL) is frequently selected for free flap transfer. Surgeons have begun to explore the utility of the plantar free flap, which offers the advantage of being harvested from a purposed weight-bearing surface. This flap may prove useful especially in paraplegic patients who no longer bear weight on their lower extremities [116].

Another important concept in pressure sore reconstruction is tissue expansion. Expanders offer the advantage of increasing the size of sensate skin that can be advanced. This is particularly useful in spinal cord injury patients, with the hopes that sensate skin will prompt pressure avoidance behavior modifications [129–131]. Tensor fasciae latae and lumbosacral fasciocutaneous flaps are two types of flaps amenable to expansion, and their donor sites can often be closed primarily [132]. The disadvantages to tissue expansion involve placing a foreign body in a chronically infected wound, which theoretically creates a nidus for infection to continue to develop. As such, the primary indication for tissue expansion is to allow for sensate coverage of shallow ulcers that require minimal dead space filling, if any at all.

Reconstruction by Anatomic Region

Sacrum

There exists a multitude of options for sacral wound reconstruction, including but not limited to wide undermining and primary closure, random skin flaps, pedicle island flaps, free flaps, gluteus myoplasty, and selected advancement flaps [117, 123, 133]. The most frequently described techniques are the musculocutaneous rotation and advancement flaps, which are based on the gluteus maximus [134]. These flaps are often advanced using V-Y technique and harvest the superior aspect of the gluteus muscle in an attempt to preserve as much muscular function as possible (Fig. 14.1). Other reported techniques include gluteal artery perforator flaps, multi-island propeller flaps, and flaps harvested from the thoracolumbar region [135–138] (Figs. 14.2 and 14.3).

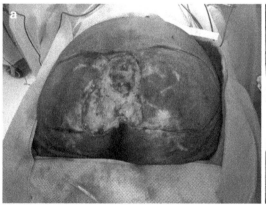
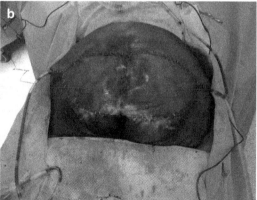
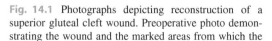

Fig. 14.1 Photographs depicting reconstruction of a superior gluteal cleft wound. Preoperative photo demonstrating the wound and the marked areas from which the flaps will be harvested (**a**). Postoperative photo demonstrating the end result of bilateral superior gluteal fasciocutaneous V-Y advancement flaps (**b**)

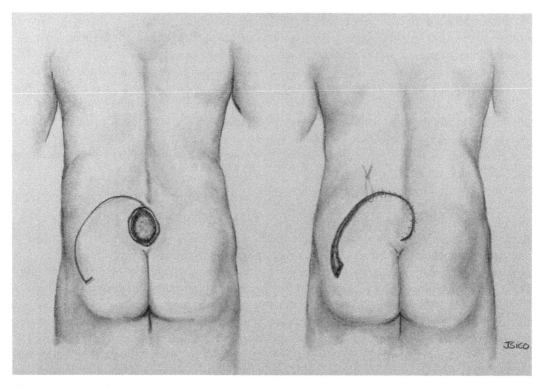

Fig. 14.2 Sacral ulcer reconstruction with rotational gluteal flap

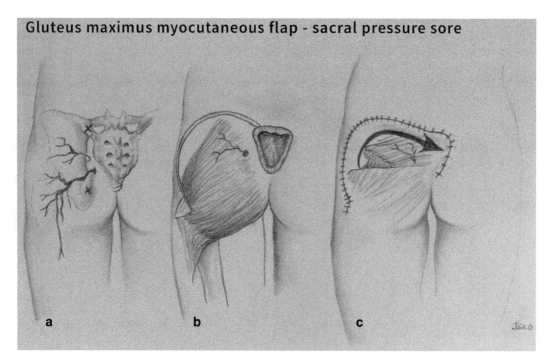

Fig. 14.3 (**a**) Vascular supply to the gluteal musculocutaneous flap. (**b**) Superior gluteal artery is preserved and rotated with the flap. (**c**) The flap is elevated and rotated medially to cover the sacral wound

Midline Defects

Lumbar perforator flaps afford an easy transposition for low posterior midline defect coverage and spare the muscles of the lower extremities. Technical advantages include a large arc of rotation, and the donor site can be closed in primary fashion [139]. Studies report no recurrence and preserved sensation at 1.5 years using innervation-sparing bilateral fasciocutaneous and myocutaneous V-Y advancement perforator flaps for large sacral wounds [140].

Ischium

Ischial ulcers are frequently reconstructed by means of a posterior V-Y advancement flap based on the biceps femoris of hamstring muscles. The biceps advancement flap is preferred in ambulatory patients and has the most successful documented outcomes [141]. The hamstring-based flap is preferred in patients with spinal cord injury. Both can be readily advanced in the event of recurrence [116]. Other options include inferior gluteal rotation flaps, gluteal thigh flaps, perforator flaps, and free flaps [142–144]. Inferior gluteus maximus island flaps and inferior gluteal thigh flaps also have shown success rates of 94 % and 93 %, respectively [144]. Some authors have advocated the use of rectus abdominis flaps. However, others believe this muscle to be especially important in paraplegics as it initiates vertebral flexion, respiration, urination, defecation, and vomiting [145–147]. Sensate tensor fasciae latae flaps, innervated by the lateral femoral cutaneous nerve, also have been shown to assist in the sensation of rectal filling [125, 128, 148] (Figs. 14.4–14.6).

Trochanter

Trochanteric ulcers are generally reconstructed by flaps based on the tensor fasciae latae (TFL) or vastus lateralis [125, 128, 148–152]. The TFL is a versatile donor and offers many options for reconstruction. It can be transferred as muscle only, skin and muscle, and as an island or free flap. TFL V-Y advancement flaps have documented success rates of 93 % in this anatomical region [144]. However, if a Girdlestone procedure, or femoral head ostectomy, is also required, the vastus lateralis becomes the muscle of choice

and can be transposed in a muscular or myocutaneous flap [153–155] (Fig. 14.7–14.10).

Prophylactic Bone Resection

Another topic that warrants mention is that of prophylactic bone resection. Some surgeons recommend prophylactic resection of bony prominences beneath the area to be reconstructed [156]. Partial ischiectomy has been associated with recurrence rates of 38 %, while extension to total ischiectomy has reduced recurrence rates to only 3 % [117]. While the results are promising for total unilateral ischiectomy, these patients frequently develop ulcers on the contralateral side due to alterations to the bony geography that, in turn, reassign the points of maximum pressure [157]. With this in mind, some authors have begun to recommend prophylactic bilateral ischiectomy. However, such resection frequently increases the risk of developing perineal ulcers, urethrocutaneous fistulas, and ulcers in the distribution of the pubic rami. Therefore, bilateral prophylactic ischiectomy should be employed only during reconstruction of deep, extensive recurrent ischial wounds [158–160].

Postoperative Management

The main goal of postoperative management is the prevention of ulcer recurrence. Care should be focused on the management of incontinence and spasticity, as well as ensuring adequate nutritional support. Relief of pressure, shear forces, friction, and moisture are paramount, and these parameters should be constantly assessed [117, 161–165]. Quite possibly the most important adjunct to postoperative physical therapy is ensuring patient understanding and compliance [166–169]. With regard to postoperative care, the ongoing debate centers on the length that a patient should remain immobilized after surgery and timing of initiation of sitting protocols. Historically, patients were kept on bed rest 6–8 weeks postoperatively based on the theory that wounds reach maximal tensile strength by this point. However, more recent studies suggest that the period of immobilization can be shortened to

Gluteal Thigh Flap

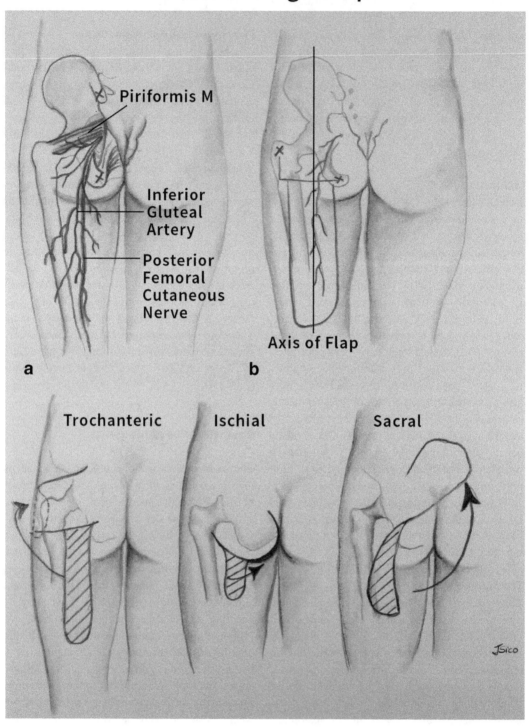

Fig. 14.4 Artist depiction of the gluteal thigh flap. The flap is based on the inferior gluteal artery and can be rotated to cover trochanteric, ischial and sacral ulcers. a. Anatomy of the posterior thigh including the dominant blood supply to the flap, the inferior gluteal artery. b. The axis of the flap is drawn showing the rotation point. The x marks the areas the flap can be rotated to cover (ischial and trochnateric ulcers)

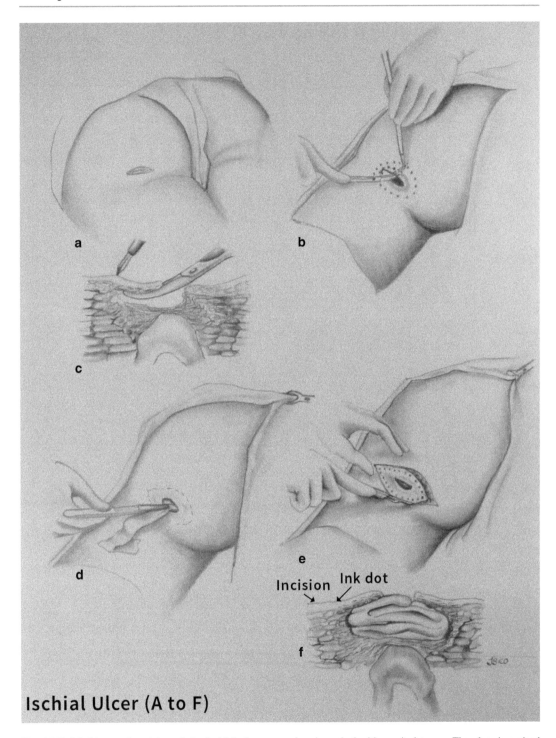

Ischial Ulcer (A to F)

Fig. 14.5 Marking and excision of the ischial ulcer a. The ulcer is shown b. Marking for proposed excision of the the ulcer c. Undermining of the ulcer is displayed. The marking is made at the edge of the undermined area d. The ulcer is packed with surgical tape e. The ulcer is excised just outside the dotted line f. The ulcer is completely excised including the undermined areas. The incision is outside the dotted line

Ischial ulcer (continued G - K)

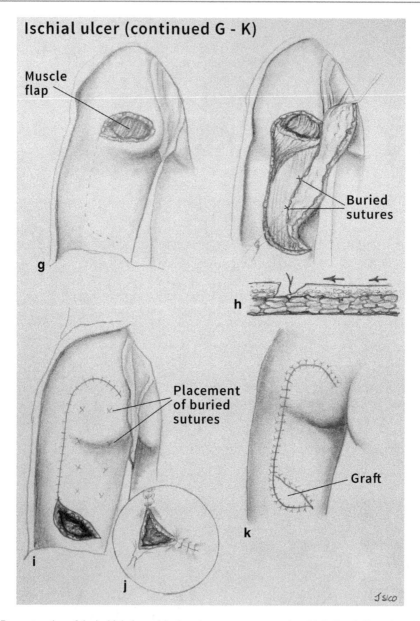

Muscle flap

Buried sutures

Placement of buried sutures

Graft

g

h

i

j

k

J SICO

Fig. 14.6 Reconstruction of the ischial ulcer with gluteal muscle flap and posterior thigh fasciocutaneous flap. g. Gluteal muscle flap covering ischium h. Quilting sutures to secure posterior thigh flap i. Posterior thigh flap has been rotated and secured j. Donor site defect k. Closure of donor site defect with skin graft

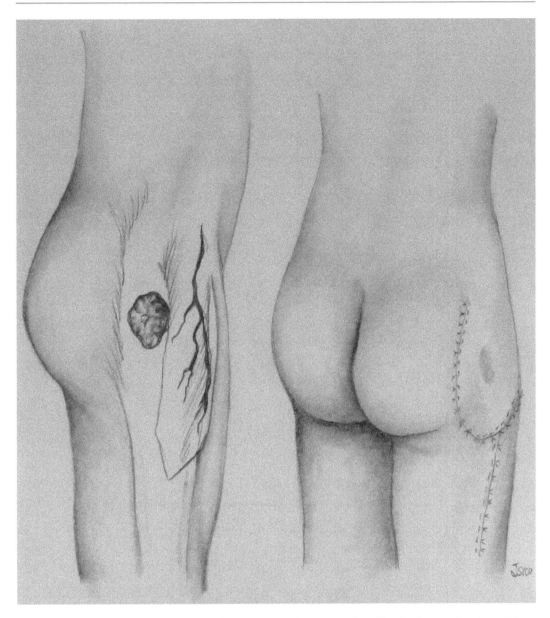

Fig. 14.7 Artist's depiction of trochanteric ulcer reconstruction using the tensor fasciae latae flap. The flap is marked preoperatively (*left*) and raised as a pedicled musculocutaneous flap. The flap is rotated on its pedicle to cover the trochanteric defect, and the donor site is closed primarily (*right*)

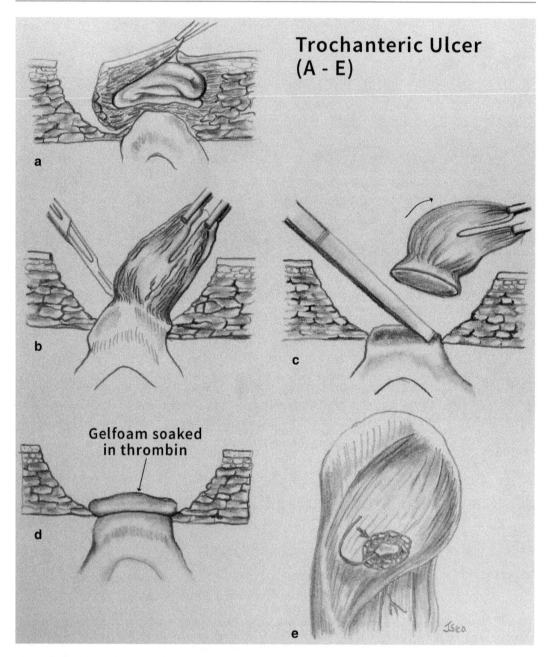

Trochanteric Ulcer (A - E)

a

b

c

Gelfoam soaked in thrombin

d

e

Fig. 14.8 Excision and trochanteric wound reconstruction with rotational musculocutaneous flap. a. Excision of ulcer to healthy tissues b. Removal of ulcer c. Excision of involved bone d. Hemostasis of wound bed e. Reconstruction of wound with rotational musculocutaneous flap

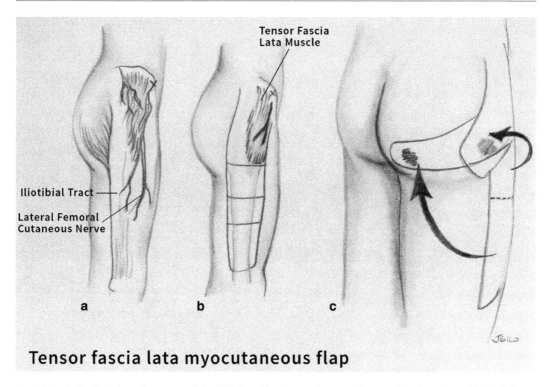

Tensor fascia lata myocutaneous flap

Fig. 14.9 Artist depiction of anatomy of the TFL flap. The flap can be rotated to cover trochanteric and ischial ulcers

2–3 weeks or even 10–14 days without significant changes in outcomes [144, 170].

Regardless of the length of postoperative immobilization, active and passive range of motion exercises of the unaffected limb should begin almost immediately, and the affected limb should be ranged only just prior to the commencement of a sitting protocol [168]. Typical sitting regimens begin at 15 min intervals once or twice a day. Frequent pressure release maneuvers are of vital importance, and surgical sites are carefully monitored for any evidence of recurrence [168]. These intervals are gradually increased until discharge [170]. Prior to discharge, patients undergo seat mapping to evalu-

ate support surfaces for potential areas of recurrence. Maximum allowable pressures are 35 mmHg for patients unable to perform pressure release maneuvers and 60 mmHg for those who can [171].

Outcomes and Complications

The principal metric of success regarding pressure sore reconstruction is the rate of recurrence. A wide range is reported in the literature, and it is therefore difficult to determine any true values [163, 165, 172–176]. In general, young, post-traumatic paraplegics and cerebrally compro-

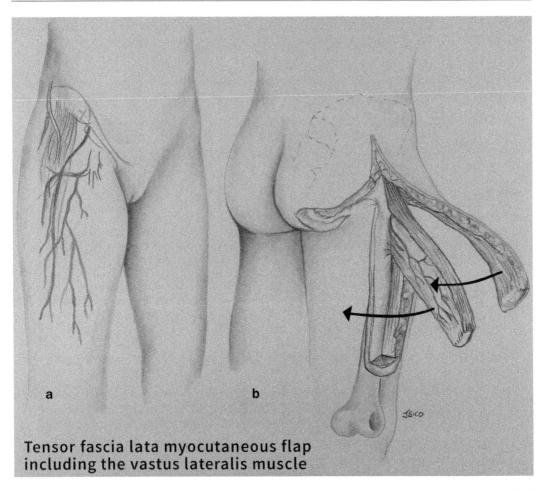

Tensor fascia lata myocutaneous flap including the vastus lateralis muscle

Fig. 14.10 Artist depiction of elevation of the TFL flap. The flap is elevated as a musculocutaneous flap with blood supply subfascial with the vastus lateralis. It is then rotated and donor site closed primarily

mised elderly patients have the highest recurrence rates at 79 % and 69 %, respectively. Given such high numbers, these preoperative conditions may preclude surgical reconstruction, as patient compliance is necessary and frequently an issue [165, 168]. As expected, children represent the other end of the spectrum and display considerably lower recurrence rates [177].

With respect to sacral wound management, success rates have been reported around 30 % for nonsurgical management and split-thickness skin grafting. However, ostectomy and ulcer excision with rotational flap reconstruction have resulted in success rates as high as 84 % [178]. Trochanteric ulcers have shown slightly higher success rates with nonsurgical management and split-thickness

skin grafts, recorded at 41 % and 33 %, respectively. However, ulcer bursa resection and reconstruction with rotational flaps have reported success rates of up to 92 % [178]. In addition to nonsurgical and grafting of ischial ulcers, primary suturing has been reported with success rates around 50 %. Nevertheless, the best outcomes result from total ischiectomy with regional rotation flaps, which have reported recurrence rates of only 35 % [178]. Even with surgical reconstruction, the best outcomes are only achieved by collaboration between plastic surgeons and physical medicine and rehabilitation physicians [177].

Complications of these procedures include hematoma, seroma, wound dehiscence, and, most importantly, ulcer recurrence. Suture line breakdown usually heals, and persistent slough from the wound is usually an indicator of inadequate preoperative debridement [111]. The same preoperative assessment for risk factors should be conducted once again, and patients should be nutritionally optimized before return to the operating room [115, 144]. Options for revision procedures include readvancing the initial flap, readvancement of a different plane of the initial flap, or harvesting a new flap from untouched territory, among others. Amputation and salvage flaps should be considered last resort options for critically ill patients with multiple confluent ulcers and/or acute life-threatening disease such as uncontrollable pelvic osteomyelitis [179, 180]. For any recurrent ulcer, biopsies should be sent for microscopic analysis to rule out malignant degeneration, also known as the development of a Marjolin's ulcer. This transformation may be preceded by a change in symptoms not limited to increasing pain and/or discharge, a foul odor, or recurrent bleeding. Latency from the initial insult has been quoted at 20 years for pressure ulcers, and early recognition with proper staging and management offers the best chance for a cure [181].

Conclusion

Pressure ulcers are a common occurrence in debilitated patients. Prevention is of the utmost importance. However, surgical reconstruction is indicated for large wounds that have failed a trial of nonoperative management. The plastic surgeon has a multitude of reconstructive options at his or her disposal. Operative approaches are generally guided by ulcer site, patient habitus, and nutritional status. Many different procedures result in acceptable outcomes at each of the common ulcer sites, and the best outcomes are achieved by regimented postoperative surveillance and physical therapy protocols.

References

1. Amlung SR, Miller WL, Bosley LM. The 1999 national pressure ulcer prevalence survey: a benchmarking approach. Adv Skin Wound Care. 2001;14:297–301.
2. VanGilder C, Amlung S, Harrison P, et al. Results of the 2008–2009 international pressure ulcer prevalence survey and a 3-year, acute care, unit-specific analysis. Ostomy Wound Manage. 2009;55:39–45.
3. Vangilder C, Macfarlane GD, Meyer S. Results of nine international pressure ulcer prevalence surveys: 1989 to 2005. Ostomy Wound Manage. 2008;54:40–54.
4. Cuddigan J, Frantz RA. Pressure ulcer research: pressure ulcer treatment. A monograph from the national pressure ulcer advisory panel. Adv Wound Care. 1998;11:294–300.
5. Smith DM. Pressure ulcers in the nursing home. Ann Intern Med. 1995;123:433–42.
6. Park-Lee E, Caffrey C. Pressure ulcers among nursing home residents: United States, 2004. NCHS Data Brief. 2009;14:1–8.
7. Holmes A, Edelstein T. Pressure ulcer success story. Provider. 2007;33:37–9, 41.
8. Capon A, Pavoni N, Mastromattei A, et al. Pressure ulcer risk in long-term units: prevalence and associated factors. J Adv Nurs. 2007;58:263–72.
9. Lindholm C, Sterner E, Romanelli M, et al. Hip fracture and pressure ulcers – the Pan-European pressure ulcer study – intrinsic and extrinsic risk factors. Int Wound J. 2008;5:315–28.
10. Baumgarten M, Margolis D, Berlin JA, et al. Risk factors for pressure ulcers among elderly hip fracture patients. Wound Repair Regen. 2003;11:96–103.
11. Baumgarten M, Margolis DJ, Orwig DL, et al. Pressure ulcers in elderly patients with hip fracture across the continuum of care. J Am Geriatr Soc. 2009;57:863–70.
12. Garber SL, Rintala DH, Hart KA, et al. Pressure ulcer risk in spinal cord injury: predictors of ulcer status over 3 years. Arch Phys Med Rehabil. 2000;81:465–71.
13. Saladin LK, Krause JS. Pressure ulcer prevalence and barriers to treatment after spinal cord injury: comparisons of four groups based on race-ethnicity. Neuro Rehabil. 2009;24:57–66.
14. Fuhrer MJ, Garber SL, Rintala DH, et al. Pressure ulcers in community-resident persons with spinal cord injury: prevalence and risk factors. Arch Phys Med Rehabil. 1993;74:1172–7.
15. Gelis A, Dupeyron A, Legros P, et al. Pressure ulcer risk factors in persons with spinal cord injury part 2: the chronic stage. Spinal Cord. 2009;47:651–61.
16. Description of NPUAP. National pressure ulcer advisory panel. Adv Wound Care. 1995;8(Suppl):93–5.
17. Russo A. Hospitalization related to pressure ulcers among adults 18 years and older, 2006. Rockville: Agency for Healthcare Research and Quality; 2008.
18. Meehan M. National pressure ulcer prevalence survey. Adv Wound Care. 1994;7:27–30, 34, 36–28.
19. Dansereau JG, Conway H. Closure of decubiti in paraplegics. Report of 2000 cases. Plast Reconstr Surg. 1964;33:474–80.
20. Landis E. Microinjection studies of capillary blood pressure in human skin. Heart. 1930;15:209.

21. Fronek K, Zweifach BW. Microvascular pressure distribution in skeletal muscle and the effect of vasodilation. Am J Physiol. 1975;228:791–6.

22. Lindan O, Greenway RM, Piazza JM. Pressure distribution on the surface of the human body. I. Evaluation in lying and sitting positions using a "Bed of springs and nails". Arch Phys Med Rehabil. 1965;46:378–85.

23. Holloway GA, Daly CH, Kennedy D, et al. Effects of external pressure loading on human skin blood flow measured by 133Xe clearance. J Appl Physiol. 1976;40:597–600.

24. Dinsdale SM. Decubitus ulcers: role of pressure and friction in causation. Arch Phys Med Rehabil. 1974;55:147–52.

25. Kosiak M, Kubicek WG, Olson M, et al. Evaluation of pressure as a factor in the production of ischial ulcers. Arch Phys Med Rehabil. 1958;39:623–9.

26. Groth K. Klinische beobachtungen and experimentelle studien über die enstehung des dekubitus. Acta ChirScand. 1942;LXXXVII(Suppl 76):1–209.

27. Husain T. An experimental study of some pressure effects on tissues, with reference to the bed-sore problem. J Pathol Bacteriol. 1953;66:347–58.

28. Nola GT, Vistnes LM. Differential response of skin and muscle in the experimental production of pressure sores. Plast Reconstr Surg. 1980; 66:728–33.

29. Daniel RK, Priest DL, Wheatley DC. Etiologic factors in pressure sores: an experimental model. Arch Phys Med Rehabil. 1981;62:492–8.

30. Gerhardt LC, Mattle N, Schrade GU, et al. Study of skin-fabric interactions of relevance to decubitus: friction and contact-pressure measurements. Skin Res Technol. 2008;14:77–88.

31. Hanson D, Langemo DK, Anderson J, et al. Friction and shear considerations in pressure ulcer development. Adv Skin Wound Care. 2010;23:21–4.

32. Gerhardt LC, Strassle V, Lenz A, et al. Influence of epidermal hydration on the friction of human skin against textiles. J R Soc Interface. 2008;5: 1317–28.

33. Reichel SM. Shearing force as a factor in decubitus ulcers in paraplegics. JAMA. 1958;166:762–3.

34. Reuler JB, Cooney TG. The pressure sore: pathophysiology and principles of management. Ann Intern Med. 1981;94:661–6.

35. Goossens RH, Zegers R, van Dijke GA H, et al. Influence of shear on skin oxygen tension. Clin Physiol. 1994;14:111–8.

36. Schubert V, Heraud J. The effects of pressure and shear on skin microcirculation in elderly stroke patients lying in supine or semi-recumbent positions. Age Ageing. 1994;23:405–10.

37. Defloor T, Grypdonck MF. Validation of pressure ulcer risk assessment scales: a critique. J Adv Nurs. 2004;48:613–21.

38. Lowthian P. The distinction between superficial pressure ulcers and moisture lesions. Skinmed. 2007;6:111–2.

39. Kottner J, Halfens R. Moisture lesions: interrater agreement and reliability. J Clin Nurs. 2010;19: 716–20.

40. Resnick NM, Beckett LA, Branch LG, et al. Short-term variability of self report of incontinence in older persons. J Am Geriatr Soc. 1994;42:202–7.

41. Saxer S, Halfens RJ, de Bie RA, et al. Prevalence and incidence of urinary incontinence of Swiss nursing home residents at admission and after six, 12 and 24 months. J Clin Nurs. 2008;17:2490–6.

42. Chassagne P, Landrin I, Neveu C, et al. Fecal incontinence in the institutionalized elderly: incidence, risk factors, and prognosis. Am J Med. 1999;106:185–90.

43. Allman RM, Goode PS, Patrick MM, et al. Pressure ulcer risk factors among hospitalized patients with activity limitation. JAMA. 1995;273:865–70.

44. Reddy M, Gill SS, Rochon PA. Preventing pressure ulcers: a systematic review. JAMA. 2006;296:974–84.

45. Guigoz Y, Lauque S, Vellas BJ. Identifying the elderly at risk for malnutrition. The mini nutritional assessment. Clin Geriatr Med. 2002;18:737–57.

46. Arnold M, Barbul A. Nutrition and wound healing. Plast Reconstr Surg. 2006;117(Suppl):42S–58.

47. Kay SP, Moreland JR, Schmitter E. Nutritional status and wound healing in lower extremity amputations. Clin Orthop Relat Res. 1987;217:253–6.

48. Dickhaut SC, DeLee JC, Page CP. Nutritional status: importance in predicting wound-healing after amputation. J Bone Joint Surg Am. 1984;66:71–5.

49. Casey J, Flinn WR, Yao JS, et al. Correlation of immune and nutritional status with wound complications in patients undergoing vascular operations. Surgery. 1983;93:822–7.

50. Cuthbertson D. Nutrition in relation to trauma and surgery. Prog Food Nutr Sci. 1975;1:263–87.

51. Wilmore DW, Aulick LH. Systemic responses to injury and the healing wound. JPEN J Parenter Enteral Nutr. 1980;4:147–51.

52. Bergstrom N, Braden B. A prospective study of pressure sore risk among institutionalized elderly. J Am Geriatr Soc. 1992;40:747–58.

53. Berlowitz DR, Wilking SV. Risk factors for pressure sores. A comparison of cross-sectional and cohort derived data. J Am Geriatr Soc. 1989;37:1043–50.

54. Green SM, Winterberg H, Franks PJ, et al. Nutritional intake in community patients with pressure ulcers. J Wound Care. 1999;8:325–30.

55. Johnson RL, Gerhart KA, McCray J, et al. Secondary conditions following spinal cord injury in a population-based sample. Spinal Cord. 1998;36:45–50.

56. Whiteneck GG, Charlifue SW, Frankel HL, et al. Mortality, morbidity, and psychosocial outcomes of persons spinal cord injured more than 20 years ago. Paraplegia. 1992;30:617–30.

57. Cardenas DD, Hoffman JM, Kirshblum S, et al. Etiology and incidence of rehospitalization after traumatic spinal cord injury: a multicenter analysis. Arch Phys Med Rehabil. 2004;85:1757–63.

58. Skold C, Levi R, Seiger A. Spasticity after traumatic spinal cord injury: nature, severity, and location. Arch Phys Med Rehabil. 1999;80:1548–57.
59. Atiyeh BS, Hayek SN. Pressure sores with associated spasticity: a clinical challenge. Int Wound J. 2005;2:77–80.
60. Gunningberg L, Stotts NA. Tracking quality over time: what do pressure ulcer data show? Int J Qual Health Care. 2008;20:246–53.
61. Voegeli D. Care or harm: exploring essential components in skin care regimens. Br J Nurs. 2010;19:810–4.
62. Held E, Lund H, Agner T. Effect of different moisturizers on SLS-irritated human skin. Contact Derm. 2001;44:229–34.
63. Hodgkinson B, Nay R, Wilson J. A systematic review of topical skin care in aged care facilities. J Clin Nurs. 2007;16:129–36.
64. Guralnik JM, Harris TB, White LR, Cornoni-Huntley JC. Occurrence and predictors of pressure sores in the national health and nutrition examination survey follow-up. J Am Geriatr Soc. 1988;36:807–12.
65. Nakagami G, Sanada H, Konya C, Kitagawa A, Tadaka E, Matsuyama Y. Evaluation of a new pressure ulcer preventive dressing containing ceramide 2 with low frictional outer layer. J Adv Nurs. 2007;59:520–9.
66. Ellis C, Luger T, Abeck D, et al. International Consensus Conference on Atopic Dermatitis II (ICCAD II): clinical update and current treatment strategies. Br J Dermatol. 2003;148 Suppl 63:3–10.
67. Schuren J, Becker A, Sibbald RG. A liquid film-forming acrylate for peri-wound protection: a systematic review and meta-analysis (3M Cavilon no-sting barrier film). Int Wound J. 2005;2:230–8.
68. Hughes S. Do continence aids help to maintain skin integrity? J Wound Care. 2002;11:235–9.
69. Cole L, Nesbitt C. A three year multiphase pressure ulcer prevalence/incidence study in a regional referral hospital. Ostomy Wound Manage. 2004;50:32–40.
70. Lyder CH, Shannon R, Empleo-Frazier O, McGeHee D, White C. A comprehensive program to prevent pressure ulcers in long-term care: exploring costs and outcomes. Ostomy Wound Manage. 2002;48:52–62.
71. Thomas DR. Prevention and treatment of pressure ulcers: what works? what doesn't? Cleve. Clin J Med. 2001;68:704–7, 710–14, 717–22.
72. Simmang C, Birnbaum EH, Kodner IJ, Fry RD, Fleshman JW. Anal sphincter reconstruction in the elderly: does advancing age affect outcome? Dis Colon Rectum. 1994;37:1065–9.
73. Colquhoun P, Kaiser R, Efron J, et al. Is the quality of life better in patients with colostomy than patients with fecal incontinence? World J Surg. 2006;30:1925–8.
74. Levi R, Hultling C, Seiger A. The Stockholm spinal cord injury study: 2. Associations between clinical patient characteristics and post-acute medical problems. Paraplegia. 1995;33:585–94.
75. St George CL. Spasticity. Mechanisms and nursing care. Nurs Clin North Am. 1993;28:819–27.
76. Parziale JR, Akelman E, Herz DA. Spasticity: pathophysiology and management. Orthopedics. 1993;16:801–11.
77. Elovic E. Principles of pharmacological management of spastic hypertonia. Phys Med Rehabil Clin N Am. 2001;12:793–816.
78. Kirshblum S. Treatment alternatives for spinal cord injury related spasticity. J Spinal Cord Med. 1999;22:199–217.
79. Gracies JM, Elovic E, McGuire J, Simpson DM. Traditional pharmacological treatments for spasticity. Part I: local treatments. Muscle Nerve Suppl. 1997;6:S61–91.
80. Barnes M. Botulinum toxin – mechanisms of action and clinical use in spasticity. J Rehabil Med. 2003;(41 Suppl):56–59.
81. Livshits A, Rappaport ZH, Livshits V, Gepstein R. Surgical treatment of painful spasticity after spinal cord injury. Spinal Cord. 2002;40:161–6.
82. Munro D. Anterior-rootlet rhizotomy; a method of controlling spasm with retention of voluntary motion. N Engl J Med. 1952;246:161–6.
83. Bliss MR, Thomas JM. Clinical trials with budgetary implications. Establishing randomised trials of pressure-relieving aids. Prof Nurse. 1993;8:292–6.
84. Ceccio CM. Understanding therapeutic beds. Orthop Nurs. 1990;9:57–70.
85. Klitzman B, Kalinowski C, Glasofer SL, Rugani L. Pressure ulcers and pressure relief surfaces. Clin Plast Surg. 1998;25:443–50.
86. Nimit K. Guidelines for home air-fluidized bed therapy, 1989. Health Technol Assess Rep. 1989;5:1–11.
87. Goldstone LA, Norris M, O'Reilly M, White J. A clinical trial of a bead bed system for the prevention of pressure sores in elderly orthopaedic patients. J Adv Nurs. 1982;7:545–8.
88. Hofman A, Geelkerken RH, Wille J, Hamming JJ, Hermans J, Breslau PJ. Pressure sores and pressure-decreasing mattresses: controlled clinical trial. Lancet. 1994;343:568–71.
89. Andersen KE, Jensen O, Kvorning SA, Bach E. Prevention of pressure sores by identifying patients at risk. Br Med J (Clin Res Ed). 1982;284:1370–1.
90. Marchand AC, Lidowski H. Reassessment of the use of genuine sheepskin for pressure ulcer prevention and treatment. Decubitus. 1993;6:44–7.
91. Jolley DJ, Wright R, McGowan S, et al. Preventing pressure ulcers with the Australian Medical Sheepskin: an open-label randomised controlled trial. Med J Aust. 2004;180:324–7.
92. McInnes E, Bell-Syer SE, Dumville JC, Legood R, Cullum NA. Support surfaces for pressure ulcer prevention. Cochrane Database Syst Rev. 2008;4:CD001735.
93. Brienza DM, Karg PE, Geyer MJ, Kelsey S, Trefler E. The relationship between pressure ulcer incidence and buttock-seat cushion interface pressure in at-risk

elderly wheelchair users. Arch Phys Med Rehabil. 2001;82:529–33.

94. Geyer MJ, Brienza DM, Karg P, Trefler E, Kelsey S. A randomized control trial to evaluate pressure-reducing seat cushions for elderly wheelchair users. Adv Skin Wound Care. 2001;14:120–9; quiz 131–2.

95. Thomas DR, Goode PS, Tarquine PH, Allman RM. Hospital-acquired pressure ulcers and risk of death. J Am Geriatr Soc. 1996;44:1435–40.

96. Pinchcofsky-Devin GD, Kaminski MV. Correlation of pressure sores and nutritional status. J Am Geriatr Soc. 1986;34:435–40.

97. Thomas DR. The role of nutrition in prevention and healing of pressure ulcers. Clin Geriatr Med. 1997;13:497–511.

98. Black J, Baharestani MM, Cuddigan J, et al. National pressure ulcer advisory Panel's updated pressure ulcer staging system. Adv Skin Wound Care. 2007;20:269–74.

99. Shea JD. Pressure sores: classification and management. Clin Orthop Relat Res. 1975;112:89–100.

100. Attinger CE, Janis JE, Steinberg J, et al. Clinical approach to wounds: debridement and wound bed preparation including the use of dressings and wound healing adjuvants. Plast Reconstr Surg. 2006;117(Suppl):72S–109.

101. Perry CR, Pearson RL, Miller GA. Accuracy of cultures of material from swabbing of the superficial aspect of the wound and needle biopsy in the preoperative assessment of osteomyelitis. J Bone Joint Surg Am. 1991;73:745–9.

102. Waldvogel FA, Medoff G, Swartz MN. Osteomyelitis: a review of clinical features, therapeutic considerations and unusual aspects (second of three parts). N Engl J Med. 1970;282:260–6.

103. Han H, Lewis Jr VL, Wiedrich TA, et al. The value of Jamshidi core needle bone biopsy in predicting postoperative osteomyelitis in grade IV pressure ulcer patients. Plast Reconstr Surg. 2002;110:118–22.

104. Lewis Jr VL, Bailey MH, Pulawski G, et al. The diagnosis of osteomyelitis in patients with pressure sores. Plast Reconstr Surg. 1988;81:229–32.

105. Huang AB, Schweitzer ME, Hume E, et al. Osteomyelitis of the pelvis/hips in paralyzed patients: accuracy and clinical utility of MRI. J Comput Assist Tomogr. 1998;22:437–43.

106. Ruan CM, Escobedo E, Harrison S, et al. Magnetic resonance imaging of nonhealing pressure ulcers and myocutaneous flaps. Arch Phys Med Rehabil. 1998;79:1080–8.

107. Stewart MC, Little RE, Highland TR. Osteomyelitis of the ilium secondary to external pelvic fixation. J Trauma. 1986;26:284–6.

108. Sugarman B. Pressure sores and underlying bone infection. Arch Intern Med. 1987;147:553–5.

109. Thornhill-Joynes M, Gonzales F, Stewart CA, et al. Osteomyelitis associated with pressure ulcers. Arch Phys Med Rehabil. 1986;67:314–8.

110. Fitzgerald Jr RH, Ruttle PE, Arnold PG, et al. Local muscle flaps in the treatment of chronic osteomyelitis. J Bone Joint Surg Am. 1985;67:175–85.

111. Marriott R, Rubayi S. Successful truncated osteomyelitis treatment for chronic osteomyelitis secondary to pressure ulcers in spinal cord injury patients. Ann Plast Surg. 2008;61:425–9.

112. Langer KG. Depression and denial in psychotherapy of persons with disabilities. Am J Psychother. 1994;48:181–94.

113. Frank RG, Kashani JH, Wonderlich SA, et al. Depression and adrenal function in spinal cord injury. Am J Psychiatry. 1985;142:252–3.

114. Akbas H, Arik AC, Eroglu L, et al. Is rational flap selection and good surgical technique sufficient for treating pressure ulcers? The importance of psychology: a prospective clinical study. Ann Plast Surg. 2002;48:224–5.

115. Foster RD, Anthony JP, Mathes SJ, et al. Ischial pressure sore coverage: a rationale for flap selection. Br J Plast Surg. 1997;50:374–9.

116. Neligan PC. Plastic surgery: volume 4, lower extremity, trunk and burns. London: Elsevier Saunders; 2013.

117. Conway H, Griffith BH. Plastic surgery for closure of decubitus ulcers in patients with paraplegia; based on experience with 1000 cases. Am J Surg. 1956;91:946–75.

118. Mathes SJ, Alpert BS, Chang N. Use of the muscle flap in chronic osteomyelitis: experimental and clinical correlation. Plast Reconstr Surg. 1982;69:815–29.

119. Mathes SJ, Feng LJ, Hunt TK. Coverage of the infected wound. Ann Surg. 1983;198:420–9.

120. Ohura T. Outcomes research-incidence and clinical symptoms of hourglass and sandwich-shaped tissue necrosis in stage IV pressure ulcers. Wounds. 2007;11:310–9.

121. Yazar S, Lin CH, Lin YT, et al. Outcome comparison between free muscle and free fasciocutaneous flaps for reconstruction of distal third and ankle traumatic open tibial fractures. Plast Reconstr Surg. 2006;117:2468–75.

122. Bruck JC, Buttemeyer R, Grabosch A, et al. More arguments in favor of myocutaneous flaps for the treatment of pelvic pressure sores. Ann Plast Surg. 1991;26:85–8.

123. Kroll SS, Rosenfield L. Perforator-based flaps for low posterior midline defects. Plast Reconstr Surg. 1988;81:561–6.

124. Higgins JP, Orlando GS, Blondeel PN. Ischial pressure sore reconstruction using an inferior gluteal artery perforator (IGAP) flap. Br J Plast Surg. 2002;55:83–5.

125. Nahai F. The tensor fascia lata flap. Clin Plast Surg. 1980;7:51–6.

126. Nahai F, Hill L, Hester TR. Experiences with the tensor fascia lata flap. Plast Reconstr Surg. 1979;63:788–99.

127. Hill HL, Hester R, Nahai F. Covering large groin defects with the tensor fascia lata musculocutaneous flap. Br J Plast Surg. 1979;32:12–4.

128. Hill HL, Nahai F, Vasconez LO. The tensor fascia lata myocutaneous free flap. Plast Reconstr Surg. 1978;61:517–22.

129. Esposito G, Di Caprio G, Ziccardi P, et al. Tissue expansion in the treatment of pressure ulcers. Plast Reconstr Surg. 1991;87:501–8.

130. Daniel RK, Terzis JK, Cunningham DM. Sensory skin flaps for coverage of pressure sores in paraplegic patients. A preliminary report. Plast Reconstr Surg. 1976;58:317–28.

131. Dibbell DG. Use of a long island flap to bring sensation to the sacral area in young paraplegics. Plast Reconstr Surg. 1974;54:220–3.

132. Kostakoglu N, Kecik A, Ozyilmaz F, et al. Expansion of fascial flaps: histopathologic changes and clinical benefits. Plast Reconstr Surg. 1993;91:72–9.

133. Koshima I, Moriguchi T, Soeda S, et al. The gluteal perforator-based flap for repair of sacral pressure sores. Plast Reconstr Surg. 1993;91:678–83.

134. Parry SW, Mathes SJ. Bilateral gluteus maximus myocutaneous advancement flaps: sacral coverage for ambulatory patients. Ann Plast Surg. 1982;8:443–5.

135. Wong CH, Tan BK, Song C. The perforator-sparing buttock rotation flap for coverage of pressure sores. Plast Reconstr Surg. 2007;119:1259–66.

136. Xu Y, Hai H, Liang Z, et al. Pedicled fasciocutaneous flap of multi-island design for large sacral defects. Clin Orthop Relat Res. 2009;467:2135–41.

137. Hill HL, Brown RG, Jurkiewicz MJ. The transverse lumbosacral back flap. Plast Reconstr Surg. 1978;62:177–84.

138. Vyas SC, Binns JH, Wilson AN. Thoracolumbarsacral flaps in the treatment of sacral pressure sores. Plast Reconstr Surg. 1980;65:159–63.

139. Kato H, Hasegawa M, Takada T, et al. The lumbar artery perforator based island flap: anatomical study and case reports. Br J Plast Surg. 1999;52:541–6.

140. Prado A, Ocampo C, Danilla S, et al. A new technique of "double-A" bilateral flaps based on perforators for the treatment of sacral defects. Plast Reconstr Surg. 2007;119:1481–90.

141. Ahluwalia R, Martin D, Mahoney JL, et al. The operative treatment of pressure wounds: a 10-year experience in flap selection. Int Wound J. 2010;7:103–6.

142. Hurwitz DJ, Swartz WM, Mathes SJ. The gluteal thigh flap: a reliable, sensate flap for the closure of buttock and perineal wounds. Plast Reconstr Surg. 1981;68:521–32.

143. Ramirez OM, Hurwitz DJ, Futrell JW. The expansive gluteus maximus flap. Plast Reconstr Surg. 1984;74:757–70.

144. Foster RD, Anthony JP, Mathes SJ, et al. Flap selection as a determinant of success in pressure sore coverage. Arch Surg. 1997;132:868–73.

145. Bunkis J, Fudem GM. Rectus abdominis flap closure of ischiosacral pressure sore. Ann Plast Surg. 1989;23:447–9.

146. Mixter RC, Wood WA, Dibbell Sr DG. Retroperitoneal transposition of rectus abdominis myocutaneous flaps to the perineum and back. Plast Reconstr Surg. 1990;85:437–41.

147. Pena MM, Drew GS, Smith SJ, et al. The inferiorly based rectus abdominis myocutaneous flap for reconstruction of recurrent pressure sores. Plast Reconstr Surg. 1992;89:90–5.

148. Nahai F, Silverton JS, Hill HL, et al. The tensor fascia lata musculocutaneous flap. Ann Plast Surg. 1978;1:372–9.

149. Dibbell DG, McCraw JB, Edstrom LE. Providing useful and protective sensibility to the sitting area in patients with meningomyelocele. Plast Reconstr Surg. 1979;64:796–9.

150. Luscher NJ, de Roche R, Krupp S, et al. The sensory tensor fasciae latae flap: a 9-year follow-up. Ann Plast Surg. 1991;26:306–10.

151. Cochran Jr JH, Edstrom LE, Dibbell DG. Usefulness of the innervated tensor fascia lata flap in paraplegic patients. Ann Plast Surg. 1981;7:286–8.

152. Withers EH, Franklin JD, Madden Jr JJ, et al. Further experience with the tensor fascia lata musculocutaneous flap. Ann Plast Surg. 1980;4:31–6.

153. Benito-Ruiz J, Baena-Montilla P, Mena-Yago A, et al. A complicated trochanteric pressure sore: what is the best surgical management? Case report. Paraplegia. 1993;31:119–24.

154. Evans GR, Lewis Jr VL, Manson PN, et al. Hip joint communication with pressure sore: the refractory wound and the role of Girdlestone arthroplasty. Plast Reconstr Surg. 1993;91:288–94.

155. Klein NE, Luster S, Green S, et al. Closure of defects from pressure sores requiring proximal femoral resection. Ann Plast Surg. 1988;21:246–50.

156. Kostrubala JG, Greeley PW. The problem of decubitus ulcers in paraplegics. Plast Reconstr Surg. 1947;2:403–12.

157. Arregui J, Cannon B, Murray JE, et al. Long-term evaluation of ischiectomy in the treatment of pressure ulcers. Plast Reconstr Surg. 1965;36:583–90.

158. Hackler RH, Zampieri TA. Urethral complications following ischiectomy in spinal cord injury patients: a urethral pressure study. J Urol. 1987;137:253–5.

159. Bors E, Comarr AE. Ischial decubitus ulcer. Surgery. 1948;24:680–94.

160. Karaca AR, Binns JH, Blumenthal FS. Complications of total ischiectomy for the treatment of ischial pressure sores. Plast Reconstr Surg. 1978;62:96–9.

161. Vasconez LO, Schneider WJ, Jurkiewicz MJ. Pressure sores. Curr Probl Surg. 1977;14:1–62.

162. Stal S, Serure A, Donovan W, et al. The perioperative management of the patient with pressure sores. Ann Plast Surg. 1983;11:347–56.

163. Hentz VR. Management of pressure sores in a specialty center. A reappraisal. Plast Reconstr Surg. 1979;64:683–91.

164. Constantian MB. Pressure ulcers: principles and techniques of management. Boston: Little, Brown; 1980.

165. Disa JJ, Carlton JM, Goldberg NH. Efficacy of operative cure in pressure sore patients. Plast Reconstr Surg. 1992;89:272–8.
166. Garber SL, Rintala DH, Holmes SA, et al. A structured educational model to improve pressure ulcer prevention knowledge in veterans with spinal cord dysfunction. J Rehabil Res Dev. 2002;39:575–88.
167. Brace JA, Schubart JR. A prospective evaluation of a pressure ulcer prevention and management e-learning program for adults with spinal cord injury. Ostomy Wound Manage. 2010;56:40–50.
168. Kierney PC, Engrav LH, Isik FF, et al. Results of 268 pressure sores in 158 patients managed jointly by plastic surgery and rehabilitation medicine. Plast Reconstr Surg. 1998;102:765–72.
169. Tavakoli K, Rutkowski S, Cope C, et al. Recurrence rates of ischial sores in para- and tetraplegics treated with hamstring flaps: an 8-year study. Br J Plast Surg. 1999;52:476–9.
170. Isik FF, Engrav LH, Rand RP, et al. Reducing the period of immobilization following pressure sore surgery: a prospective, randomized trial. Plast Reconstr Surg. 1997;100:350–4.
171. Dover H, Pickard W, Swain I, et al. The effectiveness of a pressure clinic in preventing pressure sores. Paraplegia. 1992;30:267–72.
172. Ger R, Levine SA. The management of decubitus ulcers by muscle transposition. An 8-year review. Plast Reconstr Surg. 1976;58:419–28.
173. Stevenson TR, Pollock RA, Rohrich RJ, et al. The gluteus maximus musculocutaneous island flap: refinements in design and application. Plast Reconstr Surg. 1987;79:761–8.
174. Minami RT, Mills R, Pardoe R. Gluteus maximus myocutaneous flaps for repair of pressure sores. Plast Reconstr Surg. 1977;60:242–9.
175. Yamamoto Y, Tsutsumida A, Murazumi M, et al. Long-term outcome of pressure sores treated with flap coverage. Plast Reconstr Surg. 1997;100:1212–7.
176. Relander M, Palmer B. Recurrence of surgically treated pressure sores. Scand J Plast Reconstr Surg Hand Surg. 1988;22:89–92.
177. Singh DJ, Bartlett SP, Low DW, et al. Surgical reconstruction of pediatric pressure sores: long-term outcome. Plast Reconstr Surg. 2002;109:265–9.
178. Griffith BH, Schultz RC. The prevention and surgical treatment of recurrent decubitus ulcers in patients with paraplegia. Plast Reconstr Surg Transplant Bull. 1961;27:248–60.
179. Janis JE, Ahmad J, Lemmon JA, et al. A 25-year experience with hemicorporectomy for terminal pelvic osteomyelitis. Plast Reconstr Surg. 2009;124:1165–76.
180. Peterson R, Sardi A. Hemicorporectomy for chronic pressure ulcer carcinoma: 7 years of follow-up. Am Surg. 2004;70:507–11.
181. Esther RJ, Lamps L, Schwartz HS. Marjolin ulcers: secondary carcinomas in chronic wounds. J South Orthop Assoc. 1999;8:181–7.

Acute Burn Management and Rehabilitation

15

Azra Ashraf

The Acute Burn

Epidemiology

According to the American Burn Association, in 2013 there were 450,000 burn cases requiring medical attention and 3,400 deaths, including fire/smoke/inhalation injury [1]. Approximately 69 % were male and 31 % female. Ethnic breakdown includes 59 % Caucasian, 20 % African-American, and 14 % Hispanic. In terms of location, 72 % occurred while the patient was at home, 9 % at work, 5 % in the street or highway, and 5 % while participating in recreation or sport. The breakdown of type of burn was 43 % fire/flame, 34 % scald, 4 % electrical, 3 % chemical, and 7 % other [1]. In the early 1990s, the LA_{50} (burn size lethal to 50 % of population) was 81 % total body surface area (TBSA) [2]. Current trends suggest a decreased incidence of burn deaths due to improved prevention protocols such as early excision and grafting, improved ICU care, ventilation, nutrition, and a "team approach." According to several studies, each 1 % of burn corresponded with two-day hospital stay and an overall mean cost of $39,533 [2].

Successful surgical outcomes require a multidisciplinary team approach, including therapists, nurses, psychosocial support, and nutritionists. This typically occurs in the United States in the context of a "burn unit." Some burns may reflect pediatric abuse and neglect, such as scald burns on the buttocks, and require the care provider reports the burn to appropriate authorities. Globally, burns are most common outside the United States, specifically in the developing world. Burns such as acid violence burns commonly reflect domestic violence and are more common in South Asia, in areas like India and Pakistan. Unfortunately, many of these countries have limited resources in terms of expertise, intensive care management, and appropriate follow-up to best rehabilitate their patients [3].

Rehabilitating patients may take up to several years and multiple operations. It is imperative that health-care providers have a basic understanding of the natural history of burns and techniques in their armamentarium. This chapter will present an overview of burn management and strategic reconstructive options. Details of specific procedures exceed the goals and purview of this chapter [3].

The Burn Wound and Triage

An acute wound is comprised of three zones: coagulation, stasis, and hyperemia [4] (Fig. 15.1).

Each zone exhibits specific characteristics. The zone of coagulation tends to be the central area, comprised of necrotic and nonviable tissue. The

A. Ashraf, MD
Private Practice,
Shrewsbury, NJ, USA
e-mail: Azra.ashraf@gmail.com

© Springer International Publishing Switzerland 2017
A.I. Elkwood et al. (eds.), *Rehabilitative Surgery*, DOI 10.1007/978-3-319-41406-5_15

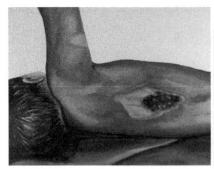

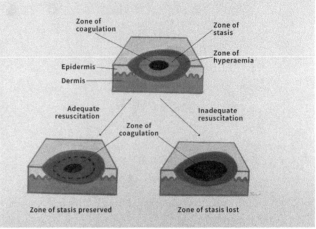

Fig. 15.1 These images depict the zones of injury in a burn wound: stasis, hyperemia and coagulation

zone of stasis surrounds the zone of coagulation and is most vulnerable to ischemia. In this zone, initially blood flow is present. However, if the patient is not appropriately resuscitated, this zone can become ischemic and nonviable. Last is the zone of hyperemia, which surrounds the zone of stasis. This zone *is* viable. Intense resuscitation efforts are targeted to salvage the zone of stasis and convert it to viable tissue.

Factors predicting the prognosis of burn wounds include extent of the burn, its age, and depth. Depth is characterized as first degree or epidermal, second degree – divided into superficial partial thickness and deep partial thickness – and full thickness also known as third degree. Determining the correct depth is most consistently based on clinical experience, though adjuncts such as dyes, fluorescein, and Doppler flow-meter assist [4].

Burn depth is important not only in predicting mortality but also in terms of rehabilitating and function. The deeper the burn, the more dermis involved and the greater the functional and/or aesthetic deficit. First-degree burns are epidermal, healing with at hyperpigment change only, and are not included in determining the percent TBSA of a burn [4]. Superficial partial thickness burns tend to be limited to the papillary dermis and typically are minor. They will often re-epithelialize with appropriate therapy

within 3 weeks. Deep partial thickness burns tend to include the reticular dermis and often do not spontaneously re-epithelialize within 3 weeks. These burns tend to form contractures and severe scars. Surgery is the mainstay of treatment for these deeper burns. Third-degree burns tend to be full thickness and extend into the fat, fascia, muscle, and/or bone. Early surgical management after appropriate resuscitation is the optimal treatment for this depth. The "rule of nines" is utilized in determining TBSA in second- and third-degree burn adult patients (Fig. 15.2).

According to the American Burn Association [1], patients who fit the following criteria should be referred to a burn center:

1. Second- and third-degree burns >10 % TBSA in patients under 10 or over 30 years of age
2. Second- and third-degree burns >10 % TBSA in patients all other age groups
3. Third-degree burn >5 % TBSA in any age group
4. Second- and third-degree burns involving the face, hands, feet, genitalia, perineum, or major joints
5. Electrical burns including lightening
6. Chemical burns with serious threat to function or cosmetic impairment
7. Inhalation injuries

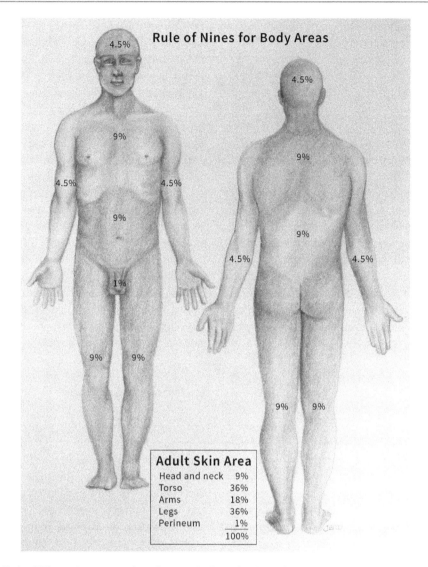

Fig. 15.2 Rule of Nines: A representation of percent body surface burns by area

8. Lesser burns in patients with preexisting medical problems which may potentially complicate management
9. Combined mechanical and thermal injury in which the burn wound poses a great risk

Care of the Acute Burn

As with all resuscitative efforts, burn resuscitation begins with the "ABC" of airway, breathing, and circulation. If suspicion for inhalation injury or inability of patient to secure the airway is high, prophylactic intubation is recommended. Fluid resuscitation is central to preventing burn shock and replacing sequestered fluid. The volume of fluid is most commonly determined by the Parkland formula: 4 ml/kg/% TBSA burn for the first 24 h. Lactated ringer is the fluid of choice and colloid is avoided the first 24 h secondary to protein leak. The best parameter of adequate resuscitation is urine output. Children have different body proportions than adults. For them, the Berkow formula is utilized to calculate TBSA. The Parkland formula should be modified to include maintenance fluid. Urine output of 1 ml/kg/h is the most reliable marker of adequate resuscitation [5].

Inhalational Injury

Inhalation injury affects about 10–20% of all hospitalized burn patients and may potentially damage the respiratory tract at multiple levels from the oropharynx to the alveolus [6]. An intense inflammatory reaction resulting in significant respiratory edema and damage can lead to bronchopneumonia and pulmonary sepsis. Management includes having a low suspicion for inhalational injury, aggressive and proactive airway management, and bronchoscopy. Singed nasal hair and carbonaceous sputum are pathognomonic for inhalational injury. Laboratory values may reflect increased carboxyhemoglobin levels (>15%) [6].

Infection

Infection is the most common cause of death in burn patients. Risk of infection increases with increasing TBSA, age (young than 16 and older than 60), environment (hot/moist), ischemia to wound, and medical comorbidities like diabetes, malnutrition, and cardiopulmonary insufficiency. Prior to the era of topical antimicrobials, partial- and full-thickness wounds often became infected and contributed to burn wound sepsis. Routine administration of prophylactic antibiotics is not indicated in burn wounds as it selects for more resistant organisms. Skin biopsy showing greater than 10^5 organisms per gram of tissue is the standard for determining if a wound is infected. Lower counts may be simple colonization not requiring treatment. The advent of silver nitrate, mafenide, and silver sulfadiazine were instrumental in controlling burn wound sepsis [6].

Burn Surgery

Escharotomy and Fasciotomy

Escharotomy and fasciotomy are performed in the acute burn setting often in patients with larger TBSA burns which are either prohibitive causing respiratory distress or compartment syndrome of an extremity. Any circumferentially burned body area is at risk of ischemia, given the fluid shifts and limitation of lung compliance. One should have a low threshold for fasciotomy if the mechanism is suggestive, i.e., electrical injury, and/or signs of numbness and tingling are present. In the upper extremity, pain on passive range of motion of the digits or increasing peak airway pressures in a circumferential chest burn may suggest impending ischemia or hypoxia and necessitate an emergent decompressive intervention [7]. In the upper extremity specifically, if evidence of an intrinsic minus hand is evident, decompression is indicated. This involves making two radial incisions in the dorsum of the hand. In the lower extremity, medial and lateral incisions are necessary. In a chest escharotomy, an "H" incision is made at the mid-axillary line [7].

Excision and Grafting

The principles of burn surgery are early excision to prevent functionally limiting contracture, prevention of infection, preservation of viable tissue, and maintenance of function. The goal of early excision is to prevent contracture that may lead to tension, resulting in hypertrophic scar formation and, depending on location, limitation of function. Earlier studies demonstrate that early excision may decrease overall mortality but does not change morbidity pattern or cause of death [8].

There is benefit to temporarily covering the wound to avoid infection and for pain relief [8]. If there is not sufficient autograft, cadaver allograft may be utilized. There are numerous physiologic dressings, including cadaver allograft and xenograft. Other dressings include amion and biobrane. Advantages of allograft include its ability to vascularize and its effectiveness in closing the wound. Allograft is, however, cost prohibitive. Examples of xenograft include porcine derivatives. Xenograft is often available in large sizes and can be rapidly applied. Its biggest limitation is lack of incorporation into the wound. Products such as amion and biobrane are not currently widely utilized.

Amion is inexpensive and widely available but due to fluid fluxes must be changed every 2–4 days. Biobrane is a synthetic comprised of nylon and silicon that is variably adherent. Autografts such as cultured epidermal cells are autografts which are harvested from the patient and expanded in vitro and are often very expensive and unstable [8].

Principles of Burn Surgery

Although significant variability exists in burn injuries, post-burn deformities have similar components, allowing for a systematic rehabilitative approach. The founding principles of burn surgery are [9]:

1. Analyze the deformity, making note of distorted and deficient tissue; identify potential donor skin sites early and protect for future use.
2. Long-term goals, including both functional and aesthetic.
3. If possible, postpone reconstruction until scars and grafts have matured (usually the 1 year point). Incorporate splints and elastic garments and compression to limit hypertrophic scarring.
4. Match donor skin to color, thickness, and texture to minimize contracture.
5. Follow relaxed skin tension lines to orient scars and regional aesthetic units to avoid scars between territories.

Burn Reconstructive Ladder

Burn reconstructive options vary from a simple excision and closure to complex flaps. Although the concept of the reconstructive ladder is fundamental to plastic surgery, it is ultimately the surgeon's discretion to customize and choose the most appropriate modality.

Direct Closure
Direct closure should be reserved for burns in aesthetically conspicuous regions which will allow for favorable orientation.

Adjacent Tissue Transfer
Z-plasty is an elegant and powerful technique fundamental to plastic surgery. The goals are scar contracture release and minimization of tension. The geometry consists of limbs that are of equal length and identical angles. Z-plasty helps lengthen scar by recruiting lax surrounding tissue redirecting the scar. Furthermore, the skin transposition decreases the angle of the scar. In effect, z-plasty results in a longer, more narrow, and less conspicuous scar while functionally releasing tension [10] (Fig. 15.3).

Skin Grafts
Skin grafts provide autologous coverage. They are harvested as either full thickness (FTSG), comprised of entire epidermis and entire dermis including hair follicles, or split thickness (STSG), comprised of entire epidermis and a portion of the dermis. STSG contract more than FTSG. STSG can also be meshed and donor sites re-harvested and are often used to cover larger burn wounds. In darker patients, STSG can hyperpigment. FTSG are more often used on the face. Given their increased thickness, they require a well-vascularized wound bed [11].

Cultured Epidermal Autografts (CEA)
In very large TBSA burns when donor skin is limited, CEA may be utilized. These are autologous cells that require culturing in specialized laboratories and may take up to 2 weeks to grow. CEAs are often unstable and cost prohibitive, limiting their clinical applicability in burn reconstruction [12].

Tissue Expansion
Tissue expansion is a modality that recruits and expands native tissue. It requires two procedures: the first being the placement of the expander with weekly visits for skin expansion; the second is the removal of the expander and local tissue rearrangements. Advantages of tissue expanders include autologous tissue and improved skin color/texture match. Disadvantages include a secondary surgical procedure and the risk of expander infection, extrusion, and temporary disfigurement. In addition in areas of limited donor skin, expanding healthy skin can create increased

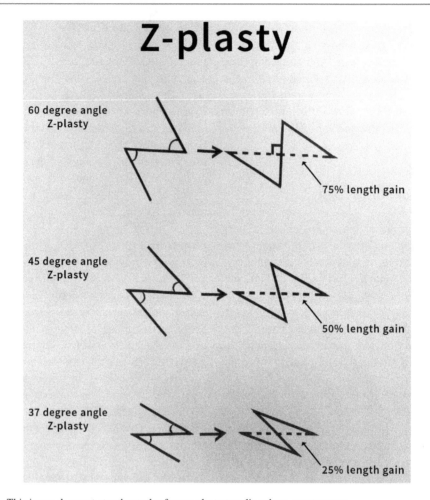

Fig. 15.3 This image demonstrates the angles for a z-plasty to relieve burn contractures

tension resulting in further contour abnormalities. Several studies report a complication rate with tissue expanders in the range of 25–50 %, limiting their use in burn reconstruction [13].

Flaps

In burns where bone, cartilage, tendon, or irradiated tissue is exposed, flaps are the choice of coverage. These may be local and pedicled flaps or free microvascular flaps. The choice of donor flaps is limited by the extent of the burn and stability of the patient [14].

Reconstruction by Anatomical Site

Scalp

Burns of the scalp can result in cicatricial alopecia. Newer modalities of hair restoration have shown benefit in hair restoration into the burn scar [15]. Although tissue expansion has a high complication rate in other regions of the body, it is a reasonable option for defects up to 50 % of the scalp. Excision and primary closure is acceptable for smaller burns. In larger burns, microvascular free flaps may need to be employed. Options for free flaps include latissimus dorsi, parascapular flap, anterolateral thigh flap, and radial forearm flap [16].

Face

Typical features of facial burns include loss of jawline definition, flat facial features, inferior displacement of lower lip and eversion, shortened and retruded upper lip, shortened nose and ala flaring, and lower eyelid ectropion. Smaller burns of the face are amenable to excision and primary closure or full-thickness skin grafts [17].

Larger burns may require local tissue transfer and the replacement of deficient tissue. For example, in burns of the eyebrow, hair micrografts may be required. Vascularized island pedicled flaps from the scalp may be used. The biggest disadvantage is misalignment of hair follicle resulting in abnormal vector of hair growth. Alternatively eyebrows may be tattooed [18].

Management of eyelid burns is of paramount importance for visual preservation. In an emergency situation, if there is adequate native upper eyelid skin, a temporary tarsorrhaphy for corneal protection may be indicated. The most common complication of eyelid burn is ectropion. Relaxing incisions may be needed to release the scar. These are often placed 1–2 mm from the ciliary margin. Full-thickness skin grafts from the contralateral upper eyelid are often utilized to replace upper eyelid skin deficiencies. Pre-auricular full-thickness skin can be used to resurface the lower eyelid [19]. Local flaps such or complete eyelid reconstruction may be warranted depending on extent of burn and visual symptoms.

Nasal burns are often complex and extensive involving the skin, mucosa, and cartilage of the nose, as well as the surrounding face. This limits local reconstructive options. Small defects can be reconstructed with composite cartilage grafts from the ear. Larger defects require free flap reconstruction. Burns of the oral commissure are usually secondary to electrical cord injuries in the pediatric population. These are amenable to oral splinting for 6–12 months. Parents need to be informed of the possibility and management of bleeding from the labial artery 7–10 days after the initial burn. Surgical reconstruction V-Y advancement flaps and transposition flaps may be indicated. Burns of the lips may result in significant oral incompetence and drooling. Local contracture release and resurfacing may be indicated. Otherwise local flap options such as the lip switch or Abbe flap may be of limited use because commonly both lips are involved [20].

Neck burns are often prone to flexion contractures. Z-plasty may be required for scar release. It is not uncommon to need to excise the entire burn skin and resurface with a thick STSG, FTSG, or microvascular free flap. A thin STSG would result in recurrence of contracture. Postoperatively splints, silicone, and compression devices are necessary to prevent contracture. In larger burns, infraclavicular tissue expanders and local deltopectoral flap may be used. Free flaps in the neck region are often cumbersome and require multiple revision procedures [21].

Breast

Burns in adolescent females may arrest breast development secondary to the intrinsic damage to progenitor cells deep to the nipple areola complex (NAC). Extrinsic developmental delay may be secondary to overlying skin contracture limiting breast development. The optimal time to reconstruct breast burns is prior to physiologic breast development. Scars should be released and skin grafts utilized for reconstruction. In postadolescent females, if the burn is extensive, including the breast parenchyma, then a more extensive procedure such as postmastectomy reconstruction such as TRAM flap from the abdomen may be warranted. Tissue expansion and implant reconstruction is difficult secondary to contracted skin [22].

Upper Extremity

Upper extremity reconstruction requires aggressive surgical care as well as occupational therapy intervention to facilitate function and prevent joint stiffness and contracture. Contractures are most successfully released from proximal to distal. Hand burns require an aggressive approach with contracture releases, early tangential excision, splinting, and physical therapy. The goal is prevention of joint stiffness. The most common post-burn complication is syndactyly, treated with z-plasty and similar scar release methods. Customized splits are essential to prevent intrinsic minus deformity [23].

Perineum

Perineal burns, like other burns, are treated initially with scar release. Surgical reconstruction of external genitalia is often complex requiring flaps and penile prosthesis [24].

Lower Extremity

As with the upper extremity, recognition and treatment of compartment syndrome is paramount. Z-plasty, skin grafts, and flaps may all be employed depending on the extent of burn. Chronic lymphedema may be treated with compression stockings [25].

Long-Term Complications

Burn patients are at an increased risk of developing Marjolin's ulcer, an aggressive ulcerating squamous cell carcinoma. These usually present as chronic, nonhealing wounds and should be biopsied [26].

Heterotopic calcification may occur in joints 1–3 months after initial injury. This more commonly affects the elbow and shoulder joints and results in joint stiffness and a limitation in range of motion. A combination of medicine and surgical intervention, focused on excision of heterotopic bone, may become necessary to preserve function [27, 28].

Conclusion

Advances in burn care have been focused on acute resuscitative efforts and the development of topical and skin substitutes. Rehabilitating patients requires a team effort and cooperation on the behalf of all health-care providers as well as long-term surveillance. Preserving function whether aesthetic or motion is integral to the patient's ultimate quality of life and well-being.

References

1. American Burn Association. www.ameriburn.org. 2014. Accessed 1 Mar 2015.
2. Saffle J, Davis B, Williams P. Recent outcomes in the treatment of burn injury in the United States: a report from the American Burn Association Patient Registry. J Burn Care Rehabil. 1995;16:219–32.
3. Brigham P, McLoughlin E. Burn incidence and medical care use in the United States: estimates, trends, and data sources. J Burn Care Rehabil. 1996;17(2):95–107.
4. Arturson M. The pathophysiology of severe thermal injury. J Burn Care Rehabil. 1985;6(2):129–46.
5. Warden GD, Kravitz M, Schnebly A. The outpatient management of moderate and major thermal injuries. J Burn Care Rehabil. 1981;2:159–61.
6. Sobel JB, Goldfarb IW, Slater H, Hammell EJ. Inhalation injury: a decade without progress. J Burn Care Rehabil. 1992;13:573–5.
7. Morehouse JD, Finklestein JL, Marano MA, et al. Resuscitation of the thermally injured patient. Crit Care Clin. 1992;8:355–65.
8. Deitch EA, Wheelahan TM, Rose MP, et al. Hypertrophic burn scars: analysis of variables. J Trauma. 1983;23:895–8.
9. Thompson PB, et al. Effect on mortality of inhalation injury. J Trauma. 1986;26:163–5.
10. Robson MC, Barnett RA, Leitch IOW, Hayward PG. Prevention and treatment of postburn scars and contracture. World J Surg. 1992;16:87–96.
11. Thompson P, et al. Effective early excision on patients with major thermal injury. J Trauma. 1987;27:205–7.
12. Atnip RG, Burke JF. Skin coverage. Curr Probl Surg. 1983;20(10):623–83.
13. Spence RJ. Experience with novel uses of tissue expanders in burn reconstruction of the face and neck. Ann Plast Surg. 1992;28:453–64.
14. Grotting J, Walkinshaw M. The early use of free flaps in burns. Ann Plast Surg. 1985;15:127–31.
15. Barrera A. The use of micrografts and minigrafts for the treatment of burn alopecia. Plast Reconstr Surg. 1999;103:581–4.
16. Platt AJ, Mckiernan MV, McLean NR. Free tissue transfer in the management of burns. Burns. 1996;22:474–6.
17. Almaguer E, Dillon BT, Parry SW. Facial resurfacing at Shriners Institute: a 16-year experience in young burned patients. J Trauma. 1985;25:1081–2.
18. Coessens B, Van Geertruyden J, DeMey A. Surgical tattooing as an aesthetic improvements in facial reconstruction with free radial forearm flap. J Reconstr Microsurg. 1995;9:331–4.
19. Kenkel JM. Eyelid reconstruction. Selected Read Plast Surg. 2000;9:1–18.
20. Pensler JM, Rosental A. Reconstruction of the oral commissure after an electrical burn. J Burn Care Rehabil. 1990;11:50–3.
21. Economides NG, Ferrell TH. Neck resurfacing with TRAM flap. Microsurgery. 1992;13:240–2.
22. Neale HW, et al. Breast reconstruction in the burned adolescent female: an 11-year, 157-patient experience. Plast Reconstr Surg. 1982;70:718–24.
23. Hunt JL, Sato R, Baxter CR. Early tangential excision and immediate mesh autografting of deep dermal hand burns. Ann Surg. 1979;189:147–51.
24. Michielsen D, Van Hee R, Neetens C, et al. Burns to the genitalia and perineum. J Urol. 1998;159:418–9.
25. Mani MM, Chhatre M. Reconstruction of the burned lower extremity. Clin Plast Surg. 1992;19:693–703.
26. Zbar RIS, Cottel WI. Skin tumors I: nonmelanoma skin tumors. Selected Read Plas Surg. 2000;9:2–19.
27. German G, Cedidi C, Hartmann B. Post-burn reconstruction during growth and development. Pediatr Surg Int. 1997;12:321–6.
28. Pruitt Jr BA. The burn patient: II. Later care and complications of thermal injury. Curr Probl Surg. 1979;16:1–95.

Part VI

Reanimation of the Paralyzed Extremity

A Global Approach to Upper Extremity Paralysis: The Role of Surgery in Limb Reanimation

Andrew I. Elkwood, Lisa F. Schneider, Deborah Yu, and Hamid Abdollahi

General Philosophy of Reanimation

The hand is the visible part of the brain. – *Immanuel Kant*

Our hands – and by extension our entire upper extremities – are the most concrete expression of our humanity. They are the means by which we do how we perform our activities of daily living and remain independent and functional. Any disruption of the link between our brain and the limb that affects its wishes has a profound impact on our ability to act and interact. This disruption exists along a spectrum from *paresis*, weakness, to *paralysis* or complete lack of movement. This motor disability may be intensified by corresponding lack of sensibility and loss of related neurofeedback as well as by chronic pain. To begin our analysis of reanimation of these deformities, we must refine our understanding of voluntary movement of the upper extremity.

A.I. Elkwood, MD, MBA (✉) • L.F. Schneider, MD
D. Yu, MD • H. Abdollahi, MD
The Plastic Surgery Center, The Institute for
Advanced Reconstruction, 535 Sycamore Ave,
Shrewsbury, NJ 07702, USA
e-mail: aelkwoodmd@theplasticsurgerycenternj.com;
lschneidermd@theplasticsurgerycenternj.com;
dyumd@theplasticsurgerycenternj.com;
habdollahimd@theplasticsurgerycenternj.com

Animation, Spastic and Flaccid Paralysis of the Upper Extremity

The impulse that drives upper extremity movement begins with the motor neurons in the cerebral cortex. These corticospinal or upper motor neurons (UMN) originate in layer five of motor cortex and descend via pyramidal tract to synapse with lower motor neurons (LMN), either directly or indirectly via interneurons [1]. The cell bodies of these lower motor neurons reside in the anterior horn of the spinal cord and transmit their signals directly to muscles [1]. The clinical pathology of this system will be determined by the level at which the disruption occurs.

Spastic Paralysis

Paralysis can be divided into two distinct categories: spastic vs. flaccid. Spasticity or spastic paralysis is defined as a disorder of the motor system that occurs after injury to the central nervous system [2] resulting in a loss of supraspinal inhibition [3]. This results in hyperactivity of muscle stretch reflexes and spastic resistance to passive movements of the affected limbs [4]. As outlined above, spastic paralysis reflects dysfunction at the level of the upper motor neuron, which inhibits movement and causes pain. This injury can occur at the level of the UMN or their axons in the cerebral cortex, subcortical white matter, internal capsule, brainstem, or spinal cord. These injuries produce weakness through decreased or lack of activation of LMN, with distal muscles

© Springer International Publishing Switzerland 2017
A.I. Elkwood et al. (eds.), *Rehabilitative Surgery*, DOI 10.1007/978-3-319-41406-5_16

more severely affected than proximal ones. Spasticity may not be present acutely [4].

Spastic paralysis is characterized clinically by muscle spasm and velocity-dependent increase in muscle tone (rigidity) or uncontrolled repetitive involuntary contractions of skeletal muscle [3]. These patients are difficult to provide care for, whether for themselves or by caregivers, and many go on to develop contractures and pressure ulcers [3]. This disorder significantly reduces quality of life and impedes patient function [5, 6]. Examples of clinical disorders that cause spastic paralysis include stroke or cerebrovascular accidents (CVA) or spinal cord injury.

These acquired disorders are a major contributor to disability across the United States. On average, nearly 800,000 patients suffer a stroke per year in the United States, roughly one every 40 s. Stroke is a leading cause of serious long-term disability with over 50 % of patients suffering residual hemiparesis and 26 % requiring assistance with activities of daily living [7]. There are an estimated over 12,000 new patients with SCI yearly [8]. The prevalence of SCI has also been increasing over time, in addition to an increased prevalence in the United States, possibly secondary to decreased mortality at the site of the initial accident. These rates are also highest for patients, often men, in their late teens and early twenties, who are in the prime of their life and have long life expectancies [8, 9].

Flaccid Paralysis

Flaccid paralysis, a very different clinical picture, presents as weakness or lack of motion resulting from progressive muscle wasting and atrophy, often with spontaneous twitching of motor units or fasciculations early after onset [4]. Demonstrated by an absence of spasticity and other signs of central nervous system motor tract disruption (hyperreflexia, clonus, or extensor plantar responses), flaccid paralysis results from the loss of contraction of voluntary muscle fibers due to the interruption of motor pathways between the cortex and muscle fibers [10, 11]. This occurs as a result of the disorder of the cell bodies of LMNs in brainstem motor nuclei and the anterior horn of the spinal cord or from

dysfunction of axons of these neurons as they pass to skeletal muscle. If LMN weakness is present, the recruitment of motor units is delayed or reduced or eliminated entirely in the case of complete paralysis [1].

Flaccid paralysis may occur following spinal cord injury, peripheral neuropathy, nerve entrapment, or injury including facial paralysis and brachial plexus injury. The incidence of traumatic brachial plexopathy is more difficult to ascertain, in part because it occurs across a wide spectrum of pathology. Roughly 1 % of all multitrauma admissions in a single center study had associated brachial plexus injury, increasing to over 4 % of all MVA and snowmobile accidents [12, 13]. Another complicating factor is the presence of concurrent injuries, including major orthopedic injuries or loss of consciousness, which may obscure the initial diagnosis. For example, we performed an arm replant on a patient who was later found to have a brachial plexopathy. There was no means, nor would it be prudent, to determine the extent of brachial plexopathy prior to attending to the patient's other severe injuries.

Treatment Options

Treatment for spastic paralysis exists along a spectrum that relates to the severity of the deformity. However, all therapies aim to reduce the reactive contractility of muscles hyperresponsive to central stimuli. For the mildest cases, physical therapy and stretching may be useful. Botulinum toxin (Botox, Allergan) has been combined with rehabilitation for the spastic conditions described above as well as for cerebral palsy [14]. However, there are a number of limitations with its use. The administration of Botox is extremely operator dependent. Furthermore, it is limited in scope of treatment. Higher doses required to treat an entire spastic limb carry higher risk of tetanus toxicity.

The next level of pharmacotherapy is baclofen. Baclofen, the most widely used antispasmodic drug, is an agonist of the inhibitory neurotransmitter gamma-aminobutyric acid (GABA) [5]. This may be administered orally or intrathecally for cases of severe or intractable spasticity [3, 5]. Intrathecal administration via pump is often the route of choice and has been widely reported in the literature. However, there are numerous potential downsides. Patients may quickly develop tolerance to the oral form. Side effects of either route of administration include drowsiness, dizziness, constipation, and muscular hypotonia, as well as the risk of seizure or drug overdose [5]. Baclofen also carries the risk of potentially fatal crises of withdrawal or overdose [15]. Baclofen pumps can be especially hazardous at the high spinal levels required to ameliorate upper extremity spasticity, where there may be a risk of respiratory depression. Furthermore, as implants, the pumps themselves are fraught with the usual limitations of all implants, including a limited half-life and infectious complications. In a recent review from a tertiary care center, mechanical complications requiring pump and/or catheter revision occurred in 19.3 % of patients and infections in an additional 21.8 % [16].

The classical, though increasingly infrequent, surgical therapy for spasticity is selective dorsal rhizotomy. Rhizotomy attempts to reduce afferent input into the reflex arc while leaving the patient with their remaining mobility. However, this reduction in afferent input occurs in an unselective way, also simultaneously reducing cutaneous and proprioceptive awareness [6]. Chronic spinal deformities, including scoliosis and abnormal kyphosis, have been noted to be long-term complications in a significant number of patients [17]. Even more concerning is the lack of predictable surgical outcome. Crilly in a *BMJ* editorial has recommended that selective dorsal rhizotomy be considered an experimental procedure for cerebral palsy patients due to lack of evidence regarding potential benefit [18]. This is coupled with a risk of severe complications, including dural leaks, infection, or spinal cord damage. Because of the unfavorable risk-benefit ratio, rhizotomy is an increasingly rare intervention. Additional classical treatments for spastic paralysis include tendon lengthening, tenotomy, and joint fusion.

Essentially, all of the treatments for spastic paralysis described above are specific techniques for reducing spasticity. However, we believe that spastic paralysis should be approached with a different perspective. In fact, spastic and flaccid paralysis are linked. It is only possible to reanimate flaccid paralysis, where the extremity is reduced to its physical components without the need to fight against spasm. If spastic paralysis can be *converted* to flaccid paralysis, it becomes possible to *reanimate* the paralyzed limb. This represents a paradigm shift in treatment, rehabilitation, and reanimation of these patients and creates new opportunities for maximizing function and minimizing pain.

This can be done in a more targeted manner in peripheral nerves as well. This new peripheral neurectomy option allows for an individual and targeted approach, e.g., to specific muscle group. This requires a more precise diagnosis of spasticity of individual muscle groups. This diagnosis may be difficult, and patients can require multiple procedures in order to appropriately denervate the muscle target. Peripheral neurectomy for relief of targeted spasticity will be discussed in more detail in a later section on treatment. It is also important to note that flaccid paralysis is *necessary but not sufficient* for reanimation. The patient's limb must be supple and have good passive range of motion, emphasizing the critical role of preoperative therapy in order to optimize outcome.

The *Garage Door* Analogy

When we are presented with a patient who has flaccid paralysis, how do we begin to approach the problem of upper extremity reanimation? For the most elegant and functional reconstructions, it is helpful to create a solution that is as close as possible to the original design and natural anatomy. An analogy may provide a basis for understanding the deficits, which is the beginning of creating a solution. Ultimately, the upper extremity can be seen as a series of pulleys and levers, motors, and muscles. Imagine that the musculoskeletal system of the upper extremity is a garage door. The central nervous system would be the wiring within the house that provides the input for the electrical system. Extending this metaphor, the nerves are the electric wires and the nerve roots, the socket for the wire. The muscle is the motor that opens the door by means of the chain or tendon. The door itself is the joint, impelled by the electrical current through the nerve wire and moved by the muscle motor through the tendon chain.

By imaging the complex injury through this simple analogy, we can better understand how to fix the problems. A damaged nerve – or shredded wire – will require a nerve graft to allow for conduction of electrical current or nerve impulses. If there is a problem with the muscle motor, the patient will require a free muscle flap. A tendon transfer is analogous to a chain to the garage next door, using the neighbor's motor to open the door. An arthrodesis or joint fusion is essentially blocking the door open permanently, while a splint is doing the same thing in a temporary way. There must be good passive range of motion – the garage door must be able to open and close easily without rust on the hinges – in order to contemplate reanimation (Fig. 16.2).

The Systematic Study of Spare Parts

There are many approaches to reanimating – literally, *to return life to* – these patients. Certainly, they present complex injuries that require challenging reconstructions with a wide variety of modalities. The initial analysis must include these four aspects:

1. Current deformities and deficits
2. "Spare parts" currently available for reconstruction
3. "Spare parts" that can be created for subsequent reconstructions
4. Bailouts and options if first or ideal plan does not work out

Furthermore, the approach to each patient must be individualized. The same injury in an octogenarian, a young mother, and a construction worker should be treated differently.

The next step is considering the correct operative procedures and sequence. Although there are many ways to approach each repair, the most elegant reconstruction is often the one that most closely approximates both original anatomy and function. A straightforward example is nerve repair, reconnecting the "wiring" but using the same anatomic structure to regain function. However, there is an inverse relationship between elegance and predictability – more elegant repairs like nerve repair are also usually the least predictable. On the other end of the spectrum would be joint fusion, which could be considered the least elegant because it succeeds by eliminating joint function, though with highly predictable results. Furthermore, each of these operations is inherently variable. The result will depend on a multitude of factors including the patient's injury, age, and their participation in rehabilitation both before and after the procedures. This variability necessitates a multi-operative approach. The surgeon must determine what functions have been successfully regained after each procedure in order to confirm the next step.

Like any problem with multiple solutions, any one of these solutions – especially any single solution – is imperfect. Just as a master chess player studies the current configuration of the pieces but plans several moves in advance, so the reanimating surgeon must provide his or her patient with a comprehensive approach to care that anticipates the steps – and possible missteps – on the road ahead. In essence, this is a "study of spare parts" – i.e., donor nerves, muscles, and tendons – in order to determine a surgical plan. Plastic and reconstructive surgery as a discipline is defined as the study of spare parts, balancing considerations of what can be gained by borrowing function or tissue from a donor versus what is lost by using that donor, i.e., the creation of donor disease. This is the "borrowing from Peter to pay Paul" principle. The reconstructive surgeon must understand not only what is functioning in each patient but also what is expendable for that particular individual.

One of the inherent difficulties of reconstructive surgery is defining the end point. A cancer surgeon may attain success by excising the cancer with clear margins or fail when tumor is left behind. Unlike this binary situation, the result of reconstructive surgery is much less clear. A patient may have sustained such severe injuries that returning "normal" function may be an impossible goal. Instead, success of reconstructive surgery slides along a spectrum defined by the patient's preoperative need and postoperative function. Not only is the treatment individualized but so too is the very definition of success or failure of the procedure in that patient. Our approach is based on maximizing functional recovery for the patient's specific circumstance. We present a global, multimodality approach for upper extremity reanimation that combines years of patient care and research with the most current understanding of surgical procedures to optimize functional reconstruction.

Surgical Planning Exam and Evaluation

Before beginning our discussion of clinical, electromyographic, and radiographic preoperative evaluation of the patient, it is important to clarify one key aspect. A *surgical planning* exam and evaluation is fundamentally different from a *diagnostic* exam and evaluation. We are not simply looking to the past injury or deficit but forward toward possible therapeutic interventions. Below we describe several examples of this distinction we which believe is an essential element of an appropriate global approach.

The initial evaluation includes a thorough determination of all deficits through a careful history and physical examination [9]. Second, the surgeon must determine which "spare parts" – functioning muscles or nerves – can be used for reconstruction. Both of these objectives are performed through a thorough history and physical exam with specific testing of relevant motor and sensory functions. We typically record muscle grading, in addition to passive and active range of motion, sensory examination, and pain threshold, on a preprinted brachial plexus diagram (see Fig. 16.1 Fig. 16.3, Fig.16.4) [9]. We also typically take videos of patients in order to document their initial exam and future progress. However, there is more to this initial analysis than simply recording muscle strength. The muscles that are not functioning normally must

be examined more closely. It is important to differentiate the function of individual muscles from the larger muscle group. If the triceps is not functioning, each individual head of the triceps must be examined on either physical exam or, if not readily apparently clinically, through dedicated super-selective electromyographic testing. If the muscle is paralyzed, is the paralysis spastic or flaccid? Neither muscle will be "functional" nor have sufficient power to resist gravity, but the treatment of these different types of paralysis will be very different.

This strategy can be summarized with these key points of analysis:

1. What functions are missing?
   For example, *arm abduction*
2. What functions are interfering with others?
   For example, *inability to flex the elbow in spastic paralysis*
3. What functions are spastic vs. flaccid?
   For example, *flaccid biceps with spastic triceps, an example of "antagonistic paralysis"*
4. What functions can be/are desirable to be restored?
   For example, pronation/supination may not be worthwhile to restore.
   For example, *wrist extension is only useful for power grip, if there is insufficient finger.*
   Flexion for power grip, it may be preferable to fuse the wrist.
5. Which donors can be used to restore function?
6. Which new donors can be created to restore function?
7. Nonneural limitations to functional restoration?
   For example, *orthopedic injury, contracture, and cognitive issues*

Assessment of Function

There are several different diagnostic maneuvers that give the surgeon insight into the possible utility of specific surgical interventions. For example, bimanual palpation can give clues to which distinct portion of the muscle is functioning by determining spasm or contraction. When

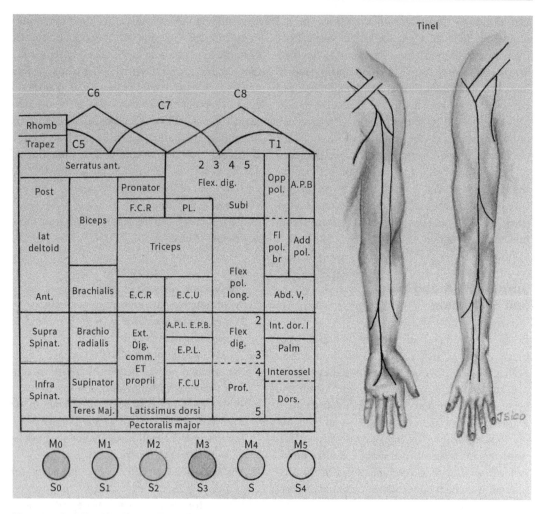

Fig. 16.1 Left Brachial Plexus (From Green's, Volume II, p. 1322) [19]

palpating a patient's deltoid muscle, abducting the arm in different directions may allow differentiation of individual muscle heads. With elbow extension, it is possible to feel the three distinct heads of the triceps. Muscles may also be differentiated based on their position during function. The biceps flexes the elbow with the hand in supination, while the brachialis flexes the elbow with the hand pronated. Another maneuver that may be used is temporary motor blockade with lidocaine or Botox. If the brachialis is iatrogenically paralyzed via the radial nerve, it is possible to determine how much the biceps itself is contributing to elbow flexion via the musculo-cutaneous nerve. It is important to note that there are limits to the physical exam. These subtle differentiations can be extremely complicated, e.g., differentiating between the ECRB (extensor carpis radialis brevis) and ECRL (extensor carpis radialis longus) muscles, and may only be performed under direct visualization in the operating room.

Assessment of Pain

The motor deficit of paresis or paralysis is the most obvious defect, but not necessarily the most important. For many patients, especially those with paralysis, the most important functional consideration is unremitting pain. This can be easily overlooked by the medical and surgical team but is often one of most central issues in patients' life and daily functioning. It is important to remember that an injury severe enough to cause paralysis may be accompanied by pain for a variety of reasons.

Pain may be secondary to four possible cases: (1) direct nerve pain, (2) neuroma, (3) joint subluxation and orthopedic derangement, and (4) phantom limb syndrome. For example, a trapezius to deltoid transfer has been well described as a technique for improving arm abduction [20–22]. However, many patients who require this procedure are in fact more greatly aided by the repositioning of the shoulder joint resulting in reduction of glenohumeral subluxation that occurs with the transfer, which ameliorates their pain, rather than simply the improved abduction [22]. This can be tested preoperatively by reducing the patient's shoulder in the office, which often provides immediate relief for a sensation described as "carrying a heavy piece of luggage and never getting to put it down."

There are also multiple potentially straightforward interventions for nerve-related pain that have the ability to significantly improve quality of life. Neuroma and phantom limb syndrome can be differentiated by injection of lidocaine into the nerve stump. If the pain resolves, it is likely secondary to neuroma, which can be treated by direct excision or other means. A patient with brachial plexopathy but without a distal limb traditionally might not be offered brachial plexus grafting because of lack of functional targets. However, these grafts have the potential to improve distal pain and therefore should be considered in the overall operative approach.

Assessment of Donors

Nerves

For the reconstructive surgeon, not all nerves are created equal. There are a number of key

considerations in selecting a donor nerve. *What loss of function will occur after nerve harvest?* One strategy to minimize this loss is using a branch of the nerve after arborization of its crucial branches. Another is to use a nerve to a muscle that is either synergistic with intact muscles or no longer functional after the patient's injury. For example, if a patient is unable to move their arm, the stabilization of the scapula by the serratus anterior via the long thoracic nerve is no longer a significant consideration. In this situation, the long thoracic becomes an excellent donor.

What is the length of the defect? This will determine whether additional nerve graft interposition is required with the neurotization, which unfortunately will decrease the success rate. For example, the spinal accessory nerve will reach the suprascapular nerve for neurotization but will require additional graft to reach the axillary nerve. *Where is the injury relative to the motor end organ?* If the nerve has to travel a long distance after neurotization, the likelihood of a successful result diminishes considerably. A classic example of this is the "baby sitting procedure," performing an anterior interosseous nerve transfer for distal ulnar nerve palsy to prevent claw hand. A more proximal neurotization would be much less likely to reinnervate the small interossei within a reasonable time frame prior to motor end plate degeneration and muscle atrophy.

Another key concept in choosing donors is that of axonal density. It is important to choose donor nerves that will allow the patient to obtain *meaningful* movement, which is more than simply movement against gravity. Part of the selection process for nerve donors must take into account *axonal density*, essentially a relatively high number of axons for the nerve diameter. The surgical result will be optimized when the donor and recipient nerve are matched in terms of total diameter and average axonal density [23–25]. In order to maximize power of nerve transfer, the donor nerve axons need to fill up as much of the cross section of engrafted nerve as possible. A loose analogy to better understand this concept is that of voltage. Much more voltage – and wiring to transmit that voltage – is needed to power the air conditioner of a house than a stereo. Similarly, if a large muscle needs to be powered, the donor nerve used to power it must have high axonal density [26].

A clinical example is a comparison between the spinal accessory and the intercostal nerve. The spinal accessory nerve has much greater axonal density than does the intercostal nerve. A rule of thumb to maximize axonal density is to choose a small nerve – like the spinal accessory nerve – that powers a large muscle, e.g., the trapezius. The intercostal nerve is similar in diameter to the spinal accessory nerve, but the intercostal muscle is much smaller than the trapezius is. A single intercostal nerve with its low axonal density would not be sufficient to power the biceps, and nerve transfer via intercostals to the biceps typically requires multiple intercostal nerves. It is also useful to consider other less, common donors that historically have been overlooked. For example, the nerves to the levator scapulae and sternocleidomastoid have good axonal density and are also synergistic. Another option to maximize axonal density is the use of cadaver nerves or living-related sources of donor nerve in order to perform multiple cable grafts [26, 27]. Muscles that require strength like the biceps or the deltoid may require the use of these adjuncts in order to maximize function, whereas a less dense nerve may be sufficient for a smaller muscle like the flexor pollicis longus (Figs. 16.5, 16.7, 16.8, 16.10)

Muscles

There are five main considerations for evaluation of muscle donors: (1) strength, (2) excursion, (3) length, (4) direction of pull, and (5) available resources, i.e., what has been spared vs. what can be created as a new donor. The surgeon needs to evaluate potential donors based on strength. Muscle strength is evaluated based on the MMT (manual muscle testing) grading system [28]. Any muscle less than M4 (holding an antigravity position against moderate resistance) is not suitable to be used for transfer. For example, the palmaris longus is a weak muscle but would be appropriate for transfer after median nerve palsy in an elderly patient who does not require much strength for thumb opposition. There is also a balance and inverse relationship between excursion length and strength, and the muscle used for transfer will depend on the requirements for function. Unipennate muscles tend to have good excursion but poor strength, while bipennate muscles have better strength but poor excursion. The direction of pull and the existing and fabricated pulleys also must be evaluated.

This muscle evaluation also must occur in the context of a larger understanding of patient function, especially planning out multiple operations in the future. One muscle that is nearly always spared, even in relatively high spinal cord injuries, is the trapezius. Its innervation, the spinal accessory nerve (CN XI), and contributions from C3 and C4 travel with the cranial nerves [22]. An injury severe enough to compromise these nerves is typically fatal. Because of this near universal availability, trapezius transfer is the most common reported transfer in adult palsy [22].

Creation of New Donors and Donor "Disease"

Using the multistaged approach, it is also possible to expand the pool of donor muscles. Muscles subsequently used as donors may not have been initially spared by the injury. For example, during an initial surgery to reconstruct arm abduction, the latissimus can be engrafted. This allows this muscle, which may not have initially been functional, to be used as a tendon transfer for biceps or triceps reanimation. It is always important to consider what new deficits or "donor disease" will be created when a donor muscle or nerve is used. What is acceptable in one patient may present too great a disability in another. For example, a patient who cannot flex their elbow is better served by using their latissimus muscle as a donor than would be a professional pitcher. The procedure needs to be personalized for the patient and their specific, unalterable limitation, e.g., inability to perform manual labor.

Some donors, although classically acceptable, create too large a deficit when appropriately understood and should not be used. The phrenic nerve has been previously recommended as a donor for restoration of elbow flexion and restoration of shoulder abduction [29–31]. However, the loss of this nerve has measurable negative consequences. Unilateral diaphragmatic paralysis has been associated with exertional dyspnea, orthopnea, sleep disturbances, and gastrointestinal reflux, all symptoms causally linked to a decrease in resting and active diaphragmatic tone [32]. The phrenic nerve should never be used as a nerve donor for transfer. In fact, we advocate phrenic nerve reconstruction in appropriately selected patients, e.g., patients' status post cardiac surgery or other iatrogenic causes with the symptoms described above. Patients who have undergone reconstruction of the phrenic nerve via neurolysis, neurotization, or interpositional nerve grafting have significant improvements in pulmonary function testing and report better scores on quality of life surveys [33].

Electromyography and Imaging

The clinical exam, however, has its own limits. It is difficult to discern muscles that (1) are synergistic, (2) are grouped, or (3) have duplicated function. For example, the deltoid needs to work synergistically with the biceps in order to stabilize the shoulder girdle during elbow flexion. Grouped muscles are those considered often as one muscle that functions together but has distinct sections or heads that may have different levels of activity after injury, like the three sections of the trapezius or three heads of the triceps. Although certain clinical maneuvers can help, muscles with duplicated function – like the extensor digitorum communis to the index and the extensor indicis proprius – may be difficult to differentiate.

Additional testing serves as a necessary adjunct to any complete physical exam but especially in situations of synergistic, grouped, or duplicated muscles. Electromyography, as mentioned above, is the cornerstone of any careful musculoskeletal evaluation. It is helpful to have a dedicated electromyographer who not only has experience in brachial plexus and peripheral nerve injuries but also an appreciation for the subtlety involved in diagnosis [9]. Minor muscles that perform the same function may have been spared by the brachial plexopathy or spinal cord injury and may function as useful donors. For example, the brachioradialis

and brachialis flex the elbow, just as the biceps does. However, if the surgeon and the electromyographer do not think to evaluate the brachialis, its suitability for use as a donor cannot be determined. Another example is determining if the muscle keeping a patient's arm in spasm is the triceps or the anconeus, which can be difficult to determine without an experienced electromyographer. In fact, the assessment of a skilled electromyography may be predictive in determining the outcome of nerve transfers [34].

Further imaging is also required. A basic chest x-ray can determine if the patient has fracture of ribs, possibly eliminating the intercostal as a donor, the clavicle or scapula. An x-ray can also demonstrate phrenic nerve paralysis with deep inspiratory and expiratory views [9]. Additional assessment of neuromuscular function using pulmonary function testing and electrodiagnostic testing can be used to further elucidate the degree of phrenic nerve dysfunction [32]. A CT myelogram should be performed in addition to an MRI of the affected brachial plexus. Traction that disrupted the brachial plexus at the initial trauma may damage the subclavian vessels or cause pseudoaneurysm formation [9]. An MRA and MRV of the subclavian and axillary arteries should also be performed to rule out any vascular injury or malformation (Fig. 16.6).

Introduction to Surgical Planning

Surgical Timing

Another difficult aspect to approaching any patient with a nerve deficit is determining the correct time for operative intervention. Many patients will improve without intervention. However, by 12–18 months after the injury, all the motor end plates will have undergone irreparable atrophy [35, 36]. How should the correct patient and correct timing of the operation be determined? If a patient has a sharp injury, e.g., a knife wound to the brachial plexus, the intervention should be performed as soon as possible. If the injury involves a gunshot wound or blunt mechanism, it can often be unclear whether the deficit is secondary to neuropraxia or a true, irremediable injury. Another complicating factor is that many injuries are mixed and may contain elements of several different Sunderland grades of nerve injury [37].

We believe that early and aggressive surgical treatment is the optimal approach in order to restore function [26]. Our practice in these injuries is to obtain a baseline electromyography (EMG) at 6 weeks, with a repeat exam at 3 months. If there has been no improvement over 3 months, the operation is performed immediately. Typically, these more severely injured patients will also have a clear, non-advancing Tinel's sign where neuropraxia patients often have no overt Tinel's [38]. What to do if some improvement is observed yet the patient has not returned to normal, baseline nerve function? If the patient is only 95 % improved by 6 months or if there is anything more than a subtle difference remaining by 9 months, we also recommend surgical intervention. These patients also require ongoing physical therapy from the time of their initial diagnosis. Patients who have inadequate therapy may develop contractures that create functional deficits [9].

The Surgical Planning Process

The most critical aspect of preoperative evaluation and surgical planning is the ability to think ahead regarding all the procedures the surgeon must perform to recreate function for the patient and minimize pain. Furthermore, the patient must understand that the surgeries themselves are a process and not an event. This process will require multiple surgeries that are necessarily fraught with trial and error without sure guarantees about what function will return. There are also practical rehabilitation rationales for operating in multiple stages. The therapy required for a flexor or extensor transfer or for a joint function will be completely different. Attempting to combine surgeries with opposing actions into one procedure necessarily prohibits optimal rehabilitation, a key component of the best possible outcome. It is also necessary to pay attention to the patient's entire

medical and surgical condition, not focusing on the injury alone. Their injuries may occur at multiple levels on the extremity in addition to being one of the multiple systems injured. For example, a patient with a brachial plexus injury combined with an orthopedic shoulder injury or a head injury will not be treated in the same way as one with the brachial plexus injury alone.

Any intervention must be planned as part of a cohesive and coherent whole. There are many different modalities that can be used to improve these patients' function, including neurotization, nerve transfer, tendon transfer, arthrodesis, and several other types of procedures. Care for these patients must be provided by either a single surgeon who is experienced and capable of performing all of these modalities or by a coordinated team of surgeons who, as a unit, serve the same purpose. It is a disservice to the patient to perform a single-nerve transfer without placing this intervention within the larger patient goals. This represents a paradigm shift in how we as physicians approach the problem of upper extremity reanimation. The specific surgical treatments will be addressed in a subsequent paper.

Targeted Muscle Reinnervation

Almost 2 million people are living in the United States with limb loss with approximately 185,000 amputations happening each year [39, 40]. Loss of the use of an upper extremity can be devastating. Prostheses have provided a solution both cosmetically and functionally for these patients. The early pioneers of the prosthesis were the Egyptians [41]. Writings as early as 424 BC describe a man amputating his own foot and replacing it with a wooden filler to continue to walk [41]. In the first century AD, tradesmen designed and created artificial limbs, even adding intricate functions using springs and gears [41]. The US Civil War forced an entrance into the field of prosthetics in America as the number of amputations increased [41]. After World War II, the United States government collaborated with military companies to improve the function of existing prostheses [41].

New advances in targeted muscle reinnervation (TMR) have enabled prostheses to function at a much higher level. Previously, patients with above-the-elbow amputations only had the options of body-powered and myoelectric prostheses that rely on functioning muscles at the level of or just proximal to the amputation level [42]. TMR allows for more coordinated movement as multiple joints can move at the same time [42]. TMR has not only allowed improved control of prostheses but also has the potential to relieve post-amputation neuroma pain [43]. The mechanism behind TMR is the use of a series of nerve transfers to provide "intuitive prosthetic control to upper extremity amputees" [43]. TMR uses transfer of transected peripheral nerves to reinnervate intact muscles and the overlying skin [44]. A pattern recognition algorithm is used to interpret the surface electromyographic signals from the reinnervated muscle [44]. These signals are used to provide control signals for the prosthetic device [44]. TMR is most often utilized in the transhumeral and shoulder disarticulation patient population [43].

Patients in whom TMR is most beneficial are those with amputations proximal to the wrist without a concomitant proximal nerve injury [43]. As with many complex procedures, TMR is most effective with interdisciplinary coordination of surgical, rehabilitative, and prosthetic teams [43].

The procedure is not technically difficult and does not require advanced instruments [43]. Thus, combined with minimal morbidity, these procedures have little downside [43]. Who is the ideal patient? TMR is entertained in patients with a proximal-to-the-wrist upper extremity amputation who wish to improve function of their prosthesis [43]. A second indication that has arisen for TMR is for post-amputation neuroma, but it is still being studied [43].

Preoperative Evaluation

It is important to keep in mind a future TMR when an initial amputation is performed in order to preserve potential donor nerves. Which nerves are transferred is dependent on the available donor nerves and muscle targets [43]. Clues to potential donor nerves are the mechanism of injury, remaining limb length, presence and location of scars, location of Tinel's signs, and presence of voluntary contracting muscles [43]. Longer residual limbs provide greater donor nerve length and more possible muscle targets as recipients [43]. Guidelines for the majority of TMR transfers are as follows: Patients should demonstrate voluntary biceps and/or triceps functions if their amputation is the transhumeral level, and they should demonstrate voluntary contraction of the pectoralis, serratus, and latissimus dorsi muscles if their amputation is at the shoulder disarticulation level [43]. Other surgical techniques can be used in combination with the TMR procedure, including, but not limited to, free flaps for soft tissue coverage and for donor muscle [43].

Transfers for Muscle Reinnervation

Transhumeral Level
For the transhumeral amputee, TMR was envisioned to create "hand close" and "hand open" control signals while preserving elbow flexion and extension signals [43]. The "hand close" signal is established with transfer of the remnant median nerve to the motor nerve of the short head of the biceps brachii [43]. The "hand open" signal is accomplished from transfer of the distal radial nerve to the motor nerve of the lateral head of the triceps [43]. In preserving the musculocutaneous innervation of the long head of the biceps and radial innervation of the long head of the triceps, elbow flexion and extension signals are respectively preserved [43]. Wrist control can be created in transferring the remnant ulnar nerve to the brachialis muscle in a patient with a long residual limb [43].

Shoulder Disarticulation Level
TMR at the shoulder disarticulation level is more difficult because of the more proximal injury and

fewer recipient muscle targets and donor nerves [43]. In most cases, there is a compromised soft tissue envelope as well [43]. It is imperative to assess what muscle and soft tissue are remaining preoperatively [43]. TMR at the shoulder disarticulation level is not as predictable and simple as a TMR in the transhumeral patient [43]. TMR at the shoulder disarticulation level may employ a variety of different nerve transfer combinations versus the same pattern used in the transhumeral patient [43, 45]. The ideal situation pairs the musculocutaneous nerve with the motor branch of the clavicular head of the pectoralis major, the median nerve and ulnar nerve are transferred to motor branches corresponding to the split segments of the sternal head, and the radial nerve is coapted to the thoracodorsal nerve [43]. The musculocutaneous nerve provides control for elbow flexion and is paired with the pectoralis clavicular head, which is a muscle target that provides the strongest and most predictable myoelectric signal [43]. Pectoralis minor and serratus anterior can be used as alternative transfer recipients [43] (Fig. 16.9).

Postoperative Care

Patients are typically observed overnight and discharged on postoperative day one [43]. It is possible to perform such procedures in the outpatient setting if the patient's pain can be adequately controlled [43]. The remaining limb is not immobilized, but compressive dressings are used to reduce postoperative swelling [43]. Approximately 4–6 weeks postoperatively, patients can resume wearing their original prosthesis, provided wound healing is uncomplicated and swelling has subsided sufficiently [43]. Patients are preemptively counseled that they will experience altered sensation in the skin overlying the reinnervated muscles [43]. Patients with preoperative phantom pain will have an exacerbation for 4–6 weeks that will typically reduce to baseline [43]. Successful reinnervation usually takes place within 3–6 months [43]. The longest reinnervation distance and time occur if the latissimus muscle is used as a target [43]. Prosthetic fitting and myoelectric testing are started at a minimum of 6 months post-TMR [43].

Future Directions

At the University of Michigan, researchers are pioneering a sensory regenerative peripheral nerve interface, whereby sensory signals are transferred from a prosthetic sensor to the residual nerve [44]. This bioartificial interface uses free muscle neurotized with the transected end of a primarily sensory nerve fascicle [44]. The muscle is stimulated with an insulated electrode and then depolarizes the afferent nerve within the muscle [44]. This loop provides sensory feedback [44].

Another approach that is being investigated is optogenetic technology [44]. Optogenetic technology uses genetically modified microbial opsins or light-sensitive ion channels specific to nerves for control of neural signaling [44]. Using this technology, particular wavelengths of light can stimulate or inhibit a nerve [44]. This approach is currently only being used in animal models [44] (Tables 16.1, 16.2, 16.3, 16.4, 16.5, 16.6, and 16.7).

Table 16.1 The Medical Research Council System

Motor recovery

M0	No contraction
M1	Return of perceptible contraction in the proximal muscles
M2	Return of perceptible contraction in both the proximal and distal muscles
M3	Return of perceptible contraction in both the proximal and distal muscles to such a degree that all *important* muscles are sufficiently powerful to act against resistance
M4	Return of function as in stage 3 with the addition that all *synergic* and independent movements are possible
M5	Complete recovery

Sensory recovery

S0	Absence of sensibility in the autonomous area
S1	Recovery of deep cutaneous pain sensibility within the autonomous area of the nerve
S2	Return of some degree of cutaneous pain and tactile sensibility within the autonomous area
S3	Return of some degree of superficial cutaneous pain and tactile sensibility within the autonomous area with disappearance of any previous overreaction
S3+	Return of sensibility as in stage 3 with the addition that there is some recovery of two-point discrimination within the autonomous area
S4	Complete recovery

From Birch et al. [46]

Table 16.3 Classification of hand function

Class	Designation	Activity level
0	Do not use	Do not use
1	Poor passive assist	Uses as stabilizing weight only
2	Fair passive assist	Can hold on to object placed in hand
3	Good passive assist	Can hold object and stabilize for use by the other hand
4	Poor active assist	Can actively grasp object and hold it weakly
5	Fair active assist	Can actively grasp object and stabilize it well
6	Good active assist	Can actively grasp object, stabilize it well, and manipulate it against the other hand
7	Spontaneous use, partial	Can perform bimanual activities easily; occasionally uses hand spontaneously
8	Spontaneous use, complete	Uses hand completely independently, without reference to the other hand

From House et al. [47]

Table 16.2 Grading of results

Motor recovery	Sensory recovery
M4 or better	Good
M3	Fair
M2	Poor
M1 and 0	Bad
S4 (normal) or S3+	Good
S3	Fair
S2	Poor
S1 and 0	Bad

From Birch et al. [46]

Note: The grades "poor" and "bad" are grouped together for the Peripheral Nerve Injury Unit of the Royal National Orthopaedic Hospital. The grade "excellent " is rarely used for results when function is almost indistinguishable from normal

Table 16.4 Clinical scale of motor control

Grade	Motor control	Description
1	Flaccid	Hypotonic, no active motion
2	Rigid	Hypertonic, no active motion
3	Reflexive mass pattern (synergy)	Mass flexion or extension in response to stimulation
4	Volitional mass pattern	Patient-initiated mass flexion or extension movement
5	Selective with pattern overlay	Slow volitional movement of specific joints; physiologic stress results in mass action
6	Selective	Volitional control of individual joints

From Wolfe et al. [48] (Figs. 16.11–16.15)

Table 16.5 Glasgow Coma Scale

Response	Score
Eye opening	
Spontaneous	4
To speech	3
To pain	2
None	1
Motor response	
Obeys	6
Localizes	5
Withdrawal	4
Abnormal flexion	3
Extension	2
None	1
Verbal response	
Oriented	5
Confused	4
Inappropriate	3
Incomprehensible	2
None	1

From Teasdale and Jennett [49]

Table 16.6 Muscle grading system: British Medical Research Council

Grade	Description
0	No contraction
1	Flicker or trace of contraction
2	Active movement with gravity eliminated
3	Active movement against gravity
4	Active movement against gravity and resistance
5	Normal power

British Medical Research Council [50] with kind permission from the UK Medical Research Council

Table 16.7 Surgical guidelines based on International Classification Group

Motor group	Author's preferred method of treatment
1	BR to ECRB
	FPL tenodesis
	Option: split FPL tenodesis
2	BR to FPL
	CMC fusion
	EPL tenodesis
	Option: split FPL tenodesis
3	BR to FPL
	CMC fusion
	EPL tenodesis
	Option: split FPL tenodesis
4 and 5	House two stages:
	Extensor phase
	EDC tenodesis (*option*: BR to EDC)
	EPL tenodesis
	Options: CMC fusion, intrinsic tenodesis
	Flexor phase
	ECRL to FDP
	BR to FPL (*option*: PT to FPL)
	Options: adduction-opponensplasty (BR or PT with FDS graft), split FPL tenodesis, lasso procedure
6	ECRL to FDP
	BR to FPL (*option*: PT to FPL)
	EPL tenodesis (option: EPL to EDC)
	Options: CMC fusion or adduction-opponensplasty (BR or PT with FDS free graft), split FPL tenodesis, lasso procedure (BR or PT to FDS)
7	ECRL to FDP
	BR to FPL (option: PT to FPL)
	Options: CMC fusion or adduction-opponensplasty (BR or PT with FDS free graft), split FPL tenodesis, lasso procedure (BR or PT to FDS)
8	FDP side to side
	BR to FPL
	Options: opponensplasty (BR or PT with FDS graft), split FPL tenodesis, lasso procedure (BR or PT to FDS)

From Wolfe et al. [48] (Figs. 16.11–16.15)

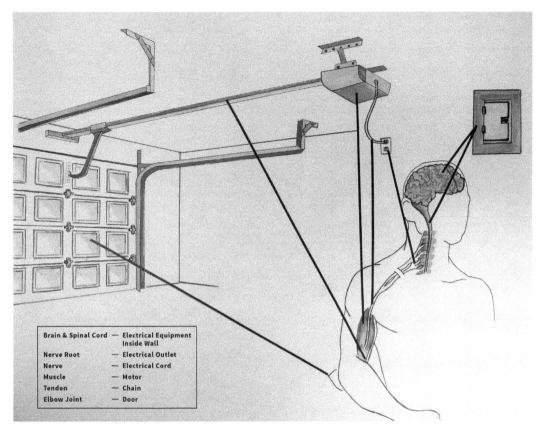

Fig. 16.2 Garage door analogy of the musculoskeletal system

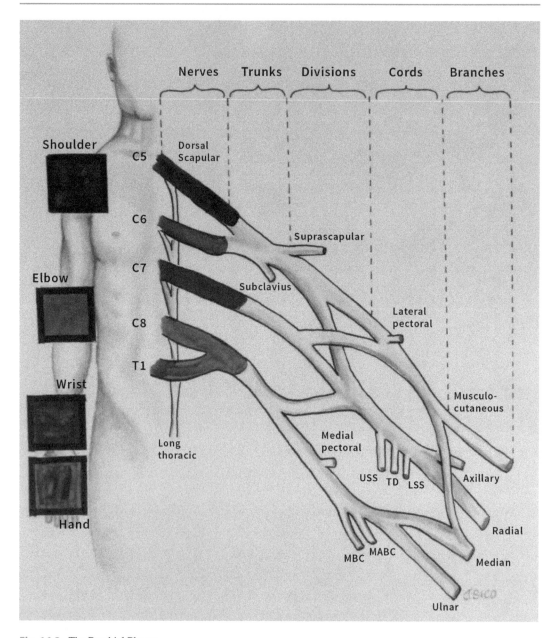

Fig. 16.3 The Brachial Plexus

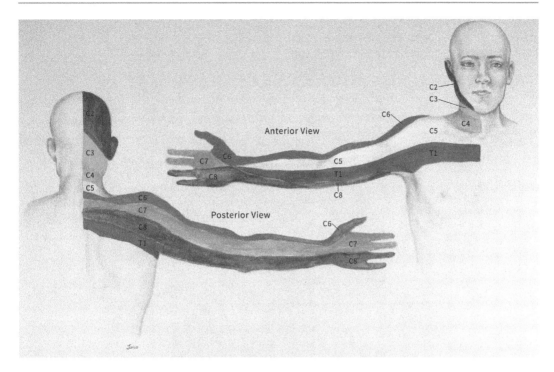

Fig. 16.4 Dermatomes of upper limb

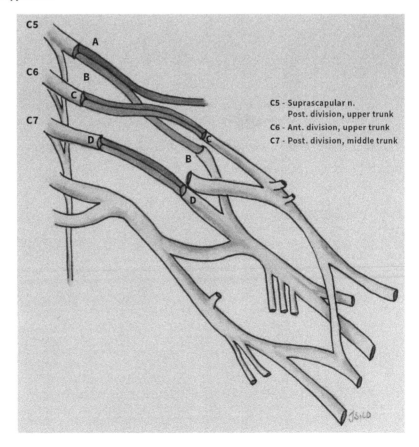

C5 - Suprascapular n.
    Post. division, upper trunk
C6 - Ant. division, upper trunk
C7 - Post. division, middle trunk

Fig. 16.5 Intraplexal
nerve grafting

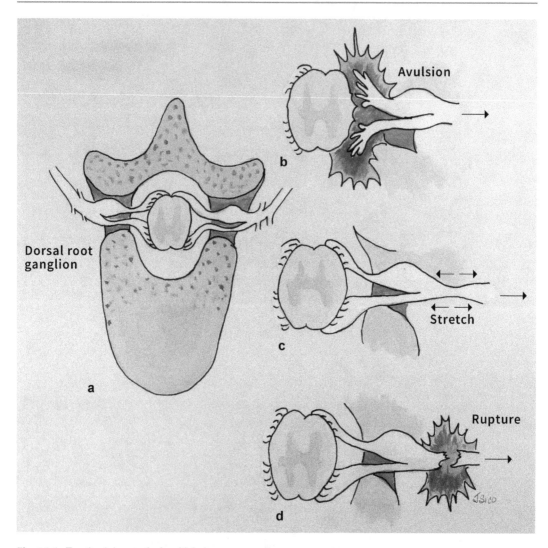

Fig. 16.6 Traction injury to the brachial plexus

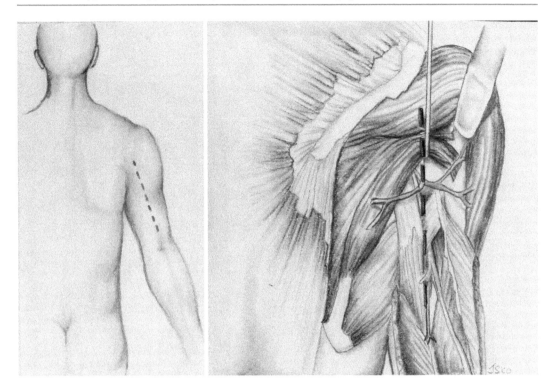

Fig. 16.7 Transfer of the right triceps branch to the axillary nerve

Fig. 16.8 Transfer
of the right triceps
branch to the
axillary nerve

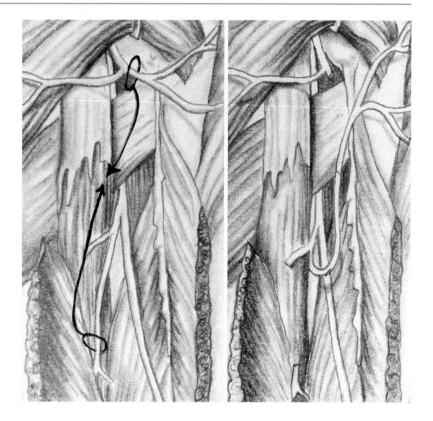

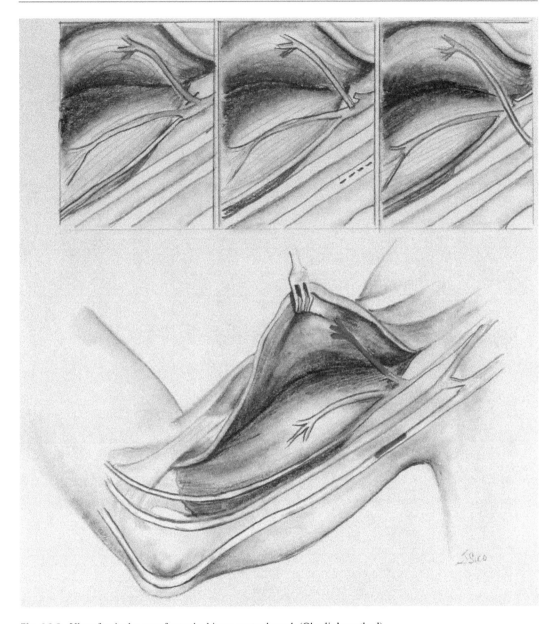

Fig. 16.9   Ulnar fascicular transfer to the biceps motor branch (Oberlin's method)

Fig. 16.10 Commonly used techniques for end-to-end flexor tendon technique

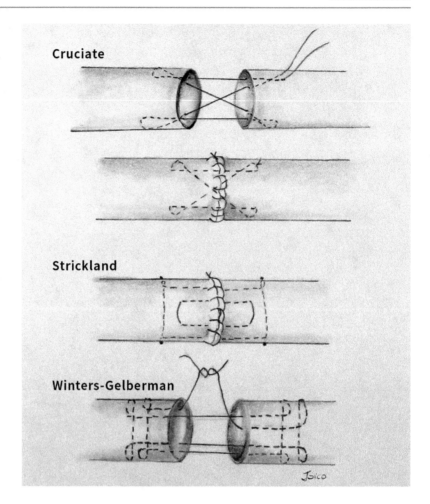

Fig. 16.11 BR transfer to ECRL and ECRB

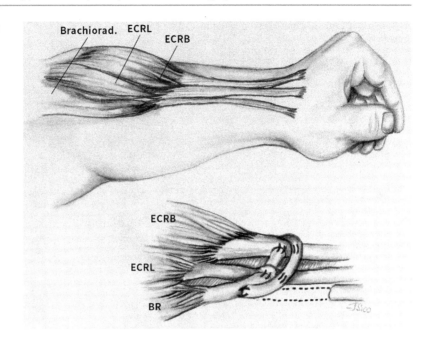

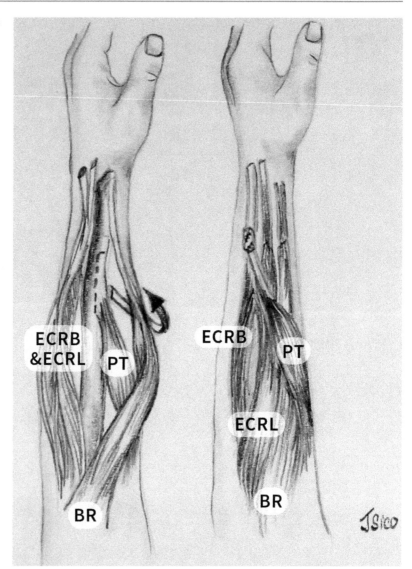

Fig. 16.12 PT to ECRB transfer

Fig. 16.13 FCU to EDC Transfer

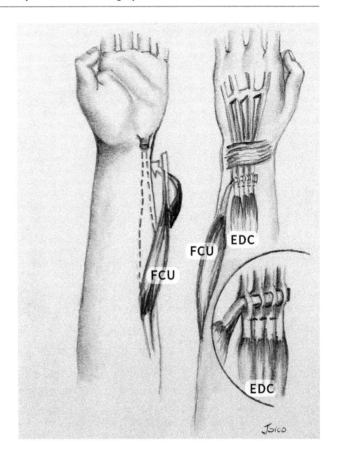

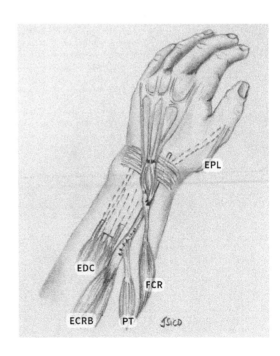

Fig. 16.14 FCR to EDC transfer

Fig. 16.15 Zancolli's lasso
operation

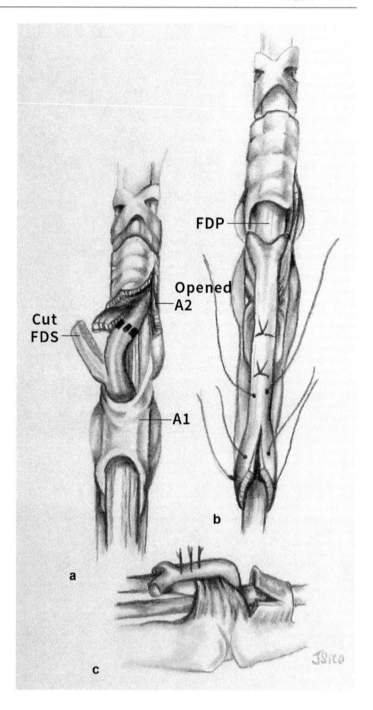

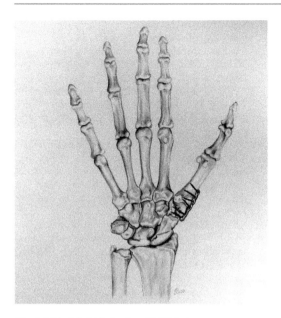

Fig. 16.16 Mini-blade plate CMC fusion

References

1. Brown Jr RH. Amyotrophic lateral sclerosis and other motor neuron diseases. In: Kasper DL, Braunwald E, Fauci AS, Hauser SL, Longo DL, Jameson JL, editors. Harrison's principles of internal medicine. New York: McGraw-Hill Book Company; 2005. p. 2424.
2. Kirshblum S. Treatment alternatives for spinal cord injury related spasticity. J Spinal Cord Med. 1999;22:199–217.
3. Korenkov AI, Niendorf WR, Darwish N, Glaeser E, Gaab MR. Continuous intrathecal infusion of baclofen in patients with spasticity caused by spinal cord injuries. Neurosurg Rev. 2002;25:228–30.
4. Olney RK. Weakness, disorders of movement, and imbalance. In: Kasper DL, Braunwald E, Fauci AS, Hauser SL, Longo DL, Jameson JL, editors. Harrison's principles of internal medicine. New York: McGraw-Hill Book Company; 2005. p. 138.
5. Ordia JI, Fischer E, Adamski E, Spatz EL. Chronic intrathecal delivery of baclofen by a programmable pump for the treatment of severe spasticity. J Neurosurg. 1996;85:452–7.
6. Roberts A. Surgical management of spasticity. J Child Orthop. 2013;7:389–94.
7. Roger VL, Go AS, Lloyd-Jones DM, Benjamin EJ, Berry JD, Borden WB, Bravata DM, Dai S, Ford ES, Fox CS, Fullerton HJ, Gillespie C, Hailpern SM, Heit JA, Howard VJ, Kissela BM, Kittner SJ, Lackland DT, Lichtman JH, Lisabeth LD, Makuc DM, Marcus GM, Marelli A, Matchar DB, Moy CS, Mozaffarian D, Mussolino ME, Nichol G, Paynter NP, Soliman EZ, Sorlie PD, Sotoodehnia N, Turan TN, Virani SS, Wong ND, Woo D, Turner MB, American Heart Association Statistics Committee and Stroke Statistics Subcommittee. Heart disease and stroke statistics – 2012 update: a report from the American Heart Association. Circulation. 2012;125:e2–220.
8. Devivo MJ. Epidemiology of traumatic spinal cord injury: trends and future implications. Spinal Cord. 2012;50:365–72.
9. Terzis JK, Papakonstantinou KC. The surgical treatment of brachial plexus injuries in adults. Plast Reconstr Surg. 2000;106:1097–122.
10. Growdon JH, Fink JS. Paralysis and movement disorder. In: Isselbacher KJ, Braunwald E, Wilson JD, editors. Harrison's principles of internal medicine. New York: McGraw-Hill Book Company; 1994. p. 115–25.
11. Marx A, Glass JD, Sutter RW. Differential diagnosis of acute flaccid paralysis and its role in poliomyelitis surveillance. Epidemiol Rev. 2000;22:298–316.
12. Jain DK, Bhardwaj P, Venkataramani H, Sabapathy SR. An epidemiological study of traumatic brachial plexus injury patients treated at an Indian centre. Indian J Plast Surg. 2012;45:498–503.
13. Midha R. Epidemiology of brachial plexus injuries in a multitrauma population. Neurosurgery. 1997; 40:1182–8.
14. Kalliainen LK, O'Brien VH. Current uses of botulinum toxin A as an adjunct to hand therapy interventions of hand conditions. J Hand Ther. 2014;27: 85–95.
15. Watve SV, Sivan M, Raza WA, Jamil FF. Management of acute overdose or withdrawal state in intrathecal baclofen therapy. Spinal Cord. 2012;50:107–11.
16. Ghosh D, Mainali G, Khera J, Luciano M. Complications of intrathecal Baclofen pumps in children: experience from a tertiary care center. Pediatr Neurosurg. 2013;49(3):138–44.
17. Steinbok P, Hicdonmez T, Sawatzky B, Beauchamp R, Wickenheiser D. Spinal deformities after selective dorsal rhizotomy for spastic cerebral palsy. J Neurosurg. 2005;102(4 Suppl):363–73.
18. Crilly MA. Selective dorsal rhizotomy remains experimental in cerebral palsy. BMJ. 2012;345:e4845.
19. Wolfe SW, Pederson WC, Hotchkiss RN, Kozin SH, editors. Green's operative hand surgery. Philadelphia: Elsevier Health Sciences; 2005.
20. Karev A. Trapezius transfer for paralysis of the deltoid. J Hand Surg Br. 1986;11:81–3.
21. Kotwal PP, Mittal R, Malhotra R. Trapezius transfer for deltoid paralysis. J Bone Joint Surg Br. 1998;80:114–6.
22. Elhassan B, Bishop A, Shin A, Spinner R. Shoulder tendon transfer options for adult patients with brachial plexus injury. J Hand Surg Am. 2010;35:1211–9.
23. Terzis J. Principles and techniques of peripheral nerve surgery. In: Daniel RK, editor. Reconstructive microsurgery. Boston: Little Brown & Co Inc; 1977.
24. Terzis JK, Strauch B. Microsurgery of the peripheral nerve: a physiological approach. Clin Orthop Relat Res. 1978;133:39–48.

25. Hadlock T, Elisseeff J, Langer R, Vacanti J, Cheney M. A tissue-engineered conduit for peripheral nerve repair. Arch Otolaryngol Head Neck Surg. 1998;124:1081–6.

26. Elkwood AI, Holland NR, Arbes SM, Rose MI, Kaufman MR, Ashinoff RL, Parikh MA, Patel TR. Nerve allograft transplantation for functional restoration of the upper extremity: case series. J Spinal Cord Med. 2011;34:241–7.

27. Mackinnon SE, Doolabh VB, Novak CB, Trulock EP. Clinical outcome following nerve allograft transplantation. Plast Reconstr Surg. 2001;107: 1419–29.

28. Palmer ML, Epler M. Principles of examination techniques. In: Palmer ML, Epler M, editors. Clinical assessment procedures in physical therapy. Philadelphia: JB Lippincott; 1990. p. 8–36.

29. Zheng MX, Xu WD, Qiu YQ, Xu JG, Gu YD. Phrenic nerve transfer for elbow flexion and intercostal nerve transfer for elbow extension. J Hand Surg Am. 2010;35:1304–9.

30. Siqueira MG, Martins RS. Phrenic nerve transfer in the restoration of elbow flexion in brachial plexus avulsion injuries: how effective and safe is it? Neurosurgery. 2009;65(4 Suppl):A125–31.

31. Sinis N, Boettcher M, Werdin F, Kraus A, Schaller HE. Restoration of shoulder abduction function by direct muscular neurotization with the phrenic nerve fascicles and nerve grafts: a case report. Microsurgery. 2009;29:552–5.

32. Kaufman MR, Elkwood AI, Colicchio AR, CeCe J, Jarrahy R, Willekes LJ, Rose MI, Brown D. Functional restoration of diaphragmatic paralysis: an evaluation of phrenic nerve reconstruction. Ann Thorac Surg. 2014;97:260–6.

33. Kaufman MR, Elkwood AI, Rose MI, Patel T, Ashinoff R, Saad A, Caccavale R, Bocage JP, Cole J, Soriano A, Fein E. Reinnervation of the paralyzed diaphragm: application of nerve surgery techniques following unilateral phrenic nerve injury. Chest. 2011;140:191–7.

34. Schreiber JJ, Feinberg JH, Byun DJ, Lee SK, Wolfe SW. Preoperative donor nerve electromyography as a predictor of nerve transfer outcomes. J Hand Surg Am. 2014;39:42–9.

35. Rb A, Naffzinger HC. The pathology of human striated muscle following denervation. J Neurosurg. 1953;10:216–27.

36. Mackinnon SE, Dvali LT. Basic pathology of the hand, wrist and forearm: nerve. In: Berger RA, Weiss APC, editors. Hand surgery, vol. 1. Philadelphia: Lippincott Williams & Wilkins; 2004. p. 37–48.

37. Sunderland S. The anatomy and physiology of nerve injury. Muscle Nerve. 1990;13:771–84.

38. Landi A, Copeland S. Value of the Tinel sign in brachial plexus lesions. Ann R Coll Surg Engl. 1979;61:470–1.

39. Ziegler-Graham K, MacKenzie EJ, Ephraim PL, Travison TG, Brookmeyer R. Estimating the prevalence of limb loss in the United States: 2005 to 2050. Arch Phys Med Rehabil. 2008;89:422–9.

40. Owings M, Kozak LJ; National Center for Health S. Ambulatory and inpatient procedures in the United States, 1996. Hyattsville: U.S. Dept. of Health and Human Services, Centers for Disease Control and Prevention, National Center for Health Statistics; 1998.

41. Norton KM. A brief history of prosthetics. inMotion. 2007 Nov/Dec; 17(7). Accessed at: http://www.amputee-coalition.org/inmotion/nov_dec_07/history_prosthetics.html. On 6 Oct 2015.

42. Bueno Jr RA, French B, Cooney D, et al. Targeted muscle reinnervation of a muscle-free flap for improved prosthetic control in a shoulder amputee: case report. J Hand Surg. 2011;36A:890–3.

43. Gart MS, Souza JM, Dumanian GA. Targeted muscle reinnervation in the upper extremity amputee: a technical road map. J Hand Surg Am. 2015;40:1877–88.

44. Ngheim BT, Sando IC, Gillespie RB, et al. Providing a sense of touch to prosthetic hands. Plast Reconstr Surg. 2015;135:1652–63.

45. Souza JM, Cheesborough JE, Ko JH. Targeted muscle reinnervation: a novel approach to post-amputation neuroma pain. Clin Orthop Relat Res. 2014;472:2984–90.

46. Birch R, Bonney G, Wynn Parry CB. Results. In: Surgical disorders of the peripheral nerves. London: Churchill Livingstone; 1998.

47. House JH, Gwathmey FW, Fidler MO. A dynamic approach to the thumb-in-palm deformity in cerebral palsy: evaluation and results in fifty-six patients. J Bone Joint Surg Am. 1981;63:216–25.

48. Wolfe SW, Hotchkiss RN, Pederson WC, Kozin SH. Green's operative hand surgery. Philadelphia: Churchill Livingston; 2011.

49. Teasdale G, Jennett B. Assessment of coma and impaired consciousness: a practical scale. Lancet. 1974;2:81–4.

50. British Medical Research Council. Reproduced from Aids to the examination of the peripheral nervous system. London: Her Majesty's Stationary Office; 1976.

Amputation Versus Limb Salvage of the Lower Extremity

David Polonet, Michael I. Rose, and D.J. Brown

Introduction

Limb-threatening conditions and actual loss of limb are complex situations that require an appreciation of the treatment options as well as potential outcomes and treatment courses associated with therapeutic interventions. Decisions about salvage and amputation have lasting effects on the patient and, in various settings, can take a patient down a pathway that can have excellent or catastrophic results. Many of these courses have no clear road map, and experience can be a caregiver's best guide. An awareness of the various options and access to skilled healthcare providers are necessary to avoid offering only a limited clinical perspective in these challenging clinical scenarios.

This chapter focuses on establishing a general understanding of the pathologic processes involved in the need for limb salvage and the decision for amputation, the treatment principles in both pathways and identifying postoperative problems that can be corrected, and how skilled and experienced care teams can achieve improved outcomes.

Salvage Versus Amputation

There are times when efforts at salvage may be unfeasible or inappropriate and other times when the practitioner must not be too quick to recommend amputation if salvage options are a reasonable alternative. The patient must understand the implications of his or her decision. When there is an attempt at salvage of a limb, there is often significant morbidity or even mortality that accompanies it that patients are unaware or unprepared for. In certain cases, limb salvage may require anticoagulation to maintain vascularity. This can lead to ongoing blood loss, require multiple transfusions, and lead to coagulopathy. Hypotension may be encountered, with metabolic acidosis affecting the patient's course. Not all hosts can tolerate this systemic burden. Rhabdomyolysis may have renal consequences, including the potential for renal failure and the need for dialysis. Hyperkalemia must be avoided due to associated cardiac risks. Infection may be a risk, both local and systemic sepses. Close

D. Polonet, MD (✉)
Jersey Shore University Medical Center,
Neptune City, NJ, USA

Rutgers Robert Wood Johnson Medical School,
New Brunswick, NJ, USA
e-mail: dpolonet@yahoo.com

M.I. Rose, MD
The Plastic Surgery Center, Institute for Advanced
Reconstruction, 535 Sycamore Ave, Shrewsbury,
NJ 07702, USA
e-mail: mrosemd@theplasticsurgerycenternj.com

D.J. Brown, MD, MPH
Department of Surgery, Rutgers Robert Wood
Johnson Medical School, New Brunswick, NJ, USA

© Springer International Publishing Switzerland 2017
A.I. Elkwood et al. (eds.), *Rehabilitative Surgery*, DOI 10.1007/978-3-319-41406-5_17

attention in patient care is necessary to avoid progression of potential complications. Pain management with narcotics, both in the setting of salvage and amputation, can have long-term effects; dependency, tolerance, and addiction are life-altering outcomes that require expert help and should be carefully avoided.

Often an amputation is presented as a definitive treatment option that will help avoid ongoing surgeries and hospitalizations in the interest of letting a patient "get on with his life." In obtaining informed consent, however, the caregiver would be wise to counsel patients that amputations may require subsequent surgical procedures and may still result in debilitating challenges related to pain and potential residual dysfunction. Commonly, wound debridement with skin grafting or flap revision and excision of heterotopic bone growth or painful neuromas may be necessary. Salvage, on the other hand, may require prolonged efforts and significant costs and may ultimately prove futile. With traumatic injuries of the extremities, even in the setting of technically "successful" limb salvage, the functional result may be unsatisfactory. In Lin's study of functional outcomes of lower-extremity fractures with vascular injury, even with salvage, every patient needed subsequent reconstructive surgery to achieve an acceptable functional result. Not surprisingly, the more severely injured limbs had poorer functional results [1].

Various factors will play important roles in the decision to choose a treatment course. These factors will include the pathologic process, the patient's general condition and goals or expectations, the treating team available, and the individual caregivers' expertise at all levels of care. Efforts have been made to help the treating team decide the predictability of salvaging a severely traumatized limb. Several amputation index scoring and rating systems were developed in attempts to try to assist the physician teams caring for severely mangled extremity injuries in deciding whether to attempt salvage or carry out primary amputations immediately after injury. These indexes were often based on the initial presentation of the extremity and often did not take into account unsuccessful salvaged limbs or functionally limiting salvaged limbs, which required a secondary amputation. There are several objective criteria which have been evaluated over the years and used to predict failure of limb salvage/high probabilities of limb amputation following lower-extremity trauma [2]. Some of the commonly utilized injury severity scoring systems include the Mangled Extremity Severity Score (MESS); the Limb Salvage Index (LSI) [3]; the Predictive Salvage Index (PSI) [4]; the Nerve Injury, Ischemia, Soft-Tissue Injury, Shock, and Age of Patient Score (NISSSA) [5]; and the Hannover Fracture Scale-98 (HFS-98) [6, 7].

Unfortunately, limb salvage scores were not shown to be successful at predicting the viability of a leg [8]. Additionally, lower-extremity scoring systems are not accurately predictive of the functional outcome of successfully salvaged limbs [9]. Ultimately, the advantages of a skilled and experienced set of caregivers produce the best option for the patient. Patients should be counseled regarding the risks and advantages associated with various treatment options.

Team management is preferable to disjointed care. Each team member should know his or her role and have a means of communication with other team members. An effective team will coordinate care in a way that involves and educates the other team members. Optimally, the team involves plastic, orthopedic, trauma, vascular, and podiatric surgeons as needed acutely. PM&R specialists, neurologists and pain management specialists, psychologists and psychiatrists, prosthetists and wound care specialists may play important roles that outlast surgical needs. Experienced nurses are invaluable. Physical therapists play a major role in optimizing the outcome. Quality care at each step is crucial, as an excellent prosthetist may be unable to compensate for suboptimal surgery, and vice versa. Outcomes and complications may be difficult to predict, and the accurate identification and treatment of secondary problems may be important in the patient's achievement of a satisfactory lifestyle. The outcomes reported from the LEAP study were similar between salvage and amputation groups [8].

There are general principles in salvage and in amputation that help guide the decisions and treatment, irrespective of the etiology. Honesty and transparency help patients make appropriate informed decisions and allow them to play an active role in achieving their goals. Acknowledgments, where appropriate, of clinical uncertainty and the explanation of realistic expectations at all times help prevent subsequent misgivings and questioning of motives. Appreciation on the part of patients and caregivers alike of the psychological and emotional impact of a life-altering situation can be helpful. The practitioner can most certainly be a crucial contributor to the psyche of the patient and will, in less optimal circumstances, contribute to potentially preventable and predictable emotional challenges.

The Pathologic Process

The disease course that leads to a limb at risk, in need of treatment and optimization, can be quite remarkably varied. The two most common causes of amputation or need for reconstructive salvage efforts are traumatic and vascular in nature. Congenital and neoplastic causes remain less common. The incidence of infection leading to the need for intervention is less well established, because it may be a secondary outcome of trauma or a multifactorial host disease, such as diabetic peripheral vascular disease, making it difficult to tease out the etiology.

There will be fundamental similarities and differences in management in these different settings. In all circumstances, the goals of eliminating disease, minimizing pain, and maximizing function must be met. Socioeconomic factors and resource availability must be taken into consideration. The speed of recovery may be more crucial in certain patient populations, such as laborers, whereas maximal tissue preservation may be a priority in younger populations at the expense of more prolonged hospital course. Upper-extremity salvage for cosmetic reasons may be preferable to some patients, even where function is limited.

Vascular Etiologies

Nontraumatic vascular pathology is usually a progressive condition that affects an older population, often with concomitant comorbidities such as diabetes mellitus. The prevention of limb loss is focused on early disease identification and correction of reversible conditions, such as smoking and control of glucose levels. Less-invasive interventions, such as stenting, have proven effective, whereas arterial bypass has become less commonly performed.

The natural history of the disease process, however, tends to be unfavorable. Twenty five percent of patients with an amputation will undergo a contralateral amputation within 3 years. Mortality rates after amputation remain high. Nonambulators undergoing amputation may be indicated for transfemoral amputations for more distal disease to avoid the need for subsequent higher-level amputation surgery. On the other hand, most transtibial amputations have the capacity to heal, and a common error is to perform amputation more proximally than necessary in ambulators.

Various diagnostic modalities related to blood flow and oxygen delivery may contribute to the surgeon's assessment of the proper level for an amputation and of the healing capacity, but none have demonstrated the ability to be independently predictive to the point of removing surgical experience and judgment. Amputations in vasculopaths are generally performed without tourniquet inflation, and postoperative compressive dressings in this patient population run the risk of causing further ischemia and catastrophic pressure necrosis.

Traumatic Etiologies

When one is considering the initial evaluation of traumatic injuries including the extremities, it is important to remember to adhere to the guidelines provided by the Advanced Trauma Life Support (ATLS) and as proposed by the American College of Surgeons (ACS), which emphasize "life over limb" by focusing on the ABC(DE)'s of care first. Other general principles with regard to the overall management of extremity injuries and salvage attempts include the general initial presentation of the patient and the extremity of concern.

Hypovolemic shock is a common occurrence with severely mangled extremities or polytrauma. This hypovolemia may compromise perfusion of the limb, whether from general global hypoperfusion or extremity-specific hypoperfusion. In the setting of extremity-specific hypoperfusion, general temporizing maneuvers to restore blood flow are used (i.e., temporary arterial shunts or definitive bypasses) depending on the estimated duration of ischemia [10]. Generally, it has been well established that after 4–8 h of "warm ischemia," efforts at limb salvage are not feasible [11–13].

Where significant limb ischemia is not a concern, skeletal fixation may be desirable to provide limb stability, allowing for the vascular and soft tissue reconstruction efforts. Any question related to injury of an extremity warrants, at a minimum, radiologic evaluation with X-rays. Likewise, any question of compromise to an extremity requires evaluation with angiography if the initial or serial physical examination or Doppler examination shows compromise. Ankle-brachial comparative pressure measurements may be predictive of a possible need for revascularization.

A few basic definitions and concepts need to be established prior to tackling the problems of traumatic extremity pathology. A mangled extremity is commonly understood to be a limb that has at least three out of the four tissue groups damaged: the soft tissue, nerves, vasculature, and bone [14]. There are several grading systems used to categorize a mangled extremity, and these grading systems have various correlations with overall outcomes with and without reconstruction and have even been used in the decision-making tree for deciding limb salvage potential versus amputation, without mandating or predicting which if either should be performed. Earlier debridement of mangled extremities is the goal for potential salvage of the best functional outcomes and limb salvage.

The general teaching of timing and sequence of acute limb salvage as taught during training is as follows: thorough debridement (as early as possible), bony stabilization and revascularization, tendon and nerve repair, and soft tissue repair and coverage [15]. There is inconclusive evidence that bony repair and fracture stabilization should precede definitive vascular reconstruction for fear of damage to the newly established vascular anastomoses. It is often preferable to perform final nerve reconstructions and transfers as well as tendon and bone grafting once wounds are clean and ready for final flap/muscle coverage.

Orthopedic Care

The management of complex limb injuries or limbs at risk for amputation requires restoration of stability and recovery of function. This can necessitate fracture fixation or stabilization after excision of compromised bone. Loss of stability can cause deformity and limb shortening under the effects of muscle contraction, which occur involuntarily. Also, an ongoing injury to the soft tissue envelope can compromise neurovascular structures, and muscle and skin necrosis can result as well. At times, reconstructive efforts may necessitate the treatment of these specific complications.

Maintaining the length of a destabilized bone or joint can be achieved in a variety of ways. Splinting and casting may be inadequate to maintain length and alignment and prohibit early range of motion following an amputation, often making internal methods preferable. Implants are selected for their ability to provide effective stability and to optimize the mechanical and biological environment. In long bones, such as the tibia or femur, the midshaft fractures can be effectively managed with intramedullary fixation. The advantages of intramedullary fixation include aligning the implant with the anatomic axis of the bone, thus diminishing forces due to bending moments. Furthermore, the surrounding soft tissues are not in contact with the implants, resulting in less potential irritation of the surrounding muscles, fascia, and skin. Periarticular fractures, on the other hand, are typically treated with plates and screws. Current implant designs are geared toward optimizing the implant fit with regard to the contour of the bone, thus minimizing irritation.

In an extremity with an elevated risk of infection, the application of metal stabilization implants may complicate matters. It is well established that infections compromise fracture stabilization implants such as plates and screws as well as prosthetic joint implants. The bacteria in this

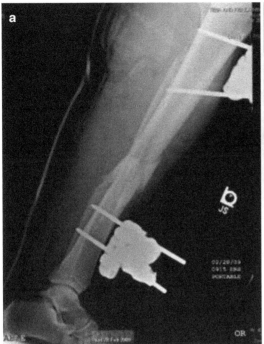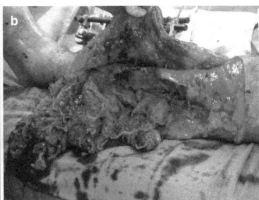

Fig. 17.1 A simple fracture with a complex associated soft tissue injury. The fracture was stabilized initially with an external fixator (a) to diminish the risk of prolonged surgery and implant-related infection. The muscular injury, however (b), resulted in extensive necrosis and the decision was made to amputate by both the patient and the surgeon. A successful transtibial amputation was performed, but soft coverage presented a technical challenge.

setting are able to establish a protective "biofilm" or glycocalyx barrier that is protective to the effects of systemic antibiotics, diminishing the efficacy of the antibiotic by a factor of 1000 [16]. In this setting, the eradication of infection often necessitates the removal of the implant, again destabilizing the extremity. Thus, introducing "permanent" implants in the setting of a compromised wound or host is highly risky.

The recommended management of a fracture or bony defect at high risk, therefore, often includes temporary or definitive external fixation. In this approach, percutaneous rigid pins and transosseous wires anchor the bone proximal to and distal to the involved region (Fig. 17.1). External to the soft tissue envelope, these pins and wires are connected by longitudinal bars and clamps. This modality commonly leaves implants more remote from the zone of injury, and if the component of the device (i.e., a pin or wire) becomes locally infected, it is easily removed or replaced. The local infection rate of the individual pins and wires can be quite high in more prolonged applications. Optimally, temporary stabilization is achieved, and the region is treated with appropriate bone and soft tissue care to optimize the local biology, allowing conversion to definitive internal fixation.

Bone defects can often be treated with bone autograft (Fig. 17.2), allograft, or, bone graft substitutes (typically osteoconductive and/or osteoinductive materials that stimulate bone growth), with various options to augment healing, such as bone marrow osteogenic cell transfer or bone morphogenetic proteins [17].

Presently, a vast industry has developed in the field of bone products and bone void filler products [18]. The user of these products should be aware of the advantages and disadvantages of the various products available and of how financial factors in this marketplace can influence decisions and cause additional confusion [19].

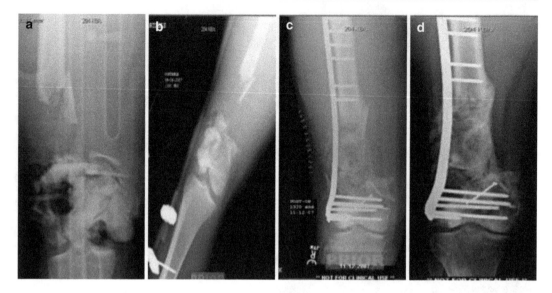

Fig. 17.2 A 26-year-old male motorcyclist sustained an open distal femur fracture dislocation with significant bone loss (**a**). External fixation (**b**) with soft tissue healing was succeeded by plate fixation and bone autografting (**c**). The patient went onto fracture union (**d**) with no additional complications

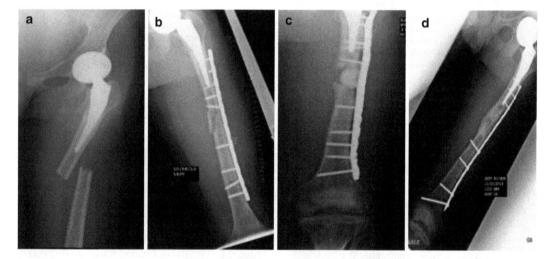

Fig. 17.3 A 29-year-old male with a history of leukemia and hip osteonecrosis following radiation. Subsequent to hip replacement for the osteonecrosis, he was assaulted and sustained a periprosthetic femoral fracture (**a**). Following plate fixation (**b**), he developed a nonunion. Upon surgical exploration, it was noted that he had dysvascular bone at the fracture site, which precluded healing. The bone was resected, the plate was revised, and a temporary cement bone spacer was placed (**c**). A vascularized fibula graft was inserted into the defect and this incorporated, enabling successful bony union (**d**)

Vascularized bone grafts may be appropriate in certain settings, where nonvascularized grafts have failed or are more susceptible to infection (Fig. 17.3). Further, vascularized bone grafts may be a component of a tissue transfer procedure that includes soft tissue coverage. Vascularized bone grafting is a technically challenging microsurgical procedure that requires expert judgment and skills and involves additional surgical risks to the patient at the donor site, typically remote from the bone defect site. This may temporarily confer additional debility to the patient (Fig. 17.3).

Finally, "bone transport" is a modality that can be very effective in bridging bony voids. This is a tech-

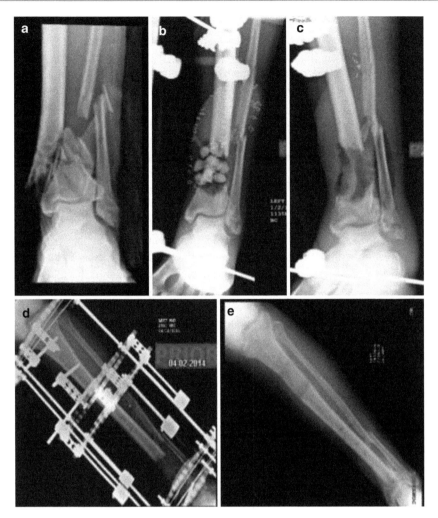

Fig. 17.4 A 54-year-old male with a history of smoking fell from a ladder with a resultant open distal tibia "pilon" fracture (**a**). He underwent initial irrigation and debridement with external fixation, but developed a deep infection with the skin and bone loss due to extensive local necrosis. This required resection of the tissue, muscle flap coverage, a cement spacer with antibiotics (**b**), and systemic antibiotics. The residual bone loss and tissue compromise were treated with a circular external fixator and bone transport. In (**c**), the external fixator components reveal the extensive nature of the device. The proximal osteotomy can be seen. Following bone transport (**d**), the proximal regenerative bone at the osteotomy site is seen, and the distal defect is eliminated with bone healing (**e**)

nique that typically uses a specially designed external fixator (although internal fixation options have been designed) to slowly move a healthy segment of the bone across a defect and grow new regenerative bone in the void. This technique can be very effective even in a compromised host or in compromised local biology but is time-consuming and labor intensive for the surgeon. Typically, the bone is moved up to 1 mm/day, and the new bone growth often takes three times as long as the "transport" of the bone takes.

This modality is very time intensive for the practitioner and may be fraught with challenges for both the surgeon and the patient. Complication rates are high, including risks of infection, neurologic injury, and joint stiffness, but success rates can be excellent when technique and judgment are good. In contrast with most temporary external fixators, the constructs assembled with definitive external fixation and bone transport are designed to last longer and may often be sturdy enough to bear weight during the process (Fig. 17.4).

A limb length discrepancy (LLD) may be treated nonsurgically, with a customized in-shoe orthosis or with shoe modification. Surgical management of LLD is usually reserved for discrepancies greater than 1 inch. In growing, skeletally immature patients, the opportunity to match limb length through surgically treating the contralateral limb exists. This is done by arresting the growth in a predictable manner on the contralateral limb through a process termed epiphysiodesis. This involves the surgical ablation of a growth plate or physis. In mature patients, this option does not exist, but selective limb shortening of bones may be an option. The amount of shortening a limb can tolerate may be 2–3 inches, depending on the bone and the size of the patient. Muscle weakness may complicate this technique due to a loss of tension generated in affected muscle groups. Limb lengthening can be performed in adults in a manner similar to the process of bone transport. To lengthen a shortened limb, the bone can be osteotomized and lengthened via a progressive distraction at the osteotomy site. This technique is known as distraction osteogenesis.

Any fracture or osteotomy site will require bony union. The amount of time a bone requires to unite is a function of many variables. Host factors, such as patient age, nutrition, prior and current medical conditions, medications, and tobacco use, often have an influence on fracture healing. Anatomic site will also be relevant. Distal tibia fractures heal notoriously slowly, whereas midshaft humeral fractures commonly heal in half the time on average. Fixation methods may also play an important role in bone growth and healing. Excessively rigid fracture fixation, for example, may inhibit the growth of the bone across any gaps. Insufficient stability, by contrast, will promote bone growth but may still result in nonunion, and alignment control may be sacrificed as well. The ideal stabilization environment may thus be an elusive concept, even for experts in the field of fracture fixation with extensive knowledge of bone biology and biomechanics.

In addition to bony sites of injury or instability, joints may develop laxity or excessive pathologic motion through traumatic, inflammatory, degenerative, or other pathologic processes. Stability is conferred through joint articular congruency and soft tissue constraints that may include the joint capsule, labral tissue, ligaments, and musculotendinous dynamic compressive forces. Our appreciation of factors affecting joint stability is continuing to evolve. Although joint laxity alone is not a limb-threatening process in most patients, when combined with other pathologic elements, this may become a serious problem. Joint instability may preclude functional recovery and may put the patient at risk for other complications, such as recurrent or further injury, or compromise other structures through reinjury or additional falls. Management of joint laxity may include nonoperative modalities such as temporary or definitive immobilization or bracing. Operative options may include external fixation options (which include hinged external fixators that allow normal motion) and soft tissue repair or reconstruction.

Loss of motion can also result in diminished function. Absent active motion with retained passive motion implies altered motor function, resultant from weakness or paralysis. In this setting, a neuromuscular etiology should be considered. Loss of sensation in a neurologic or dermatomal distribution may help establish the source of the deficit. EMG/NCV studies can help elucidate the pathologic process. Specific causes may include spasticity, contracture, or weakness. Spasticity or contracture may be treated with physical therapy, sometimes coupled with botulinum toxin injection. Muscle lengthening or tenotomy should be performed with caution. Joints may also develop stiffness that can adversely affect function. Various etiologies may be contributory, in isolation or in combination. Joint manipulation under anesthesia, with or without arthroscopic lysis of peri- and intra-articular adhesions, may have a role for selected refractory cases.

Plastic Surgery Care

Coverage of injured extremities generally follows the same principles regardless of whether salvage or amputation is being pursued. However, if salvage is being considered, the surgeon must consider the fact that the attempt at salvage may fail, an amputation might be needed, and thus donor sites for initial salvage attempts should be chosen carefully so they do not compromise future amputation needs, i.e., incisions where future amputation flaps might be and "spare parts" from the potentially amputated limb [20]. All of the reconstructive options and the technical details of each are beyond the scope of this chapter, but the principles that stand behind the decisions are addressed herein, and these principles are what guides the reconstructive plastic surgeon more than any particular surgical procedure.

The basic principles for soft tissue reconstruction revolve around a reconstructive "ladder." The ladder has rungs of increasing complexity as one moves up the ladder. In this scheme, the simplest procedure (the lowest "rung") is considered first, and progressively more complicated procedures are only considered once the less complicated ones are considered and discarded as insufficient. This thought process progresses up the ladder until the least complicated, but surgically sufficient, technique is happened upon.

At the bottom of the ladder is simple closure. Rarely is this the answer in an injury as severe as being considered in this chapter. However, often portions of the wound can be directly closed, making a more complicated injury less complicated, and thus amenable to a somewhat less aggressive overall treatment. Specifically, the first priority for areas of direct closure is areas over critical tissues (the bone, tendon, nerve, vascular) or hardware. When this can be accomplished, closure of the remaining soft tissue envelope is rendered significantly simpler. Nonetheless, swelling, soft tissue loss, and the presence of hardware – which takes up space – coupled with the paucity of soft tissue in the lower extremity, all render a direct closure to a distinct minority of lower-extremity trauma repairs.

Skin grafts are considered the next most complex form of reconstruction. Skin grafts must have a suitable, viable bed to receive them. They cannot be placed directly on the bone, cartilage, vascular tissues, tendons, or hardware/implants. These situations require vascularized tissue (flaps) to be brought in either as a pedicled or free tissue transfer. However, skin grafts are often needed to cover a muscle or facial flap as these

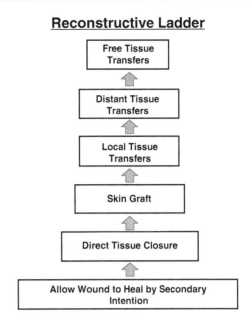

Reconstructive Ladder

Fig. 17.5 Reconstructive ladder

are typically transposed without the overlying, bulky skin and subcutaneous fat. So in the setting of limb salvage, skin grafting often has an important but secondary role of simply putting the "roof" on top of a well-vascularized muscle or facial flap which is actually doing the work of covering, nourishing, and revascularizing the injured area (Fig. 17.5).

Next on the list is local tissue rearrangement. This includes Z-plasty, unilobed and bilobed flaps, rhomboid flaps, and other local rotational or advancement flaps (Fig. 17.6) [21]. Figure 17.7 shows a summary of a variety of commonly used options for flap reconstruction for the salvage of lower extremities after trauma [22]. The benefits of locally based flaps and pedicle flaps over free tissue transfers include the lack of complicated and tenuous microvascular anastomoses. Sural neurofasciocutaneous pedicle flaps are another example used in ankle reconstruction and have the added benefit of bringing sensation to the lateral aspect of the hindfoot [22]. Unfortunately in the lower extremity, there is a paucity of extra tissue to use for such a rearrangement. These local flaps utilize a random blood supply to nourish the tissues being rearranged. This renders them fairly susceptible to failure as they are nec-

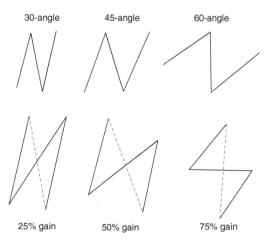

30-angle   45-angle   60-angle

25% gain   50% gain   75% gain

Fig. 17.6 Classic 3-incision Z-plasty theory is to create 3 incisions of equal lengths of varying degree angles to allow movement and rearrangement of equilateral triangular flaps to reconstruct tissue loss defects. From Aasi SZ [21]. Z-Plasty Made Simple. Dermatol Res Pract. 2010.

essarily in the zone of injury and are thus not the healthiest tissues to be transposed.

More distal tissue transfers are considered next, such as gastrocnemius or soleus flaps, sural flaps, and propeller perforator flaps. Other microvascular free flaps include the latissimus dorsi free flap, anterolateral thigh flap, and rectus abdominis muscle flap. These flaps utilize known vascular flow patterns to safely incise and transfer tissue to a new area based upon the vascular supply to that tissue [23, 24]. The vascular supply is preserved in the pedicle of the flap, and thus the range of the flap reach is limited by the length of the vascular pedicle. A good analogy is an astronaut who is tethered to his spaceship can only explore space as far as the reach of his oxygen hose will let him go.

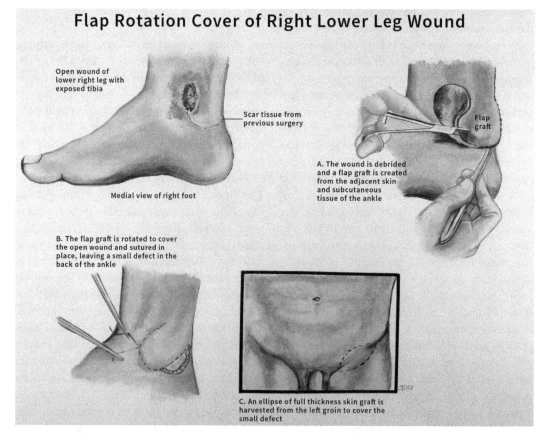

Flap Rotation Cover of Right Lower Leg Wound

Open wound of lower right leg with exposed tibia

Scar tissue from previous surgery

Medial view of right foot

Flap graft

A. The wound is debrided and a flap graft is created from the adjacent skin and subcutaneous tissue of the ankle

B. The flap graft is rotated to cover the open wound and sutured in place, leaving a small defect in the back of the ankle

C. An ellipse of full thickness skin graft is harvested from the left groin to cover the small defect

Fig. 17.7 Images retrieved from soft tissue management of war wounds to the foot and ankle by summary from an atlas of flaps of the musculoskeletal system and the atlas of microvascular surgery

The pinnacle of the reconstructive ladder is the free tissue transfer [25]. Often considered the gold standard in lower-extremity reconstruction, this is a highly technical procedure that has the advantage of bringing new, uninjured tissue to the area for coverage purposes. Free tissue transfer can bring in tissues of different thicknesses and tissue types including the muscle, skin, fat, fascia, bone, or any or all of the above. There are even flaps with nerves and blood vessels in them to restore sensation and/or blood flow to an injured area [26]. The reach of the free tissue flap is not limited by anything as it is completely detached from the donor site and then reattached via arterial and venous anastomoses at the recipient site. Once flow has been reestablished, the transferred tissues (typically a muscle) can be inset and sutured into the area of deficiency. As mentioned previously, these flaps are typically transferred without the overlying skin, and a skin graft is then harvested to cover the flap in its new position.

The injured extremity has to be evaluated, and form and function deficits have to be assessed. A realistic plan for reconstruction/coverage needs to be created, but the patient and reconstructive surgeon have to be flexible as the plan will often change as the injury evolves or complications arise. The most important is the coverage of vital structures to preserve function and prevent infection. Many functional deficits can be addressed later with therapy, tendon or nerve transfers, and joint fusions. Still, consideration should always be made with regard to what technique is going to have the best form in the area being reconstructed and whether there are any options that fulfill more than one role. An example of this would be using a free anterolateral thigh flap (ALT) with attached tensor fascia lata (TFL) as a combined free flap to reconstruct an Achilles tendon defect [27]. The skin/fat portion of the flap can cover the vital structures and span the skin defect, while the TFL can span the Achilles tendon defect and reconstruct the functional aspect of the wound.

As mentioned above, the reconstructive principles are the same, regardless of whether salvage or amputation attempts are being dealt with. However, a frequent problem in this population is

an impending amputation that will have a paucity of the soft tissue at the below-knee level. Since a prosthesis will have to sit on the end of a stump ("residual limb"), durable soft tissue is preferable, but often not available. Skin grafting to the end of a stump directly over the muscle is a poor option but has been employed in an effort to preserve length and maintain a joint. Extra care in these cases is needed to avoid wounds on the end of the stump once ambulation is considered. Skilled prosthetic professionals can modify and customize prostheses to overcome these challenging stumps.

To recap and to give more of a long-term overview of the process involved in the reconstruction and rehabilitation of the injured extremity, initial concerns are stabilization of the fractures, restoration of vascular continuity, and debridement of nonviable tissues. Next, attention is turned toward the coverage of the fractures and exposed vital structures and hardware. These first two steps represent the acute phase of the reconstructive process. It is during this time that the feasibility of the salvage efforts becomes clearer, and a decision for continued salvage efforts versus amputation is made. Assuming salvage efforts continue, functional issues are addressed next such as motor deficits and sensory deficits. These functional reconstructions are addressed elsewhere in this book. Typically these functional reconstructions take place in the 6–12-month time frame after injury, but exceptions in both temporal directions are not uncommon. Finally, long-term issues such as chronic pain need to be managed over the long term. Phantom limb pain, neuromas, and complex regional pain syndrome (CRPS) are a few of the neurologic causes of pain after lower-extremity trauma, but other sources such as muscular pain and painful joints are also common causes of pain after trauma in this area.

Phantom limb pain is pain perceived in the area where a limb has already been amputated. This happens when the nerve stump continues to send pain signals to the brain and confuses the brain into thinking the limb is still there and in pain. It can range from mild to severe and can be temporary or chronic. In addition, there can be "real" stump pain in the amputation stump. The course may be variable, with potential for spontaneous progressive improvement or worsening or for therapeutic interventions that can alter the course. Treatments are similar for both and include desensitization therapy, TENS therapy, stretching, medications (including antidepressants, gabapentin or pregabalin, and narcotics), and complementary modalities such as acupuncture and biofeedback. If these fail to ameliorate the pain, surgery to remove entrapping scar tissue and/or excision of a painful neuroma can be helpful. Pain management modalities can include percutaneous ablation of the offending nerve. Insertion of spinal stimulators can be considered as well in severe cases [28].

Neuromas typically form at the end of the nerve that is cut in the course of an amputation. Not all neuromas cause pain, but they can be very painful. They can complicate a salvaged limb as well as amputated limbs. Treatment starts similarly to that for phantom limb pain with physical therapy modalities and pain management techniques, including medication and noninvasive ablation techniques. Ultimately, many cases require reoperation to find the offending neuroma and dissect it more proximal and bury the end of the nerve into a "quiet" area such as into a muscle belly or into a hole burred into a nearby bone [29]. In these places, the nerve is much less likely to be stimulated and thus less likely to send pain signals. Also, surgical techniques, such as avoiding traction and electrocautery near the nerve, and sharp nerve transection (scalpel rather than scissors, which cause shear), are recommended.

A possibly related issue is that of complex regional pain syndrome – a poorly understood pain condition that results from central or peripheral nerve dysfunction, typically after a trauma. Somehow pain receptors become hypersensitive and send excess nerve impulses that result in pain, warmth, swelling, and erythema of the affected area. One of the hallmarks of the condition is that the amount of pain experienced seems to be higher (and more chronic) than that expected by the injury. As with phantom pain, treatment starts with noninvasive techniques such as physical therapy, medications, and surgery including neu-

roma removal, intrathecal drug pumps, spinal cord stimulators, and others [30].

Psychosocial Aspects

Such difficult clinical scenarios introduce challenging emotional circumstances that require the clinician to extend his or her patience, communication techniques, and empathy to meet the needs of the patient. Devastating limb injury and amputation surgery are life-altering events requiring caregiver patience and empathy [31]. The salvage of complex extremity injuries must set out to have realistic goals and expectations from the very beginning. Protracted limb salvage attempts may adversely affect a person physically, psychologically, and financially, affecting the entire family as well as the care providers and medical team [1]. However, according to some research, the majority of patients (92%) involved in attempted salvage of their lower extremity preferred their salvaged leg to an amputation at any stage of their injury, and none would have preferred primary amputation at the time of injury [32].

Overall Outcomes

More than 95% of patients and families want accurate details, even though the information may be upsetting [33]. This is true both in the disclosure of medical errors and even in the delivery of information which may be indicating a poor prognosis. Therefore, in discussing compromised extremities, it is important to keep in mind that not all severely injured or diseased extremities can be technically salvaged. More importantly, not all technically salvaged extremities can be rehabilitated to achieve adequate function. Because of the complexities of each situation and individual, the decision to attempt salvage, amputate, and even reconstruct is highly individualized.

It has been suggested in several studies that because of the lack of correlation between the amputation indexes and functional outcomes, the clinical judgment should be the primary determinant used in deciding between an attempt at salvage and primary amputation [32]. Secondary amputations are also not always a failure, but an eventual outcome of an unsalvageable limb, which required delayed amputation. Delayed amputations or secondary amputations often occur secondary to infection, delay in revascularization, thrombosis of distal vascular beds or lack of establishing collateral flow, infected nonunion, persistent nonunion, gangrene, or sepsis (Fig. 17.8).

The major goal of any reconstructive team when attempting to salvage a severely damaged extremity is to achieve a functional level, which allows a reasonable return to daily activities and/ or return to work in a reasonable time frame. Preinjury well-being and quality-of-life measures are the new norms.

the worse initial extremity injury which motivated patients to pursue legal action as opposed to those who would think there was a greater psychological component to the disability. It is likely also that this greater physical disability impairs earlier return to work, if ever any return at all. It is important that physicians understand potential causes for unanticipated outcomes, including (1) unreasonable patient expectations, which exist despite pretreatment counseling, (2) biologic variations, (3) occurrence of low-probability risks and adverse side effects, (4) wrong medical judgments made without negligence, and (5) individual, team, or system errors and equipment failures, which involve negligence [31].

Litigation and Outcomes

Patients who undertook litigation had worse physical outcome scores but not mental or pain outcome scores, indicating that it is the poorer physical function and disability and possibly

Financial Considerations

The more severe an injury, the greater the cost to the worker and society in general [34]. According to the 2013 National Safety Council data and reports, the total costs of unintentional injuries in

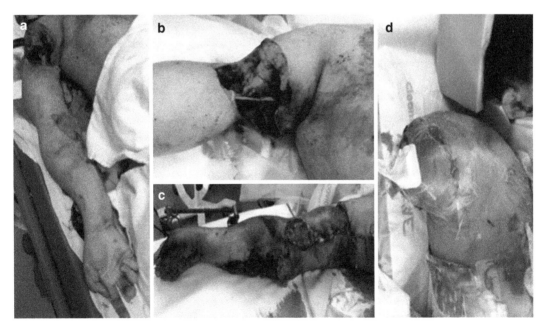

Fig. 17.8 A high subtotal (dominant) arm traumatic amputation left a 25-year-old woman with almost no tissue in continuity (**a, b**). Though there were slim hopes for replantation, an effort was made. Revascularization of the brachial artery and fixation of the humerus, forearm, and wrist fractures resulted in a dysvascular limb in spite of extensive efforts to maintain perfusion (**c**). A delayed amputation was performed before the patient was aware of her situation (**d**)

2011 cost more than $753 billion. When considering the loss of wages and productivity, quality of life, medical expenses, and impact on caregivers and families, a staggering additional $3,611 billion has been estimated as the cost to the healthcare system, GDP, and patients themselves. In 2003, the comprehensive cost of occupational injuries in the United States was estimated to be greater than $156 billion [35]; this is an exponential increase in merely a decade, possibly reflecting the inflation of healthcare costs. Typically falls are the most common cause of injury in the workplace, with fractures of the extremities being the most common type of injury. These work-related injuries (WRIs) represent a significant economical and logistical burden to healthcare systems [36]. They not only cost more in the acute setting secondary to increased ICU stays, OR costs, and procedures but more commonly affected younger working-aged males without significant comorbidities.

Despite these findings of increased acute care needs and resource utilizations, data show that many of these injured patients in general on average use less rehabilitation facilities and home care support services, likely because of their relative lower comorbidity index. Wage and productivity loss represent the greatest percentage of costs, approximately 48%, followed by direct healthcare costs, which measure about 26% (Fig. 17.9) [36].

Obesity is a costly, difficult, and increasingly prevalent challenge facing orthopedic care. The financial implications of treating patients who are obese will continue to challenge surgeons [37]. The medical costs of obesity-related illnesses were estimated to be $209.7 billion in 2008 [38]. Patients who are obese and have multiple comorbidities are more likely to experience surgical complications and worse outcomes after surgery. These comorbidities include but are not limited to diabetes, peripheral vascular disease, pulmonary disease, sleep apnea, peripheral neuropathy, and venous thromboembolic disease [37], all of which can

Costs of unintentional Injuries by component, 2011

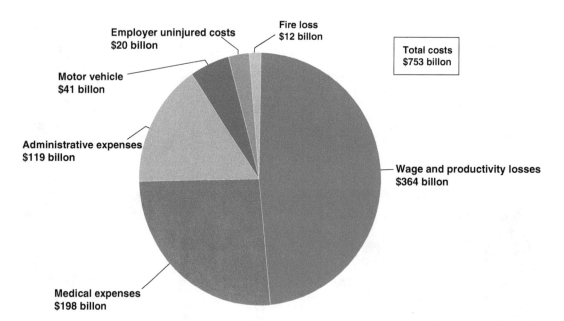

Fig. 17.9 Costs of unintentional injuries by component, 2011. National Safety Council. (2013). Injury Facts®, 2013 Edition. Itasca, IL: Author. [35])

impact the success of attempts at salvaging severely traumatized extremities.

Summary

Limb-threatening conditions and actual loss of limb are complex and expensive endeavors which require an appreciation of all of the treatment options and the potential outcomes associated with these attempts at therapeutic intervention. Decisions about salvage versus amputation are not to be taken lightly because they have both significant financial costs to the patient, the healthcare system as a whole, and the long-term quality-of-life issues.

Patients and families need to be prepared for multiple invasive procedures both in the acute setting during the initial hospitalization and even later after discharge. Indirect complications in the long term including those related to therapeutic anticoagulation after revascularization or chronic pain syndromes are also important points to communicate to families. It is important that surgeons and these multidisciplinary healthcare provider teams keep honest and open communication at the forefront of disclosure and pain realistic outcomes as treatment proceeds. Although attempts at generating high-quality scoring systems for anticipating limb salvage success/failure and quality-of-life estimates have been made, there currently is no perfect system available.

Each patient and mangled extremity is unique, and although basic principles are used in salvage attempts, their courses have no clear road map, and the experienced multidisciplinary teams are often the best advocate for the patient. Despite best efforts, there can be times when attempts at salvage are unfeasible and even inappropriate. On the other hand, the decision to recommend amputation can be made too quickly if the provider has limited experience or knowledge when salvage options might be available at specialized centers or other departments. An awareness of the various options and access to skilled healthcare providers are necessary for the early identification of postoperative problems that can be corrected for overall improved outcomes.

References

1. Lin CH, Wei FC, Levin LS, Su JI, Yeh WL. The functional outcome of lower-extremity fractures with vascular injury. J Trauma. 1997;43:480–5.
2. Johansen K, Daines M, Howey T, Helfet D, Hansen Jr ST. Objective criteria accurately predict amputation following lower extremity trauma. J Trauma. 1990;30:568–72; discussion 572–3.
3. Russell WL, Sailors DM, Whittle TB, Fisher Jr DF, Burns RP. Limb salvage versus traumatic amputation. A decision based on a seven-part predictive index. Ann Surg. 1991;213:473–80; discussion 480–1.
4. Howe Jr HR, Poole Jr GV, Hansen KJ, et al. Salvage of lower extremities following combined orthopedic and vascular trauma. A predictive salvage index. Am Surg. 1987;53:205–8.
5. McNamara MG, Heckman JD, Corley FG. Severe open fractures of the lower extremity: a retrospective evaluation of the Mangled Extremity Severity Score (MESS). J Orthop Trauma. 1994;8:81–7.
6. Tscherne H, Oestern HJ. A new classification of soft-tissue damage in open and closed fractures (author's transl). Unfallheilkunde. 1982;85:111–5.
7. Helfet DL, Howey T, Sanders R, Johansen K. Limb salvage versus amputation. Preliminary results of the Mangled Extremity Severity Score. Clin Orthop Relat Res. 1990:80–6.
8. Bosse MJ, MacKenzie EJ, Kellam JF, et al. An analysis of outcomes of reconstruction or amputation after leg-threatening injuries. N Engl J Med. 2002;347:1924–31.
9. Ly TV, Travison TG, Castillo RC, Bosse MJ, MacKenzie EJ, Group LS. Ability of lower-extremity injury severity scores to predict functional outcome after limb salvage. J Bone Joint Surg Am. 2008;90:1738–43.
10. Scully RE, Hughes CW. The pathology of ischemia of skeletal muscle in man; a description of early changes in muscles of the extremities following damage to major peripheral arteries on the battlefield. Am J Pathol. 1956;32:805–29.
11. Scully RE, Shannon JM, Dickersin GR. Factors involved in recovery from experimental skeletal muscle ischemia produced in dogs: I. Histologic and histochemical pattern of ischemic muscle. Am J Pathol. 1961;39:721–37.
12. Harman JW, Gwinn RP. The recovery of skeletal muscle fibers from acute ischemia as determined by histologic and chemical methods. Am J Pathol. 1949;25:741–55.

13. Sanderson RA, Foley RK, McIvor GW, Kirkaldy-Willis WH. Histological response on skeletal muscle to ischemia. Clin Orthop Relat Res. 1975:27–35.

14. Gregory RT, Gould RJ, Peclet M, et al. The Mangled Extremity Syndrome (M.E.S.): a severity grading system for multisystem injury of the extremity. J Trauma. 1985;25:1147–50.

15. Thorne CHM G, Chung K, Gosain A, Mehrara B, Rubin P, Spear S. Grabb and Smith's plastic surgery. 7th ed. In: Wilkins LWa, editor. Grabb and Smith's plastic surgery. 7th ed. 13 ed. Philadelphia: Lippincott Williams & Wilkins; 2013.

16. Shirwaiker RA, Springer BD, Spangehl MJ, et al. A clinical perspective on musculoskeletal infection treatment strategies and challenges. J Am Acad Orthop Surg. 2015;23(Suppl):S44–54.

17. Urist MR. Bone: formation by autoinduction. Science. 1965;150:893–9.

18. Gelberman RH, Samson D, Mirza SK, Callaghan JJ, Pellegrini Jr VD. Orthopaedic surgeons and the medical device industry: the threat to scientific integrity and the public trust. J Bone Joint Surg Am. 2010;92:765–77.

19. Mirza SK. Folly of FDA-approval studies for bone morphogenetic protein. Spine J Off J North Am Spine Soc. 2011;11:495–9.

20. Weinberg MJ, Al-Qattan MM, Mahoney J. "Spare part" forearm free flaps harvested from the amputated limb for coverage of amputation stumps. J Hand Surg. 1997;22:615–9.

21. Aasi SZ. Z-Plasty made simple. Dermatol Res Pract. 2010;2010:982623.

22. Baechler MF, Groth AT, Nesti LJ, Martin BD. Soft tissue management of war wounds to the foot and ankle. Foot Ankle Clin. 2010;15:113–38.

23. Gir P, Cheng A, Oni G, Mojallal A, Saint-Cyr M. Pedicled-perforator (propeller) flaps in lower extremity defects: a systematic review. J Reconstr Microsurg. 2012;28:595–601.

24. Chaput B, Herlin C, Espie A, Meresse T, Grolleau JL, Garrido I. The keystone flap alternative in posttraumatic lower-extremity reconstruction. J Plast Reconstr Aesthet Surg JPRAS. 2014;67:130–2.

25. Bunkis J, Walton RL, Mathes SJ. The rectus abdominis free flap for lower extremity reconstruction. Ann Plast Surg. 1983;11:373–80.

26. Sonmez A, Bayramicli M, Sonmez B, Numanoglu A. Reconstruction of the weight-bearing surface of the foot with nonneurosensory free flaps. Plast Reconstr Surg. 2003;111:2230–6.

27. Kuo YR, Yeh MC, Shih HS, et al. Versatility of the anterolateral thigh flap with vascularized fascia lata for reconstruction of complex soft-tissue defects: clinical experience and functional assessment of the donor site. Plast Reconstr Surg. 2009;124:171–80.

28. Nikolajsen L, Christensen KF, Haroutiunian S. Phantom limb pain: treatment strategies. Pain Manag. 2013;3:421–4.

29. Pet MA, Ko JH, Friedly JL, Mourad PD, Smith DG. Does targeted nerve implantation reduce neuroma pain in amputees? Clin Orthop Relat Res. 2014;472:2991–3001.

30. Bruehl S. Complex regional pain syndrome. BMJ. 2015;351:h2730.

31. Marks MR, Phillips D, Halsey DA, Wong A. Difficult conversations in orthopaedics. Instr Course Lect. 2015;64:3–9.

32. Dagum AB, Best AK, Schemitsch EH, Mahoney JL, Mahomed MN, Blight KR. Salvage after severe lower-extremity trauma: are the outcomes worth the means? Plast Reconstr Surg. 1999;103:1212–20.

33. Gallagher TH, Waterman AD, Ebers AG, Fraser VJ, Levinson W. Patients' and physicians' attitudes regarding the disclosure of medical errors. JAMA. 2003;289:1001–7.

34. Friedman LS, Forst L. Occupational injury surveillance of traumatic injuries in Illinois, using the Illinois trauma registry: 1995-2003. J Occup Environ Med. 2007;49:401–10.

35. Council NS. National Safety Council. Injury Facts: 2013 Edition. 2013.

36. Robertson-More C, Wells BJ, Nickerson D, Kirkpatrick AW, Ball CG. The economic and logistical burden of care for severe work-related injuries in a level 1 tertiary care trauma referral center. Am J Surg. 2015;210:451–5.

37. Bergin PF, Russell GV. The effects of obesity in orthopaedic care. Instr Course Lect. 2015;64:11–24.

38. Apovian CM. The clinical and economic consequences of obesity. Am J Manag Care. 2013;19(11 Suppl):s219–28.

Surgical Rehabilitation of the Tetraplegic Upper Extremity

18

Andreas Gohritz, Istvan Turcsányi, and Jan Fridén

Abbreviations

APB   Abductor pollicis brevis
APL   Abductor pollicis longus
BR   Brachioradialis
CMC   Carpometacarpal
DIP   Distal interphalangeal
ECU   Extensor carpi ulnaris
EDC   Extensor digitorum communis
EDM   Extensor digiti minimi
ECRB   Extensor carpi radialis brevis
ECRL   Extensor carpi radialis longus
EPL   Extensor pollicis longus
FDP   Flexor digitorum profundus

FDS   Flexor digitorum superficialis
FPL   Flexor pollicis longus
MCP   Metacarpophalangeal
PIP   Proximal interphalangeal
PNI   Peripheral nerve injury
PT   Pronator teres
SCI   Spinal cord injury

Introduction

Tetraplegia means paralysis of all four extremities due to cervical spinal cord injury (SCI). It is profoundly disabling, mainly because of the lost arm and hand function.

Epidemiology

Global incidence of spinal cord injury (SCI) has been estimated 10–80 new cases per million annually which means that about 12,000 in the USA alone and 250,000–500,000 people worldwide become newly paralyzed every year [1]. This population represents often otherwise healthy and active individuals aged between 20–40 years. In about 50 %, SCI occurs at cervical level leading to tetraplegia [2].

Etiology

Causes of SCI differ between countries but worldwide most commonly occur due to motor vehicle accidents, falls, violence, and sports and

A. Gohritz, MD (✉)
Department of Hand Surgery, Swiss Paraplegia Centre, Guido A. Zäch-Str. 1, Nottwil CH-6207, Switzerland

Department of Plastic, Reconstructive and Aesthetic Surgery, Hand Surgery, University Hospital, Spitalstr. 21, Basel CH-4031, Switzerland
e-mail: andreas_gohritz@yahoo.com

I. Turcsányi, MD
Department of Orthopaedics, Szabolcs-Szatmár-Bereg County Hospitals and University Hospital, Szent István u. 68, Nyíregyháza H-4400, Hungary

J. Fridén, MD, PhD
Centre of Advanced Reconstruction of Extremities (C.A.R.E.), and Department of Hand Surgery, Institute of Clinical Sciences, Sahlgrenska University Hospital, Göteborg, SE-41345, Sweden

Department of Hand Surgery, Swiss Paraplegia Centre, Guido A. Zäch-Str. 1, Nottwil CH-6207, Switzerland

© Springer International Publishing Switzerland 2017
A.I. Elkwood et al. (eds.), *Rehabilitative Surgery*, DOI 10.1007/978-3-319-41406-5_18

leisure activities. Nontraumatic causes include tumors, infection, and degenerative or vascular disorders – it can happen to anyone of us any day [1–4].

Upper Extremity Functional Surgery

Besides the brain, upper extremity function is the most important functional resource of tetraplegic patients and judged to be the most desirable to regain, before bowel, bladder, sexual function, or walking ability. Anderson reports that 49 % of surveyed tetraplegic individuals ranked rehabilitation of arm and hand function as first priority, with no other goal surpassing 13 % [2]. Similarly, another study reports that 77 % of 565 tetraplegic patients expected important or very important improvement in quality of life if their hand function improved [5].

Tendon and nerve transfers, tenodeses, and joint stabilizations reliably restore upper extremity abilities, reduce muscle imbalance and pain in spasticity, and prevent joint contractures. Restored elbow extension improves reaching capabilities and stabilizes the elbow, allowing for further reconstruction of grasping, swimming, and driving [3, 6, 7]. Reconstructed grip eliminates the need for adaptive equipment; allows to groom, self-feed, self-catheterize, manipulate objects, write, and perform productive work; markedly improves autonomy and spontaneity; and thus enhances self-esteem for tetraplegic persons [8].

Current Utilization of Upper Extremity Surgery

Regrettably, despite highly positive results, tetraplegia surgery is profoundly underutilized. In the USA with over 100,000 tetraplegic citizens, fewer than 400 receive upper extremity functional surgery annually – less than 10 % of appropriate candidates. This rate may be even lower in other industrial nations and nearly nil in developing countries. Reasons explaining this paradox are complex but may relate to inadequate

information causing skepticism of patients, therapists, and rehabilitation physicians and inadequate referral networks [9].

Clinical Picture: Symptoms and Physical Findings

1. *Muscle testing*: Planning depends on upper extremity evaluation regarding muscle strength tests according to the British Research Council system and International Classification of Surgery of the Hand in Tetraplegia (ICSHT) (Tables 18.1 and 18.2) [3]. Donor muscles must be healthy, of adequate strength (M 4), preferably not injured or reinnervated, yet with limited available donors, weaker muscles (M3) may be used. Donors should be similar in architecture, be synergistic, and have adequate soft tissue bed along their transfer route [3, 8, 10, 11].

2. *Joint range of motion*: Passive joint motion, above all in the shoulder, elbow, forearm, wrist, MCP, and PIP joints, is prerequisite for reconstruction. Tenodesis effect during wrist extension (hand closure) and flexion (hand opening) and joint stability (primarily thumb CMC joint) is preferable but not required for reconstruction.

3. *Sensibility testing:* Sensory examination focuses on cutaneous afferences with a 2-point discrimination of 10 mm or better in the thumb for cutaneous control (Cu); otherwise ocular control (O) is required [10].

Table 18.1 Muscle function according to British Research Council system

Muscle strength grade	Muscle function
M0	No active range of motion, no palpable muscle contraction
M1	No active range of motion, palpable muscle contraction only
M2	Reduced active range of motion – not against gravity, no muscle resistance
M3	Full active range of motion, no muscle resistance
M4	Full active range of motion, reduced muscle resistance
M5	Full active range of motion, normal muscle resistance

Table 18.2 International classification of surgery of the hand in tetraplegia – with additional resources for nerve transfers

Group	Spinal cord segment	Possible muscle transfers	Possible axon sources for nerve transfers
0	≥ C5	No transferable muscle below elbow	Musculocutaneous nerve branches to coracobrachialis and brachialis muscle
1	C5	Brachioradialis (BR)	Axillary nerve branches to deltoid and teres minor muscles
2	C6	+ Extensor carpi radialis longus (ECRL)	Radial nerve branches to supinator or ECRB muscles
3	C6	+ Extensor carpi radialis brevis (ECRB)	
4	C6	+ Pronator teres (PT)	
5	C7	+ Flexor carpi radialis (FCR)	
6	C7	+ Extensor digitorum	
7	C7	+ Extensor pollicis longus	
8	C8	+ Flexor digitorum	
9	C8	No intrinsic hand muscles	
10 (X)		Exceptions	

4. *Special aspects:* Neuromuscular examination also considers brachial plexus lesions, entrapment neuropathies, spine deformity, thoraco-scapular stability, spasticity, and contractures. Pain and swelling are relative contraindications and need to be treated before surgery [3, 12].

Therapeutic Options

Nonoperative Treatment

Dedicated physiotherapy and occupational therapy including splinting optimize preoperative circumstances and postoperative function. It provides the "other half" of rehabilitation by patient motivation, retraining of transferred tendons, edema control, and contracture prevention and is, besides input from rehab specialists and the patients themselves, essential for successful rehabilitation [3, 13, 14].

Surgical Treatment

Indications for Surgery

Specific requirements must be met preoperatively (Table 18.3).

Table 18.3 Preoperative requirements in tetraplegia surgery

1 Neurological functional plateau – no further recovery expected

2 Emotional stability – accepting the consequences of injuries

3 Realistic expectations and postoperative goals

4 No open wounds or pressure sores (decubitus), no infections (e.g., bladder)

5 Motivation and ability of the patient to cooperate actively in aftertreatment

6 Treatment plan based on clinical examination and counseling of the patient

7 Available donor muscles (muscle strength grade ≥M4)

8 Free passive joint mobility [3, 8, 10, 25]

Time Management

The abovementioned conditions are usually achieved after completing the first rehabilitation, yet strict time rules (e.g., no operations before 1 year since injury) are not appropriate. Neurological stability may be achieved after 3–6 months in complete tetraplegia. Early surgery has many advantages, such as faster reintegration. Often, however, financial, family, or work-related problems must be solved first. Notably, a tendon transfer reconstruction remains feasible even decades after SCI. In incomplete SCI, functional recovery takes longer so that treatment plans should be developed only after complete regeneration spasticity control [12].

Regarding nerve transfers, muscles in SCI can be categorized into:

1. Still functional muscles innervated by the supralesional segment
2. Muscles with damaged anterior horn cells and lower motor neuron denervation
3. Paralyzed muscles innervated by infralesional segment

The first group represents potential donor nerves; the nerves to the latter two groups are potential recipients. Early surgery (within 1 year) is critical, as neuromuscular end-plate degeneration makes the denervated muscle refractory to eventual reanimation (after about 2 years). In upper motoneuron lesions, neuromuscular degeneration is slowed which may extend the time window for successful nerve transfers [15, 16].

Goals of Surgery

Surgical operations aim at better daily life performance (Table 18.4).

Reconstructive algorithms depend on the level of paralysis (Table 18.5).

Surgical Techniques

Reconstruction of Elbow Extension

Elbow extension is critical for overhead activities, weight shifting, and transfers and greatly increases wheelchair propulsion and workspace

Table 18.4 Surgical procedures (excluding nerve transfers) to achieve patients' ability goals

Ability goal	Functional goal	Procedure
Stabilizing elbow in space, reaching overhead objects, propelling wheelchair, stabilizing trunk	*Elbow extension*	*Reconstruction of triceps function* Posterior deltoid-triceps Biceps-triceps
Use of utensils, hand writing, propelling wheelchair	*Hand closure*	*Reconstruction of grip*
		Reconstruction of passive key pinch BR-ECRB FPL-radius CMC 1 arthrodesis *Reconstruction of active key grip* BR-FPL CMC I arthrodesis Split FPL-EPL tenodesis *Reconstruction of finger flexion* ECRL-to-FDP 2–4
Reaching for objects, e. g., glass, thumb and finger positioning for improved grasp control	*Hand opening*	*Reconstruction of thumb and finger extensors*
		Passive opening CMC I arthrodesis EPL to extensor retinaculum attachment *Active opening* PT-EDC and EPL/APL *Thumb stabilization* ELK procedure, CMC 1 arthrodesis *Reconstruction of intrinsics* Zancolli-Lasso tenodesis House tenodesis EDM-APB

Table 18.5 Surgical algorithms according to International Classification (IC)

IC group	Recommended surgical procedure
0	Abducted shoulder (anterior deltoid muscle transfer) Flexion contracture of the elbow (biceps tendon Z-tenotomy) Supinated but not contracted forearm (Zancolli biceps rerouting – check presence of supinator muscle!) Fixed supination contracture – osteotomy of radius
1	BR-to-ECRB for active wrist extension Moberg's key pinch procedure ELK procedure
2	BR-to-FPL (active key pinch) CMC 1 fusion ELK procedure EPL tenodesis to dorsal forearm fascia
3	BR-to-FPL ECRL-to-FDP 2–4 ELK procedure House intrinsic procedure CMC 1 fusion EPL tenodesis
4	BR-to-FPL ECRL-to-FDP 2–4 ELK procedure House intrinsic procedure CMC 1 fusion EPL tenodesis
5	BR-to-FPL ECRL-to-FDP 2–4 ELK procedure House intrinsic procedure CMC 1 fusion EPL tenodesis
6	BR-to-FPL ECRL-to-FDP 2–4 ELK procedure House intrinsic procedure EDM-to-APB transfer EDC-to-EPL
7	BR-to-FPL ECRL-to-FDP II-IV ELK procedure (if required) House intrinsic procedure EDM-to-APB or EIP-to-APB
8	BR-to-FPL ECRB-activated ADPB Opponens plasty (EIP, EDM, FCU) Active Zancolli lasso procedure (ECU) House intrinsic procedure
9	House intrinsic procedure
10	Pathological postures (MP joints fixed in hyperextension, lack of any functioning intrinsic muscles, wrist fixed either in flexion or extension, etc.) Release of contracted muscles, joint capsules, tendon lengthenings

of the hand by 800 %. Elbow restoration should precede grip reconstructions because:

- Use of a hand that cannot reach out is limited.
- Elbow extension stabilizes the trunk in the wheel chair.
- Stability enables more controlled hand use.
- Tendon transfer functions (e.g., using brachioradialis) improve with antagonistic elbow extension.

Procedures to restore triceps function include:

1. *Tendon transfer* (posterior deltoid-to-triceps or biceps-to-triceps transfer) [7, 8, 17]
2. *Nerve transfer* (axillary or musculocutaneous nerve fascicles) [15, 16]

Posterior deltoid transfer reliably restores triceps function in C5/C6 tetraplegia (Fig. 18.1a, b). Candidates for biceps transfer usually demonstrate intact and functional brachialis and supinator muscles and elbow flexion contracture exceeding approximately 20°. Both techniques are time proven and provide improved arm control useful in many daily activities. Alternatively, triceps reanimation is possible by transferring fascicles of axillary (branches to posterior portion of deltoid or teres minor muscle) or musculocutaneous (brachialis branch) nerve [15, 16].

Reconstruction of Forearm Pronation

Supination contracture due to imbalance between the functional biceps brachii and supinators and weak or paralyzed pronators seriously impairs hand function and increases the risk of gravity-induced wrist extension contracture. Restoration of forearm pronation re-enabling key pinch is possible by:

1. *Distal biceps tendon rerouting*, if necessary with interosseous membrane release [17]
2. *Dorsal brachioradialis transfer* during BR-to-FPL transfer to achieve simultaneous thumb flexion and forearm pronation [3]
3. *Derotation osteotomy of the radius* [18]

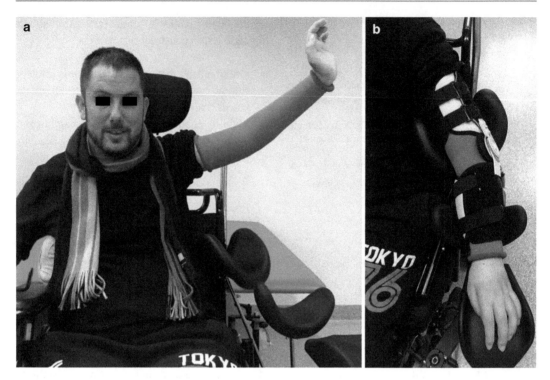

Fig. 18.1 (**a**) C5–C6 tetraplegic patient demonstrates his restored elbow extension after posterior deltoid-to-triceps reconstructions. (**b**) After reconstruction of elbow extension by posterior deltoid-to-triceps muscle transfer, the operated arm is immobilized in an arm rest between train- ing sessions in elbow extension and 30° of shoulder abduction to protect the tendon attachment, e.g., from excessive shoulder adduction. Elbow flexion is then increased by 10–15° per week using an adjustable orthosis until full flexion is allowed

Reconstruction of Wrist Extension

1. BR-to-ECRB tendon transfer

    Reconstruction of active wrist extension is highly important to enable wrist-related tenodesis effect. If wrist extension is absent (IC group 0 and 1), the brachioradialis (only IC group 1) can be transferred onto the ECRB for wrist extension-driven key pinch after additional FPL-to-radius tenodesis (Moberg procedure) [7].

2. Nerve transposition from above the elbow

    If antigravity wrist extension is absent and cannot be restored by tendon transfer because donors lack below elbow (group 0) in C5 tetraplegia, tenodesis grip can be restored by brachialis motor nerve transfer to the ECRL motor branch and FPL-to-radius tenodesis [19].

Positioning and Stabilization of the Thumb

Interphalangeal (IP) joint hyperflexion disturbs thumb function if extrinsic flexor function is preserved or reconstructed (e.g., by FPL reanimation) but intrinsic or extrinsic thumb extensors are paralyzed. The EPL-loop-knot (ELK) procedure has advantages compared to FPL split tenodesis or arthrodesis (Fig. 18.2) [20].

Reconstruction of Grip Function

Tetraplegic patients usually have a spontaneous weak pinch depending on wrist extension (tenodesis grip). To produce a useful grip, preoperative planning considers patient's goals, hand muscle function, sensibility, and spasticity. In IC group

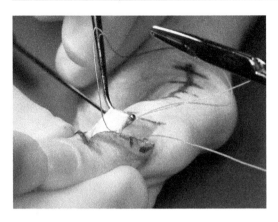

Fig. 18.2 EPL-loop-knot (*ELK*) procedure to stabilize the thumb interphalangeal joint and prevent it from hyperextension: The EPL tendon is mobilized and elevated with a hook and then duplicated by forming a loop of the tendon and suturing this loop onto the tendon itself proximally

2, ECRL is the only reliable wrist extensor and is unavailable for a transfer. In IC 3 and higher groups with two strong radial wrist extensors, ECRL is expedient for active transfers [3, 42].

1. Reconstruction of key pinch

    Lateral key pinch grip depends on hand opening by wrist flexion and closing by wrist extension whereby the thumb pulp ideally meets the index middle phalanx radially. Prerequisites are M3 wrist extension, forearm pronation, and acceptable relationship between thumb and fingers. Stabilizing procedures are ELK distal thumb tenodesis and CMC 1 arthrodesis. Active key pinch is preferably achieved by BR-FPL tendon transfer (Fig. 18.3a–c) [3, 8].

2. Reconstruction of power grip – ECRL-to-FDP tendon transfer

    Active whole hand closure is powered by ECRL tendon transfer on the deep finger flexors 2–4 excluding the little finger to prevent hyperflexion (Fig. 18.4) [3, 8].

3. Nerve transfer to restore interosseous anterior nerve function

    Transferring the brachialis motor branch (musculocutaneous nerve) to the interosseous anterior nerve (median nerve) can reanimate finger and thumb flexion [15].

Reconstruction of Intrinsics

Interossei/lumbrical reconstruction can secure MCP joint flexion and PIP and DIP extension and optimize index position and flexion to meet the thumb and also create support by digits 3–5. Extension of the PIP joints is essential for grasp and release and provides a more normal hand opening compared to EDC reconstruction giving an intrinsic minus type of opening. The House procedure has proven superior to the formerly used Zancolli lasso plasty in experimental and clinical experience [21, 22].

1. *Passive interossei function using passive tenodesis by tendon grafts into lumbrical canals (House procedure)* [22].
2. *Reconstruction of active interossei function by tendon transfer, e.g., FDS 4 with four tendon slips into lumbrical canals (Brand procedure)*
3. *Restoration of palmar abduction of the thumb*

    Transferring extensor digiti minimi (EDM) to the insertion of abductor pollicis brevis (APB) restores thumb palmar abduction. Notably, M3 power of the EDM is usually sufficient to increase first web space opening and position the thumb radially along the index [11].

Reconstruction of Hand Opening (Extensor Phase)

Reconstruction of hand opening facilitates coming around objects during grasp (Table 18.3) which is frequently impossible due to adhesions of flexors and insufficient finger stretching even with good passive wrist flexion. Improved hand opening of the hand is particularly necessary when gravity or remaining finger extension strength cannot overpower the finger flexion spasticity [12].

1. *Passive opening of the first commissure* by EPL tenodesis to forearm fascia (powered by active or passive wrist flexion)
2. *Active opening by tendon transfer* by transferring PT to EPL, APL, and EDC

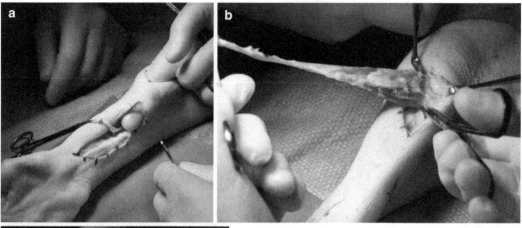

Fig. 18.3 Intraoperative view of BR-to-FPL transfer, (a): Creating a subcutaneous tunnel between donor and recipient site, (b): Mobilization of the BR from its proximal adhesions to enable an adequate excursion of the donor muscle for its new function as a thumb flexor (4–5 cm), (c): BR-to-FPL site-to-site tendon suture

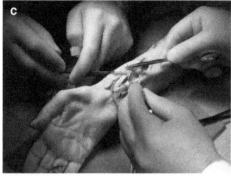

Fig. 18.4 Intraoperative view of ECRL-to-FDP 2–4 tendon transfer for restoration of finger flexion. The ECRL tendon is transferred obliquely (direct line of pull) into the deep finger flexor tendons (FDP 2–4); the little finger is usually excluded due to its early excessive flexion which may impede hand closure

3. *Nerve transfer of the supinator motor branches (C6) to the posterior interosseous nerve (C7–Th1) (Bertelli S-PIN procedure)*

As supinator is always C6 innervated and redundant when biceps is intact, the posterior interosseous nerve roots that are C7/C8 innervated can be restored by transferring the expendable supinator motor branches to reanimate finger and thumb extension as well as ECU function (Fig. 18.5a–c) [16, 17].

ECU Tenodesis for Wrist Alignment

Wrist radial deviation often occurs due to lack of ulnar deviation muscle action, especially in groups 0 and 1 where only ECRL is strongly present. By suturing of a tendon loop onto the ECU tendon itself, the gripping force doubles, compared to unbalanced hands, and due to more ergonomic hand function, the shoulder is not compensatory externally rotated as in the radially deviated wrist [23, 24].

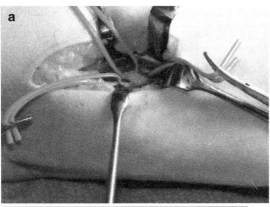
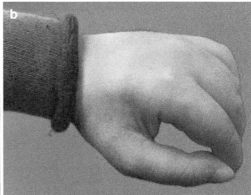
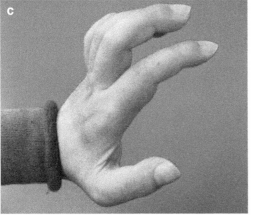

Fig. 18.5 Nerve transfer of supinator-to-posterior interosseous nerve (S-PIN procedure by Bertelli) in a patient grouped IC 1 (brachioradialis M4, wrist extension M3) – (a): intraoperative picture of donor branches to both C6 supinator muscle branches (*blue slings*) and C7-/C8-recipient posterior interosseous nerve (*red sling*) and postoperative resting position (b) and extension function showing restored finger, thumb, and increased wrist extension (by ECU) (c)

Additional Procedures to Reduce Spasticity

Spasticity, if present, can be very important. It is not a contraindication per se, but severe spasticity must be treated first depending in which muscle groups it is present. Spasticity can be treated with Botox® or myotomies. In some cases, spastic tone can be useful to facilitate hand grasp and grip. Harmful spasticity that does not respond to medication or surgical treatment is a contraindication. The shoulder muscles, pectoralis major, and latissimus dorsi must be evaluated. The shoulder must not only have good motor condition but also good proprioceptive control. The trophicity and articular condition of the upper limb must also be considered. A poor condition requires a preoperative rehabilitation program [3].

Before any hand surgery is performed, the patient should be able to actively extend the elbow. Therefore, if there is no active elbow extension, elbow extension reconstruction surgery should precede any hand surgery. A contraindication specifically for posterior deltoid-to-triceps transfer is a flexion contracture of the elbow; biceps-to-triceps transfer might then be a possible transfer for elbow extension reconstruction. The contraindications for biceps-to-triceps transfer relate to the muscle balance surrounding the elbow. The m. supinator and m. brachialis function is a prerequisite for this surgery. If one of these muscles is nonfunctional, the patient will lose forearm supination and elbow flexion if the tendon is transferred.

As incomplete tetraplegia increased, more patients demonstrate more complex functional

Table 18.6 Surgical management of spasticity in the tetraplegic upper extremity

Spasticity	Affected muscles	Surgical procedure	Function
Forearm	Pronator teres	Release	Supination possible
Wrist	FCR, FCU	Tendon lengthening	Wrist extension possible
Thumb	FPL, AdP	Tendon lengthening	Thumb extension and opening of first web space possible
Fingers	FDS / FDP	Tendon lengthening	Hand opening
Fingers	Interossei	Release	Reduction of intrinsic tightness, better grip

Table 18.7 Advanced Balancing Combined Digital Extension Flexion Grip (ABCDEFG) Reconstruction

	Procedure	Type	Function	Effect
1	ELK procedure	Tenodesis[a]	Stabilize IP joint	Prevent hyperflexion of IP, increase contact surface to index
2	CMC 1 stabilization	Arthrodesis	Fusion of basis of the thumb and correct deformity	Secure thumb's approach against index during key pinch
3	BR-to-FPL	Tendon transfer	Thumb flexion	Key pinch
4	ECRL-to-FDP 2–4	Tendon transfer	Finger flexion	Power grasp
5	Free tendon transplant at (FDS4, PL, plantaris) → extensor hood digits 2–3 and 4–5	Tenodesis[b]	Interossei [3]	Opening hand
6	EPL-to-dorsal forearm fascia	Tenodesis[c]	Extend thumb	Opening hand
7	ECU-to-ulnar head	Tenodesis	Prevent radial deviation of wrist	Balance hand position at all types of grips

[a]Powered by BR-to-FPL
[b]Powered by MCP flexion, PIP / DIP extension
[c]Powered by wrist flexion

losses with spastic muscle joint deformities that can frequently be corrected by muscle release and/or tendon lengthening and release (Table 18.6). Flexor tenotomies are performed about 5 cm proximal to the carpal canal using a stair-step incision of 6–8 cm in length which achieves a parallel sliding of both tendon stumps and subsequent prolongation of 2–3 cm [12].

Combined Procedures: Active Flexor and Passive Extensor Phase with Intrinsic Reconstruction (Alphabet Operation)

Traditionally, operations for flexors and extensors were separated, yet we developed a reliable one-stage combination of active key pinch and

finger flexion together with passive hand opening in C6 tetraplegia (Table 18.7).

To reduce adhesions after extensive surgery and facilitate relearning, activation of transferred muscles with new functions requires early active postoperative training. Overall, this simultaneous reconstruction saves time and limits need for immobilization and effort compared to standard 2-stage reconstructions without increased complications; functional results are very rewarding (Fig. 18.6a, b) [23, 24].

Nerve Transfers

Nerve transfers have been seldom applied in tetraplegia until recently. Extra-anatomical short circuit between expendable donor nerve fascicles from above the SCI and the motor branch of

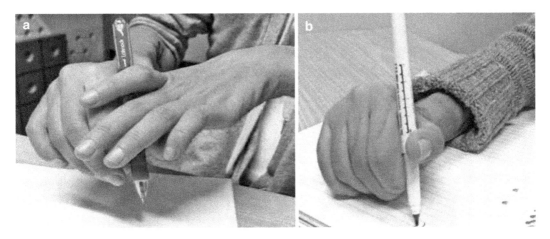

Fig. 18.6 Clinical example of patient with C6 tetraplegia showing handwriting technique before (**a, b**) and about 4 weeks after (**b**) one-stage complete grip reconstruction (Alphabet procedure [56, 57])

Table 18.8 Options of nerve transfer in tetraplegia (C6/7 level)

Donor nerve / muscle branch	Recipient nerve	Restored function
Brachialis (musculocutaneous nerve)	Median nerve/anterior interosseous nerve	Finger and thumb flexion (FDS, FDP, FPL)
	ECRL (radial nerve)	Wrist extension
	Triceps (radial nerve)	Elbow extension
Teres minor/posterior deltoid (axillary nerve)		Elbow extension (triceps)
Supinator C6 (radial nerve)	Posterior interosseous nerve C7/C8 (radial nerve)	Finger, thumb, and wrist extension, thumb extension (EDC, EPL, ECU, APL)
ECRB (radial nerve)	FPL (median nerve)	Thumb flexion

a paralyzed muscle underneath is effective. In SCI recipient muscles with intact lower motoneuron and preserved reflex arcs should not become refractory to reinnervation / external stimulation after 18–24 months, like after peripheral palsy. Axon transfer to the intact donor nerve may allow highly selective neurotization by intraoperative fascicle stimulation of the intact recipient nerve, with minimized distance between donor and recipient and regeneration time. Furthermore, natural biomechanics, force, and excursion of the original muscle are preserved, and scar-induced motion restrictions are prevented without the need for extended immobilization – a primary factor why appropriate candidates refuse muscle transfers. Axon transfers also provide options for patients not amenable to conventional tendon transfers, including IC group 0 (Table 18.8) [3, 15, 16] .

Further research should be directed at combining traditional algorithms with these new approaches, as Bertelli et al. restoring elbow extension, finger extension (MCP joint), thumb extension, and pinch [25, 26] .

Postoperative Protocol

Immediate Activation of Transferred Tendons

Immediate postoperative activation of transferred muscles means that the day after surgery, a removable splint replaces the cast, and intermittent exercises start by activating the donor muscles with slight external resistance. Early activation not only prevents adhesions but facilitates voluntary recruitment of motors before swelling, and

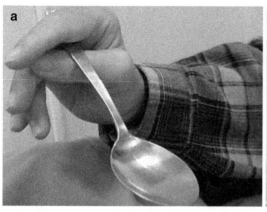
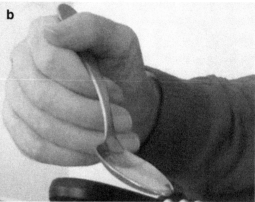

Fig. 18.7 Comparison of weak ability holding a spoon before (**a**) and firm and stable grip pattern after (**b**) Alphabet procedure in a C6 tetraplegic patient

immobilization-induced stiffness restrains muscle contractions. Additionally, the patient experiences a very motivating effect during the often demanding initial postoperative period. This approach requires reliable tendon-to-tendon attachments using side-to-side attachments with crossed sutures along both sides over a minimum of 5 cm (Fig. 18.5). This technique is extremely safe, as, e.g., the maximum passive tendon tension in a cadaver model was only about 20 N, while the failure strength of this specific repair exceeded 200 N (Fig. 18.7a, b) [25] .

Complications

Complications are related to candidate selection, surgery, and rehabilitation (Table 18.9). Tendon rupture with sudden loss or drop in function during rehabilitation phase should be carefully evaluated. Upon the suspicion of transfer/tenodesis failure, the patient should be brought back to the operating room for revision, and the surgeon should be prepared to augment the revised transfer/tenodesis with tendon graft. Transfers and tenodeses also may stretch over time, mostly due to overuse.

Thumb/index positioning during pinch reconstruction is important for effective pinch. Problems arise if the thumb CMC is fused in too much flexion or too much extension. There are times where the index finger fails to flex enough

to meet the pulp of the thumb about the level of the middle phalanx/DIP. We have attempted FDP tenodesis, Zancolli lasso, and even MCP capsulodesis to improve index finger posturing. Unfortunately, none are truly satisfactory, yet individuals ultimately learn to adjust to this difficulty by using a surface to help flex their fingers during the acquisition phase of pinch.

Strict adherence to postoperative therapy is critical. Surgeons and therapists should watch for signs indicating stretch of the transfer and modify aftertreatment or use protective splinting. Finally, dissatisfaction may occur despite good objective results, resulting from poor candidate selection, inadequate information, and thus unrealistic expectations. Preoperative patient-to-patient contacts and good documentation with written and video documentation of the functional status and goals may minimize this risk.

Clinical Results

Tendon Transfers

Historically, results have been measured in terms of grasp and pinch strength and activity of daily living performance [3, 8]. A meta-analysis of the literature from over 500 cases in 14 studies revealed a mean increase of Medical Research Council score for elbow extension from 0 to 3.3 after reconstruction and a mean postoperative

Table 18.9 Complication management in tetraplegia surgery

Complication	Measure/therapy
Preoperative	
Lack of donor muscles, e.g., due to additional brachial plexus (rare)/lower motoneuron injury (more frequent)	Exact preoperative muscle testing, simplified operative technique, e.g., passive key pinch reconstruction
Doubt if both ECRL/ECRB are present with M4 strength (Groups 2 or 3?)	Distinction often difficult, e.g., by visible muscle groove between extensor muscle origins, safely possible if pronator teres muscle function is present, preservation of both radial wrist extensors and reconstruction of passive key pinch (Moberg operation) and active finger flexion (BR-pro-FDP 2–4)
Intraoperative	
Nerve or vessel injury	Immediate microsurgical reconstruction
Insufficient tendon tension	Intraoperative testing (tenodesis effect) with test suture
Postoperative	
Swelling, edema (increased risk for postoperative adhesions, wound healing problems)	Preservation of dorsal veins, elevation of the upper extremity, lymph drainage, early mobilization
Insufficient or slack tendon suture	Operative revision, new suture, tenodesis
Tendon elongation or rupture	Stable side-to-side technique
Hematoma	Evacuation
Slackening of tendon suture	Information and education of patients (e.g., transfer techniques – not on flat hand but on fist)
Infection, wound healing problems	Antibiotics, conservative wound care, operative revision
Nerve and vessel compression	Operative revision and decompression
Tendon tension too high (with impaired motion, e.g., impaired hand closure)	Operative revision
Elbow contracture	Splinting Operation (arthrolysis, muscle release, tendon lengthening, tenotomy)
Impaired movement caused by adhesions, scarring of transferred tendons	Early mobilization and protection by splints controlled by hand therapy
Impaired wrist extension and opening (clenched fist)	Conservative therapy (splints) and operative opening, e.g., tendon lengthening, release, or tenotomy (e.g., adductor pollicis, pronator teres, wrist extensor muscles)
Loss of wrist extension, e.g., due to mixing up ECRL and ECRB or transfer of ECRL in case of weak ECRB (strength grade below M3)	Reoperation and re-transfer of split ECRL tendon for wrist extension (while the other half remains for finger flexion)
Problems after arthrodesis, above all thumb IP joint (e.g., hyperflexed position, nonunion, migration of K-wires, hardware failure, etc.)	Tenodesis
Unsatisfied patients despite good objective results, e.g., due to unrealistic expectations	Realistic information preoperatively, contact with already operated patients, good documentation (functional status, goals preoperative)

pinch strength of 2 kg which markedly improved upper extremity usability [27]. More recently, reconstructive procedures have been evaluated regarding improved independence as evidenced by patient-perceived satisfaction and performance of preoperatively prioritized daily activity goals [12–15]. Upper extremity surgery affects body function, activity, participation, and personal and environmental factors, and improve-

ments are not just seen in basic ADL activities, such as eating, but in more complex activities, such as domestic life and leisure activities [13].

The Canadian Occupational Performance Measure (COPM) is used to measure a tetraplegic patient's performance and satisfaction before and after upper limb surgery, and a positive change is seen in patient-perceived performance and satisfaction with self-identified goals after tendon transfers. In a recent interview study by Wangdell et al., patients summarized their gains as "enhanced independence" which meant autonomy, freedom from control, self-reliance, and acting for oneself and to participate more actively in social situations. Psychological aspects included feelings of greater management in daily life, less dependence on people and environment, and greater self-efficacy in hand control [14]. Mohammed et al. presented their results of surgical restoration in large patient series reporting improved quality of life in 84 % [29]. Individuals with stable nontraumatic tetraplegia benefit similarly from surgical rehabilitation of their upper extremities as traumatic cohorts [4]. The sustainability of these benefits has been established [28].

Neuroprosthetic Devices (Functional Electrical Stimulation (FES))

Results from neuroprosthesis reported improved ability to perform functional tasks, as well as allowed patients to perform many activities without adaptive equipment [30]. Although no longer commercially available but still studied in academic centers, the functional benefits of implanted neuroprostheses may serve selected subpopulations in the future [30].

Nerve Transfers

Nerve transfers have been used for elbow, wrist, and finger extension and digital grasp including over 70 procedures with two double nerve and triple transfers and overall rate of postoperative M3 and M4 functions exceeding 80 %, mostly in young patients (under 25 years) who were operated early (until 6–12 months after their accident). Notably, results in patients aged over 40 years or operated beyond 12 months after trauma were significantly worse [15, 16, 31, 32].

Conclusions

Patients with tetraplegia have the main goal of more mobility and independence from foreign aid that can be realistically achieved by surgical rehabilitation of arm and hand function.

Every person with tetraplegia should be assessed and informed concerning possible reconstructive options. This form of hand surgery is reliable, and results are rewarding from the perspective of patients and surgeons, possibly more than in any other field of hand surgery. Combining traditional muscle with innovative nerve transfer will expand the indications in the future. Reconstruction remains possible, even decades after a cervical spinal cord paralysis. Improved communication between the disciplines, who care for these patients, therapists, patients, and their relatives should contribute in the future to ensure that more patients benefit from these options to at least partially "take their lives into their own hands" again.

Declaration of Conflicting Interests The authors have no financial disclosures.

References

1. Bickenbach J, editor. International perspectives on spinal cord injury. Geneva: World Health Organization; 2013.
2. Anderson KD. Targeting recovery: priorities of the SCI population. J Neurotrauma. 2004;21:1371–83.
3. Fridén J, Gohritz A. Novel concepts integrated in neuromuscular assessments for surgical restoration of arm and hand function in tetraplegia. Phys Med Rehabil Clin N Am. 2012;23:33–50.
4. Fridén J, Reinholdt C, Wangdell J, Gohritz A. Upper extremity reconstruction in non-traumatic spinal cord injuries: an under-recognized opportunity. J Rehabil Med. 2014;46:33–8.
5. Snoek GJ, Ijzerman MJ, Hermens HJ, Maxwell D, Biering-Sorensen F. Survey of the needs of patients with spinal cord injury: impact and priority for improvement in hand function in tetraplegics. Spinal Cord. 2004;42:526–32.
6. Fridén J, Gohritz A. Tetraplegia management update. J Hand Surg Am. 2015;40:2489–500.
7. Moberg E. The upper limb in tetraplegia. A new approach to surgical rehabilitation. Stuttgart: Thieme; 1978.
8. Hentz V, Leclercq C. Surgical rehabilitation of the upper limb in tetraplegia. New York: WB Saunders; 2002.
9. Curtin CM, Gater DR, Chung KC. Upper extremity reconstruction in the tetraplegic population, a national epidemiologic study. J Hand Surg Am. 2005;30:94–9.
10. Kozin SH, Zlotolow DA, Abzug JM. Upper limb reconstruction in persons with tetraplegia. In: Abzug JM et al.,

editors. The pediatric upper extremity. New York: Springer; 2015.

11. Fridén J, Gohritz A, Turcsanyi I, Ejeskar A. Restoration of active palmar abduction of the thumb in tetraplegia by tendon transfer of the extensor digiti minimi to abductor pollicis brevis. J Hand Surg Eur Vol. 2012;37: 665–72.

12. Fridén J, Reinholdt C. Current concepts in reconstruction of hand function in tetraplegia. Scand J Surg. 2008;97:341–6.

13. Wangdell J, Carlsson G, Fridén J. Enhanced independence: experiences after regaining grip function in people with tetraplegia. Disabil Rehabil. 2013;35: 1968–74.

14. Wangdell J, Fridén J. Activity gains after reconstructions of elbow extension in patients with tetraplegia. J Hand Surg Am. 2012;37:1003–10.

15. Van Zyl N, Hahn JB, Cooper CA, et al. Upper limb reinnervation in C6 tetraplegia using a triple nerve transfer. J Hand Surg Am. 2014;39:1779–183.

16. Bertelli JA, Ghizoni MF. Nerve transfers for elbow and finger extension reconstruction in mid-cervical spinal cord injuries. J Neurosurg. 2014; 24:1–7.

17. Zancolli E. Structural and dynamic bases of hand surgery. 2nd ed. Philadelphia: Lippincott; 1979.

18. Coulet B, Boretto JG, Allieu Y, Fattal C, Laffont I, Chammas M. Pronating osteotomy of the radius for forearm supination contracture in high-level tetraplegic patients: technique and results. J Bone Joint Surg Br. 2010;92:828–34.

19. Fridén J, Gohritz A. Brachialis-to-extensor carpi radialis longus selective nerve transfer to restore wrist extension in tetraplegia: case report. J Hand Surg Am. 2012;37:1606–8.

20. Fridén J, Reinholdt C, Gohritz A. The extensor pollicis longus-loop-knot (ELK) procedure for dynamic balance of the paralyzed thumb interphalangeal joint. Tech Hand Up Extrem Surg. 2013;17:184–6.

21. Muzykewicz DA, Arnet U, Lieber RL, Fridén J. Intrinsic hand muscle function, part 2: kinematic comparison of 2 reconstructive procedures. J Hand Surg Am. 2013;38:2100–5.

22. McCarthy CK, House JH, Van Heest A, et al. Intrinsic balancing in reconstruction of the tetraplegic hand. J Hand Surg Am. 1997;22:596–604.

23. Fridén J, Reinholdt C, Turcsanyí I, Gohritz A. A single-stage operation for reconstruction of hand flexion, extension, and intrinsic function in tetraplegia: the Alphabet procedure. Tech Hand Up Extrem Surg. 2011;15:230–5.

24. Reinholdt C, Fridén J. Outcomes of single-stage grip-release reconstruction in tetraplegia. J Hand Surg Am. 2013;38:1137–44.

25. Bertelli JA, Ghizoni MF. Single-stage surgery combining nerve and tendon transfers for bilateral upper limb reconstruction in a tetraplegic patient: case report. J Hand Surg Am. 2013;38:1366–9.

26. Brown SH, Hentzen ER, Kwan A, Ward SR, Fridén J, Lieber RL. Mechanical strength of the side-to-side versus Pulvertaft weave tendon repair. J Hand Surg Am. 2010;35:540–5.

27. Hamou C, et al. Pinch and elbow extension restoration in people with tetraplegia: a systematic review of the literature. J Hand Surg Am. 2009;34:692–9.

28. Mohammed KD, Rothwell AG, Sinclair SW, Willems SM, Bean AR. Upper-limb surgery for tetraplegia. J Bone Joint Surg Br. 1992;74:873–9.

29. Vastamäki M. Short-term versus long-term comparative results after reconstructive upper-limb surgery in tetraplegic patients. J Hand Surg Am. 2006;31:1490–4.

30. Keith MW, Peljovich A. Surgical treatments to restore function control in spinal cord injury. Handb Clin Neurol. 2012;109:167–79.

31. Krasuski M, Kiwerski J. An analysis of the results of transferring the musculocutaneous nerve onto the median nerve in tetraplegics. Arch Orthop Trauma Surg. 1991;111:32–3.

32. Cain S, Gohritz A, Fridén J, van Zyl N. Review of upper extremity nerve transfer in cervical spinal cord injury. J Brach Plex Peripher Nerve Inj. 2015;10: e34–42.

Andrew I. Elkwood, Lisa F. Schneider,
and Michael I. Rose

Approach to the Lower Extremity of Patients

The legs are the wheels of creativity. Albert Einstein

There are clear analogies and similarities between the approach to rehabilitative surgery of the lower extremity and that of the upper extremity. As with the upper extremity, the three basic issues to be addressed are motion, sensibility, and pain. However, even within these similar issues, there are differences in the priorities of the approach. For example, in the lower extremity overall, the ability to bear weight is a key factor in any reconstruction. Although the position of the extremity is important, the relative importance of weight bearing is greater than it is in the upper extremity because the leg is required to support the entire weight of the body. This contrasts with the upper extremity, where positioning has greater relative value because of the finer movements it must execute. In some instances, the ability to position the leg without supporting the body's weight may have value in transferring, supine positioning, and directing an extremity sup-

ported by a brace, but is likely of limited value. One exception to this is foot drop. Dorsiflexion of the foot requires very little strength but is crucial to "re-cocking" the foot to achieve a normal gait. Foot drop will be discussed in detail below.

With regard to sensibility, at least partial sensibility – protective and proprioceptive – is necessary to ambulate properly and to avoid injury and breakdown. For the most part, such sensibility is only absolutely necessary in the sole of the foot. Overall, sensibility to other areas of the leg is of minimal importance. Two-point discrimination is far less important in the lower extremity than it is the hand, as fine dexterity is not required. However, protective sensibility and the ability to feel pain or pressure can have significant importance in the development or prevention of pressure ulcers. This is especially true over bony prominences like the ischium and sacrum, common sites of pressure ulcers in paraplegic and quadriplegic patients. New procedures have allowed for re-sensitization of these areas with the goal of prevention of pressure ulcers through the patient's own perception of pain. This is covered in detail in the chapter on "Pressure Ulcers."

Lastly, although nerve pain in the legs is not as common as it is in the upper extremity, many compression syndromes do exist and, unfortunately, often go undiagnosed. This is especially the case with regard to peripheral diabetic neuropathy. The lack of accurate diagnosis may be attributed to the lack of specificity of the sensory distribution and therefore cloudy symptomatology.

A.I. Elkwood, MD, MBA (✉) • L.F. Schneider, MD
M.I. Rose, MD
The Plastic Surgery Center, Institute for Advanced
Reconstruction, 535 Sycamore Ave,
Shrewsbury, NJ 07702, USA
e-mail: aelkwoodmd@theplasticsurgerycenternj.com;
lschneidermd@theplasticsurgerycenternj.com;
mrosemd@theplasticsurgerycenternj.com

© Springer International Publishing Switzerland 2017
A.I. Elkwood et al. (eds.), *Rehabilitative Surgery*, DOI 10.1007/978-3-319-41406-5_19

Anatomy

Compartments of the Leg

The lower extremity can be thought of as two separate units, the upper and lower leg. Each unit contains a series of fascial compartments that define a precise relationship between muscles, nerves, and blood vessels. The thigh contains three compartments, anterior, medial, and posterior, named for their relationship to the femur. The anterior compartment contains the sartorius as well as the iliopsoas, pectineus, and quadriceps, which includes four muscles: the rectus femoris, vastus medialis, vastus lateralis, and vastus intermedius. This region is supplied by the femoral artery and the femoral nerve (L2–4). The next compartment is the medial compartment which contains the adductor longus, brevis, and magnus, obturator externus, and gracilis. These muscles are supplied by the profunda femoris artery and the obturator nerve (L2–4). The final posterior compartment contains the biceps femoris, semitendinosus, semimembranosus, and adductor magnus muscles. It is also supplied by the profunda femoris artery but differently by the sciatic nerve (L4–S3).

The lower leg is divided into four compartments, also named in relation to tibia and fibula. The anterior compartment contains the tibialis anterior, extensor hallucis longus, extensor digitorum longus, and peroneus tertius muscles. The arterial supply is the anterior tibial artery, and the motor nerve is the deep peroneal nerve (L4–5). The lateral compartment contains only two muscles: peroneus longus and peroneus brevis. The arterial supply is the peroneal artery and the nerve, the superficial peroneal nerve (L4–S1). The posterior aspect of the leg is divided into two separate compartments, superficial and deep. The superficial posterior compartment contains the gastrocnemius, the soleus, and the plantaris, which may be absent in 10–15% of patients. The deep posterior compartment contains the tibialis posterior, flexor hallucis longus, flexor digitorum longus, and popliteus muscles. The blood supply to both compartments is a combination of the posterior tibial and peroneal arteries. Both compartments are innervated by the tibial nerve (S1–2) (Figs. 19.1, 19.2, 19.3).

Innervation

For our purposes within the text, especially with our emphasis on nerve compression and neurotization, a different way to conceptualize the anatomy is by visualizing the leg from a purely nervous perspective. This begins superiorly with the lumbar and sacral plexi, a collection of nerve roots that form the source of the nerves to the leg. The lumbar plexus is anterior to the transverse processes of the lumbar vertebrae and is formed from L1–L4 as well as contributions from T12. The most superior branches are the iliohypogastric (T12–L1) and ilioinguinal (L1) nerves, which innervate the transversus abdominis and internal oblique muscles before continuing as sensory nerves innervating the skin of the gluteal region, hypogastrium, and the anterior scrotum or labia. The next is the genitofemoral (L1–2) nerve, which after innervating the cremaster muscle continues on to the femoral and genital rami, supplying sensation to the skin of the anteromedial thigh as well as the scrotum or mons pubis. Next is the lateral femoral cutaneous (L2–3) nerve, a purely sensory nerve that supplies the lateral thigh. The motor innervation of the next two subsequent divisions, the obturator (L2–4) and femoral (L2–4), has been described above. Both of these nerves have sensory terminations in the medial and anterior thigh, respectively. This portion of the femoral nerve is known as the anterior femoral cutaneous (L2–3) nerve. A separate, more inferior portion of the femoral nerve continues inferiorly as the saphenous (L3–4) nerve, which supplies sensation to the medial aspect of the leg.

The sacral plexus is formed from the spinal roots S1–S4. The anterior rami of these nerve roots combine with contributions from L4 and L5 to form the lumbosacral trunk. The first branch is the superior gluteal nerve (L4–S1), which innervates the gluteus minimus, gluteus medius, and tensor fascia latae. This exits the pelvis above the piriformis muscle, while the inferior gluteal nerve (L5–S2) exits below the piriformis and innervates the gluteus maximus alone.

The major offshoot of the lumbosacral trunk is the sciatic nerve, which spans contributions from

L4–S3. It is a major motor and sensory nerve. The tibial portion of the nerve innervates all the muscles of the posterior compartment of the thigh, the posterior compartment of the leg, and the sole of the foot (see above for specific muscles innervated). It terminates as a sensory nerve innervating primarily the sole of the foot, as well as the posterolateral and medial surfaces. The nerves innervating the sole of the foot are known as the medial and lateral plantar nerves.

The common fibular or peroneal portion innervates the short head of the biceps femoris, all muscles in the anterior and lateral compartments of the leg, and the extensor digitorum brevis. This branch also terminates as a sensory nerve innervating the anterolateral surface of the leg and dorsal aspect of the foot. Specifically, the nerve innervating the lateral aspect of the leg is known as the sural nerve. The first webspace is innervated by the deep peroneal nerve while the rest of the dorsal foot is innervated by the superficial peroneal nerve.

The posterior femoral cutaneous nerve (S1–3) is the next major branch of the lumbosacral trunk, also passing inferiorly to the piriformis muscle. This nerve, however, is exclusively sensory, innervating the posterior surface of the thigh and leg as well as the perineum. These sensory branches are called the perineal branches and inferior cluneal nerves. The last major branch is the pudendal nerve (S2–4), which has both motor and sensory functions. It innervates the muscles of the perineum, the external urethral and anal sphincters, as well as the levator ani muscle. It also provides sensation to the penis, clitoris, and most of the perineum. Additional direct branches from the plexus innervate the piriformis (S1–2), obturator internus (L5–S1), and quadratus femoris (L4–S1) muscles.

Compression Syndromes

Pudendal Neuralgia

For nearly every major nerve of the lower extremity, there is a corresponding compression syndrome. We will begin superiorly and continue our description inferiorly. The first compression syndrome we will discuss is pudendal nerve compression. Pelvic pain is an extremely complex and heterogenous group of diagnoses. These patients often present emotionally distraught, are ashamed of their problem, and are with little hope of improvement. However, in patients who fit specific criteria, nerve compression syndromes may be the cause of the pelvic pain. In these patients, intervention can provide some hope of relief for this extremely disabling and embarrassing problem.

The pudendal nerve is derived from sacral roots S2–4, though it is primarily derived from S3 in anatomical studies [1]. It is a mixed nerve, containing motor, sensory, and autonomic fibers [2]. After originating from these sacral roots, the pudendal nerve enters the gluteal region through the infra-piriform canal. At this level, it exits between the sacrospinal ligament ventrally and the sacrotuberous ligament dorsally [1]. The nerve then enters the perineal region through the lesser sciatic foramen and then continues into Alcock's canal [1]. The site of compression is often at the site where the nerve passes between the sarcospinal and sacrotuberous ligaments. Another possible location of entrapment is within the fascia of the obturator externus, through which the nerve passes to enter Alcock's canal [1].

During this terminal section, the pudendal nerve divides into three branches: the inferior anal nerve, the perineal nerve, and the dorsal nerve of the penis or clitoris [3]. In some patients, the inferior anal nerve may arise more proximally from the pudendal plexus itself [1]. The symptoms of pudendal neuralgia correspond directly to the function of these three branches. These symptoms may include unilateral or bilateral pain in the female vulva, vagina, or clitoris or, in the male, the scrotum, testes, or penis [3]. Patients may describe the pain as burning, torsion, or heaviness or the sensation of a foreign body in the rectum or vagina [1]. In severely affected patients, urgency or incontinence of urine or stool may also be part of the presentation [4].

Many cases are idiopathic. However, there are some known inciting factors. The compression from cycling, especially in competitive or long-range cyclist, has been shown to cause pudendal neuralgia in some patients [5]. Diabetes is also another known risk factor. Certainly, regional surgery – whether urologic, gynecologic, or anorectal – may also create or exacerbate an existing problem [1].

There is no absolute agreement about the exact diagnostic criteria for pudendal neuralgia. However, a group of urologic surgeons, neurologists, and pain specialists in Nantes, France, who have published extensively on this disorder have proposed a five-part set of diagnostic criteria, now known as the "Nantes Criteria." This includes the following: (1) there is pain in the anatomic territory of the pudendal nerve; (2) pain is worsened by sitting; (3) the patient is not woken at night by the pain; (4) there is no objective sensory loss on clinical examination; and (5) the patient has a positive response to an anesthetic pudendal nerve block [6]. Some of these criteria bear more discussion. Patient will not only complain of difficulty sitting, they can often be observed to be uncomfortable in a sitting position during the interview and clinical exam. Length of time sitting has been used as criteria in some studies to demonstrate postoperative improvement in nerve function. In some patients, sitting on a toilet relieves the discomfort due to a lack of compression on the nerve [6].

In patients who present with sensory loss in the distribution of the superficial perineal nerve, it is mandatory to rule out the presence of a sacral nerve root lesion, including the cauda equina nerve roots or a sacral plexus lesion [6]. In our protocol, patients undergo a CT-guided injection of a steroid-anesthetic combination. These injections are not only diagnostic but potentially therapeutic. The only patients considered for surgery are those who have a temporary but no sustained benefit from these injections. A small percentage of patients improve from this injection alone. In a study by Mamlouk et al., 2 of 31 patients improved with CT-guided injection alone. 14 patients had improvement in symptoms with nerve block, and all 14 patients had improvement postoperatively [7]. On rectal exam, the patients have exquisite tenderness at the region of the ischial spine [1].

There is both surgical and nonsurgical treatment for pudendal neuralgia. The nonsurgical treatment is generalized treatment for neuropathic pain. Therapies include topical lidocaine gel, amitriptyline, and tramadol [2]. However, all of these therapies are nonspecific and have side effects. In patients who meet the criteria described above, especially having temporary relief with the anesthetic block, we recommend surgical release of the nerve. This is performed with the patient in a prone position. We use a nerve stimulator as an adjunct to determine the identity of the nerve as well to verify its function at every point during the procedure. We also do not perform bilateral nerve releases simultaneously out of concern for possible temporary or in rare cases permanent nerve dysfunction after extensive release. The nerve is primarily trapped in two locations: in between the sacrospinous and sacrotuberous ligaments, in Alcock's canal, and/or the fascia of the obturator internus muscle [8].

We confirm the site of the patient's Tinel sign preoperatively. We then make a diagonal incision over the medial third of the buttock, extending from superior-lateral to inferior-medial. This is typically over the site of the Tinel. The dissection proceeds down through the soft tissue to reach the level of the nerve. The nerve is most easily identified directly lateral to the anus. We then perform an extensive release and neurolysis of the nerve, confirming its freedom from as far proximally and distally as can be observed through this posterior approach.

During release of this passage in symptomatic patients, we have directly observed the nerve to be often scarred and with abnormal clinical morphology. In some patients with venous stasis disease or dilation of the veins, this venous engorgement itself may be the cause of the compression syndrome. A randomized controlled trial by Robert et al. demonstrates the benefit of the release. 32 patients who had perineal pain and a positive response to a pudendal nerve block at the ischial spine and Alcock's canal were randomized to either surgery ($n = 16$) or control ($n = 16$) groups. At 12 months, 71.4% of the surgery group reported improvement in their pain vs. 13.3% of the control group ($p = 0.0025$) [8].

Piriformis Syndrome

Piriformis syndrome (PS) is defined by sciatica caused by the direct compression of the sciatic nerve by the piriformis muscle as it exits the pelvis. PS is often misdiagnosed as disc disease and therefore may be diagnosed late. PS is often idiopathic but may be associated with gluteal trauma and posttraumatic scarring [9]. It has been associated specifically with pregnancy, competitive cycling, and certain medications [10–12]. Anything that expands muscle or compresses the sciatic nerve at that level – including lipomas, hematomas, and inflammation of the muscle – can contribute to the development of PS [13–15].

The patient will present with complaints of pain running down the leg, particularly in the gluteal region and posterior leg, exacerbated with sitting or prolonged periods of standing [9, 16, 17]. This may be positional and may radiate to the groin. In patients with long-standing or severe disease, associated foot drop has been reported [18]. Unlike disc disease, there is no associated back pain [17]. On exam, the patient will have pain with leg flexion, adduction, and internal rotation. They will also have a tender sciatic notch and piriformis muscle [9]. The Freiberg sign is specifically associated with this diagnosis. The patient's hip is placed in extension and internal rotation, and the patient is asked to externally rotate the hip against resistance. Positive findings include pain at the piriformis and reproduction of sciatica symptoms. An additional clinical maneuver is the Pace sign in which the patient is asked to resist abduction and external rotation of the hip while in the seated position, increasing stress on the piriformis muscle [9]. PS is a diagnosis of exclusion, and patients must be ruled out for other causes of sciatica including lumbar radicular compression, inflammatory or mechanical sacroiliac problems, or inflammatory, infectious, or tumor-related pelvic disease [17]. Preoperative imaging includes radiographs of the hip and pel-

vis, EMG of the sciatic nerve, MRI of the lumbar spine and pelvis, and MR neurography.

Conservative therapy with medication, such as muscle relaxants and physiotherapy may aid a considerable number of patients [9, 17]. In a recent study, conservative therapy significantly ameliorated symptoms in 51.2% of 250 patients who presented with PS [17]. In patients who do not respond to conservative management after a period of 6–12 weeks, pain management specialists may also attempt therapy with either anesthetic or a combination of anesthetic and corticosteroid. In a prospective, randomized controlled trial comparing these two therapies, there was no significant difference in outcome, indicating that the syndrome is mostly muscular in origin [16]. Ultrasound-guided injection improves accuracy of locating the piriformis muscle [19]. Nonsurgical therapy with botulinum toxin can also be attempted in order to decrease the size and thickness of the muscle and then its compression of the nerve. In a case control study, MRI was used to evaluate 12 patients with PS after botox injection vs. eight controls with PS who were not injected. The patients who had been injected demonstrated a significant decrease in the thickness and volume of the muscle as well as an increase in fatty infiltration [20].

In patients with recalcitrant disease, we recommend surgical release. We typically perform this release through a short incision with partial resection (tenotomy) of the piriformis and superior gemellus muscles. The nerve is freed from the scar tissue surrounding it and an extensive neurolysis is performed. Many patients present with both piriformis syndrome and pudendal neuralgia concurrently. Simultaneous releases can easily be performed.

Femoral and Obturator Nerve Compression

As with other compression neuropathies, femoral and obturator neuralgia can present with vague symptoms of pain, weakness, and numbness. However, specific diagnostic considerations can allow for appropriate differentiation. Femoral neuralgia presents with numbness of the anterior thigh and weakness of knee extension. Patients may complain of a subjective feeling of knee instability [21]. The two most common sites of femoral nerve injury are in the retroperitoneal space or under the inguinal ligament [21]. This may occur during urologic or gynecologic surgery, especially when using a large retractor called a Bookwalter [22]. The nerve can also be injured during anterior approaches to hip surgery and even from prolonged lithotomy positioning [21].

In obturator neuralgia, numbness extends down the medial thigh. On exam, the patient will have weakness of hip adduction. Obturator pathology may be associated with an obturator hernia. This can be identified by pain of the medial thigh on internal rotation of the hip, known as a Howship-Romberg sign. Obturator compression may be caused by pelvic fractures, especially those involving the sacroiliac joint, and prolonged labor as well as many of the same causes of femoral compression [21]. It may be related to inferior pubalgia or entrapment within the adductor canal of the medial thigh.

Electrodiagnostic and nerve conduction studies of the involved nerve, as well as the contralateral normal side, are recommended [21]. For example, if the femoral nerve has axonal loss less than 50% of the normal, contralateral nerve, these patients would be expected to have return of functioning within 1 year. However, if axonal loss is greater than 50%, half of these patients showed no improvement [23]. No nerve conduction studies can be performed of the obturator nerve, though EMG studies may have some utility if the diagnosis is uncertain [21].

The treatment for either obturator or femoral nerve compression is initially conservative, using methods such as physical therapy and steroid injections. In select patients who do not improve with conservative management, surgical treatment may be indicated. A neurolysis or nerve release may be combined with a local nerve transfer. For example, if the femoral nerve is not functioning normally, we perform a transfer from one of the branches of the obturator nerve to the quadriceps to the femoral nerve in addition to a neurolysis.

Peroneal Nerve Compression

The peroneal nerve can be compressed at the fibular head, clinically presenting as foot drop. Idiopathic cases are common, but typically there is a recent or remote history of surgery or trauma. Foot drop may also be the first presenting symptom of central nerve disorders, including L4/L5 spinal disc disease and neurologic syndromes such as Charcot-Marie-Tooth disease, which should be ruled out before embarking on surgical treatment. Potential donor muscles, e.g., tibialis posterior and peroneus longus, should be examined for strength during initial evaluation. If the donor muscles are weak, then a central lesion should be considered. Electromyography (EMG) and nerve conduction studies (NCS) can also be helpful in localizing the lesion. Long-standing compression may result in an irreversible denervation of the tibialis anterior muscle. This must be taken into account when planning a treatment strategy [24].

Ideally, surgical nerve decompression should result in spontaneous functional recovery [25]. However, long-standing compression may not recover after simple decompression. In these cases, tendon transfer should be considered. The most common transfer is tibialis posterior to tibialis anterior. The tendon is passed through the interosseous membrane and then either woven into the tibialis anterior tendon or anchored to the midfoot, just lateral to the tibialis anterior [26].

If a central lesion is identified, nerve transfers can be used to reinnervate the tibialis anterior distal to the central lesion. Typical transfer donors are branches of the tibial nerve.

The functional deficits resulting form treatment failures and untreatable etiologies may be mitigated with an AFO splint or ankle fusion.

Tarsal Tunnel Syndrome

Tarsal tunnel syndrome occurs when the tibial nerve and its branches are compressed within the tarsal tunnel of the medial ankle. Symptoms include numbness, burning, pain, and tingling of the foot and heel and ankle. In addition to idiopathic cases, known causes include direct compression from tumors or cysts, swelling from trauma, and varicose veins in the tarsal tunnel. Most commonly, the syndrome occurs in patients who suffer from diabetes or spinal disc disease, rendering the nerve far more susceptible to compression symptoms. The diagnosis is primarily clinical, but imaging studies can rule out a space-occupying lesion. Nerve conduction studies, while not diagnostic, may confirm the clinical suspicions [27].

Nonsurgical treatments include stretching, physical therapy, steroid injections, weight loss, and changes to lifestyle, such as eliminating high-velocity loading such as with basketball or volleyball. Surgical treatment is recommended when nonsurgical strategies fail. In a classical tarsal tunnel release, the flexor retinaculum is simply divided. Success rates can be dramatically improved from 50% to nearly 80% success rates if the tibial nerve branches are followed into their individual tunnels in the porta-pedis of the foot and decompressed individually [28]. Any space-occupying lesions can be removed at surgery as well (Fig. 19.4).

Lower Extremity Neuropathy

Neuropathy of the lower extremities has myriad causes, including diabetes, chemotherapy, alcoholism, and trauma. There is no universal definition of "neuropathy" nor is there a diagnostic test for it. It is thus a diagnosis of exclusion and a clinical diagnosis. The clinical diagnosis can be difficult because symptoms vary from patient to patient and may change over time in the same patient. Typically, the symptoms consist of varying degrees and combinations of numbness, tingling, burning, and pain of the lower extremity. It is often symmetrical, but one side may be "worse" than the other. Not all patients report pain, and every patient with pain reports it to varying degrees. Some complain of numbness and tingling, while others have crampy pain or shooting pains. Some are affected at night, others during the day. Some feel better lying down, some standing up and walking. Some feel like there is some-

thing stuck in their shoe (like walking on sand, or that their sock is bunched up) while others notice that they can't feel all or part of their foot at all, despite the pain they feel. Similar presentations may occur in other, unrelated conditions such as Charcot-Marie-Tooth disease, lumbar disc disease, and spinal stenosis [29].

Diagnosis

Often, the patient will be sent for an expensive and painful EMG and NCS. Unfortunately, electrodiagnostic studies are notoriously unreliable in distal extremity neuropathy diagnosis. Furthermore, expense and patient discomfort precludes these modalities as a screening test or one that can be used to follow the course of disease over time. Once a patient is clinically diagnosed with neuropathy, they may be sent for electrodiagnostic tests to rule out another cause and possibly illuminate the current disease process. However, Dellon and others advocate noninvasive neurosensory testing as a modality to quantify and follow the progression of disease of time as well as after surgical therapy [30, 31]. In most cases, clinical examination coupled possibly with noninvasive sensory threshold testing is adequate to make a decision to move forward with treatment, including surgery.

Medical Therapy

Like most systemic problems, initial treatments for neuropathy are aimed at systemic amelioration of symptoms. Medical treatments such as Gabapentin and Pregabalin are commonly prescribed along with SSRIs such as Duloxetine. Narcotics are frequently needed to control the pain, resulting in escalating doses to maintain efficacy. This often leads to chronic dependence on narcotics. While many of these treatments offer some degree of symptomatic efficacy, what they all have in common is that they simply cover up the pain or make it more tolerable. Unfortunately, these treatments do little or nothing to reverse or treat the underlying cause.

Furthermore, while pain is the main symptom that drives the patient to seek help, it is not the symptom that is most dangerous to the patient. The resulting lack of protective sensation in the neuropathic extremity is a major cause of ulcers, infections, and subsequent amputations.

Surgical Therapy

Despite the limited efficacy of current medical treatments, and the fact that they only treat the most "obvious" aspects, until recently there has been little interest in exploring surgical therapies for this condition. This is not at all surprising, because at first blush, it would seem that there is no rationale for a surgical approach to a symptom of a systemic issue, e.g., diabetes or chemotherapy. This resulted in a long lag between the recognition of the cause of diabetic neuropathy, which was the first and most extensively studied type of neuropathy, and the application of a successful surgical treatment to alleviate its effects on the extremities. The lessons learned from the success in the treatment of diabetic neuropathy allowed for investigations into the feasibility of transferring similar techniques into the realm of other forms of neuropathy. These surgical techniques have proven to be valuable adjuncts to available medical therapies for this disabling and painful condition [29].

In 1991, Dellon published the seminal paper demonstrating the efficacy of nerve decompression on both the symptoms and natural course of diabetic neuropathy. Not only were the symptoms improved in 85% of treated patients, but treated extremities no longer had the ulcers, infections, and subsequent amputations characteristic of neuropathy, unlike the remaining untreated extremities which still suffered from the classic associated problems. This indicated that the decompression was protective against future neuropathy-derived morbidity. This phenomenon was further discussed in a paper in 2004 [32]. To date, there are 13 clinical studies demonstrating the efficacy of the nerve decompression approach to the treatment of diabetic neuropathy. Nevertheless, the surgical approach

to the treatment of diabetic peripheral neuropathy has its critics.

Over time, clinicians with experience in surgical approaches to diabetic neuropathy began to expand their indications for this treatment. First, it was diabetic neuropathy, then it was "idiopathic" neuropathy, and eventually chemotherapy-induced neuropathy became a valid target for this treatment [33]. In fact, this approach has been successfully applied to neuropathies associated with alcoholism, lead, and even Hanson's disease (A.L. Dellon, personal communication). The cause of the neuropathy becomes less relevant because of a common pathologic pathway that renders the nerves susceptible to compression at known sites of anatomic narrowing. This allows for nerve decompressions to treat the effects of many variations of neuropathy.

The crux of the problem, and the reason that surgery can be effective, relates to the double-crush phenomenon. While the exact mechanism for the development of neuropathy after chemotherapy is not known, there is evidence for direct neuronal toxicity as well as a component of intracellular and extracellular edema as a response to that neurotoxicity. The slow component of axoplasmal transport appears diminished in most forms of chemotherapy-induced neuropathy, a pathophysiologic mechanism also found in diabetes-induced peripheral neuropathy. The resulting stiffening of tissues and swelling of nerves may result in neurocompressive symptoms caused at the known sites of anatomic narrowing (carpal tunnel, tarsal tunnel, etc.). The direct effect of the toxic agent causes decreased function of the nerve, but more importantly, that decreased function leads to swelling, and in predisposed individuals that results in nerve compression at the anatomic tunnels.

A loose analogy would be if a man who wore the same suit and tie every day gained 30 lb. He would certainly be less healthy for the weight gain, but it would be his belt and his collar, i.e., sites of fixed anatomic narrowing, that would be most likely to cause him pain and distress. After loosening his belt and unbuttoning his collar, he will feel considerably better, even though the underlying problem is still there. So the weight gain is one "crush" but the presence of fixed-diameter tunnels provides the second "crush" that ultimately leads to the distress.

Basic Science

Most of the work in the surgical treatment of or neuropathy has been done in the diabetes model, with some additional study in a chemotherapy-induced model. In 1994, Dellon et al. found that rats made diabetic with Streptozotocin developed a neuropathic walking-tract pattern. This pattern could be prevented by pretreating the rats with decompression of their tarsal tunnels [34]. This study was duplicated by Kale et al. in 2003 [35]. Similar rat studies were performed in a model of cisplatin neuropathy in adult rats. In that study, rats administered cisplatin developed neuropathic walking patterns, yet rats that had tibial nerve decompressions concurrent with the commencement of cisplatin therapy did not develop these abnormal walking patterns. This indicated that similar to the diabetic model, tibial nerve decompression was protective against the development of neuropathic walking patterns in the adult rat [36].

One issue that remains is the ability to reliably predict outcomes from surgery preoperatively. Multiple factors determine who will or will not be helped by the surgical decompressions, but no reliable test exists to select the best candidates for the procedure. Interestingly, the diabetic neuropathy literature presents evidence that the presence of a positive Tinel-Hoffman (often simply called a Tinel sign) sign is a strongly positive predictor of a good outcome [37]. Simply put, if you tap in the known areas of anatomic narrowing and the patient reports electric sensations (tingling, vibrations, etc.) along the expected sensory distribution of the nerve being tapped, then you have a positive Tinel sign (similar to hitting your "funny bone" (ulnar nerve) at the elbow and feeling the electrical sensation down at your fifth finger. Anecdotal evidence in the two published human papers regarding the surgical treatment of chemotherapy-induced neuropathy also find a positive Tinel-Hoffman sign a good predictor of outcomes in this population, but larger and higher level of evidence studies are needed to confirm this.

Typically, a patient will have a stocking or glove distribution of their symptoms, though isolated mono-neuropathies have been reported. A Tinel sign should be present at the site of anatomic narrowing to establish a high chance of clinical success after surgery. The typical sites on the upper extremity to be examined are (1) the cubital tunnel, (2) the carpal tunnel, (3) Guyon's canal at the wrist, and (4) the radial nerve in the dorsal forearm. On the lower extremity, it is typical to examine (1) the tarsal tunnel, (2) the common peroneal nerve's tunnel just below the lateral condyle of the fibular neck, and (3) the deep peroneal nerve as it passes underneath the extensor hallucis brevis tendon in the mid-dorsum of the foot. If Tinel signs are positive at these sites with positive symptoms in the distribution covered by that nerve, then surgical decompression has a high likelihood of success.

Both peripheral sensory and motor nerves can regenerate at any time after injury. However, the motor nerves terminate at motor endplates on the muscles that irreversibly atrophy sometime between 6 and 12 months after impulses stop being received at the motor endplate. This physiologic fact makes the timing of intervention with motor neuropathy more critical. Since there is a lag between the time of nerve decompression and the resumption of motor impulses on the order of several months, it behooves the surgeon to consider surgery for motor symptoms well prior to the 6–12 month window where the endplates begin to stop functioning forever.

Prior to surgery, the patient should be examined and worked up to eliminate more central causes for the neuropathic symptoms, including disc compressions and spinal stenosis. Furthermore, vascular compromise of the lower extremity can alter healing capacity and mimic neuropathy symptoms. Any vascular deficit should be ruled out and corrected prior to surgical intervention for neuropathy. The patient's general health should be evaluated prior to surgery as well.

There are a number of specific surgical interventions that are performed in order to release lower extremity nerves at classic points of entrapment. Common peroneal nerve compression is treated by release of the nerve as it passes through the peroneus longus fascia. Deep peroneal nerve decompression involves resecting a segment of the extensor hallucis brevis tendon as it passes over the deep peroneal nerve in the dorsum of the foot. Finally, the tarsal tunnel as well as the four medial ankle tunnels should be decompressed to improve symptoms attributable to the tibial nerve. Surgery is generally performed as an outpatient procedure, with follow-up typically 1 week after the surgery.

Coverage of the Diabetic Foot Wound

This is a difficult reconstructive problem as there are alterations in the sensibility of the foot and alteration of foot mechanics coupled with a susceptibility to infection. These issues are often seen in patients with poor circulation, further compounding the problem and increasing the complexity. Standard wound care is implemented with debridement, serial assessment, and analysis of the wound. Inflow should be assessed and corrected if deficient. Infection should be treated and consideration for amputation should be made when appropriate. A team approach is preferred as vascular, neurologic orthopedic, podiatric, plastic surgical, and rehabilitation considerations are all part of the salvage of the extremity.

Clinical Evaluation and Surgical Planning

The location of the wound on the foot is noted, along with the size and depth. Etiology is important as things such as pressure can be corrected. Generally the simplest reconstructive method,

such as a skin graft, should be initially considered. However, a complex reconstructive methodology, such as a local rotational flap or free tissue transfer, is the best option even as a first choice, depending on the characteristics of the wound and patient. Some wounds that might traditionally only be a candidate for local or free tissue transfer because of exposed tendon or bone can be converted to a wound treatable with a skin graft after judicious use of advanced wound care methods such as negative pressure dressings and biologic dressings such as Epicel, Integra, and Apligraf, among others. Considerations include the location on the foot and what the weight-bearing status of that portion of the foot as well as bulk of the proposed reconstructive technique. The technique must provide a surface that is durable enough for the zone of the foot and the pressure and shearing loads it will encounter.

Reconstructive Options

Hindfoot and mid-plantar defects can be reconstructed with skin grafts and sural flaps. The sural flap is interesting as it utilizes retrograde arterial flow up the leg along the fascia overlying the sural nerve. The flap is thus based distally and can be utilized to cover defects of the ankle and foot as far as the middle of the foot in many cases. Flexor digitorum brevis muscle flaps can be used along with instep fasciocutaneous flaps (Fig.19.5). Larger defects require free tissue transfer. Non-weight-bearing portions of the foot can be reconstructed with grafts, rotation flaps, and intrinsic foot muscle flaps. More recently perforator "propeller" flaps have been popularized to cover distal leg/foot defects.

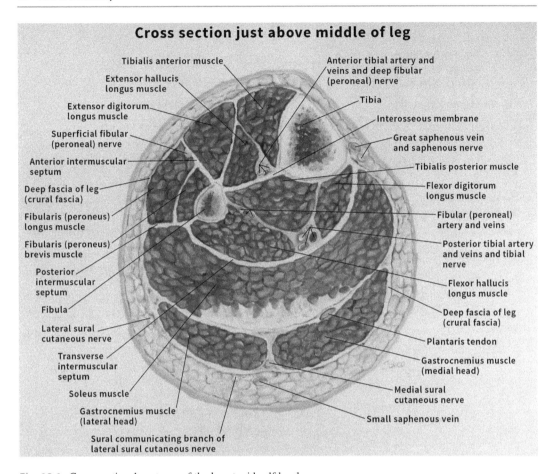

Cross section just above middle of leg

Tibialis anterior muscle

Extensor hallucis
longus muscle

Extensor digitorum
longus muscle

Superficial fibular
(peroneal) nerve

Anterior intermuscular
septum

Deep fascia of leg
(crural fascia)

Fibularis (peroneus)
longus muscle

Fibularis (peroneus)
brevis muscle

Posterior
intermuscular
septum

Fibula

Lateral sural
cutaneous nerve

Transverse
intermuscular
septum

Soleus muscle

Gastrocnemius muscle
(lateral head)

Sural communicating branch of
lateral sural cutaneous nerve

Anterior tibial artery and
veins and deep fibular
(peroneal) nerve

Tibia

Interosseous membrane

Great saphenous vein
and saphenous nerve

Tibialis posterior muscle

Flexor digitorum
longus muscle

Fibular (peroneal)
artery and veins

Posterior tibial artery
and veins and tibial
nerve

Flexor hallucis
longus muscle

Deep fascia of leg
(crural fascia)

Plantaris tendon

Gastrocnemius muscle
(medial head)

Medial sural
cutaneous nerve

Small saphenous vein

Fig. 19.1 Cross sectional anatomy of the leg at mid calf level

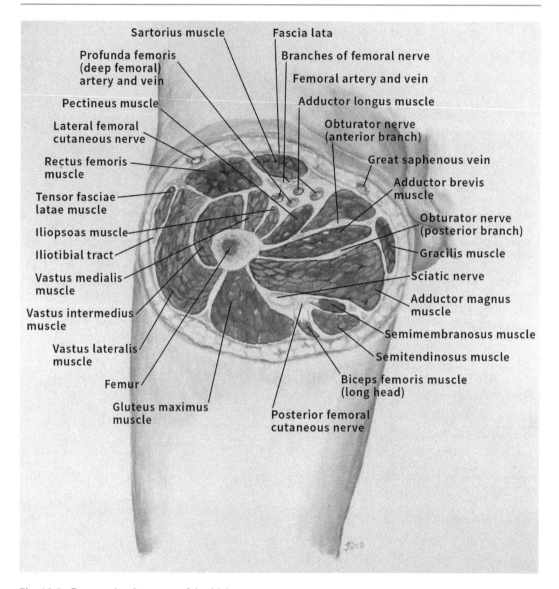

Sartorius muscle

Profunda femoris
(deep femoral)
artery and vein

Pectineus muscle

Lateral femoral
cutaneous nerve

Rectus femoris
muscle

Tensor fasciae
latae muscle

Iliopsoas muscle

Iliotibial tract

Vastus medialis
muscle

Vastus intermedius
muscle

Vastus lateralis
muscle

Femur

Gluteus maximus
muscle

Fascia lata

Branches of femoral nerve

Femoral artery and vein

Adductor longus muscle

Obturator nerve
(anterior branch)

Great saphenous vein

Adductor brevis
muscle

Obturator nerve
(posterior branch)

Gracilis muscle

Sciatic nerve

Adductor magnus
muscle

Semimembranosus muscle

Semitendinosus muscle

Biceps femoris muscle
(long head)

Posterior femoral
cutaneous nerve

Fig. 19.2 Cross sectional anatomy of the thigh

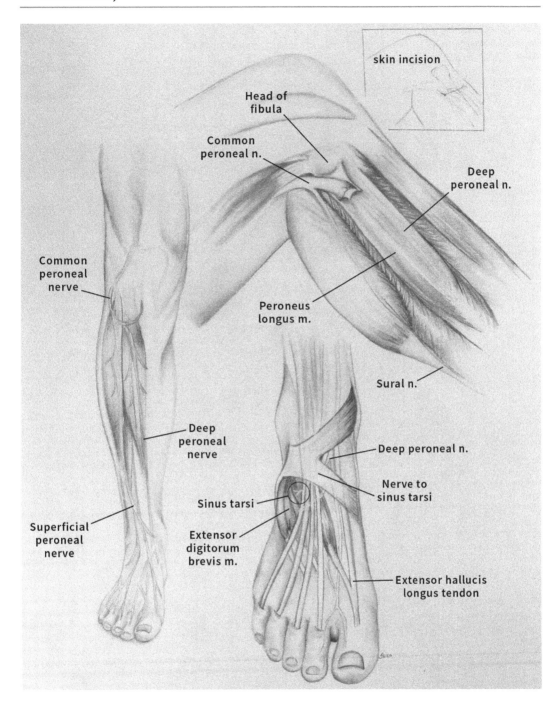

Fig. 19.3 Anatomy of the peroneal nerve

Fig. 19.4 Tarsal
Tunnel Release

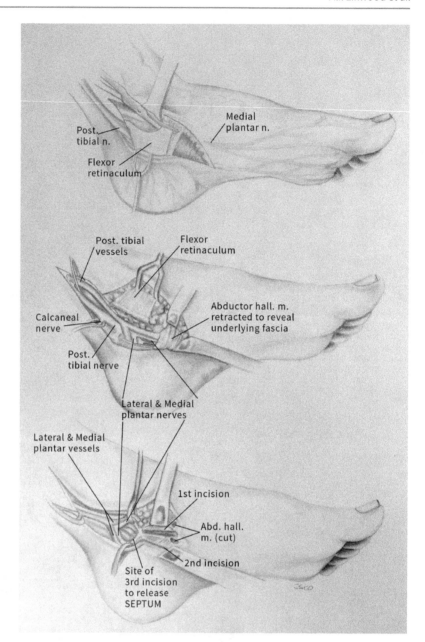

Fig. 19.4 Tarsal Tunnel Release

Flexor digitorum brevis muscle flap

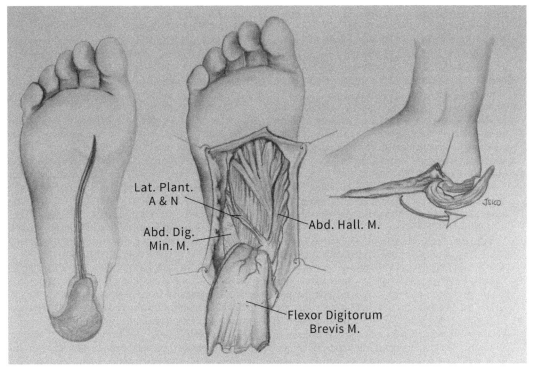

Lat. Plant.
A & N

Abd. Dig.
Min. M.

Abd. Hall. M.

Flexor Digitorum
Brevis M.

Fig. 19.5 Flexor digitorum brevis muscle flap for heel coverage

References

1. Robert R, Raoul S, Leborgne J, Prat-Pradal D, Labat J, Bensignor M, Thiodet J. Anatomic basis of chronic perineal pain: role of the pudendal nerve. Surg Radiol Anat. 1998;20:93–8.
2. Pereira A, Pérez-Medina T, Rodríguez-Tapia A, Rutherford S, Millan I, Iglesias E, Ortiz-Quintana L. Chronic perineal pain: analyses of prognostic factors in pudendal neuralgia. Clin J Pain. 2014;30:577–5.
3. Hibner M, Desai N, Robertson LJ, Nour M. Review Article: pudendal neuralgia. J Minimally Invasive Gynecology. 2010;17:148–53.
4. Possover M, Forman A. Voiding Dysfunction Associated with Pudendal Nerve Entrapment. Curr Bladder Dysfunct Rep. 2012;7:281–5.
5. Leibovitch I, Mor Y. Review: the vicious cycling: bicycling related urogenital disorders. Eur Urol. 2005;47:277–87.
6. Labat J, Rigaud J, Riant T, Robert R, Amarenco G, Lefaucheur J. Diagnostic criteria for pudendal neuralgia by pudendal nerve entrapment (Nantes Criteria). Neurourol Urodyn. 2008;27:306–10.
7. Mamlouk MD, VanSonnenberg E, Dehkharghani S. CT-guided nerve block for pudendal neuralgia: diagnostic and therapeutic implications. AJR Am J Roentgenol. 2014;203:196–200.
8. Robert R, Labat J, Bensignor M, Glemain P, Deschamps C, Raoul S, Hamel O. Decompression and transposition of the pudendal nerve in pudendal neuralgia: a randomized controlled trial and long-term evaluation. Eur Urol. 2005;47:403–8.
9. Cass SP. Piriformis syndrome: a cause of nondiscogenic sciatica. Curr Sports Med Rep. 2015;14:41–4.
10. Sivrioglu AK, Ozyurek S, Mutlu H, Sonmez G. Piriformis syndrome occurring after pregnancy. BMJ Case Rep. 2013;26:2013.
11. Hamdi W, Ghannouchi MM, Kaffel D, Kchir MM. Piriformis muscle syndrome: an unusual adverse effect of atorvastatin. J Clin Rheumatol. 2013;19:156–7.
12. Menu P, Fouasson-Chaillou A, Dubois C, Dauty M. Piriformis syndrome diagnosis: on two professional cyclists. Ann Phys Rehabil Med. 2014;57:268–74.
13. Drampalos E, Sadiq M, Thompson T, Lomax A, Paul A. Intrapiriformis lipoma: an unusual cause of piriformis syndrome. Eur Spine J. 2014;24:551–4.

14. Kitagawa Y, Yokoyama M, Tamai K, Takai S. Chronic expanding hematoma extending over multiple gluteal muscles associated with piriformis syndrome. J Nippon Med Sch. 2012;79:478–83.

15. Toda T, Koda M, Rokkaku T, Watanabe H, Nakajima A, Yamada T, Murakami K, Nakajima H, Murakami M. Sciatica caused by pyomyositis of the piriformis muscle in a pediatric patient. Orthopedics. 2013;36:e257–9.

16. Misirlioglu TO, Akgun K, Palamar D, Erden MG, Erbilir T. Piriformis syndrome: comparison of the effectiveness of local anesthetic and corticosteroid injections: a double-blinded, randomized controlled study. Pain Physician. 2015;18:163–71.

17. Michel F, Decavel P, Toussirot E, Tatu L, Aleton E, Monnier G, Garbuio P, Parratte B. Piriformis muscle syndrome: diagnostic criteria and treatment of a monocentric series of 250 patients. Ann Phys Rehabil Med. 2013;56:371–83.

18. Yildirim P, Guler T, Misirlioglu TO, Ozer T, Gunduz OH. A case of drop foot due to piriformis syndrome. Acta Neurol Belg. 2015;115(4):847–9.

19. Jankovic D, Peng P, van Zundert A. Brief review: piriformis syndrome: etiology, diagnosis, and management. Can J Anaesth. 2013;60:1003–12.

20. Al-Al-Shaikh M, Michel F, Parratte B, Kastler B, Vidal C, Aubry S. An MRI evaluation of changes in piriformis muscle morphology induced by botulinum toxin injections in the treatment of piriformis syndrome. Diagn Interv Imaging. 2015;96:37–43.

21. Craig A. Entrapment neuropathies of the lower extremity. PMR. 2013;5(5 Suppl):S31–40.

22. Maneschi F, Nale R, Tozzi R, Biccirè D, Perrone S, Sarno M. Femoral nerve injury complicating surgery for gynecologic cancer. Int J Gynecol Cancer. 2014;24:1112–7.

23. Kuntzer T, van Melle G, Regli F. Clinical and prognostic features in unilateral femoral neuropathies. Muscle Nerve. 1997;20:205–11.

24. Mackinnon SE, Dellon AL. Surgery of the peripheral nerve, Chapter 13. New York: Thieme Pub; 1988. p. 320–36.

25. Mont MA, Dellon AL, Chen F, Hungerford MW, Krackow KA, Hungerford DH. Operative treatment of peroneal nerve palsy. J Bone Joint Surg. 1996;78A:863–9.

26. Steinau HU, Tofaute A, Huellmann K, Goertz O, Lehnhardt M, Kammler J, Steinstraesser L, Daigeler A. Tendon transfers for drop foot correction: long-term results including quality of life assessment, and dynamometric and pedobarographic measurements. Arch Orthop Trauma Surg. 2011;131:903–10.

27. Mackinnon SE, Dellon AL, Tarsal tunnel syndrome, surgery of the peripheral nerve, Chapter 12. New York: Thieme Pub; 1988.

28. Mullick T, Dellon AL. Results of treatment of four medial ankle tunnels in tarsal tunnels syndrome. J Reconstr Microsurg. 2008;24:119–26.

29. Dellon AL. Treatment of symptoms of diabetic neuropathy by peripheral nerve decompression. Plast Reconstr Surg. 1992;89:689–97.

30. Valdivia JMV, Dellon AL, Weinand MD, Maloney Jr CT. Surgical treatment of peripheral neuropathy: outcomes from 100 consecutive decompressions. J Am Podiatr Med Assoc. 2005;95:451–4.

31. Aszmann OC, Kress K, Dellon AL. Results of decompression of peripheral nerves in diabetics: a prospective, blinded study utilizing computer-assisted sensorimotor testing. Plast Reconstr Surg. 2000;106:816–22.

32. Aszmann OC, Tassler PL, Dellon AL. Changing the natural history of diabetic neuropathy: incidence of ulcer/amputation in the contralateral limb of patients with a unilateral nerve decompression procedure, accepted. Ann Plast Surg. 2004;53(517):22.

33. Dellon AL, Swier P, Levingood M, Maloney CT. Cisplatin/Taxol neuropathy: treatment by decompression of peripheral nerve. Plast Reconstr Surg. 2004;114:478–83.

34. Dellon AL, Dellon ES, Seiler IV WA. Effect of tarsal tunnel decompression in the streptozotocin-induced diabetic rat. Microsurgery. 1994;15:265.

35. Kale B, Yuksel F, Celikoz B, et al. Effect of various nerve decompression procedures on the functions of distal limbs in streptozotocin-induced diabetic rats: further optimism in diabetic neuropathy. Plast Reconstr Surg. 2003;111:2265.

36. Tassler P, Dellon AL, Lesser GJ, Grossman S. Utility of decompressive surgery in the prophylaxis and treatment of cisplatin neuropathy in adult rats. J Reconstr Microsurg. 2000;16:457.

37. Lee CH, Dellon AL. Prognostic ability of Tinel sign in determining outcome for decompression surgery in diabetic and nondiabetic neuropathy. Ann Plast Surg. 2004;53:523.

Adam Saad, Matthew Pontell

Introduction

The aims of the following chapter are to discuss the pathophysiology and management of *athletic pubalgia* (AP) and inguinal neuralgia. Both clinical entities encompass a variety of syndromes involving a multitude of structures located in and around the groin area. Both share a common presentation of refractory groin pain, and surgical repair results in excellent outcomes.

Athletic Pubalgia

Among other names, this condition is also commonly referred to as the "sports hernia." This is an unfortunate misnomer as AP is not associated with the development of a hernia. This name was likely acquired secondary to the fact that AP and inguinal hernias commonly present with groin pain. By definition, a hernia is a protrusion of tissue through a wall which it is normally enclosed by. AP is neither

---

The original version of this book was revised. An erratum to this chapter can be found at DOI 10.1007/978-3-319-41406-5_28

A. Saad, MD (✉)
The Plastic Surgery Center, Institute for Advanced Reconstruction, 535 Sycamore Ave, Shrewsbury, NJ 07702, USA
e-mail: asaadmd@theplasticsurgerycenternj.com

M. Pontell, MD
Department of Surgery, Drexel University College of Medicine, Philadelphia, PA, USA

a hernia, nor is it a single clinical entity. On the contrary, AP is a collection of injuries to the abdominopelvic musculature that presents with pelvic and/or groin pain. These injuries may be isolated to a single muscle or may involve multiple, and they may be either unilateral or bilateral. It is critical to understand that AP is not related to hernia formation, nor is it related to pathology of the femoroacetabular joint or its supporting structures [1].

Pathophysiology

In order to properly discuss the pathophysiology of AP, it is imperative to understand the complex musculoskeletal anatomy of the pelvis, as well as the concept of the "pubic joint" [1]. The "pubic joint" is distinct from the femoroacetabular and pubic symphyseal joints. It refers to the entire right and left pubic rami and the pubic symphysis serving as a point of attachment of many soft tissue structures, as well as a convergence point for several, multidirectional forces. In a non-pathologic setting, the forces exerted by the soft tissue attachments are symmetrically distributed around the pelvic brim and exert both oppositional and supportive forces. When one of these soft tissue structures is injured or weakened, a disruption in these forces transmitted across the pubic joint results. The resultant pubic joint instability manifests in the lower abdominal and/or groin pain known as *athletic pubalgia*. Thus, these injuries are conceptualized by defining which of these tissues are injured and which are overcompensating [1].

© Springer International Publishing Switzerland 2017
A.I. Elkwood et al. (eds.), *Rehabilitative Surgery*, DOI 10.1007/978-3-319-41406-5_20

All of these muscular and ligamentous tissues of the pubic joint are subject to injury, especially when they are subjected to the tremendous amount of torque that is commonplace in professional athletics. The "torque" that is responsible for many cases of AP results from a combined hyperextension of the abdominal wall and hyperabduction of the thighs. This pattern of force commonly results in a tear or a series of micro-tears of the pubic soft tissue attachments as they insert onto the cartilaginous plate of the pubis. The tissues frequently subjected to this injury pattern are the soft tissue components of the anterior abdominopelvic region, specifically the rectus abdominis (RA), adductor longus, pectineus, and iliopsoas. The most common constellation of injuries is an RA with concomitant adductor muscle injury [1].

Clinical Presentation and Physical Examination

The diagnosis of AP relies primarily on a high clinical suspicion and a thorough history and physical examination. As the name suggests, athletic pubalgia frequently presents with pain in the groin, lower abdomen, or proximal adductor region [2] (Fig. 20.1). The pain may also be associated with coughing and may radiate to the groin, thigh, or testicle [3]. Historically, AP has been more prevalent in the male population; however, an increasing number of females are being diagnosed [1]. More often than not, the pain is chronic in nature, and by the time of diagnosis, patients may have already sought out treatment and been subsequently misdiagnosed. Occasionally, AP patients present with persistent pain after a surgically repaired "hernia" [3]. AP is found more frequently in athletes engaging in sports that require "cutting" and/or pivoting, as well as rapid acceleration and deceleration [4–6]. Less commonly, AP can present acutely and, as such, is usually the result of extreme trunk hyperextension and lower extremity hyperabduction [1, 2, 7]. These maneuvers can lead to partial or complete ruptures of the distal RA and/or adductor aponeuroses [1, 2, 7]. In the acute setting, the pain is reproducible with activity and will resolve with time off from stren-

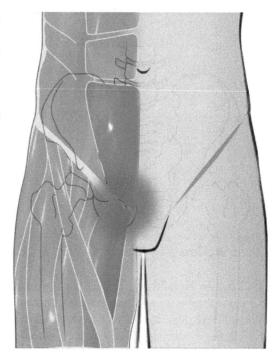

Fig. 20.1 Athletic pubalgia: a representation of the important pain generators in *AP* and the direction of forces they apply to the pubic joint

uous activity; however, it frequently recurs [3]. The pain of AP may also vary in location and laterality depending on patterns of muscular compensation and the number of soft tissues involved [8]. It is important to differentiate hip-related pain, which may present with anterolateral groin pain associated with minimal activity, prolonged sitting and/or flexion, lower extremity abduction, or torsional activities [9, 10]. Formal hip joint pathology is often more sporadic and less predictable, yet it is crucial to remember that it may also coexist with AP [9, 10].

Physical exam in these patients will elicit tenderness to palpation in the areas of injury, but correlation to the area of reported pain is important as athletes frequently have concomitant soft tissue and/or hip injuries that fall outside the realm of AP [3]. Muscular palpation can also be combined with a series of resistance tests targeted at the muscles that cross the pubic joint [2, 11, 12]. A positive test results in pain in the area of the muscle at which activity is restricted. At this time, it is imperative to also conduct a formal hernia evaluation, as well as an evaluation of the femoroacetabular joint to rule out coexisting pathologies [9, 10, 13]. Diagnostic injections can be a useful adjunct to physical exam with respect to identifying the primary pain-generating muscles as well as defining associated pathology of the hip joint [3]. Fluoroscopic and/or ultrasound-guided anesthetic injections are used in the diagnosis of femoroacetabular disease [3]. Persistent pain despite injection is suggestive of AP, and the origins/insertions of commonly implicated muscles can also be anesthetized for confirmation [3].

Diagnostic Imaging

Over the past 10 years, significant advancements in medical technology have made diagnostic imaging an invaluable complement to physical examination in the evaluation of AP [8]. Magnetic resonance imaging (MRI) has been reported to be 98 % sensitive and 89–100 % specific in diagnosing AP syndromes involving the RA and adductor tendon origins [7]. MRI has become a critical adjunct, and current studies are examining the use of specific MRI-based protocols in conjunction with clinical injury grading scales [8, 14] (Table 20.1). MRI is also useful in ruling out and/or identifying coexisting pathology involving the femoroacetabular joint [1]. Incidental intra-articular hip pathology is common in athletes, which underscores the importance of correlating clinical and radiographic findings [15]. Conventional X-rays are of limited use in the diagnosis of AP; however, they do assist in ruling out other pathologies that may present similarly, including osteitis pubis, pelvic avulsion fractures, apophyseal injury/inflammation, and/or degenerative hip disease [3].

Table 20.1 AP MRI grading

Grade	MRI Findings
I	Single or multiple small identifiable soft tissue tears
II	Partial soft tissue avulsion or detachment
III	Complete soft tissue avulsion or detachment

From Meyers et al. [8]

Surgical and Postoperative Management

The initial treatment of AP includes a trial of nonoperative management. Such interventions are targeted toward restoring core stability and posture while normalizing the forces transmitted across the pubic joint by the musculature of the hip and pelvis [3]. At this time, patients are advised to refrain from activity resulting in deep hip flexion, lower extremity hyperabduction, and any heavy strength training [3]. Nevertheless, studies on nonoperative management are not promising, and surgical intervention is usually required to obtain acceptable outcomes [3].

Surgical management of AP is centered on restoring the balance of forces that cross the pubic joint. These procedures are designed to tighten and/or broaden soft tissue attachments that are acting on and causing instability of the pubic joint [1]. Frequently, surgery is also performed on the side contralateral to the region of pain to help restore a balance of forces above and below the pubic joint and on either side of the pubic symphysis [1]. To date, there have been over 20 different types of surgical procedures performed alone or in combination on over 15 different musculoskeletal structures implicated in AP [1]. Repair techniques reported in the literature include open, laparoscopic, and "minimally" open. Some surgeons reinforce their repairs with mesh, and some advocate for contralateral muscular releases and/or neurectomies [1, 2, 16–23]. Regardless of the type of repair performed, on average, these procedures result in an 80–100 % return-to-play rate, and prospective studies report rates as high as 95 % [1, 2, 11, 17–24]. Not only are these procedures successful in restoring functionality, but return-to-play times average as early as 3 months postoperatively [1]. In order to maximize outcomes, surgery is frequently complemented by postoperative core stabilization programs, designed to maintain the rebalanced forces across the pubic joint [1]. Postoperative complications are infrequent and are usually limited to minor bruising or clinically insignificant hematoma formation. The most common indication for reoperation in certain studies was the development of pain on the contralateral side, which supports the decision to perform a bilateral repair at the time of the first operation [1].

Inguinal Neuralgia

The groin is a complex area of musculoskeletal anatomy, but it is also an area rich in neural innervation derived from the lumbar plexus. The ilioinguinal, iliohypogastric, and the genitofemoral nerves are a few of the major nervous structures in the region and they are all subject to entrapment. These entrapment syndromes also commonly present with refractory groin pain. Inguinal neuralgia is frequently regarded as a postoperative complication and the overall incidence remains unknown [25]. They are most commonly seen after herniorrhaphy, but also have been reported after appendectomy, abdominoplasty, iliac bone graft harvest, blunt trauma, and many gynecological procedures involving Pfannenstiel or paramedian incisions [26].

Pathophysiology

The inguinal, iliohypogastric, and genitofemoral nerves can be injured anywhere along their course (Fig. 20.2); however, the point of injury is usually associated with the inciting operation. The mechanisms of injury may involve partial or complete section, stretch, contusion, crush, or electrocoagulation [26]. Secondary damage may also occur

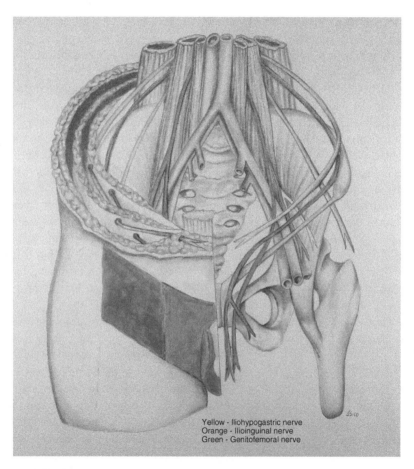

Yellow - Iliohypogastric nerve
Orange - Ilioinguinal nerve
Green - Genitofemoral nerve

Fig. 20.2 Lumbar plexus: a diagram showing the course of the ilioinguinal, iliohypogastric, and *GFN* and where they exit on the anterior abdominal wall/pelvis

from scar and/or neuroma formation or irritation by an adjacent inflammatory process, i.e., suture granuloma [27]. The procedure that most commonly results in postoperative inguinal neuralgia is the inguinal hernia repair, and the two most commonly affected nerves are the ilioinguinal and iliohypogastric [26]. The ilioinguinal nerve is most at risk for entrapment as it courses immediately beneath the external oblique fascia [25]. Here, it is subject to inclusion by suture, adherence to incorporated mesh, or encasement by scar [25]. The iliohypogastric nerve is also at risk for mesh adherence due to its close proximity, and both nerves are subject to stretching during transposition at the time of hernia sac dissection [25, 28]. Low Pfannenstiel incisions are also implicated in inguinal neuralgia for some of the same reasons [26]. The genitofemoral nerve is less commonly involved but may also be injured by suture inclusion, mesh adherence, or excessive tightening of the internal ring during herniorrhaphy [25]. Although these patterns of injury are likely responsible for the associated neuralgia, postoperative histological examination of the excised nerve segments frequently shows normal nervous architecture [25]. Occasionally, microscopic examination will reveal perineural fibrosis, cicatricial neuroma formation, and/or evidence of foreign bodies, i.e., suture material [25, 26].

Clinical Presentation

Entrapments of these nerves present similarly with chronic, disabling postoperative pain that is out of proportion to findings on clinical exam [26]. The pain is usually characterized as burning and constant with associated hyperesthesia [26]. It is exacerbated by forcible stretching of the hip joint, twisting of the torso, and movements that increase intra-abdominal pressure [25, 26]. Some patients even adopt a position of hip flexion with a slight forward truncal bend to alleviate the symptoms [26]. The time of presentation varies from immediately post-op to months or even years after surgery [25, 29]. Radiation of pain, however, is what helps to distinguish which nerves are involved. The pain

from inguinal neuralgia will frequently radiate along the associated area of innervation (Fig. 20.3); however, neuroanatomic variability can complicate the diagnosis [30]. Pain from ilioinguinal or iliohypogastric neuralgia may be localized to the area of a hernia repair or radiate down to the medial thigh [26, 30]. Perceived deep pelvic pain, rectal, and even proximal vaginal pain may be referred from entrapment of the iliohypogastric nerve [31]. The genitofemoral nerve innervates the testicle and labia and thus may have associated pain in those areas [30]. Pain with deep pressure at the external ring or palpation of the spermatic cord/round ligament against the pubic bone may also elicit pain consistent with genitofemoral neuralgia [30]. Obviously, the differential diagnosis of groin/pelvic pain is vast, and additional imaging modalities are frequently employed to rule out other causes [29, 32]. Nevertheless, groin pain 1–2 months post-op should be further investigated for consideration of inguinal neuralgia.

Diagnosis

The diagnosis of inguinal neuralgia relies heavily on history and physical, with special attention to be paid to the presenting symptoms mentioned previously [25]. The diagnostic triad of nerve entrapment or postoperative neuroma formation is as follows: (1) burning or lancinating pain near the precipitating operation's incision site that radiates is the sensory distribution of that particular nerve, (2) clear evidence of impaired sensory perception in the involved nerve territory, and (3) pain that is relieved by infiltration with anesthetic [33–35]. Inguinal neuralgia can also be reproduced and confirmed in some patients by truncal hyperextension and torso rotation in either direction [25]. As per the triad, subcutaneous anesthetic nerve blocks result in at least temporary relief for most patients [26]. These blocks can be used to target the culprit nerves; however, anatomic variation and cross innervation may complicate the diagnostic process [25]. The inguinal and iliohypogastric nerves can usually be blocked with local anesthetic superomedially to the ante-

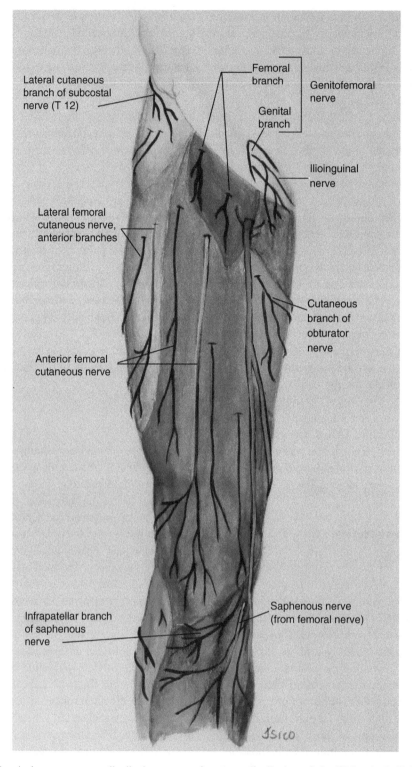

Fig. 20.3 Inguinal nerve sensory distribution: areas of sensory distribution of the ilioinguinal, iliohypogastric, and *GFN*

rior superior iliac spine [25]. Pain not relieved by this block may suggest genitofemoral neuralgia, which some surgeons confirm with a paravertebral block at L1/L2 [36]. Few studies report the use of electromyography, mainly to assess denervation of the pyramidalis muscle, which is specific for ilioinguinal nerve injury [26]. However, the utility of electromyography is still a matter of debate [37–39].

Management

Most authors recommend a trial of nonoperative management for all patients diagnosed with inguinal neuralgia [37]. Nonoperative techniques include biofeedback, neuropathic oral analgesics, transcutaneous electrical nerve stimulation, and repeated nerve blocks with either steroids, anesthetics, phenol, or alcohol [25, 26]. In many cases, the pain from nerve entrapment will resolve within 4–6 months; however, in some patients, the progression is crippling, and surgical intervention is warranted [26]. The best surgical outcomes are achieved by targeted neurectomy [25, 26]. Some surgeons advocate for the "triple neurectomy" due to the cross innervation between three aforementioned nerves; however, preoperative nerve block frequently allows for identification and excision of the implicated nerve [40]. Excisional techniques vary; however, most surgeons advocate for neurectomy at the exit of the internal oblique near the anterior superior iliac spine or at the level of the inguinal ring with regard to the genitofemoral nerve [25]. Others advocate for a more proximal excision in the retroperitoneum to avoid entrapment of the remaining nerve trunk in the abdominal wall musculature [30]. At the time of excision, all foreign bodies are removed, including mesh, screws, tacks, sutures, etc. [25]. Nerve dissection and rerouting have also been described, but results are not as promising as neurectomy [32]. After the nerve segment has been removed, pure alcohol or phenol solution may be injected into the surgical bed to prevent neuroma formation [25].

Inguinal neurectomy results in excellent outcomes, and the majority of patients are able to resume their occupation, as well as other daily activities [25]. Studies have reported over 90 % pain relief in patients with ilioinguinal and iliohypogastric nerve excision [26, 30]. Genitofemoral nerve excision results in slightly worse outcomes, and patients with scar encasement at the time of surgery also frequently have painful relapses as these areas are prone to scar renewal [26, 34, 35]. As expected, the most common postoperative complications include persistent numbness in the distribution of the excised nerve and loss of the cremasteric reflex [26]. Other less common complications include surgical site infections and the development of seromas or hematomas [25]. Division and excision of nerves also carry a risk of neuroma development which may be responsible for "recurrent" pain [25]. Prophylactic measures at the time of the initial surgery are being explored and include electrofulguration of the nerve bed, YAG laser, end-to-side nerve anastomosis, epineural ligation and coverage with flap, and inserting the nerve end into the muscular tissue [41–43].

Summary

Inguinal neuralgia and *athletic pubalgia* are the two complex and frequently misunderstood conditions that share a presenting symptom of refractory groin pain. Their diagnosis may be complicated by the multitude of conditions that also present with groin pain; however, both of these conditions can most often be identified with a thorough history and physical. A trial of nonoperative management is always warranted, but surgical repair offers excellent results for both syndromes, and few patients are unable to achieve their pre-injury level of functioning.

References

1. Meyers WC, McKechnie A, Philippon MJ. Experience with "sports hernia" spanning two decades. Ann Surg. 2008;248:656–64.
2. Meyers WC, Foley DP, Garrett WE, et al. Management of severe lower abdominal or inguinal pain in high-

performance athletes. PAIN (Performing Athletes with Abdominal or Inguinal Neuromuscular Pain Study Group). Am J Sports Med. 2000;28:2–8.

3. Larson CM. Sports hernia/athletic pubalgia: evaluation and management. Sports Health. 2014;6:139–44.

4. Gilmore J. Groin pain in the soccer athlete: fact, fiction, and treatment. Clin Sports Med. 1998;17:787–93.

5. Irshad K, Feldman LS, Lavoie C, et al. Operative management of "hockey groin syndrome: 12 years experience in National Hockey League players. Surgery. 2001;130:759–64.

6. Minnich JM, Hanks JB, Muschaweck U, et al. Sports hernia: diagnosis and treatment highlighting a minimal repair surgical technique. Am J Sports Med. 2011;39:1341–9.

7. Zoga AC, Kavanagh EC, Omar IM, et al. Athletic pubalgia and the "sports hernia": MRI imaging findings. Radiology. 2008;247:797–807.

8. Meyers WC, Yoo E, Devon ON, et al. Understanding "sports hernia" (athletic pubalgia): the anatomic and pathophysiologic basis for abdominal and groin pain in athletes. Oper Tech Sports Med. 2012;20:33–45.

9. Hammoud S, Bedi A, Magennis E, et al. High incidence of athletic pubalgia symptoms in professional athletes with symptomatic femoroacetabular impingement. Arthroscopy. 2012;28:1388–95.

10. Larson CM, Pierce BR, Giveans MR. Treatment of athletes with symptomatic intra-articular hip pathology and athletic pubalgia/sports hernia: a case series. Arthroscopy. 2011;27:768–75.

11. Farber AJ, Wilckens JH. Sports hernia: diagnostic and therapeutic approach. J Am Acad Orthop Surg. 2007;15:507–14.

12. Williams PR, Thomas DP, Downes EM. Osteitis pubis and instability of the pubic symphysis. When nonoperative measures fail. Am J Sports Med. 2000;28:350–5.

13. Martin RL, Enseki KR, Draovitch P, et al. Acetabular labral tears of the hip: examination and diagnostic challenges. J Orthop Sports Phys Ther. 2006;36:503–15.

14. Khan W, Zoga AC, Meyers WC. Magnetic resonance imaging of athletic pubalgia and the sports hernia: current understanding and practice. Magn Reson Imaging Clin N Am. 2013;21:97–110.

15. Silvis ML, Mosher TJ, Smetana BS, et al. High prevalence of pelvic and hip magnetic resonance imaging findings in asymptomatic collegiate and professional hockey players. Am J Sports Med. 2011;39:715–21.

16. Brannigan AE, Kerin MJ, McEntee GP. Gilmore's groin repair in athletes. J Orthop Sports Phys Ther. 2000;30:329–32.

17. Gilmore OJ. Gilmore's groin: ten years experience of groin disruption–a previously unsolved problem in sportsmen. Sports Med Soft Tissue Trauma. 1991;1:12–4.

18. Hackney RG. The sports hernia: a cause of chronic groin pain. Br J Sports Med. 1993;27:58–62.

19. Brown RA, Mascia A, Kinnear DG, et al. An 18-year review of sports groin injuries in the elite hockey player: clinical presentation, new diagnostic imaging, treatment and results. Clin J Sports Med. 2008;18:221–6.

20. Kluin J, den Hoed PT, Van Linschoten R, et al. Endoscopic evaluation and treatment of groin pain in the athlete. Am J Sports Med. 2004;32:944–9.

21. Gentisaris M, Goulimaris I, Sikas N. Laparoscopic repair of groin pain in athletes. Am J Sports Med. 2004;32:1238–42.

22. Muschaweck U, Berger L. Minimal repair technique of sportsmen's groin: an innovative open suture repair technique to treat chronic inguinal pain. Hernia. 2010;14:27–33.

23. Jakoi A, O'Neill C, Damsgaard C, et al. Sports hernia in National Hockey League players: does surgery affect performance? Am J Sports Med. 2013;41:107–10.

24. Ingoldby CJ. Laparoscopic and conventional repair of groin disruption in sportsmen. Br J Surg. 1997;84:213–5.

25. Madura JA, Madura II JA, Copper CM, et al. Inguinal neurectomy for inguinal nerve entrapment: an experience with 100 patients. Am J Surg. 2005;189:283–7.

26. Kim DH, Murovic JA, Tiel RL, et al. Surgical management of 33 ilioinguinal and iliohypogastric neuralgias at Louisiana State University Health Sciences Center. Neurosurgery. 2005;56:1013–20.

27. Kennedy EM, Harms BA, Starling JR. Absence of maladaptive neuronal plasticity after genitofemoral-ilioinguinal neurectomy. Surgery. 1994;116:665–71.

28. Salama J, Sarfati E, Chevrel JP. The anatomical basis of nerve lesions arising during the reduction of inguinal hernia. Clin Anat. 1983;5:75–81.

29. Stulz P, Pfeiffer KM. Peripheral nerve injuries resulting from common surgical procedures in the lower portion of the abdomen. Arch Surg. 1982;117:324–7.

30. Lee CH, Dellon AL. Surgical management of groin pain of neural origin. J Am Coll Surg. 2000;191:137–42.

31. Liszka TG, Dellon AL, Manson PN. Iliohypogastric nerve entrapment following abdominoplasty. Plast Reconstr Surg. 1994;93:181–3.

32. Hp K, Thompson WA, Postel AH. Entrapment neuropathy of the ilioinguinal nerve. New England J Med. 1962;266:16–9.

33. Rab M, Ebmer J, Dellon AL. Anatomic variability of the ilioinguinal and genitofemoral nerve: implications for the treatment of groin pain. Plast Reconstr Surg. 2001;108:1618–23.

34. Starling JR, Harms BA, Schroeder ME, et al. Diagnosis and treatment of genitofemoral and ilioinguinal entrapment neuralgia. Surgery. 1987;102:581–6.

35. Starling JR, Harms BA. Diagnosis and treatment of genitofemoral and ilioinguinal neuralgia. World J Surg. 1989;13:586–91.

36. Harms BA, Dehaas Jr DR, Starling JR. Diagnosis and management of genitofemoral neuralgia. Arch Surg. 1984;119:339–41.

37. Hahn L. Treatment of ilioinguinal nerve entrapment– a randomized controlled trial. Acta Obstet Gynecol Scand. 2011;90:955–60.

38. Arcocha guirrezabal J, Irimia Sieira P, Soto O. Ilioinguinal neuropathy: usefulness of conduction studies. Neurologia. 2004;19:24–6.

39. Benito-Leon J, Picardo A, Garrido A, et al. Gabapentin therapy for genitofemoral and ilioinguinal neuralgia. J Neurol. 2001;248:907–8.

40. AMid PJ. A 1-stage surgical treatment for postherniorrhaphy neuropathic pain: triple neurectomy and proximal end implantation without mobilization of the cord. Arch Surg. 2002;137:100–4.

41. Aszmann OC, Korak KF, Rab M, et al. Neuroma prevention by end-to-side neurorrhaphy: an experimental study in rats. J Hand Surg. 2003;28:1022–8.

42. Yuksel F, Kislaoglu E, Durak N, et al. Prevention of painful neuromas by epineural ligatures, flaps and grafts. Br J Surg. 1997;50:182–5.

43. Martini A, Fromm B. A new operation for the prevention and treatment of amputation neuromas. J Bone Joint Surg Br. 1989;71:379–82.

Hand Transplantation and Rehabilitation

21

Eric G. Wimmers and Justin M. Sacks

Introduction

Approximately 1.7 million Americans live with a limb loss, and an estimated 1 in 200 Americans has had an amputation [1]. As technology and scientific research advance, the possibilities for people who have lost a limb become seemingly endless. From bionic limbs that move with a person's brain and hand transplants that graft a donated hand, a new world of life after amputation is emerging. The need for occupational therapy following a hand transplant surgery, for example, is enormous—some patients receive more than 8 h of occupational therapy a day.

E.G. Wimmers, MD (✉)
The Plastic Surgery Center, Institute for Advanced Reconstruction, 535 Sycamore Ave, Shrewsbury, NJ 07702, USA
e-mail: ewimmersmd@theplasticsurgerycenternj.com

J.M. Sacks, MD, FACS
Department of Plastic and Reconstructive Surgery, Johns Hopkins School of Medicine,
Baltimore, MA, USA

Vascularized Composite Allograft Transplant Laboratory, Carey School of Business, Johns Hopkins Outpatient Center, Johns Hopkins University,
601 North Caroline Street Suite 2114C,
Baltimore, MA 21287, USA
e-mail: jmsacks@jhmi.edu

Unique Aspects

The first successful hand transplant was performed in 1998, opening up a new possibility for patients who have suffered mutilating hand injuries. Since then, more than 80 such procedures have been performed throughout the world. In the case of mutilating hand injuries, surgeons often cannot replant the severed parts, requiring patients to be treated with amputation and fitted for a prosthetic limb. Because upper-limb prostheses do not provide sensation and fine motor control, they are an inadequate replacement for the lost hand or arm for many patients, particularly those with bilateral amputations. Hand transplantation is a new option for patients in which the missing part is replaced, allowing for reestablishment of sensation and fine motor control [2, 3].

Despite their obvious advantages, the adverse effects of prolonged immunosuppression necessary for graft survival have limited the routine clinical use of these procedures. These risks include infection, cancer, and metabolic derangement and greatly affect recipient quality of life, alter the risk profile, and jeopardize the potential benefits of upper extremity transplantation [4]. Unlike solid-organ transplants, clinical success requires not only graft acceptance and survival but also nerve regeneration, which determines ultimate functional outcomes. There are emerging strategies, such as cellular and biologic therapies that integrate the concepts of immune regulation with those of nerve regeneration, that have shown promising results in small and large animal models [5, 6]. Clinical translation of these insights to upper extremity reconstructive transplantation could further minimize the need of immunosuppression and optimize functional outcomes, enabling greater feasibility and wider application of these procedures as an option for upper extremity amputees.

Upper Extremity Allotransplantation

The human hand consists of 27 bones, 28 muscles, 3 major nerves, 2 major arteries, multiple tendons, veins, and soft tissue. This complex surgery can last from 8 to 10 h. It involves bone fixation, reattachment of arteries and veins, and repair of tendons and nerves. Upper extremity transplants are vascularized composite allografts (VCA) because they are modules of distinct tissues, including the skin, muscle, ligament, tendon, nerve, blood vessel, bone, joint and cartilage, bone marrow, and lymph nodes [7].

Donor and Recipient Selection

In contrast to the case of identifying an organ donor, selecting a donor for a hand transplant must involve additional and careful emphasis on matching skin color, skin tone, gender, ethnicity and race, and the size of the hand. Decades of experience with solid organs have allowed us to establish criteria for donor and recipient selection. In a novel field like hand transplantation, parameters for inclusion and exclusion of donors and recipients have not yet been conclusively defined nor standardized [8].

Medical screening of recipients includes a complete medical history and physical examination, routine laboratory studies, blood typing and cross matching, human leukocyte antigen (HLA) typing, testing for panel reactive antibodies, and serology for Epstein–Barr virus, *Cytomegalovirus*, HIV, and viral hepatitis. Other tests include radiography (to plan for osteosynthesis), angiography (to exclude abnormal vascular patterns), electromyography,

nerve conduction velocity, and functional magnetic resonance imaging (fMRI) [2].

Donor Limb Procurement

The organ procurement organization will ensure that the selection of potential hand donors is completely in accordance with study criteria. If the donor is unstable, the hand dissection is performed following organ dissection. However, before cross clamping of aorta, the hand team commences dissection and retrieves the limb prior to organ retrieval. The limb is perfused under isolated tourniquet by cold histidine–tryptophan–ketoglutarate (HTK, Custodiol) solution through a brachial artery cannula prior to disarticulation [9]. Upon completion of hand retrieval, the donor stump is closed, and the body can be fitted with a cosmetic prosthesis.

Recipient Surgery

Hand transplantation does not differ greatly from replantation. Instrumentation and technique are similar. A twoteam approach is used. The donor team prepares the donor limb once received on the back table, tailoring the graft to the needs of the recipient and tagging the structures. The sequence of tissue repair is to minimize ischemia time and could depend on surgical preference. Commonly, it includes bony fixation → artery repair → vein repair (revascularization) → tendon repair → nerve repair → skin closure [10].

Maintenance Immunosuppression

The current immunosuppressive protocols are derived from regimens used in solid-organ transplantation. The overall amount of immunosuppression required to ensure graft survival is comparable with that used in renal transplantation. Such conventional immunosuppression has resulted in 100 % patient and graft survival at 1 year after upper extremity transplantation, an outcome that has not been achieved in any other field of transplantation [11]. Despite immunosuppression, acute rejection episodes occur in 85% of patients within the first year [11]. The International Registry on Hand and Composite Tissue Allotransplantation reports that all episodes of acute rejection have been controlled with modification of immunosuppressive medications.

Acute rejection, in cases of hand transplantation, is evaluated through skin biopsies. Rejection episodes usually display a rash or dermatitis. Skin biopsies show evidence of lymphocytic infiltration in cases of acute rejection. Rejection episodes in hand transplant patients should be handled similar to the management of rejection in solid-organ transplant patients. Hand transplant patients appear to have better survival rates than patients who have received solid organs when immunosuppressive protocols are followed properly [12]. The majority of acute rejection episodes may be managed with topical or systemic corticosteroids and topical Tacrolimus®.

Rehabilitation

Patients are encouraged to start moving the hand early, within 24–48 h, to reduce edema and stiffness. Therapy after hand transplant is long and intensive, and patients are educated before surgery on the critical importance of rehabilitation in improving functional outcome after the procedure.

Functional Assessment

Rehabilitation and functional assessment are integral components of successful upper extremity allotransplantation [13]. The hand therapist is involved in the entire process from initial screening of prospective patients through final discharge. The goal is functional integration of the transplanted hand into the patient's daily activities. Successful rehabilitation for the hand transplant patient follows guidelines similar to replant protocols. There are several significant differences, however, such as screening for an ideal candidate and monitoring for signs of rejection.

During the preoperative evaluation, occupational therapy will perform tests to assess the patient's baseline functionality and will be performed annually posttransplantation:

- *Carroll Test*: This test quantifies functional capabilities of upper extremities on a scale of 0–99, with a score of less than 50 being considered "poor" and greater than 85 as "excellent" [14]. The test assesses what basic upper extremity functions you are able to do prior to transplant.
- *Michigan Hand Outcomes Questionnaire*: This questionnaire is designed to assess one's perceived and actual hand function and is employed yearly to assess for improvement or regression. Sections of the questionnaire assess for the following: activities of daily living, overall function, work performance, visual appreciation of the hand, and overall satisfaction of functionality [15].
- *DASH (Disabilities of the Arm, Shoulder, and Hand)*: This questionnaire assesses the patient's ability to perform certain upper extremity activities [16]. After listing, the patient is expected to receive therapy on an outpatient basis 1–3 times a week, to strengthen the upper extremities, in preparation for upcoming transplantation.

The goals of postoperative therapy, bracing, and splinting are similar to replantation. The planning of the splinting therapy relies on the knowledge of the exact level of the nerve repair, type of osteosynthesis used, and details of tendon repairs. Uniquely, the hand therapist can help monitor for signs of rejection as the patient spends considerable time in rehabilitation after surgery.

During the first 3–6 months, an intense rehabilitation protocol has to be implemented in all patients with 3–6 h of supervised occupational therapy 5 days a week, depending on the nature and level of the transplant. Therapy must consist of both passive and active range of motion (ROM) exercises with appropriate static and dynamic splinting to allow gentle active flexion/extension and limit adhesions and promote healing. All patients should use hand splints, such as dynamic extension outrigger splints and anticlaw splints. Constant tension is produced by the outrigger throughout the range of controlled motion; the outrigger allows for an intrinsicplus position and protects flexors and extensors. Compression gloves are useful in patients with lymphedema.

Rejection Assessment

Rejection can appear as a rash that could be spotty, patchy, or blotchy. It could appear anywhere on the transplant and is usually painless. As rejection almost always appears first in the skin, patients are encouraged to carefully watch for the signs and report to the physician for timely biopsy and treatment. The therapist plays a crucial role in identifying a rejection episode early, since he or she most closely examines the patient's hands on a daily basis. Unlike internal organ transplants, where rejection is difficult to spot early, it is easy to detect and monitor in the hand, allowing for early medical intervention.

In 2007, the Banff working classification was published as an international standard for classifying rejection of vascular composite allografts [17]. Any rash on the transplanted graft should be immediately reported to the plastic surgeon managing the patient (Fig. 21.1). According to the Banff 2007 working classification of skin-containing composite tissue allografts, visible skin changes should be reported as follows: no signs, <10 %, 10–50 %, and >50 % [17]. Most frequently, lesions are located at the dorsal and volar aspects of the forearm and wrist with the dorsum of the hand affected in some cases [17, 19, 20]. This pattern has been referred to as the "classical" pattern of rejection. The skin of the palm and nail beds are usually spared.

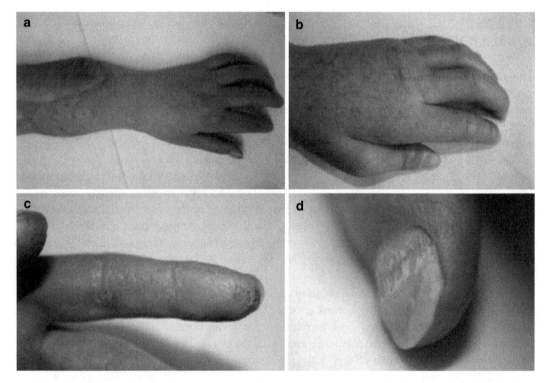

Fig. 21.1 Clinical presentation of skin rejection. The macroscopic changes may be heterogeneous. In mild cases, skin lesions most often appear in a spotted pattern (**a**). Rejection may be associated with limb and hand edema (**b**). In rare cases, the volar aspect of the hand may show signs of rash, dryness, and scaling (**c**). Dystrophy (**d**) and other nail changes may be observed during rejection of a hand allograft (From Hautz et al. [18]. This material is reproduced with permission of John Wiley & Sons, Inc.)

Overall, lesions indicating skin rejection in VCA are not very specific and mimic several inflammatory, infectious, and rarely neoplastic dermatoses. The most important finding in the differential diagnosis between VCA skin rejection and inflammatory dermatoses is the absence of skin lesions on the recipient's own skin [21].

Outcomes

Current long-term graft survival among patients in Europe and the United States is better than 94 % [22]. Immune-mediated rejection has been the primary cause of graft loss [23]. The first case of graft loss occurred in 1998 in Lyon, France, with the first unilateral hand transplant patient; pathologic specimens of the rejected hand showed evidence of lichenoid-like lesions, which can also be seen in cases of graft versus host disease [22, 23]. Rejection occurred after the patient stopped taking his immunosuppression medications. The only case of graft loss in a US patient was the result of ischemia caused by fibro-intimal hyperplasia. Fibro-intimal hyperplasia is thought to be a form of chronic rejection similar to that which has been described in heart transplant recipients [24].

Functional outcomes have been very encouraging, with all patients recovering protective sensibility, 90 % recovering tactile sensibility, and 82.3 % recovering discriminative sensibility [22]. Muscle recovery begins with the extrinsic flexor and extensor groups, allowing some patients to perform grasp-and-pinch activities shortly after transplantation. The recovery of intrinsic muscles can take up to 15 months. Recovery of intrinsic muscle function has been confirmed by electromyographic studies in several hands [12, 25]. Extrinsic and intrinsic muscle function has allowed patients to perform most daily activities, including eating, driving, grasping objects, riding a bicycle or motorbike, shaving, using the telephone, and writing [3]. In addition, functional MRI has demonstrated that after transplantation, hand representation is regained within the sensory and motor cortex of the brain [26, 27].

Cortical Plasticity and Neurointegration

A unique phenomenon occurs after upper extremity transplantation in which portions of the recipient's brain are reassigned to control the limb. This plasticity of cortical organization has been demonstrated to occur after amputation as well as after limb transplantation [26]. After a hand is amputated, the area of the brain that was receiving signals from the hand is gradually lost and is taken over by other functions. However, after an upper extremity transplant, that area of the brain can reestablish its original function, and the signals from the new hand go back to the area of the brain that was used to control the original hand [28].

Summary

The progressive increase in worldwide hand transplantation will lead to common rehabilitation protocols and data collection. That being said, it is important to remember that every patient will require his or her own unique treatment plan. Therapy guidelines should consider the level of transplantation, bilateral versus unilateral, and any lower extremity issues. Ultimately a successful hand transplant is dependent on the involvement of an occupational therapist, during candidate selection and postoperatively.

References

1. Ziegler-Graham K, MacKenzie EJ, Ephraim PL, Travison TG, Brookmeyer R. Estimating the prevalence of limb loss in the United States: 2005 to 2050. Arch Phys Med Rehabil. 2008;89:422–9.
2. Kvernmo HD, Gorantla VS, Gonzalez RN, Breidenbach WC. Hand transplantation. A future clinical option? Acta Orthop. 2005;76:14–27.
3. Brandacher G, Ninković M, Piza-Katzer H, et al. The Innsbruck hand transplant program: update at 8 years after the first transplant. Transplant Proc. 2009;41:491–4.
4. Gorantla VS, Brandacher G, Schneeberger S, et al. Favoring the risk-benefit balance for upper extremity transplantation- the Pittsburgh Protocol. Hand Clin. 2011;27:511–20.
5. Wachtman GS, Wimmers EG, Gorantla VS, et al. Biologics and donor bone marrow cells for targeted

immunomodulation in vascularized composite allo-transplantation: a translational trial in swine. Transplant Proc. 2011;43:3541–4.

6. Ibrahim Z, Cooney DS, Shores JT, et al. A modified heterotopic swine hind limb transplant model for translational vascularized composite allotransplantation (VCA) research. J Vis Exp. 2013;(80):1–8.

7. Shores JT, Brandacher G, Schneeberger S, Gorantla VS, Lee WPA. Composite tissue allotransplantation: hand transplantation and beyond. J Am Acad Orthop Surg. 2010;18:127–31.

8. Hollenbeck ST, Erdmann D, Levin LS. Current indications for hand and face allotransplantation. Transplant Proc. 2009;41:495–8.

9. Jones JW, Gruber SA, Barker JH, Breidenbach WC. Successful hand transplantation. One-year follow-up. Louisville Hand Transplant Team. N Engl J Med. 2000;343:468–73.

10. Brandacher G, Gorantla VS, Lee WPA. Hand allotransplantation. Semin Plast Surg. 2010;24:11–7.

11. Petruzzo P, Dubernard JM. The international registry on hand and composite tissue allotransplantation. Clin Transpl. 2011;247–53.

12. Breidenbach WC, Gonzales NR, Kaufman CL, Klapheke M, Tobin GR, Gorantla VS. Outcomes of the first 2 American hand transplants at 8 and 6 years posttransplant. J Hand Surg. 2008;33:1039–47.

13. Hodges A, Chesher S, Feranda S. Hand transplantation: rehabilitation: case report. Microsurgery. 2000; 20:389–92.

14. Petit F, Minns AB, Dubernard J-M, Hettiaratchy S, Lee WPA. Composite tissue allotransplantation and reconstructive surgery: first clinical applications. Ann Surg. 2003;237:19–25.

15. Chung KC, Hamill JB, Walters MR, Hayward RA. The Michigan Hand Outcomes Questionnaire (MHQ): assessment of responsiveness to clinical change. Ann Plast Surg. 1999;42:619–22.

16. Hudak PL, Amadio PC, Bombardier C. Development of an upper extremity outcome measure: the DASH (disabilities of the arm, shoulder and hand) [corrected]. The Upper Extremity Collaborative Group (UECG). Am J Ind Med. 1996;29:602–8.

17. Cendales LC, Kanitakis J, Schneeberger S, et al. The Banff 2007 working classification of skin-containing composite tissue allograft pathology. Am J Transplant. 2008;8:1396–400.

18. Hautz T, Weissenbacher A, Jablecki J, et al. Standardizing skin biopsy sampling to assess rejection in vascularized composite allotransplantation. Clin Transplant. 2013;27:E81–90.

19. Hautz T, Engelhardt TO, Weissenbacher A, et al. World experience after more than a decade of clinical hand transplantation: update on the Innsbruck program. Hand Clin. 2011;27:423–31.

20. Kanitakis J, Petruzzo P, Jullien D, et al. Pathological score for the evaluation of allograft rejection in human hand (composite tissue) allotransplantation. Eur J Dermatol. 2005;15:235–8.

21. Kanitakis J. The challenge of dermatopathological diagnosis of composite tissue allograft rejection: a review. J Cutan Pathol. 2008;35:738–44.

22. Petruzzo P, Lanzetta M, Dubernard J-M, et al. The international registry on hand and composite tissue transplantation. Transplantation. 2010;90: 1590–4.

23. Lanzetta M, Petruzzo P, Dubernard J-M, et al. Second report (1998–2006) of the International Registry of Hand and Composite Tissue Transplantation. Transpl Immunol. 2007;18:1–6.

24. Michaels PJ, Espejo ML, Kobashigawa J, et al. Humoral rejection in cardiac transplantation: risk factors, hemodynamic consequences and relationship to transplant coronary artery disease. J Heart Lung Transplant. 2003;22:58–69.

25. Dubernard J-M, Petruzzo P, Lanzetta M, et al. Functional results of the first human double-hand transplantation. Ann Surg. 2003;238:128–36.

26. Giraux P, Sirigu A, Schneider F, Dubernard JM. Cortical reorganization in motor cortex after graft of both hands. Nat Neurosci. 2001;4:691–2.

27. Vargas CD, Aballéa A, Rodrigues EC, et al. Re-emergence of hand-muscle representations in human motor cortex after hand allograft. Proc Natl Acad Sci U S A. 2009;106:7197–202.

28. Frey SH, Bogdanov S, Smith JC, Watrous S, Breidenbach WC. Chronically deafferented sensory cortex recovers a grossly typical organization after allogenic hand transplantation. Curr Biol. 2008;18: 1530–4.

Targeted Reinnervation Strategies to Restore Upper Limb Function

Victor W. Wong and Richard J. Redett

Introduction

In 2005, approximately 1.6 million people in the United States were missing a limb. This number is expected to more than double by 2050 [1]. Military personnel are disproportionately affected by limb loss, and limb amputation rates remain high with the active conflicts in the Middle East [2, 3]. Trauma is the leading cause of upper extremity amputation which results in considerable loss of function in an otherwise healthy patient population [4]. Limb amputees also commonly suffer from chronic pain and psychological impairments as a result of limb loss [5, 6]. Several options exist for upper limb amputees, each with their own set of advantages and disadvantages.

Prostheses aim to restore form and function to the missing limb. The earliest known prosthesis is the "Cairo toe," a wooden and leather device dating from 950 BC which was found on the mummified foot of an Egyptian noblewoman. During the American Civil War, prostheses powered by body motion were developed to treat amputees. Prosthetic technology continued to advance throughout both World Wars [7]. Externally powered hydraulic prostheses were introduced in the early 1900s. Myoelectric

designs, using muscle-generated electric signals to control a motorized joint, were also developed in this period [8]. Modern prosthetic designs continue to be based on these early concepts.

Vascularized composite *allotransplantation* (a medical term that includes "arm transplant") offers the potential of replacing the missing tissue with similar functional tissue. As of 2014, over 107 hand or upper extremities have been transplanted around the world. The early experience has been promising in properly selected patients [9]. The transplanted limb has the potential to provide greater function, integration, and compliance compared to prosthetics [10]. However, lifelong immunosuppression, high costs, surgical complexity, and the complications of rejection currently limit its widespread acceptance.

Targeted muscle reinnervation (TMR) was developed to combine surgical and engineering approaches to restoring function for people with proximal upper limb amputations, specifically transhumeral or shoulder dislocation amputations [11]. The remainder of this chapter focuses on TMR concepts and techniques with particular emphasis for rehabilitation specialists.

Targeted Muscle Reinnervation: Basic Concepts

Targeted muscle reinnervation (TMR) aims to restore intuitive control of limb function. In simple terms, the brain (control center) initiates

V.W. Wong, MD • R.J. Redett, MD (✉)
Department of Plastic and Reconstructive Surgery, Johns Hopkins Medical Institutions, Baltimore, MD 21287, USA
e-mail: rredett@jhmi.edu

© Springer International Publishing Switzerland 2017
A.I. Elkwood et al. (eds.), *Rehabilitative Surgery*, DOI 10.1007/978-3-319-41406-5_22

muscle contraction (effector) through nerves (electrical conduit), allowing for movement across a particular joint. By simultaneously integrating numerous nerve signals from the brain to upper extremity muscles, complex movements can be precisely orchestrated. After amputation, there is variable loss of muscle effectors, but the *control center* (cortical system) and *electrical conduits* (peripheral motor nerves) remain intact up to the amputation site (Fig. 22.1). Control signals can still be initiated and propagated, but the terminal effectors are either absent or dysfunctional. By rerouting nerves to new muscle targets, the electrical signal can be amplified and transmitted across the skin surface as electromyogram (EMG) signals at the amputation site (Fig. 22.2). Surface electrodes within the myoelectric prosthesis detect these signals and activate prosthetic function. This reconstructive approach theoretically allows for more instinctive control of increasingly complex robotic prostheses.

By reorganizing the orientation of terminal branches of the brachial plexus, a greater number of myoelectric control signals can be distinctly activated to mimic the original functions of those nerve/muscle units. The musculocutaneous, median, ulnar, and radial nerves are all present at a transhumeral amputation site and could theoretically generate unique EMG signals to control different prosthetic motors. The musculocutaneous nerve normally controls elbow flexion via the biceps brachii, brachialis, and coracobrachialis. Redirection of the musculocutaneous nerve to generate a surface EMG signal could be used to activate prosthetic elbow flexion, similar to its native function. Likewise, a rerouted radial nerve could activate prosthetic elbow or hand extension via surface EMG signals, similar to its original role as an extension signal in an intact limb.

Animal and human studies have demonstrated that in newly created nerve motor units (e.g., cross-innervated muscle), motor control is dominated by the original function of the nerve, not the function of the muscle [11–13]. By exploiting the nerve's intrinsic motor programming, the prosthetic control mechanisms can be made more intuitive and natural which ultimately translates into greater function. Importantly, functional muscle–nerve units are left intact during TMR procedures, and only

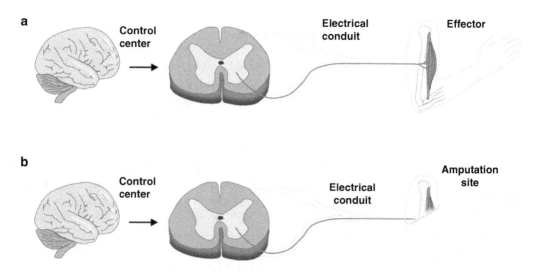

Fig. 22.1 Targeted muscle reinnervation concepts. (**a**) In an uninjured limb, the cortical system serves as the control center and initiates voluntary movement. Motor nerves function as an electrical conduit and transmit the signal to a target effector (muscle). Contraction of the muscle results in movement across a particular joint. (**b**) After amputation, there is variable loss of muscle effectors and terminal motor nerves. However, the control center and proximal ends of the electrical conduits remain intact and functional

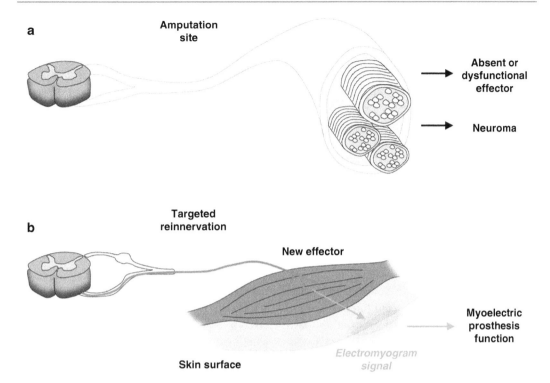

Fig. 22.2 Targeted muscle reinnervation schematic. (**a**) In the setting of amputation, distal motor nerves are variably injured, innervate absent or dysfunctional muscle effectors, and/or are prone to painful neuroma formation. (**b**) With targeted muscle reinnervation, select motor nerves of the brachial plexus are rerouted to new func- tional muscle effectors. By surgically redirecting these nerves, independent electromyogram signals can be gen- erated via voluntary contractions by the patient. Skin sur- face electrodes then detect these signals and initiate myoelectric prosthesis function, allowing for more intui- tive control of advanced robotic arms

residual nerves are used to minimize additional morbidity. It is also critical to preserve shoulder biomechanics so that body-powered functions are not lost.

For TMR to be successful, three require- ments have been described [11]. First, multiple nerves need to adequately reinnervate distinct areas of the muscle and skin consistently. Second, independent signals with minimal sur- rounding interference (i.e., muscle cross talk) must be detected from each myoelectric control area (i.e., patch of the skin). Third, a prosthesis must be able to receive myriad EMG inputs, integrate multiple motor functions, and provide sensory feedback. Early experience with TMR highlights the feasibility and potential of this treatment paradigm for proximal upper limb amputees [14].

Integration with Bioprostheses

Modern prostheses can be "cosmetic" and appear quite similar to a normal upper limb at the expense of minimal function. Conversely, "functional" prostheses aim to restore upper limb movements using body power (e.g., shoulder movement), external (e.g., electric) power, or both in a "hybrid" approach. Body-powered prostheses use harnesses and cables to convert shoulder motion to prosthetic function and rely on patient strength. Only one component of the prosthesis can be acti- vated at a time and must be locked into place before a different component can be activated, resulting in "sequential" control.

External prostheses are generally based on electric power and use motors to create move- ment. Most are myoelectric, i.e., they use EMG signals from terminal muscles at the amputated limb to control motorized components. Complex movements are limited based on the number of independent control signals. Similar to body-powered systems, only sequential control is able to operate separate prosthetic functions. Ideally, antagonistic flexion and extension muscle pairs would be used to control a joint with independent feedback mechanisms and minimal adjacent muscle cross talk. This approach is more useful for distal amputations such as transradial but difficult with high-level proximal amputations because there are fewer physiologically appropriate muscle groups.

TMR has been shown to improve control and function of myoelectric prostheses in validated functional tests [14]. Patients demonstrated markedly improved gross hand function in block movement and clothespin relocation tests. Patients also reported subjective improvements in hand control and lesser disability after TMR surgery. However, the nerves transferred during TMR transmit signals far more complex than just an "on–off" cue to a single muscle [15]. Conventional myoelectric systems can only receive defined EMG amplitudes at specific control sites, thus failing to incorporate more nuanced information needed to perform more complex tasks.

One approach to better capture this neural information is via pattern recognition algorithms that utilize machine learning to predict intended movements [11, 16]. TMR patients provide sample contractions for each of their myoelectric prosthesis movements. A computer algorithm then "learns" the EMG patterns and can facilitate future motions over time, allowing for improved coordination and greater complexity of movement. EMG patterns, including more than just signal amplitude, are detected over both native and reinnervated muscles to capture patterns in regional activity with each motion.

Myoelectric control systems are largely limited by the difficulty in detecting adequate EMG signals and the scarcity of information needed to control multiple functions. To address these challenges, new technologies are being developed to improve the nerve–prosthesis interfaces [7].

Implantable electrodes have been designed to record myoelectric signals directly from the muscle, thus obviating the need for skin surface conduction which is affected by environmental factors [17]. Implantable devices would need to be powered for long-term recording and be compatible with telemetry systems that function in deeper tissues.

Direct access to peripheral nerves is another strategy to improve the resolution of cortical signals. However, these signals are almost a thousand times smaller than EMG signals, thus requiring sensitive electrodes for recording and stimulation [7]. Electrodes can be extraneural or intraneural, the latter demonstrating greater precision and sensitivity. Current limitations include the risk of nerve damage with intraneural electrodes and inconsistent results, because only a fraction of a nerve's individual action potentials can be captured by a single electrode.

Researchers have also explored capturing electric potentials directly from the brain. Neuronal activity can be recorded from inside, on the cortex surface (electrocorticogram), or over the scalp (electroencephalogram) [18]. The motor and somatosensory cortices contain a topographical map of the human body and thus represent a potential interface to detect neuronal activity. Research in these areas is actively ongoing but requires significantly more investigation before widespread clinical testing and adoption.

Surgical Considerations

Successful application of TMR is based on an understanding of brachial plexus and upper extremity peripheral nerve anatomy. Briefly, it is a plexus of somatic nerves formed by the ventral roots of the lower four cervical nerves (C5–C8) and the first thoracic nerve (T1). It innervates all muscles of the upper extremity except for the trapezius and levator scapula. The brachial plexus is subdivided into roots, trunks, divisions, cords, and branches. The major terminal branches innervate muscle groups with distinct functions and include the median, ulnar, musculocutaneous, and radial nerves. By rerouting these motor nerves to defined muscle skin areas, surface electrodes can detect independent signals that activate prosthetic functions aligned with the "original" nerve function.

Another important anatomic concept underlying TMR is agonist–antagonist muscle groups. For arm movement, nerve activation of a muscle agonist (e.g., the biceps brachii for elbow flexion) requires inactivation of the corresponding muscle antagonist (e.g., the triceps brachii for elbow extension). For example, in an intact arm, elbow flexion would be activated by musculocutaneous nerve stimulation of the biceps brachii, whereas radial nerve stimulation of the triceps brachii would be absent. During TMR surgery, the musculocutaneous and radial nerves would be rerouted to distinct areas so that they could activate opposing movements of the prosthesis, similar to a normal arm.

As part of the process in evaluating patients for TMR, reconstructive surgeons assess the amputation site for evidence of adequate healing and durable soft tissue coverage. Certain areas of the limb may have an excess of subcutaneous fat or scar that may dampen the myoelectric signal at the skin surface. This may require subcutaneous thinning procedures or excision of the scar tissue. Surgeons have developed techniques to place flaps of adipose tissue between adjacent muscle segments to isolate myoelectric signals and minimize muscle cross talk [19]. Areas of heterotopic ossification (ectopic bone formation in the soft tissues) may be present from the initial injury and may interfere with prosthetic fitting. Skin graft coverage may have been used initially for reconstruction but may not be ideal for long-term prosthetic wear. Pedicled flaps or free tissue transfer may help to deliver thick vascularized tissues to the amputation site to establish a more durable stump or prosthetic fitting site. Free muscle flaps can even be innervated to provide functional motor units and new targets for TMR.

The level of upper limb amputation is also critical in surgical planning to facilitate TMR. For elbow disarticulations or long transhumeral amputations, the limb may need to be shortened and/or angulated for prosthesis wear. TMR should be considered at the time of elective amputation or revision so that nerves can be protected and transferred earlier in the recovery process [20]. The following technique has been described by Dumanian and Cheesborough [19, 20]. Two incisions, both dorsal and ventral, are made in the upper arm to identify motor nerves using a nerve stimulator. The median nerve is transferred to the motor nerve of the short head of the biceps brachii to activate prosthetic hand closure. The long head of the biceps brachii remains intact for prosthetic elbow flexion via the native musculocutaneous nerve. Via the dorsal incision, the long head of the triceps brachii remains intact for prosthetic elbow extension via the native radial nerve. The distal radial nerve is transferred to the motor nerve of the lateral head of the triceps brachii to activate prosthetic hand opening. The ulnar motor nerve can also be transferred to the brachialis to provide an additional myoelectric control point.

TMR for shoulder disarticulation patients is extremely challenging for multiple reasons, including the short nerve lengths, the paucity of muscle targets, and the severe soft tissue defects associated with the injury. However, the prosthetic goals are identical to those for more distal level amputations: elbow flexion/extension and hand opening/closing. Trunk muscles available for reinnervation include the pectoralis major and minor, serratus anterior, and latissimus dorsi. Additionally, the pectoralis major may have muscular subdivisions (clavicle, superior sternal head, inferior sternal head) that can be individually reinnervated. Specific techniques have been previously published, but particular emphasis should be placed on transfer of the musculocutaneous nerve for prosthetic elbow control and the median nerve for prosthetic hand closing [20, 21].

Targeted Sensory Reinnervation

Despite the use of advanced robotic arms capable of reproducing complex human motor functions, the ability to provide physiologic sensory feedback remains lacking. Approaches including peripheral nerve stimulation and cortical electrodes have been examined, but the clinical viability of implanted devices remains a major challenge [22]. TMR techniques have enabled some proximal arm amputees to regain missing limb sensation over the reinnervated muscle, suggesting that afferent nerves can regrow at the amputation site and prompting the development of sensory reinnervation techniques.

Three main approaches have been described to improve sensory reinnervation during TMR surgery. First, the skin overlying the target reinnervated muscle is denervated during the procedure, thus allowing for sensory nerve regrowth into the skin area [23]. Sensation may be restored 4–6 months after the initial surgery, but the referred sensations are highly variable and lack somatotopic organization. A second approach involves performing an end-to-side connection between a cutaneous sensory nerve and a main nerve trunk during the traditional TMR. In one case report, partial reinnervation was established at 6 months post-surgery. However, normal pressure sensation was deficient, and there was no somatotopic organization [24].

The third and most selective approach employs end-to-end nerve fascicle reinnervation with intraoperative nerve stimulation to aid in sensory fascicle selection. Because the median and ulnar nerves have distinct motor and sensory fascicles, the use of somatosensory evoked potentials (SSEPs) can help identify sensory fascicles from the main nerve trunk that can be coapted to cutaneous sensory target nerves [22]. The remaining motor fascicles are left intact for the standard TMR procedure. In one case report, this procedure produced unique sensory areas of the ulnar and median nerve distributions that did not overlap. By combining microsurgical techniques with peripheral nerve surgery concepts, targeted sensory reinnervation appears to be a powerful adjunct to traditional TMR. Future studies are needed to determine its reproducibility and long-term viability.

Clinical Applications

Clinical reports have demonstrated that TMR can produce functional recovery in transhumeral amputees and shoulder disarticulation patients [11, 19, 20, 25]. In an earlier study, five patients

who underwent TMR were shown to produce sufficient EMG signals to operate advanced prosthetic arms [25]. By employing pattern recognition algorithms, these TMR patients were able to demonstrate improved performance during a series of functional tests. Another study of six TMR patients with transhumeral amputations displayed evidence of reinnervation at 8–12 weeks after surgery and pain levels similar to preTMR levels at 2 months post-surgery [19]. Patients were able to wear a myoelectric prosthesis by 1–2 months post-surgery and could simultaneously control elbow and hand prosthetic functions after only a few rehabilitation therapy sessions.

Cases of bilateral TMR procedures have also been reported [20, 25]. For example, a 41-yearold male with severe upper extremity burn injuries underwent a staged reconstructive approach 1 year after his initial injury. His surgeries included tissue expansion of the chest wall skin, multiple neuroma excisions, excision of heterotopic ossification from the scapula, and pedicled (latissimus dorsi) and free (gracilis) tissue flaps to prepare the amputation sites for TMR [20]. This patient was eventually fitted with bilateral myoelectric prostheses and able to perform multiple functional tasks independently.

Up to one-quarter of limb amputees develop chronic pain in the amputation stump, often due to neuroma formation [26]. This disorganized regeneration of axons within the scar tissue can result in chronic pain that is extremely difficult to treat and may complicate or prevent prosthesis wear. TMR techniques have the potential to alleviate this problem by providing an end-organ target for injured nerves [27]. Additionally, animal models of neuroma formation have demonstrated improved nerve morphology when nerve stumps are implanted into the muscle [28, 29]. In TMR, injured nerve stumps are connected to motor nerves, thus providing a more physiologic context for regeneration and theoretically preventing the random regrowth of nerve stumps that produces a neuroma.

In addition to utilizing TMR for late-stage reconstruction, TMR has also been employed during the early management of a traumatic amputation [21]. A 54-year-old lady sustained devastating crush injuries to her left upper arm that precluded replantation. Seventy-two hours after her initial washout, she underwent shoulder disarticulation and TMR with the goal of preventing neuroma formation, rerouting nerves before intense scarring occurred, and preparing the soft tissues for eventual prosthesis wear. Eight months after surgery, she demonstrated control of four separate myoelectric control sites and no neuroma pain, highlighting the potential of TMR in the acute trauma setting for select patients.

Future Directions

TMR has moved beyond proof of concept and has been successfully performed at several centers around the United States. Based on the pioneering work of Kuiken and others, above-elbow amputees now have the ability to regain intuitive control of increasingly advanced myoelectric prostheses. Continued research in multifunctional prosthetics and improved pattern recognition algorithms will allow patients to achieve a greater range of complex multi-joint functions. Moreover, advances in manufacturing, device design, and neural-prosthesis interface technologies will permit better biointegration of these prosthetic systems. The collaborative effort of surgeons, bioengineers, and rehabilitation specialists has made TMR a clinical reality with a promising future for upper limb amputees.

References

1. Ziegler-Graham K, MacKenzie EJ, Ephraim PL, Travison TG, Brookmeyer R. Estimating the prevalence of limb loss in the United States: 2005 to 2050. Arch Phys Med Rehabil. 2008;89:422–9.
2. Stansbury LG, Lalliss SJ, Branstetter JG, Bagg MR, Holcomb JB. Amputations in U.S. military personnel in the current conflicts in Afghanistan and Iraq. J Orthop Trauma. 2008;22:43–6.
3. Krueger CA, Wenke JC, Ficke JR. Ten years at war: comprehensive analysis of amputation trends. J Trauma Acute Care Surg. 2012;73(6 Suppl 5): S438–44.

4. Tintle SM, Baechler MF, Nanos 3rd GP, Forsberg JA, Potter BK. Traumatic and trauma-related amputations: part II: upper extremity and future directions. J Bone Joint Surg Am. 2010;92:2934–45.
5. Hanley MA, Ehde DM, Jensen M, Czerniecki J, Smith DG, Robinson LR. Chronic pain associated with upper-limb loss. Am J Phys Med Rehabil. 2009;88:742–51; quiz 752, 779.
6. McKechnie PS, John A. Anxiety and depression following traumatic limb amputation: a systematic review. Injury. 2014;45:1859–66.
7. Schultz AE, Kuiken TA. Neural interfaces for control of upper limb prostheses: the state of the art and future possibilities. PM R. 2011;3:55–67.
8. Childress DS. Closed-loop control in prosthetic systems: historical perspective. Ann Biomed Eng. 1980;8:293–303.
9. Shores JT, Brandacher G, Lee WA. Hand and upper extremity transplantation: an update of outcomes in the worldwide experience. Plast Reconstr Surg. 2014;135:351e–60.
10. Elliott RM, Tintle SM, Levin LS. Upper extremity transplantation: current concepts and challenges in an emerging field. Curr Rev Musculoskelet Med. 2014;7:83–8.
11. Kuiken TA, Li G, Lock BA, et al. Targeted muscle reinnervation for real-time myoelectric control of multifunction artificial arms. JAMA. 2009;301: 619–28.
12. Luff AR, Webb SN. Electromyographic activity in the cross-reinnervated soleus muscle of unrestrained cats. J Physiol. 1985;365:13–28.
13. Nagano A, Tsuyama N, Ochiai N, Hara T, Takahashi M. Direct nerve crossing with the intercostal nerve to treat avulsion injuries of the brachial plexus. J Hand Surg Am. 1989;14:980–5.
14. Miller LA, Stubblefield KA, Lipschutz RD, Lock BA, Kuiken TA. Improved myoelectric prosthesis control using targeted reinnervation surgery: a case series. IEEE Trans Neural Syst Rehabil Eng. 2008;16: 46–50.
15. Zhou P, Lowery MM, Englehart KB, et al. Decoding a new neural machine interface for control of artificial limbs. J Neurophysiol. 2007;98:2974–82.
16. Scheme E, Englehart K. Electromyogram pattern recognition for control of powered upper-limb prostheses: state of the art and challenges for clinical use. J Rehabil Res Dev. 2011;48:643–59.
17. Weir RF, Troyk PR, DeMichele GA, Kerns DA, Schorsch JF, Maas H. Implantable myoelectric sensors (IMESs) for intramuscular electromyogram recording. IEEE Trans Biomed Eng. 2009;56: 159–71.
18. Schwartz AB, Cui XT, Weber DJ, Moran DW. Brain-controlled interfaces: movement restoration with neural prosthetics. Neuron. 2006;52:205–20.
19. Dumanian GA, Ko JH, O'Shaughnessy KD, Kim PS, Wilson CJ, Kuiken TA. Targeted reinnervation for transhumeral amputees: current surgical technique

and update on results. Plast Reconstr Surg. 2009;124:863–9.

20. Cheesborough JE, Smith LH, Kuiken TA, Dumanian GA. Targeted muscle reinnervation and advanced prosthetic arms. Semin Plast Surg. 2015;29:62–72.

21. Cheesborough JE, Souza JM, Dumanian GA, Bueno Jr RA. Targeted muscle reinnervation in the initial management of traumatic upper extremity amputation injury. Hand (N Y). 2014;9:253–7.

22. Hebert JS, Olson JL, Morhart MJ, et al. Novel targeted sensory reinnervation technique to restore functional hand sensation after transhumeral amputation. IEEE Trans Neural Syst Rehabil Eng. 2014;22:765–73.

23. Kuiken TA, Miller LA, Lipschutz RD, et al. Targeted reinnervation for enhanced prosthetic arm function in a woman with a proximal amputation: a case study. Lancet. 2007;369:371–80.

24. Kuiken TA, Marasco PD, Lock BA, Harden RN, Dewald JP. Redirection of cutaneous sensation from the hand to the chest skin of human amputees with targeted reinnervation. Proc Natl Acad Sci U S A. 2007;104:20061–6.

25. Kuiken T. Targeted reinnervation for improved prosthetic function. Phys Med Rehabil Clin N Am. 2006;17:1–13.

26. Pierce Jr RO, Kernek CB, Ambrose 2nd TA. The plight of the traumatic amputee. Orthopedics. 1993;16:793–7.

27. Souza JM, Cheesborough JE, Ko JH, Cho MS, Kuiken TA, Dumanian GA. Targeted muscle reinnervation: a novel approach to postamputation neuroma pain. Clin Orthop Relat Res. 2014;472:2984–90.

28. Kim PS, Ko JH, O'Shaughnessy KK, Kuiken TA, Pohlmeyer EA, Dumanian GA. The effects of targeted muscle reinnervation on neuromas in a rabbit rectus abdominis flap model. J Hand Surg Am. 2012;37: 1609–16.

29. Ko JH, Kim PS, O'Shaughnessy KD, Ding X, Kuiken TA, Dumanian GA. A quantitative evaluation of gross versus histologic neuroma formation in a rabbit forelimb amputation model: potential implications for the operative treatment and study of neuromas. J Brachial Plex Peripher Nerve Inj. 2011;6:8.

David Polonet and Howard Bar-Eli

Principles of Acute Orthopedic Injury Treatment

Understanding the nature of orthopedic injuries and the basis of orthopedic care allows for interdisciplinary management of patients with musculoskeletal injuries or deficits. Optimal care of the patient with musculoskeletal pathology requires close collaboration between orthopedists and specialists in the rehabilitative arena. Where interaction is inadequate, the patient may have limited access to various diagnostic and therapeutic options and modalities. The outcome will thus likely be adversely affected without the benefit of a coordinated team providing specialized care.

The goals of orthopedic care are straightforward conceptually but challenging to achieve in the setting of pathologic processes. Musculoskeletal optimization includes minimization of pain and maximization of function. Outcomes such as motion and strength are of paramount importance. Interventions should be considered in terms of the

likelihood of success in the context of risks assumed. Even nonoperative or conservative management has inherent risks, such as failing to achieve a satisfactory outcome where more aggressive treatment might have achieved greater results.

On the other hand, surgery can have more dramatic complications at times. The potential risks and benefits of various treatment options should be considered by the caregiver and by the patient in the decision process, and a treatment plan agreed upon by both parties. Experience and attention to detail enables caregivers to educate patients appropriately regarding anticipated outcomes. Furthermore, it is important for patients to understand that it is not always possible to avoid complications.

Orthopedic problems may have widely variable etiologies. As with other organ systems, we may encounter congenital and developmental conditions; degenerative processes; neoplastic challenges; traumatic, iatrogenic, acquired, or inherited metabolic conditions; and inflammatory and infectious disease states. Often, predictable outcomes are not well established or evidence-based medicine is lacking. Levels of evidence in orthopedic care tend to be underwhelming. Appreciating the merits of evidence-based medicine, practitioners must learn to properly interpret studies and evaluate literature critically. Establishing a working diagnosis, understanding the natural course of a disease or injury condition, and the likelihood of improving

D. Polonet, MD (✉)
Jersey Shore University Medical Center,
Neptune City, NJ, USA

Rutgers Robert Wood Johnson Medical School,
New Brunswick, NJ, USA
e-mail: dpolonet@yahoo.com

H. Bar-Eli, MD
Rutgers Robert Wood Johnson Medical School,
New Brunswick, NJ, USA
e-mail: chambareli@gmail.com

© Springer International Publishing Switzerland 2017
A.I. Elkwood et al. (eds.), *Rehabilitative Surgery*, DOI 10.1007/978-3-319-41406-5_23

the results should be appreciated. As opposed to evolving surgical techniques, which may not have longer-term outcome studies, more conservative treatment methods will often have more predictable courses.

Still, where the natural course of a given disorder may be generally characterized, individual host nuances in pathology, medical comorbidities, and expectations may prove crucial to helping establish an individual care algorithm. While the nature of a pathologic condition will often establish some "ground rules" specific to that condition, particular patient populations will have needs that may not apply to other patients. Treating pediatric populations must include an understanding of the immature physiology (e.g., open growth plates, rapid healing, immature pain response, and psychological effects). In mature populations, a fracture should be understood in the context of potential conditions like metastatic carcinoma, osteoporosis, or diabetes, medications that may affect the patient's course (such as steroids or bisphosphonates), pre-injury function and independence, social support, cultural implications, financial concerns, and emotional characteristics. A practitioner treating cancer-related problems must be sensitive to the various concurrent or sequential modalities involved in care, immunologic and healing challenges, unique psychosocial elements, and specific prognosis (among other issues).

Timing of interventions may be important. Early intervention in the management of developmental hip dysplasia may dramatically alter the progression of disability [1]. Infection, unrecognized or untreated, can progress. Planned, staged interventions may improve outcomes [2]. The treatment of muscle tightness or contracture differs from that of joint contracture or arthrofibrosis, and untreated tightness will often lead to fixed deformity and loss of function [3]. A predictable post-injury or postoperative deficit can thus result in loss of function that may be treated successfully only with surgical intervention, or worse, may be permanent. Delays in the initiation of postoperative rehabilitative therapy should be avoided [4]. Orthopedic surgeons must clearly establish postoperative instructions and restrictions. Where questions remain, direct communication and clarification are crucial.

Common Orthopedic Complications and Treatments

Acute Blood Loss and Vascular Injury

Acute complications of musculoskeletal pathology may be manifested as pain and dysfunction. Following injury, hemorrhage and inflammation are typical. While life-threatening bleeding is uncommon, the population continues to age, and the use of anticoagulants has become quite prevalent [5]. This presents practitioners with the concerns of hemorrhage acutely and with the potential need to interrupt anticoagulant therapy to allow for safe surgical intervention. Intraoperatively, hemostasis must be achieved or ongoing blood loss coupled with wound complications may result. Drains may be utilized to decrease the risk of postoperative hematoma, although no statistical advantage to the use of drains has been proven [6]. Finally, the postoperative restarting of anticoagulants raises challenges as the subsequent risk of surgical site hematoma or wound drainage may compromise the outcome of an otherwise successful procedure. These concerns must be balanced with the risk of thrombosis [7].

Arterial injury is a rare complication of orthopedic procedures and may manifest as bleeding and/or ischemia. Outcomes may be severely affected. Bleeding may require transfusion and secondary procedures, such as arterial repair, embolization or ligation, grafting, or bypass. Failure to adequately identify and control bleeding can be a life-threatening complication. Resultant hematoma formation may result in secondary complications, such as infection, neurologic compromise, compartment syndrome, and wound complications. Ischemia and reperfusion may result in neuromuscular deficits, limb loss, and renal and metabolic complications.

Venous Thromboembolic Disease

Venous thromboembolic disease (VTED) is a known complication of both orthopedic conditions and interventions. Obstruction of deep veins in the extremities, or proximally, may compromise outflow with local or regional swelling and pain. Chronic sequelae, known as post-thrombotic syndrome, may be significant. Thrombi may embolize and risk migrating to the pulmonary arteries causing potentially fatal hypoxia. In patients with a patent foramen ovale, this may manifest as stroke [8]. Multiple risk factors for VTED have been identified. Host-related factors merit consideration of patient risk prior to interventions; these include history of previous deep-vein thrombosis or varicose veins, age, use of oral contraceptives, pregnancy, cancer, myocardial infarction, and stroke [9, 10].

Injury and surgery-related risk factors also exist, including increased surgical duration, arthroplasty, or proximal lower extremity fracture surgery [10, 11]. Studies have shown that in the absence of thromboprophylaxis, the incidence of proximal deep-vein thrombosis in patients undergoing total knee arthroplasty ranges from 5 to 22%, while in patients undergoing total hip arthroplasty the range is from 16 to 36% [9–13]. The incidence of fatal pulmonary embolism was estimated to be 0.1–1.7% in patients undergoing total knee arthroplasty and 0.1–4% in those undergoing total hip arthroplasty. In patients undergoing hip fracture surgery, although the incidence of proximal deep-vein thrombosis is 23–30%, comparable with those in patients undergoing hip or knee arthroplasty, the incidence of fatal pulmonary embolism is markedly higher, estimated to be between 2.5 and 13% of patients [9–13].

Clinical trials have shown thromboprophylaxis to reduce the risk of deep-vein thrombosis in patients undergoing total hip arthroplasty by between 23 and 78%, with lower but significant risk reductions after knee arthroplasty or hip fracture surgery [14–17]. Preventative modalities that have been shown to be efficacious include mechanical interventions such as compressive stockings and pneumatic compression pumps. Chemical modalities may be orally, intravenously, or subcutaneously administered. The agent, dosage, schedule, and route may differ for particular indications.

Fat Embolism Syndrome (FES)

Fat embolism syndrome (FES) is the obstruction of vessels by particulate marrow debris, with inflammatory mediators exacerbating the clinical picture. This can manifest as tachycardia, hypoxia, and altered mental status. This phenomenon is clinically important and may be seen in the acute setting of fracture and intramedullary instrumentation of bones. FES can affect the course of recovery of a patient vis-à-vis pulmonary compromise, with a mortality rate of up to 20%; the most common and significant clinical sequelae are usually acute, and ultimately good recovery is seen in survivors.

Neurologic Injury

Any orthopedic injury or procedure can be accompanied by focal neurologic injury, such as traction neuropraxia or generalized sensorimotor compromise, as is seen in the setting of compartment syndrome. It is appropriate for surgeons to know the rate of postsurgical neurologic deficit a patient is at risk for with any relevant procedures, as the end result is typically dissatisfactory to a patient in this setting.

For example, nerve injuries are reported to occur in 1–2% of patients undergoing rotator cuff surgery, 1–8% of patients undergoing surgery for anterior shoulder instability, and 1–4% of patients undergoing prosthetic shoulder arthroplasty [18]. The prevalence of major nerve injuries during THA has been reported to be around 1% [19]. The nerves at risk are dependent on the surgical approach, with sciatic nerve injury most commonly seen. While this may seem like a low incidence, it should be appreciated that this is equivalent to the incidence of infection after THA, and infection gets considerably more attention. Recovery of normal function is seen in only

35–40 % of cases [20]. Pelvic and acetabular fractures are high-energy injuries, and concomitant neurologic deficits have been reported in up to 20–25 % of cases [21, 22]. Full recovery of function is infrequent in this setting.

Managing neurologic injury or compromise begins with the identification of the deficit and subsequent assessment. Characterizing the injury requires a detailed and focused history and examination, with incorporation of nerve studies such as EMG and NCV as indicated. Acutely, identifying ongoing insults and removing them may be helpful. Acute nerve exploration and decompression or transposition may be useful in select circumstances. Splinting and rehabilitating an extremity affected by neurologic injury may be very important in preventing debilitating contractures. This can, in turn, help a patient avoid additional and preventable surgery. The treatment of neurologic deficits is addressed in greater detail in other chapters.

Acute Infection and Chronic Osteomyelitis

Infection is always a concern, and the sterile environment within an operating room or even during a minimally invasive procedure that can be performed in the emergency department should be treated with the highest regard. Infections can be managed in several ways from as simple as a course of oral antibiotics to serial operations for irrigation and debridement coupled with a prolonged course of parenteral antibiotics in order to eradicate the infection. Complications can range from altered outcomes, loss of function, loss of limb, to sepsis and death if treatment is delayed.

A laboratory workup of an infection usually starts with a CBC, ESR, and CRP [23]. If a patient is presenting with systemic symptoms, blood cultures may be drawn and are helpful in isolating an organism in cases of joint sepsis or osteomyelitis. Imaging starts with plain radiographs [24], which may show a periosteal reaction (*involucrum*) in the setting of chronic osteomyelitis, or a walled off abscess in bone

(*sequestrum*). In the event that plain radiographs are negative, MRI with and without contrast, Technetium-99 (Tc-99) bone scan, and Indium tagged WBC scan are other options.

Treatment for a septic joint or musculoskeletal abscess (bone and/or soft tissue) is irrigation and debridement of nonviable tissue with intraoperative cultures. An infectious disease consultation is warranted so the appropriate antibiotic can be administered. Local antibiograms should be referenced when choosing antibiotics, as rates of resistance can vary based on geographic location. Antibiotics are usually delivered through a peripherally inserted central catheter (PICC) line for approximately 6 weeks. The treatment of a septic prosthetic joint can vary from irrigation and debridement with partial component exchange to explanting the prosthesis with insertion of a temporary antibiotic-impregnated cement spacer in addition to systemic antibiotics [25] (Figs. 23.1 and 23.2).

Acute and Chronic Soft Tissue and Wound Complications

Since there is a natural inflammatory process during wound healing, it may be challenging to differentiate an actual infection from the natural healing process. Normal tissue healing and repair undergoes an inflammatory stage where immune cells such as macrophages consume bacteria and necrotic tissue. This is followed by a stage where precursor cells differentiate into the appropriate cells in the healing of the soft

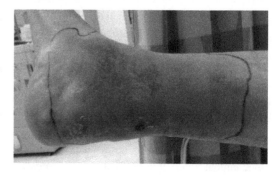

Fig. 23.1 Cellulitis of medial ankle

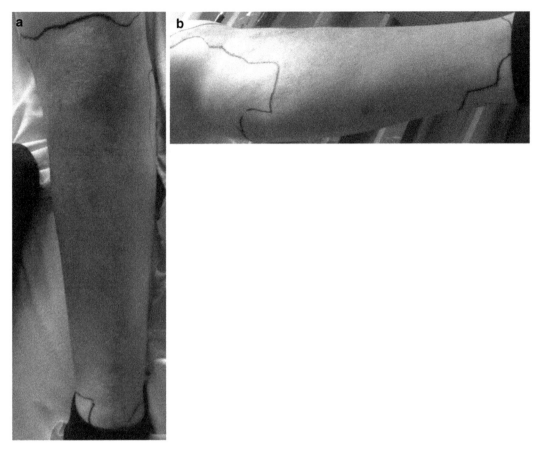

Fig. 23.2 (**a, b**). Recurrent cellulitis in a patient who had undergone fixation for a tibial plateau fracture. The patient developed osteomyelitis and required implant removal

tissue layer. Lastly, the new tissue needs to mature and become stronger through a process known as remodeling, which may take over a year. Clinically, the skin may appear warm and erythematous, have a scab or *eschar* over the incision or wound, feel indurated, and be tender to palpation. The method of skin closure itself may cause local skin irritation seen more commonly with skin staples as opposed to suture material. The erythema in this case is usually confined to the area around the staples and there is a sharp demarcation between color of the irritated skin and normal surrounding skin. There is also no associated drainage with this condition as may be the case with an infection. In the case of a cellulitis, the erythema is more diffuse and has less of a distinct border in the vicinity of the incision.

Another complication that may be seen acutely is wound edge necrosis. Patient-based factors such as poor nutrition or diabetes may impair the body's ability to heal an incision leading to wound dehiscence. In this scenario, the body cannot heal from the trauma caused to the skin even in a controlled setting. An extrinsic cause would be tissue strangulation and ischemia from sutures being tied too tightly or having too much tension across the incision or wound. This can lead to wound dehiscence if the necrosis is severe enough (Fig. 23.3).

In such a case, or if the dehiscence is from another cause, it is important to determine the depth of the dehiscence, whether it is superficial and above the fascia or deep extending beyond the fascia. If the dehiscence is superficial, then monitoring the wound and providing local wound

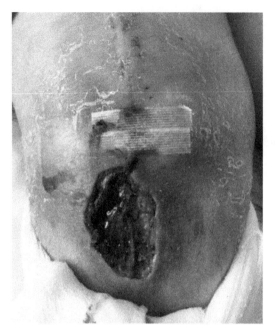

Fig. 23.3 Wound dehiscence and necrosis within 2 weeks of a primary knee arthroplasty

effect, and seromas may become secondarily infected. If located near the spine, it can cause spinal cord compression.

Both collections will be difficult to see on plain radiographs and warrant more advanced imaging such as ultrasound, CT scans, or MRI with and without contrast. The clinician must take into account the patients presenting symptoms such as systemic signs of infection during the workup of this collection. Labs such as CBC with differential, ESR, and CRP are a good start to check if an inflammatory process is occurring in the body and, at the very least, can serve as a baseline for future trending. If the lab values are elevated, once treatment is initiated, the CRP usually decreases first, within 48–72 h, if the treatment was correct. Radiographically guided percutaneous drainage of abscesses can decompress some of these fluid collections and save the patient a formal irrigation and debridement in the operating room with general anesthesia.

care or negative pressure wound therapy to assist in wound closure via secondary intention healing will suffice. If the fascia is involved, wound exploration and revision closure may help avoid prolonged healing and infection.

When the fascial layer is not closed properly or if the closure fails, a hernia can develop. This complication is known to occur after iliac crest bone graft harvest [26]. It can also occur in the thigh or lower leg. This may cause localized pain to the patient and it may be cosmetically displeasing depending on the location and the person's body habitus.

Additional complications involving soft tissues include walled off fluid collections. One is a collection of serous fluid that superficial, known as a seroma, and the other is an abscess, which implies a collection of purulent material. A seroma may develop around a foreign body or fill in a void in soft tissues that may be created surgically or after trauma. The body may not reabsorb the reactive fluid or a foreign body may irritate the local surrounding tissues and cause the fluid to accumulate as the body protects itself. Both types of fluid collections can cause pain or a mass

Nonunion or Fixation Failure

Most fractures heal when treated appropriately, but some fractures will fail to heal and develop what is termed a "nonunion." Certain features are typically necessary for fractures to heal, such as sufficient stabilization, vascularity (or blood flow), absence of infection with appropriate soft tissue coverage, and sufficient host nutrition. On the other hand, there may be risk factors for nonunion as well. These include hypothyroidism, diabetes mellitus, smoking, vitamin D deficiency, and chemotherapeutic agents. The point at which a slowly healing fracture is distinguished from a nonunion can be a function of a clinician's discretion and may vary from bone to bone. As an example, a typical description of a humeral shaft nonunion is "no evidence of radiographic healing 6 months after an injury" [27].

Three types of nonunion are described: hypertrophic, atrophic, and oligotrophic. A hypertrophic nonunion demonstrates callus around the fracture site. However, the callus does not bridge the fracture site. This scenario is attributed to a lack of stability. The body has the biological capacity to form new bone demonstrated by the callus, but excessive fracture motion prevents the bone from uniting across the fracture site. With an atrophic nonunion, the exact opposite is true. The stability may be adequate, but the local or systemic biologic response to form new bone is lacking, therefore no callus forms. The host's nutritional status may be inadequate and unable to provide the necessary factors for new bone generation [28]. Oligotrophic nonunions show some capacity to heal, but is insufficient given the needs at the fracture site. One example would be a poor reduction or alignment of a fracture that may be solved by revision of the fracture reduction and more stability.

When fractures do not unite, under physiologic stresses, any metallic implant will mechanically fatigue over time. If the bone does not fail at the bone-implant interface, ultimately the implant will fail. Identifying a failure to progress toward union may allow a surgeon to intervene prior to fixation failure and correct the problem preemptively. Thus, the determination of a "delayed union" may allow fixation implant retention, and a less extensive surgical intervention may allow for successful fracture healing.

Deformity/Malunion

"Deformity" is a broader term when describing how a bone did not heal properly. "Deformity" includes leg-length discrepancy, whereas "malunion" encompasses varus, valgus, rotation, procurvatum, and recurvatum. When reconstructing a bone or a limb, it is important to restore its proper alignment, length, and rotation. Restoring these three factors restores the normal mechanics to the bone with the muscles attached to and acting upon it; the joints above and below that particular bone will consequently be affected.

If, for example, someone sustains a tibia or femur fracture that heals in varus, there are increased joint forces through the medial compartment of the knee, which already sustains 70–80 % of the weight-bearing load of the knee. In order to enable gait, the patient will compensate at the ankle joint, causing a valgus deformity

and predisposing the ankle to osteoarthritis from abnormal wear of its cartilage. Gait can also be affected by a sagittal plane deformity such as recurvatum (apex posterior) or procurvatum (apex anterior) deformity of the tibia because the knee cannot fully extend for a proper heel strike or may not generate enough power during toe-off entering the next stride.

Certain bones and joints may tolerate greater levels of deformity. The humerus can tolerate 4–6 times the acceptable deformity of a tibia with acceptable functional outcomes. One such reason has to do with the ability of the glenohumeral joint (shoulder) to compensate for deformity of the humerus since it has such a large range of motion and will still be able to accomplish the goal of positioning the hand where it is necessary in space. Altered forces in the lower extremity, by contrast, rapidly manifest in problems due to the increased demands of weight-bearing during ambulation.

Long-term consequences of deformity and malunion can lead to pain, joint contractures, ligamentous instability or imbalance (contractures and laxity on opposite sides of the joint), and ultimately joint degeneration. Uncorrected deformity with persistent pain and dysfunction may be treatable with joint replacement (arthroplasty). In the setting of joint arthroplasty, the surgery may be more technically difficult if ligaments are imbalanced, and the joint may not perform well without the use of special equipment and possibly customized implants.

Arthritis and Avascular Necrosis

There are several types of arthritis: inflammatory, osteoarthritis, posttraumatic, and septic. Osteoarthritis has four characteristic radiographic signs, which are asymmetric joint space narrowing, subchondral sclerosis, osteophytes, and subchondral cysts. Patients may present with complaints of pain, limited motion, stiffness, especially after periods of immobilization, and limited function. On exam the patient may have an erythematous, warm, edematous, tender joint, with an effusion. The most important condition to rule out in this circumstance is an acutely septic joint. Fevers are typically absent in the setting of an osteoarthritic or posttraumatic arthritic flare and inflammatory markers can be normal. If the patient's history and clinical picture are unclear, performing a joint aspiration and sending the synovial fluid for gram stain and culture, crystals (to rule out gout), and cell count can rule out infection.

Part of the radiographic workup in posttraumatic arthritis and osteoarthritis especially in the lower extremity weight-bearing joints are weight-bearing radiographs. Avascular necrosis (AVN) results from a vascular insult to the bone's blood supply. Risk factors include hypercoagulable disorders, chronic alcohol usage, steroids, chemotherapeutic agents, HIV/AIDS, and excessive soft tissue stripping from a trauma or iatrogenic soft tissue stripping. The use of alendronate ® delayed subchondral bone collapse in the femoral head for 2 years with findings of AVN on MRI and bone scan [29]. However, only 10 % of members of the American Association of Hip and Knee Surgeons (AAHKS) treat pre-collapse hip AVN with bisphosphonates [30].

There is questionable efficacy of bisphosphonates for shoulder and knee AVN as well as unknown effects in smaller areas and bones such as scaphoid, lunate, and capitellum. Presenting symptoms of avascular necrosis can be swelling, pain at rest, pain with motion, and restricted motion due to abnormal mechanics of the joint containing the bone with AVN. Treatment consists of identifying reversible causes or underlying disorders and rendering the proper treatment for those. Immobilization or at least decreasing the stress on the affected bone is another initial step of treatment. MRI is more sensitive in detecting avascular necrosis compared to plain radiographs.

Heterotopic Ossification

Bone may form in areas not associated with normal growth or fracture healing. This pathologic condition is known as heterotopic ossification (H.O.). The abnormal bone usually forms in areas of muscle issue, creating painful or limited joint motion. It is most well known for formation about the hip and elbow after trauma or surgery. Risk factors include head or spinal cord trauma and soft tissue damage (i.e., iatrogenic from surgery or from the trauma itself) and in the setting of burn injuries.

There are two methods employed prophylactically to decrease the risk of heterotopic ossification formation in high-risk patients. The first is with nonsteroidal anti-inflammatory drug (NSAID) therapy, and the second is radiation therapy [31, 32]. Indomethacin is commonly administered for 6 weeks. Radiation therapy is performed within a day preoperatively or the first 48–72 h postoperatively (at least in the setting of acetabular surgery).

Workup of heterotopic ossification is performed with plain radiographs and bone scan at times. In the event of surgery, a CT scan of the affected area can help with surgical planning.

When heterotopic ossification causes significant pain or functional limitations, surgical excision is indicated. Outcomes are generally very favorable, but may vary depending on anatomic location. H.O. may involve or abut other crucial structures, such as skin, neurovascular structures, and ligaments. In complex cases, an experienced practitioner must approach surgery cautiously and with careful consideration of risks and anticipated outcomes. Heterotopic ossification can take 6 months to a year or more to fully "mature" before it is excised, or the risk of recurrence may be high (Fig. 23.4).

Contracture and Arthrofibrosis

Joint contractures can lead to deformity and affect function by causing limb length discrepancy, altering gait, and preventing motion necessary for activities of daily living. Causes can be subdivided into intrinsic or extrinsic factors. Intrinsic factors that limit joint motion leading to contracture are due to irregularities in the joint itself, such as osteophytes, degenerative cartilage, pannus formation in the setting of inflammatory arthritides, or intra-articular adhesions.

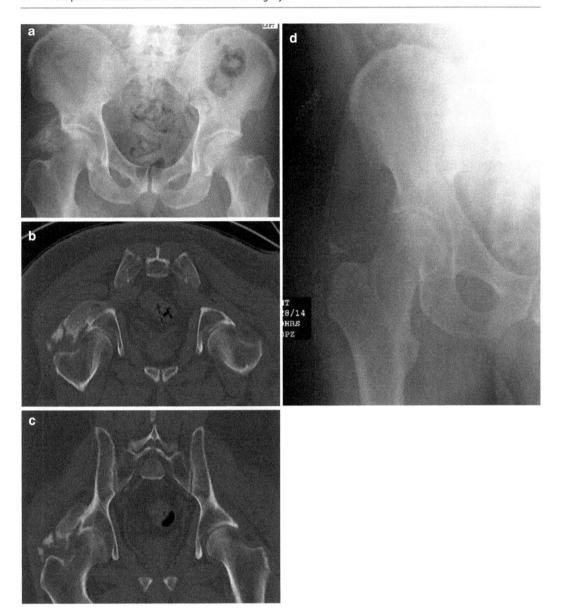

Fig. 23.4 (**a–d**) Following cardiac arrest with resuscitation and prolonged intubation, this patient had an excellent recovery but developed right hip heterotopic ossification (**a–c**). The resultant hip flexion/adduction deformity made sitting, lying supine, and walking very difficult. Range of motion was very restricted and pain was severe. Following excision (**d**), his quality of life was dramatically improved

Extrinsic causes to joint contracture limit joint mobility from tissues surrounding the joints such as muscular, capsular, or ligamentous tightness, heterotopic ossification, and skin contractures.

In order to regain motion, the treatment arm is split into nonoperative and surgical modalities. Almost universally, nonsurgical modalities should precede invasive interventions. Conservative and nonoperative measures include therapy, either physical or occupational, on a rigorous schedule to increase and regain motion. The therapy is a painful process, as muscles and periarticular soft tissues are being stretched and expanded on a daily basis by a therapist. In addition, a home exercise program that requires strict compliance is needed to continue with the progress the therapist achieves.

In the shoulder, in cases of adhesive capsulitis, NSAIDs are recommended if the patient tolerates the side effects.

Another modality to regain motion in the setting of a joint contracture is static progressive splinting. This splint is used commonly for elbow contractures because it can be done in the patient's home and under a controlled setting. The patient secures the splint to his/her elbow and turns a dial that stretches the elbow. When the stretching sensation is felt, the patient stops turning the dial to allow the elbow to acclimate to its new position. After a period of rest, the dial is turned again thereby increasing the amount of extension across the elbow. The same process can be performed to increase flexion. Dynamic splinting involves braces with an adjustable spring preload that exerts forces across a targeted joint.

Depending on the joint involved and the cause for the stiffness, timing for surgical intervention will vary. In the shoulder, arthroscopic capsular release with manual manipulation can be effective for adhesive capsulitis and contracture. In the knee, a manipulation under anesthesia (MUA) can be performed usually 6 weeks after a total knee arthroplasty if satisfactory flexion (90°) is not achieved. In contrast, after an ACL reconstruction, if >90° of flexion is not achieved between 4 and 12 weeks, then an MUA can be performed [33].

If the patient presents in an even more delayed fashion, beyond 6 weeks, a combined procedure of arthroscopic lysis of adhesions and MUA will be of benefit to the patient [34]. In the setting of a healing fracture, such as a tibial plateau fracture, an MUA is typically delayed until the fracture has healed. Arthroscopy of the knee for a lysis of adhesions for intrinsic contractures may be indicated. Elbow contractures are initially managed with static progressive or dynamic splinting, but if no improvement is noticed over time, arthroscopic or open contracture releases can be performed. Each procedure type, whether open or arthroscopic, has its own set risks and benefits. Risks of surgery include nerve injuries from portal placement, postoperative nerve entrapment within scar tissue, infection, hematoma, or wound healing complications (the latter two more likely

with open procedures) [35–38]. Extrinsic causes of contracture may be treated with muscle lengthening or release, depending on the site and severity of involvement.

Instability*

Instability of a joint can be caused by genetic factors leading to ligamentous laxity as in Ehlers-Danlos syndrome (collagen defect), degenerative or chronic overuse as in thumb CMC arthritis (degenerative tearing of volar oblique "beak" ligament) or "gamekeeper's thumb" (attenuation of ulnar collateral ligament of thumb MCP joint), or acutely traumatic like an ACL tear [39]. Symptoms of instability include pain (especially if acutely traumatic), clicking, locking, catching, and giving way. On physical exam this can manifest as an incongruent range of motion of a joint because of abnormal motion secondary to a damaged structure. Instability can also be assessed if a patient is apprehensive during a physical exam maneuver such as abduction/external rotation after a shoulder dislocation or lateral displacement of a patella after a patellar dislocation (stressing the damaged structures in each of these situations).

Imaging should start with plain x-rays of the involved joint. Sometimes instability can be suspected if a certain bone is broken (ulnar styloid, tibial spine) or based on how the joint is aligned (lateral displacement of thumb metacarpal in CMC arthritis, medial clear space in the ankle mortise). If plain films do not reveal the answer, because they capture a moment in time, then stress radiographs can be obtained. In the scenario of a distal fibular ankle fracture, first internally rotating the tibia 15° and then simultaneously dorsiflexing and externally rotating the foot to stress the deltoid ligament in the medial clear space of the ankle (tibiotalar) joint. A second example is a weight-bearing film to rule out a Lisfranc ligament (medial cuneiform to base of second metatarsal) injury. CT scans and MRIs may provide additional insight to the extent of the damaged structures (Fig. 23.5).

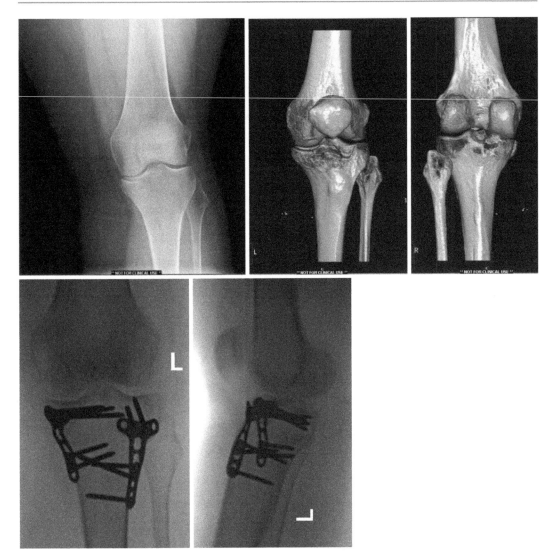

Fig. 23.5 This obese patient had a low-energy knee dislocation. Following initial closed reduction, plain radiographs suggested a medial tibial plateau irregularity that was better depicted on CT scan. The CT scan also demonstrated an anterolateral tibial plateau impaction and a PCL insertional avulsion posteriorly on the tibia. The patient exceeded the MRI scanner's weight limitation. The anterior bony injuries were treated surgically, but residual hyperextension laxity was noted. Additional stabilization with an external fixator was deemed necessary until the posterior bony/capsuloligamentous injury healed

Treatment options range from bracing and physical therapy rehabilitation to surgical repair or reconstruction of a ligament. In addition to fixing the damaged structure, an underlying cause for the injury should be sought. An example can be derived from a patient with recurrent patellar dislocations due to abnormal alignment of the lower extremity, which can be solved with a tibial tubercle osteotomy in some cases.

References

1. Guille JT, Pizzutillo PD, MacEwen GD. Developmental dysplasia of the hip from birth to six months. J Am Acad Orthop Surg. 2000;8: 232–42.
2. Sirkin M, Sanders R, DiPasquale T, Herscovci Jr D. A staged protocol for soft tissue management in the treatment of complex pilon fractures. J Orthop Trauma. 2004;8(Supp):S32–8.

3. Robinson CM, Seah KT, Chee YH, Hindle P, Murray IR. Frozen shoulder. J Bone Joint Surg Br. 2012;94:1–9.

4. McGregor AH, Probyn K, Cro S, Doré CJ, Burton AK, Balagué F, Pincus T, Fairbank J. Rehabilitation following lumbar surgery for spinal stenosis. Cochrane Database Syst Rev. 2013;12:CD009644.

5. Kirley K, Qato DM, Kornfield R, Stafford RS, Alexander GC. National trends in oral anticoagulant use in the United States, 2007–2011. Circ Cardiovasc Qual Outcomes. 2012;5:615–21.

6. Quinn M, Bowe A, Galvin R, Dawson P, O'Byrne J. The use of postoperative suction drainage in total knee arthroplasty: a systematic review. Int Orthop. 2015;39:653–8.

7. Douketis JD, Spyropoulos AC, et al. Perioperative bridging anticoagulation in patients with atrial fibrillation. N Engl J Med. 2015;373:823–33.

8. Chun KJ. Patent foramen ovale and cryptogenic stroke. Korean Circ J. 2008;38:631–7.

9. Geerts WH, Pineo GF, Heit JA, et al. Prevention of venous thromboembolism. Chest. 2004;126:338S–400.

10. Kahn SR. The clinical diagnosis of deep venous thrombosis: integrating incidence, risk factors, and symptoms and signs. Arch Intern Med. 1998;158:2315–23.

11. Nicholaides AN, Breddin HK, Fareed J, et al. Prevention of venous thromboembolism. International Consensus Statement. Guidelines compiled in accordance with the scientific evidence. Int Angiol. 2001;20:1–37.

12. Edselberg J, Ollendorf D, Oster G. Venous thromboembolism following major orthopedic surgery: review of epidemiology and economics. Am J Health Syst Pharm. 2001;58 Suppl 2:S4–57.

13. Gillespie W, Murray D, Gregg RJ, Warwick D. Risks and benefits of prophylaxis against venous thromboembolism in orthopaedic surgery. J Bone Joint Surg Br. 2000;82:475–9.

14. Freedman KB, Brookenthal KR, Fitzgerald RH, Lonner JH. A meta-analysis of thromboembolic prophylaxis in total hip arthroplasty. J Bone Joint Surg Am. 2000;82A:929–38.

15. Brookenthal KR, Freedman KB, Lotke PA, Fitzgerald RH, Lonner JH. A meta-analysis of thromboembolic prophylaxis in total knee arthroplasty. J Arthroplasty. 2001;26:293–300.

16. Westrich GH, Haas SB, Mosca P, Peterson M. Meta-analysis of thromboembolic prophylaxis after total knee arthroplasty. J Bone Joint Surg Br. 2000;82:795–800.

17. Zufferey P, Laporte S, Quenet S, et al. Optimal low-molecular-weight heparin regimen in major orthopaedic surgery. A meta-analysis of randomized trials. Thromb Haemost. 2003;90:654–61.

18. Boardman 3rd ND, Cofield RH. Neurologic complications of shoulder surgery. Clin Orthop Relat Res. 1999;368:44–53.

19. Farrell CM, Springer BD, Haidukewych GJ, et al. Motor nerve palsy following primary total hip arthroplasty. J Bone Joint Surg Am. 2005;87:2619–25.

20. Schmalzried TP, Noordin S, Amstutz HC. Update on nerve palsy associated with total hip replacement. Clin Orthop Relat Res. 1997;344:188–206. Letournel E, Judet R. Fractures of the acetabulum. 2nd ed. New York: Springer; 1993.

21. Giannoudis PV, Da Costa AA, Raman R, et al. Double-crush syndrome after acetabular fractures. A sign of poor prognosis. J Bone Joint Surg Br. 2005;87(3):401–7.

22. Wright R, Barrett K, Christie MJ, et al. Acetabular fractures: long-term follow-up of open reduction and internal fixation. J Orthop Trauma. 1994;8(5):397–403.

23. Neumaier M, Scherer MA. C-reactive protein levels for early detection of postoperative infection after fracture surgery in 787 patients. Acta Orthop. 2008;79(3):428–32.

24. Calhoun JH, Manring MM. Adult osteomyelitis. Infect Dis Clin North Am. 2005;19(4):765–86.

25. Zalavras CG, Patzakis MJ, Holtom P. Local antibiotic therapy in the treatment of open fractures and osteomyelitis. Clin Orthop Relat Res. 2004;427:86–93.

26. Ahlmann E, Patzakis M, Roidis N, et al. Comparison of anterior and posterior iliac crest bone grafts in terms of harvest-site morbidity and functional outcomes. J Bone Joint Surg Am. 2002;84A:716–20.

27. Cadet ER, Yin B, Schulz B, et al. Proximal humerus and humeral shaft nonunions. J Am Acad Orthop Surg. 2013;21:538–47.

28. Brinker MR, O'Connor DP, Monla YT, et al. Metabolic and endocrine abnormalities in patients with nonunions. J Orthop Trauma. 2007;21:557–70.

29. Lai K-A, Shen W-J, Yang C-Y, et al. The use of alendronate to prevent early collapse of the femoral head in patients with nontraumatic osteonecrosis. A randomized clinical study. J Bone Joint Surg Am. 2005;87:2155–9.

30. McGrory BJ, York SC, Iorio R, Macaulay W, et al. Current practices of AAHKS members in the treatment of adult osteonecrosis of the femoral head. J Bone Joint Surg Am. 2007;89:1194–204.

31. McLaren AC. Prophylaxis with indomethacin for heterotopic bone after open reduction of fracture of the acetabulum. J Bone Joint Surg Am. 1990;72:245–7.

32. Bosse M, Poka A, Reinert CM, et al. Heterotopic ossification as a complication of acetabular fracture. J Bone Joint Surg Am. 1988;70:1231–7.

33. Noyes FR, Berrios-Torres S, Barber-Westin SD, et al. Prevention of permanent arthrofibrosis after anterior cruciate ligament reconstruction alone or combined with associated procedures: a prospective study in 443 knees. Knee Surg Sports Traumatol Arthrosc. 2000;8:196–206.

34. Magit D, Wolff A, Sutton K, Medvecky M. Arthrofibrosis of the knee. J Am Acad Orthop Surg. 2007;15:682–94.

35. Dumonski ML, Arciero RA, Mazzocca AD. Ulnar nerve palsy after elbow arthroscopy. Arthroscopy. 2006;22:577.e1–3.

36. Haapaniemi T, Berggren M, Adolfsson L. Complete transection of the median and radial nerves during arthroscopic release of post-traumatic elbow contracture. Arthroscopy. 1999;15:784–7.

37. Ruch DS, Poehling GG. Anterior interosseus nerve injury following elbow arthroscopy. Arthroscopy. 1997;13:756–8.

38. Kelly EW, Morrey BF, O'Driscoll SW. Complications of elbow arthroscopy. J Bone Joint Surg Am. 2001;83:25–34.

39. Pellegrini Jr VD. The ABJS 2005 Nicolas Andry Award: osteoarthritis and injury at the base of the human thumb: survival of the fittest? Clin Orthop Relat Res. 2005;438:266–76.

Upper Extremity Neuromuscular Disorders

24

Kenneth R. Means, Christopher L. Forthman,
W. Hugh Baugher, Ryan D. Katz,
Raymond A. Wittstadt, and Keith A. Segalman

Upper Extremity Basic Orthopedic Principles

Normal bone healing occurs not with scarring but rather through replacing the injured bone with new bone, making it a unique human tissue. Bone healing occurs via a gradual progression through four different stages. The same basic stages of bone healing occur following a fracture or a surgical trauma, such as an osteotomy or fusion procedure.

The initial stage is the *inflammatory stage* when inflammatory cells migrate to and hematoma forms at the site of injury. The second stage is called the *soft callus stage*. Here, cartilage cells enter the injured area and create a cartilage matrix. This matrix is moderately stable mechanically but not yet calcified. The third stage is the *hard callus stage*, in which the matrix becomes calcified and is removed slowly while osteoblasts replace it with osteoid, or bone substance. At this stage definitive

mechanical stability is established, and the fracture is clinically healed. The final stage is *remodeling* in which osteoclasts and osteoblasts work to remove and replace bone, respectively. This final stage can occur for several years and seeks to return the injured bone to its native shape and biomechanical characteristics as well as possible.

Bone healing is sometimes also described as either primary or secondary. Secondary bone healing is the process that has just been described above and occurs for all bones that heal without rigid fixation. Clinical examples include healing in a splint, cast, or with surgical pinning or intramedullary rods. In these instances, the bone is said to have relative stability or fixation during the healing process. Primary bone healing has traditionally been thought to occur when bone fractures are fixed with plates and screws or interfragmentary compression screws. This type of stabilization is termed absolute, or rigid, fixation. Primary bone healing has classically been thought to occur without callous formation and instead via direct extension of "cutting cones" containing osteoclasts and followed by osteoblasts and other cells from one side of the fracture into the other side of the fracture. There is recent evidence to suggest that even rigid internal fixation of fractures leads to secondary bone healing but that the amount of callous formed is much smaller than that for less rigid methods of bone stabilization.

Tendon healing occurs primarily via fibroblast proliferation and subsequent collagen synthesis

K.R. Means, MD (✉) • C.L. Forthman, MD
W.H. Baugher, MD • R.D. Katz, MD
R.A. Wittstadt, MD • K.A. Segalman, MD
The Curtis National Hand Center, MedStar
Union Memorial Hospital, 3333 N. Calvert St., JPB
2nd Floor, Johnston Professional Building # 200,
Baltimore, MD 21218, USA
e-mail: kennethrmeans@yahoo.com;
clforthman@chesapeakehand.com;
w.hugh.baugher@gmail.com; ryankatz1@gmail.com;
rwittstadt@chesapeakehand.com;
ksegalman@comcast.net

© Springer International Publishing Switzerland 2017
A.I. Elkwood et al. (eds.), *Rehabilitative Surgery*, DOI 10.1007/978-3-319-41406-5_24

between/within and around the two cut tendon ends, which is termed intrinsic and extrinsic healing, respectively. Extrinsic tendon healing contributes to the tendency for adhesions to form between the healing tendon and the surrounding environment, which can subsequently lead to decreased range of motion. Specific tendon repair techniques and post-tendon injury therapy protocols have been devised in an effort to allow tendon healing to occur while limiting motion-restricting adhesion formation as best as possible.

Peripheral nerve healing occurs via a process that is distinct from central nervous system healing following an injury. When a peripheral nerve is completely lacerated or ruptured, it is termed *neurotmesis*. Without surgical repair of this injury, the ends of the cut nerve will not reestablish a meaningful connection and will instead form scar at each cut end, termed a *neuroma* at the cut end of the proximal nerve stump and termed a *glioma* at the cut end of the distal nerve stump. After peripheral nerve transection, the proximal nerve stump undergoes a process termed Wallerian, or retrograde, degeneration. During this process the nerve cell body sends out signals for cells to clear the internal parts of the peripheral nerve away but to keep the scaffold of the nerve intact. The cell body then sends out new sprouting axons that grow distally within the scaffold of the nerve toward the site of injury. Schwann cells help to coordinate this process. When these new axons reach the area of injury, they will grow into the distal nerve stump as long as the two ends are in close proximity via surgical repair, and there is no blockage to growth across the repair site [1]. Although surgical repair techniques for peripheral nerve injuries have advanced significantly over the past century, we still have not been able to reliably achieve excellent clinical outcomes following treatment of peripheral nerve injuries. Following repair, there is an initial approximately 1 month of no peripheral nerve growth, and subsequently the nerve regenerates at the rate of approximately 1 mm per day or 1 inch per month.

Although sensory targets can remain viable for several years following a peripheral nerve injury, motor nerve targets typically only remain viable for approximately 18 months following a peripheral nerve injury. There is thus a race between nerve regeneration and viability of the distal sensory and motor targets. If the distance from the site of nerve injury is too far from the distal targets to allow meaningful recovery following nerve repair, then other options, such as nerve or tendon transfers, are considered. Most surgeons now think that the answer to improving peripheral nerve repair outcomes for patients will come in the form of a biological solution. For example, younger patients (<25 years old) have significantly better outcomes following peripheral nerve repair compared to older patients.

Knowledge about some basic bone fixation techniques will be helpful for the later sections of this chapter. Lag screw fixation is a technique by which surgeons are able to apply compression between two apposed bone surfaces. Lag screw fixation may be performed with either a standard fully threaded screw using "lag screw technique" or it may be achieved via a specifically designed lag screw. Lag screw technique with a standard fully threaded screw is performed by drilling the near bone surface drill hole so that it is large enough for the screw to simply slide through the hole without purchasing the bone with the screw threads. The near hole must still be small enough so the screw head will not fall into the hole. The far bone surface is drilled to create a smaller hole, which does allow the screw threads to engage the bone. The screw is then inserted from the near bone into the far bone, and once the screw head abuts the near bone surface while the screw threads are engaging the far bone drill hole, then compression is created between the near and far bone apposing surfaces. Specially designed lag screws allow for use of a single drill size for both the near and far bone surfaces. The lag screw only has threads toward the tip of the screw while the area toward the head of the screw is smooth in order to glide through the drill hole in the near bone [2].

Plate-and-screw technique also allows for compression between two bone surfaces, if desired. The plate is placed so that an equal number of screws may be placed on either side of the bone-to-bone interface, if possible. Classic teaching is to obtain three screws of fixation on either side of the bone-to-bone interface for a total of six screws in the construct, although the need for this many screws in all situations has recently been challenged by authors of biomechanical and clinical studies [3]. If compression between the bone surfaces is desired, one screw is placed on one side of the bone-bone interface, and then a second screw is placed on the other side of the bone-bone interface. This second screw hole is drilled at the end of the chosen hole in the plate so that the drill is eccentric within the plate hole, away from the bone-bone interface. Then, when the screw is inserted into the drilled hole in the bone and is tightened down, the screw head will contact the plate hole away from the bone-bone interface and will drag the plate toward this second screw. Because the first screw purchased the bone on the opposite side of the bone-bone interface, the opposite bone will also be dragged toward the second screw, thus achieving compression across the bone-bone interface.

Screws that are part of a plate-and-screw formation are often described as being bicortical. This means that each screw engages both cortices of the bone. The cortex of a tube-shaped bone, such as the metacarpals, phalanges, radius, humerus, etc., is the outer surface of the bone. A bicortical screw will engage one cortical area at the outer surface of the tubular bone, traverse the inner or intramedullary portion of the bone, and then exit and engage the cortex on the other side of the bone.

A unicortical screw engages only one cortex of the bone. With the recent advent of locking plate-and-screw technology, some screws are purposefully placed with a unicortical technique. For example, if a screw is near a joint, tendon, or other structure where bicortical purchase might cause the screw tip to penetrate the structure and cause harm, a unicortical locking screw can be used instead of using bicortical technique.

Locking screws have threads on the periphery of their heads that lock into matching threads in the screw hole of the plate [4]. Because of this, there is no toggle between the screw head and the plate, in essence creating a fixed-angle device that is very stable even with the use of a unicortical

screw technique. A transcortical screw is one that cuts through the side of a tubular bone rather than going through the inner or intramedullary portion of the bone. This creates a notch in the bone and is never desired as it creates a weak point in the bone and obtains poor screw-bone purchase. Surgeons try to avoid this technical error, formerly known as a "unicortical screw" since it only purchases one cortex of the bone. However, with today's use of locking technique and often purposeful use of unicortical screws as described above, the more appropriate term for undesired notching via drilling on the side of the bone is transcortical. Other bone fixation techniques are addressed elsewhere throughout this chapter for specific upper extremity neuromuscular issues.

Shoulder Reanimation: Tendon and Nerve Transfers

The shoulder girdle allows for positioning of the upper extremity. Shoulder motion is determined by a complex interplay between multiple joints and a host of muscles anchored to the chest wall, neck/back, scapula, clavicle, and humerus. The scapulothoracic joint where the scapula meets the chest wall provides a remarkable one-third of arm elevation motion, though often forgotten by clinicians. The remaining motion comes via the glenohumeral joint, the ball-and-socket joint of the shoulder. Neuromuscular disorders about the shoulder can have devastating consequences on global arm function because the hand cannot be placed in the correct position for the simplest activities of daily living (ADLs), like combing hair, brushing teeth, or eating with a fork.

The scapula, or shoulder blade, is normally anchored firmly to the chest wall by the strong trapezius and serratus anterior muscles. Failure of either muscle will allow the scapula to drift, or "wing," away from the chest wall. The trapezius receives innervation from the spinal accessory nerve. The spinal accessory nerve may be damaged during neck surgery, resulting in wasting of the normally robust trapezius muscle and an often dramatic movement of the medial scapula away from the chest wall, known as "lateral winging" (lateral scapular winging figure). While some patients can cope with this loss of function, those with profound loss of overhead use may benefit from the Eden-Lange procedure [5]. This procedure involves rerouting the levator scapulae and rhomboid major and minor to more lateral positions on the scapula. These new insertion sites provide a mechanical advantage for keeping the scapula pulled to the chest wall medially.

The serratus anterior may also fail to maintain scapular position resulting in a less apparent but more common "medial winging." The serratus may fatigue with certain activities (e.g., swimming), or its nerve supply, the long thoracic, may be damaged by trauma or other means such as viral neuritis. Given the variety of causes for serratus dysfunction, a long trial of nonoperative treatment is usually appropriate. If symptoms are persistent and impede functioning, patients may benefit from a pectoralis major transfer to the inferior angle of the scapula. Most surgeons only use the sternal head of the pectoralis so the clavicular head can function normally (medial scapular winging and tendon transfer figure; medial scapular winging post-op figure).

The glenohumeral joint or shoulder joint proper is best described as a large ball (the humeral head) sitting on a shallow platter (the glenoid), much like a golf ball sitting on a golf tee. The joint is balanced and remains congruent largely because a cuff of four muscles pulls the humeral head snug into the glenoid during activity. Failure of this "rotator cuff" is the most frequent etiology of lost shoulder function. The large powerful deltoid muscle envelops the glenohumeral region and normally provides great strength to rotate the humeral head about the glenoid and elevate the arm. When the smaller rotator cuff muscles fail to keep the humeral head centered on the glenoid, the humerus tends to slide superiorly, limiting elevation of the arm.

Tears in the rotator cuff can occur acutely with trauma in the young, gradually with degeneration in the old and, most often, through a combination of minor trauma and normal age-related change. Rotator cuff tears are exceedingly common, and many patients function well and are comfortable despite this problem. Large tears, especially in younger patients, will typically benefit from surgical repair. The tendon or tendons can be sewn back onto the humerus with the help of anchors often placed arthroscopically.

Sometimes the tendons are excessively degenerated or the muscles severely atrophied, making repair futile. This is especially the case in neuromuscular disorders or following brachial plexus injury. In these situations, other tendons, if functional, can be transferred to compensate for the most deficient portion of the rotator cuff [6]. For example, the latissimus dorsi tendon can be harvested from the axilla and transferred to the greater tuberosity in the setting of a dysfunctional infraspinatus (posterosuperior cuff). In children with brachial plexus birth palsy, the teres major is often transferred with the latissimus to improve abduction and external rotation of the arm. A less common cuff deficiency involves the anterior rotator cuff tendon, the subscapularis. In this case, one half or more of the pectoralis major, usually at least the clavicular head, can be detached from the humerus and rerouted to the lesser tuberosity region so as to provide an internal rotation and downward force.

The most common peripheral neuromuscular cause of loss of shoulder function is brachial plexus injury. Other sources of neuromuscular disorder about the shoulder include a direct peripheral nerve injury secondary to an open wound or during surgeries such as shoulder arthroplasty, fracture fixation, or neck dissections. Stroke, or cerebrovascular accident (CVA), and brachial plexus neuritis (Parsonage-Turner syndrome) can also cause significant shoulder dysfunction. The etiology, extent, and mechanism of the neuromuscular condition will determine the chance of spontaneous recovery and the possible need for nerve transfers. There are few studies comparing nerve transfers to tendon transfers, but there is recent evidence for improved recovery for double nerve transfer compared to nerve grafting for isolated musculocutaneous nerve injuries. Unfortunately, like all nerve transfers, the muscle(s) must be reinnervated within 18 months of injury to get useful motor recovery. There is no definitive patient age limit for nerve transfer, but the results are poorer in progressively older patients. To be a candidate, the patient must have good passive motion of the shoulder, normal bony architecture, and intact donor nerves.

The primary goal of nerve transfer surgery about the shoulder is to regain shoulder abduction and flexion. This requires nerve transfer to the suprascapular and axillary nerves to allow reinnervation of their motor targets. The donor choices include the distal branch of the spinal accessory, the medial motor branch from the triceps, intercostal nerves, and the contralateral C7 nerve root. Most authors choose not to use contralateral C7 due to the resulting deficit in the contralateral arm and lack of improved results compared to other less morbid options. Our experience has also been poor with use of the intercostal nerves, encountering too many residual shoulder weakness issues due to poor regeneration following nerve transfer. Our preference is, whenever possible, to use the distal branch of the spinal accessory transferred to the suprascapular nerve and the distal nerve branch from the medial head of the triceps transferred to the axillary nerve (spinal accessory to suprascapular nerve transfer figure). Typically, no nerve grafts are required for either of these transfers. As with all nerve transfers, every effort is made to have the donor nerve be transferred to the shortest possible recipient nerve stump in order to decrease the amount of distance needed to achieve muscle reinnervation.

Postoperatively the patient is immobilized in a sling for 3 weeks, and then active and passive range of motion is begun. One advantage to nerve transfer(s) compared to tendon transfer(s) is there is less reeducation required, although certain forms of feedback during therapy can be helpful in training newly reanimated muscles. Reinnervation should occur within 6 months, but maximum recovery can take more than a year. If the patient does not show clinical signs of regeneration by 6 months after surgery, we typically recommend follow-up neurodiagnostics in an effort to determine whether there is any subclinical evidence of reinnervation in which case waiting longer for clinical recovery may be beneficial.

Scapulothoracic and Glenohumeral Fusions

Soft tissue surgery such as tendon and/or nerve repair or transfer may fail to provide a stable yet mobile shoulder. In these situations, a joint fusion will create a stable and comfortable platform upon which the remainder of the upper extremity can function [7]. By definition, joint fusion eliminates motion so this surgical option is often reserved for the most challenging problems.

Scapulothoracic fusion can be used for failed tendon transfers, in cases of muscular dystrophy and in the setting of other uncommon traumatic and developmental conditions. The goal of the surgery is to achieve a bony union between the front of the scapula and multiple posterior ribs. Once the scapulothoracic joint is stable, a functioning rotator cuff and glenohumeral joint can serve to elevate the arm. In fact, a key contraindication to scapulothoracic fusion is glenohumeral joint dysfunction from arthritis, rotator cuff disease, or nerve damage about the shoulder.

Fusing the thin sheet of scapular bone to a handful of thin ribs can be a technical challenge. As the risks are high, the typical candidate is profoundly limited at baseline preoperatively with maximal active elevation below the horizon. The incision is made along the medial border of the scapula with exposure of both sides of the scapular body. After preparation of multiple fusion sites between the ribs and the scapula, the scapula is secured to the underlying ribs with 18 gauge wire wrapped around the ribs, through the scapula and over a plate placed posteriorly to reinforce the thin scapular bone. Bone graft is harvested from the iliac crest to minimize the nonunion rate, which has been reported to be as high as 25 %.

Facioscapulohumeral dystrophy (FSHD) is the primary dystrophic condition associated with scapular winging. FSHD is a genetic disorder that usually begins during adolescence. Most patients have a progressive disease, presenting first with weakening of the muscles of the face, shoulders, and upper arm and then ultimately weakening of other muscle groups in the lower leg, abdominal girdle, and elsewhere. Patients with FSHD typically have a normal expected lifespan. Scapulothoracic fusion is used commonly in this patient population to relieve pain associated with shoulder motion. Progressive weakening in the upper arm muscles such as the deltoid will gradually diminish the elevation gains obtained with scapulothoracic fusion.

Like scapulothoracic fusion, glenohumeral joint fusion is reserved for the most challenging shoulder problems. In the past, glenohumeral fusion was done for severe arthrosis and rotator cuff dysfunction, but modern shoulder replacements such as the "reverse" prosthesis allow potential reconstruction of even the worst arthritic and rotator cuff-deficient situations. Hence, glenohumeral joint fusion is usually employed in management of the paralyzed shoulder with absent rotator cuff and deltoid function. A functioning scapulothoracic joint with functioning trapezius and serratus anterior is a prerequisite for glenohumeral joint fusion.

The paralyzed or so-called "flail" shoulder typically results from nerve injury, tumor resection, infection, or failed arthroplasty. In addition to frustration with instability, patients with a flail arm often have a constant pain from the weight of the arm pulling the humerus inferiorly off the glenoid and causing traction to the brachial plexus. Fusion can eliminate this pain and provides stability. The ideal alignment for fusion is controversial and must be individualized as patients commit to a life with the arm in a fixed and sometimes awkward position.

Glenohumeral fusion can be accomplished with a large plate spanning the scapular spine, acromion, and proximal humerus. Ideally, fusion occurs at the glenohumeral and acromiohumeral bone interfaces. As with scapulothoracic fusion, the nonunion rate is not insignificant and can be minimized with good postoperative immobilization. Patients are placed in a shoulder spica cast or adjustable shoulder brace for up to several months after surgery.

Elbow Reanimation: Tendon and Nerve Transfers

Spinal cord injuries and stroke are the two most common causes of global loss of upper extremity function. Other traumas such as brachial plexus birth palsies, brachial plexus traumatic injuries, and other high nerve injuries may also cause limited use of the hand and arm. Restoration of upper extremity function is a critical component of improving individual independence with dressing, eating, wheelchair mobility, and other ADL tasks. Authors of a recent study reported that 90 % of spinal cord injury patients felt that improving their arm and hand function would improve their quality of life [8]. In addition, 80 % were willing to spend 2–3 months with less independence in order to eventually improve their independence.

Priority of functional reconstruction for these patients has changed little over time. Restoration of elbow flexion is the first priority, with shoulder stability/function being a close second priority. Improving elbow function starts with a history, detailed physical examination, and appropriate ancillary studies such as focused MRIs and neurodiagnostics (EMG) as needed. Four muscles are specifically checked during examination and/or neurodiagnostic studies: the supraspinatus, infraspinatus, deltoid, and biceps. Responsible for shoulder and elbow function, these muscles act synergistically to bring the hand to the mouth and away from the body. With this information, patients can be grouped according to the International Classification of Surgery of the Hand in Tetraplegia (ICSHT). The ICSHT can be used to categorize individuals with tetraplegia into surgically meaningful categories. With consultations from rehab specialists, physical and occupational therapists, nurses, and other care team members, a comprehensive plan for restoration of upper extremity function can be undertaken.

Surgical treatment to restore elbow motion may include attempts at primary reconstruction with nerve repair, neurolysis, nerve grafting, and transfers. These can be combined with secondary reconstructive procedures such as tendon transfers, functioning free muscle transfers (FFMT), tendon or muscle releases, or bony stabilization of joints to achieve an optimal functional outcome. While the traditional techniques of nerve repair, nerve grafting, and tendon transfers have been the mainstays of treatment, over the past two decades the development of nerve transfer techniques has provided important functional gains. With advances in microsurgery, nerve transfer(s) to restore elbow flexion is now a viable option. Although the recovery process is longer than with tendon or muscle transfers, sacrificing or weakening one function for another is avoided, and the chance for normal or near-normal function seems to be increased. Optimal outcomes may be improved with a combination of techniques.

Tendon transfers to restore elbow flexion include the Steindler flexorplasty, triceps-to-biceps transfer, latissimus dorsi transfers, and the pectoralis major transfer. The Steindler flexorplasty attempts to restore elbow flexion by transferring the common flexor-pronator origin from the medial epicondyle to a more proximal and radial position on the humerus. This increases the lever arm of the transferred muscle-tendon units at the elbow joint, thus improving elbow flexion. This is best utilized to augment preexisting elbow flexion after reconstruction of the nerves to biceps/brachialis (Steindler flexorplasty figures). The triceps-to-biceps transfer is a reliable means of producing elbow flexion but at the cost of losing active elbow extension.

If the transfer of local muscle "motors" is not an option, as can be the case in global trauma or with a systemic or regional neurologic process, the surgeon should consider remote alternatives. A classic example of this principle is use of the latissimus dorsi (LD) muscle in a pedicled fashion for restoration of elbow flexion. This transfer requires no microsurgery and keeps the muscle attached to its blood supply and nerve throughout the transfer and inset process. Thus, the muscle is alive with the potential to provide elbow motion even in the immediate postoperative setting. When used as a pedicled flap to restore motion, the LD flap has the obvious limitation of a restricted arc of motion. It therefore could not be used in this manner to restore motion to muscle groups below the elbow. The latissimus dorsi transfer to restore elbow flexion can be done with a monopolar (transfer of insertion) or bipolar (transfer of origin and insertion) modalities. Bipolar transfer is generally preferred for its bio-

mechanical advantages. The pectoralis major muscle can also be utilized to regain elbow flexion, again with a unipolar or bipolar transfer.

The external macroanatomy of the brachial plexus has been known for decades. Recent advances in the knowledge of the internal topographical anatomy of the brachial plexus fascicles has allowed the transfer of specific motor fascicles from functioning nerves to nonfunctioning nerves. Both intra-plexal and extra-plexal nerve transfers have been developed. Intra-plexal nerve transfers are the result of a new understanding of the intraneural topography of the median and ulnar nerves with the possibility of being able to accurately locate the motor fascicles to the flexor carpi radialis (FCR) and flexor carpi ulnaris (FCU) muscles, respectively. These can then be transferred to the musculocutaneous nerve (MCN) to the brachialis and biceps muscles to restore elbow flexion (musculocutaneous nerve transfer figure). Extra-plexal nerve transfers to the MCN using the intercostal, spinal accessory, medial pectoral, thoracodorsal, and rarely the phrenic nerves have been utilized. In general, intra-plexal donors have shown better results than extra-plexal donors [9].

Strong active elbow extension is crucial for overhead activities, transfers, and weight shifting and greatly enhances wheelchair propulsion. Posterior deltoid to triceps tendon transfer has previously been the operation of choice for restoration of active elbow extension, but this required a tendon graft and functional antigravity strength was not often achieved. Superior results have been achieved by transferring the biceps to the triceps in order to restore true functional antigravity strength [10].

Functioning free muscle transfers can also be used to restore both elbow flexion and extension, generally using extra-plexal nerves to reinnervate the free muscle transfer. In these cases the donor muscle, usually the gracilis from the inner thigh, is harvested and transferred as a free flap to the upper extremity where it is revascularized and reinnervated with microsurgery techniques using the vessels and nerves in the recipient upper extremity and vessel or nerve grafts as needed.

Elbow Fusion

Elbow fusion has been described by one of our colleagues as a procedure that is dissatisfying to both the patient and the surgeon. Because at least some degree of elbow motion is required for most activities of daily living, fusion is again reserved for extreme cases. Elbow fusion may be considered following severe neuromuscular conditions where nerve/tendon function about the elbow is unable to be restored and the instability and pain at the elbow are unable to be improved by other means. Fusion is also considered for those patients with prior infections or failed joint replacements where joint reconstruction is not possible or advisable. Perhaps one of the best indications for elbow fusion is a Charcot joint in which the elbow joint is destroyed due to a loss of protective sensation within and around the joint, usually from a neurological cause such as a spinal cord mass or defect. For these patients, the elbow joint can become dysfunctionally unstable and progressively destroyed. In this situation, joint replacement or other motion-sparing reconstructions usually fail.

Elbow fusion involves fusing the distal humerus to the proximal ulna. An incision is made on the back of the elbow. Any cartilage between the humerus and the ulna is removed until fresh and healthy bone surfaces are created. The humerus and ulna are then joined, typically via a combination of screws and a plate. The elbow is classically fused in an approximately 90° flexed position. However, especially for patients with neuromuscular disorders, a multidisciplinary approach involving the patient and other caregivers can help determine the most functional fusion position for the patient [11]. Local bone or harvested bone graft can be used to fill any gaps between the humerus and ulna and to provide bridging bone on the outer bone surfaces to encourage union. A prolonged period of immobilization is required until the fusion is confirmed to be clinically and radiographically healed.

Even after healing of the fusion site, there can be tremendous stresses at the ends of the plate on the humerus and ulna which can lead to later fractures at these locations, especially in patients who use the extremity for heavy activities. Another potential issue with elbow fusion is the relatively thin skin and soft tissue envelope on the back of the elbow. This is especially a concern for patients with neuromuscular disorders who may have poor volitional upper extremity control and/or protective sensation. Skin and soft tissue breakdown and loss in this area can be difficult to heal and may require regional or free soft tissue flap coverage.

Wrist Reanimation: Tendon and Nerve Transfers

Loss of wrist range of motion following neurologic injury or associated with neuromuscular disorders can lead to significant dysfunction and/or pain. Loss of wrist extension is much more functionally debilitating than loss of wrist flexion because the hand typically functions with the wrist extended, especially for power grip activities. Even just splinting the wrist in extension can have a significant positive impact on patient function and comfort in the setting of loss of active wrist extension.

The most common neurological cause of decreased active wrist motion is radial nerve pathology. Radial nerve injury or palsy will lead to a wrist-drop in which patients are unable to actively extend their wrist. This can be seen with isolated radial nerve injury or may be part of a more proximal brachial plexus condition. The entire radial nerve can be involved or just a distal motor branch, the posterior interosseous nerve (PIN), can be affected. The PIN innervates all of the wrist and digital extensors except for the brachioradialis, the extensor carpi radialis longus (ECRL), and the extensor carpi radialis brevis (ECRB), all of which are known collectively as the mobile wad. If the entire radial nerve is involved, the entire wrist will lose active extension. If just the PIN is affected, the patient will still maintain the ability to extend the wrist in a radial-deviated position because the ECRL and ECRB will still be functional.

Nerve and tendon transfers to restore wrist extension are considered whenever normal return of wrist extension is not expected following neurological compromise. The recent advent of several nerve transfer options to restore upper extremity motor and sensory function is one of the most exciting developments in upper extremity surgery [12]. These nerve transfers have the potential to restore near-normal independent nerve function without the biomechanical drawbacks and intense physical therapy retraining associated with tendon transfers. Having said that, there is still certainly a strong role for tendon transfers for loss of wrist motion and nerve transfer is not usually considered for isolated loss of wrist motion.

Nerve and tendon transfers to restore wrist extension both typically focus on the ECRB, the central wrist extensor that can provide the most pure wrist extension without associated radial or ulnar deviation. Nerve transfer involves use of a branch or branches of the median nerve to flexor digitorum superficialis, flexor carpi radialis, and/or pronator teres that are transferred to the radial nerve branch to the ECRB or a combination of the other wrist and finger extensors. The most common tendon transfer to restore wrist extension is transfer of the median-innervated pronator teres to the ECRB, but other static or dynamic tendon transfers are possible if pronator teres is not available or functional. For both nerve and tendon transfers that seek to restore wrist extension, the loss of function from the median-innervated donors is minimal as long as the correct branches are carefully isolated and the remainder of the median nerve and its branches are protected.

Wrist Fusion

Total wrist fusion is performed relatively commonly for patients with significant neuromuscular disorders. Wrist replacement arthroplasty is typically not appropriate for patients with neuromuscular disorders as those procedures do not reliably provide a stable platform for upper extremity weight bearing or other high-demand activities that these patients often need to perform. Also, the neuromuscular imbalances across the patient's wrist that have necessitated fusion in the first place would put any replacement arthroplasty at high risk for early failure and unacceptably high complication rates.

The most commonly seen diagnoses requiring total wrist fusion are cerebral palsy and stroke, although certainly other diagnoses may necessitate wrist fusion as well. The most common reasons for recommending wrist fusion are pain and severe flexion or extension deformity that cannot be reliably corrected with soft tissue procedures. Often in neuromuscular disorders, the wrist will be held in a rigidly flexed or extended position that cannot be corrected actively by the patient or passively by care providers. In these cases, the severe position of the wrist can cause pain and eventual articular cartilage degeneration. These severe wrist positions can also be significantly dysfunctional for patients. Fusing the wrist in a better position can help with pain and function for the patient [13].

There are certain things that should be considered when discussing possible wrist fusion with patients and any involved caregivers. One is in which position the wrist should be fused. The most commonly used functional position for wrist fusion is slight extension. However, personal hygiene and other activities of daily living should be considered for the individual patient being treated. The wrist should be placed in whichever position will make these activities easiest for the patient and any caregivers. Another consideration is the patient's contralateral wrist and whether it will also need to be fused in the near future or has already been fused. Typically if one wrist is fused, then the contralateral wrist is placed in a complementary position. For example, if the other wrist is in slight extension, then the wrist to be fused is placed in slight flexion.

There are some technical considerations for the wrist fusion surgical procedure. The surgical approach is typically through the dorsal wrist and hand. The extensor tendons to the digits are protected, and the wrist joint is opened. Some surgeons routinely remove the proximal carpal row of the wrist, which includes the scaphoid, lunate, and triquetrum bones, at the time of fusion to simplify the procedure. Other surgeons routinely maintain these bones during fusion to try to increase the amount of bone mass for fusion.

For neuromuscular disorder patients, the usual consideration in this regard is how much shortening of the wrist is necessary in order to place it in the most functional position and allow the best digit positions and function. Due to contracted flexor or extensor tendons which have placed the wrist in its baseline dysfunctional position, it may be necessary to remove carpal bones and even some of the distal radius in order to achieve a functional wrist fusion position. Once the correct position is achieved, any articular cartilage remaining at the planned fusion site is removed. The goal is to achieve healthy bleeding cancellous bone on both sides of the fusion site to encourage healing.

Surgeons often use a metal plate and screws to span the fusion site, which provides stability until the bones have fused together. The wrist is placed in the desired position of flexion or extension and radial or ulnar deviation. The plate is contoured to match the desired wrist fusion position. Then the plate is applied to the dorsum of the radius proximally and whichever finger metacarpal distally will allow maintenance of the desired wrist position, which is usually the index or long finger metacarpal. The first two screws are placed through the plate in a compression mode on either side of the fusion site. A check of the clinical and radiographic position is made to ensure satisfactory fusion and plate/screw position. Next the remaining screws are inserted through the plate as needed, typically with at least three screws proximal and three screws distal to the fusion site (Wrist Fusion X-rays Figure).

Bone graft can be placed around the fusion site using either the local bone graft taken from the wrist previously during the procedure or from another site if needed. The deep soft tissue and skin are closed, and the patient is placed in a splint if possible. If the patient's neuromuscular condition necessitates use of a cast, ample padding should be applied and the cast should be placed as loosely as possible to allow for swelling of the patient's wrist postoperatively.

If possible, postoperatively the patient should do open/close fist 20 times per hour for the operative hand while awake, either actively or passively using the other hand or a caregiver to assist. This helps prevent digital stiffness and promotes good edema control for the patient's digits, hand, and wrist. Elevation above heart level at all times as possible is also recommended. The fusion is typically protected for the first 6 weeks until clinical and radiographic healing are confirmed before allowing weight bearing and other increases in activities.

Digital Reanimation: Tendon and Free Muscle Transfer

For the hand to function as a useful tool, both sensation and motion are prerequisites. When one or both are absent, the hand becomes dysfunctional and may even be an impediment to the patient's quality of life. It is the surgeon's primary goal when evaluating the neuromuscular patient with a flaccid, spastic, or dysfunctional hand to determine the overall potential of the hand. This will serve as the foundation upon which a surgical plan can be built.

Before any surgical intervention to improve hand function for neuromuscular patients, several questions must be answered: If the dysfunction is the result of a neurologic insult, has the insult ceased? Has the patient's recovery plateaued? Is the patient at imminent risk for further insult? Is the patient at an unacceptably high risk for surgery? Does the patient have volitional control of some upper extremity musculature, and if so, what is the strength of the working muscle groups?

Assuming the patient's neuromuscular insult has passed and the patient's recovery has plateaued, reconstruction to restore hand function can be considered. From a motor standpoint, it is worthwhile to consider and make a list of poorly or nonfunctioning musculotendinous groups and the resultant specific deficit. Consideration should then be given to those musculotendinous groups still in working order. These can be local (on the same hand or arm) or remote, involving free muscle transfer from a site distant from the deficit, e.g., gracilis muscle transferred from the leg to restore hand function.

A classic example of a set of local transfers to restore motion is the "brand transfer" for a patient with radial nerve palsy. This set of tendon transfers can illustrate the power of using working, strong muscles to restore function lost as the result of a neurologic deficit. Since the radial nerve palsy patient lacks wrist extension, finger extension, and thumb extension, restoration of these three actions becomes the surgeon's goal. To accomplish this task, the surgeon can harvest median nerve innervated muscle-tendon units and reroute them to the dorsal forearm to restore lost radial nerve function. Ideally, these muscle-tendon units can be harvested with minimal functional deficit to the patient. Such relatively expendable units include the pronator teres (PT), the flexor carpi radialis (FCR), and the palmaris longus (PL).

In the brand transfer, wrist extension is regained by transferring the PT to the extensor carpi radialis brevis (ECRB), finger extension is regained by transferring the FCR to the extensor digiti communis (EDC), and thumb extension is regained by transferring the PL to the extensor pollicis longus (EPL). Though these transfers usually work well, there are certainly other muscle-tendon units which can be transferred to achieve a similar function. Every muscle-tendon unit is unique with what it can bring to a transfer. For example, transferring an expendable flexor digitorum superficialis (FDS) to the EDC affords the patient more tendon excursion than the classic FCR to EDC transfer and is especially considered for patients with wrist fusions who cannot use wrist range of motion to aid the tendon transfers in regaining finger extension.

Overcoming the constraints of local or regional muscle-tendon unit transfer distances can be accomplished only with free tissue transfer. This microvascular procedure requires an intricate understanding of muscle anatomy and involves separating a muscle from its blood supply and motor nerve, transferring it to the dysfunctional extremity, and anastomosing it to a new blood supply and new nerve. Because it involves sectioning the muscle's motor nerve, this technique does not deliver immediate or early restoration of motor function. Such function can only be regained once the muscle becomes reinnervated. The classic example of the muscle used to restore upper extremity function

is the gracilis muscle [14]. This muscle has a dominant and reliable pedicle (blood supply), a reliable motor nerve (obturator nerve), excellent excursion, and a favorable tendon that can be used to suture into the digital flexors or extensors to reanimate the digits.

Whether performing a tendon transfer, pedicled muscle transfer, or free muscle transfer, the surgeon would be wise to adhere to the following principles:

1. The donor muscle should be expendable and not result in obvious loss of function.
2. The donor muscle should have adequate excursion and length.
3. The donor muscle-tendon unit should be inset with a direct line of pull.
4. The joints upon which the donor muscle-tendon unit is acting should be supple.
5. The donor muscle should work synergistically with the motion to be restored.

Digital Fusion

Digital fusion is an option for patients with neuromuscular disease who have digital joint deformities which are causing pain and dysfunction and which cannot be corrected by therapy, splints, medications, or other soft tissue or bone/joint procedures. Neuromuscular disorders can lead to an imbalance in flexion and extension forces across digital joints. For the thumb, abduction, adduction, pronation, and supination imbalances are also possible. These conditions can lead to flaccid, spastic, or rigid finger joints, which in turn can lead to pain, degeneration, and dysfunction [15]. Rigid hardware fixation is usually chosen for digital fusion in neuromuscular disorder patients in order to maintain the corrected joint position until fusion has occurred.

For the thumb, the carpometacarpal (CMC), metacarpophalangeal (MCP), and/or interphalangeal (IP) joints may be fused. For the fingers, the proximal or distal IP joints may be fused. It is unusual to consider fusion of the MCP joints except for perhaps the index finger. This is because MCP joint fusion significantly hampers functional use of the hand. However, it can be considered for the index finger where pinch activities are still possible following metacarpophalangeal fusion and the loss of finger flexion is less disabling. The only other times MCP fusion might be considered for the other fingers is for patients with inadequate volitional control who require better finger positioning to prevent skin/soft tissue breakdown or for intractable pain control.

For finger and thumb MCP fusions and finger proximal IP fusions, dorsal incisions are made over the joint. The digital extensors are surgically mobilized and protected, and the articular cartilage surface is removed down to healthy, bleeding cancellous bone on both sides of the fusion. Most finger and thumb MCP and finger proximal IP fusions are placed in 20–30° of flexion, but again patient activity and other upper extremity involvement are considered in determining optimal fusion placement. If the patient does not have rigid joints, several trial-and-error splints in different degrees of joint position can be used preoperatively to help guide ultimate fusion position at the time of surgery.

For patients with neuromuscular disorders, most surgeons prefer to use either a tension-band or plate-and-screw construct to hold the fusion in position, as these are the most robust stabilization options available. Tension-band technique involves placing two wires longitudinally across the fusion site. The fusion site is then checked clinically and radiographically to confirm proper fusion and hardware position. A drill hole is then placed transversely at the dorsal proximal base of the bone distal to the fusion site. A steel wire is placed through this hole and is curved in a figure-of-8 fashion and secured under the proximal aspect of the previously placed longitudinal wires. The figure-of-8 wire is tightened down until the fusion site is secure (*see PIP Fusion Figures*). For plate-and-screw technique, an appropriate size and length plate is chosen to span the fusion site and permit placement of sufficient screws proximal and distal to the fusion site. The plate is contoured to match the desired fusion position and one screw is placed on either side of the fusion site in compression mode if possible. Clinical and radiographic fusion and hardware position are confirmed and the remaining screws are placed in neutral position.

Finger distal IP and thumb IP fusions are typically positioned in neutral or slight flexion, depending on functional needs. Again dorsal incisions are used, the extensor tendon is either split or transected, and the articular cartilage surfaces are removed to healthy bleeding cancellous bone. Many surgeons prefer to use intramedullary screw fixation for these fusions because the skin and soft tissue is thinner and more vulnerable to breakdown and infection when larger implants external to the bone are used. If an internal screw is to be used, a guide wire is placed across the fusion site and the clinical and radiographic position of the fusion and wire are confirmed. The screw is then placed through a stab incision at the tip of the digit, over the guide wire, across the fusion site, and into the bone proximal to the fusion site (*See DIP Fusion figures*). Appropriate final clinical and radiographic fusion and hardware position are confirmed, and the patient is placed in a splint postoperatively. Weight bearing, lifting, pinching, and strengthening are avoided at the fusion site for at least 6 weeks in addition to clinical and radiographic healing confirmation.

Thumb CMC, or trapeziometacarpal, fusion can be difficult to achieve without complication. Just as with finger MCP joints, thumb carpometacarpal fusion is typically avoided as well as it severely limits functional thumb range of motion. However, for patients with neuromuscular conditions, it is not unusual to need to place the thumb in a more functional position so that tip-pinch with the fingers is at least possible and when soft tissue balancing options may not be reliable or possible. For this fusion, a dorsal incision is made, and cutaneous nerve branches are protected. The interval between the thumb extensors is opened, the dorsal radial artery branch is protected, and the joint between the thumb metacarpal base and the trapezium is opened. The articular cartilage of the thumb metacarpal base and distal aspect of the trapezium is removed and healthy bleeding cancellous bone surfaces are prepared. The planned fusion position is temporarily pinned and checked clinically and radiographically. Most surgeons use a T-type plate, staples, or similar rigid fixation option to stabilize the fusion. Protection from weight bearing, lifting, pinching, or strengthening is continued for at least 6 weeks and until clinical and radiographic healing.

Cerebral Palsy Involving the Upper Extremities

Cerebral palsy can be defined as a static, irreversible, perinatal brain injury that affects the musculoskeletal system. The central lesion, the brain injury, defines the "static" portion of the pathology. Although the musculoskeletal manifestations may appear to change over time, this in fact is due to a peripheral progression of unbalanced forces. It is important to remember that there are often other neurologic problems besides those involving the musculoskeletal system. Most often cerebral palsy is classified by type (spastic, flaccid, athetoid, or mixed) and limb involvement (hemiplegia, diplegia, or quadriplegia). An early preference for hand dominance and inability to develop a pulp-to-pulp thumb pinch pattern by 1 year of age may be signs of milder cerebral palsy. Spasticity, often with weakness in the reciprocal muscles, is the most common form of cerebral palsy. Muscle imbalance leads to decreased motion and, if not monitored and treated, can lead to secondary fixed contractures of the affected joints.

At its earliest stages, cerebral palsy should be treated by passive range of motion and splinting to maintain motion and prevent contractures. Medications often play a significant role but are not in the scope of this discussion. Surgical treatment is usually not pursued until the child has reached 5 or 6 years of age. This is because it is difficult to assess a younger child regarding surgical needs and prognosis. In addition, a child at this age begins to develop the ability to cooperate with treatment. Depending on the severity of the disease, the goal of surgery can range from an attempt to improve function to facilitating care to simply allowing better hygiene and preventing skin breakdown. In milder cases, improving cosmesis may also be considered [16]. Broadly speaking, all of these goals can be accomplished by decreasing a spastic deforming force, increasing the strength of a weak motor unit, and releasing fixed contractures.

As an example of how to approach this problem, let us consider the most typical upper extremity deformity seen in cerebral palsy. Imagine a 6-year-old hemiplegic child with reasonable cognitive ability who presents with the more classic deformity of internal rotation at the shoulder, flexion at the elbow, pronation of the forearm, a flexed wrist and fingers, and a thumb-in-palm deformity. For the sake of simplicity, assume that the child has reasonable ability to place the arm in space and has had their shoulder problems adequately managed by a stretching and range of motion program.

In addressing the elbow, note that the deforming forces are the biceps, the brachialis, and possibly the brachioradialis. In this situation, the elbow extensors are usually present but weak, and elbow extension is augmented by gravity. Therefore, one usually addresses only the deforming forces. The biceps is surgically lengthened, usually by a Z-plasty of the tendon. The brachialis is lengthened or a tenotomy can be considered. At the time of surgery, the surgeon may wish to include release of the brachioradialis from its bony origin on the humerus. A postoperative dressing augmented with plaster to hold the correction is applied. This may be changed for a thermoplastic splint at a later date. The correction is protected for 3–6 weeks, depending on the patient's ability to cooperate. After this point in time, night splinting is often continued, and range of motion and active use exercises may commence.

In patients who are more cognitively impaired and for whom the procedure is done simply to address hyperflexion of the elbow and allow greater ease in skin care and dressing, simple tenotomies are more typically performed and passive stretching can proceed at an earlier time postoperatively. Often in severe cases, the limit of achievable elbow extension is determined by the tightness of the neurovascular bundle at the anterior elbow at the time of surgery.

Forearm pronation is caused by weakness of the supinators coupled with overactivity of the pronators, in particular the pronator teres. The milder pronation deformities can sometimes be addressed with a flexor carpi ulnaris (FCU) transfer. The more severe deformities are addressed by release of the pronator and occasionally transfer of the pronator teres to diminish its deforming force and redirect it to a correcting force. If the pronator alone is released, immobilization is continued only to hold the correction and early remobilization can be considered. However, if a tendon transfer is carried out, the transfer has to be protected for 3–6 weeks until remobilization and strengthening can be attempted.

Wrist and finger flexion are related and usually have to be addressed simultaneously because correcting a flexion contracture of the wrist may require lengthening of the finger flexors. One tries to predict preoperatively whether placing the wrist in an extended position will make the fingers tight enough to require lengthening of the finger flexors. The deforming forces at the wrist are the flexor carpi radialis (FCR) and FCU, the latter typically being more critical. The deforming force of the FCU can be removed by tenotomy, but frequently the tendon is brought around the ulnar border of the wrist and sutured dorsally into a wrist extensor or the finger extensors. This relieves a deforming force and at the same time augments weakened muscles. If the tendon transfer option is performed, once again 3–6 weeks of protection is indicated prior to mobilization.

Decision-making regarding correction of the thumb-in-palm deformity requires one to identify extrinsic causes of deformity (mainly the flexor pollicis longus (FPL)) versus intrinsic causes (the abductor pollicis, the flexor pollicis brevis, and the first dorsal interosseous) or a combination. The intrinsic muscles are usually released in the palm. The FPL is lengthened when necessary. Frequently the forces about the thumb need to be rebalanced by rerouting the EPL as a tendon transfer. Sometimes the MCP joint has to be addressed as well with a capsulodesis or arthrodesis. These are smaller muscle-tendon units and are usually protected for 4–6 weeks before allowing mobilization. An arthrodesis is usually solid enough at 6 weeks to discontinue immobilization.

We recommend that physical, occupational, and/or hand therapists be provided with the operative procedure note and specific instructions as to how long splinting should be maintained and as to when simple active motion can be initiated and when it is safe for strengthening. It is also important to realize that in the above examples, we have discussed a minimally involved child. Often, there are multiple other neuromuscular conditions that are quite difficult to care for outside of a children's specialty medical center.

Heterotopic Ossification: Traumatic Brain and Neurological Injury

Heterotopic ossification refers to the development of bone in locations where it would not normally be found. This means that muscle and soft tissue can become ossified and cause bony blocks to joint motion or even ankylosis, i.e., complete motion loss, across the joint. Heterotopic ossification can be a significant issue about the large joints of the upper extremity for patients with neuromuscular disorders. Patients most likely to develop heterotopic ossification are those with a recent traumatic brain injury or significant upper extremity trauma. The joints most commonly affected are the elbow and the forearm axis although the condition may also develop about the shoulder.

Typical treatment is aimed at trying to maintain range of motion via gentle therapy until the heterotopic ossification has stopped developing. This stopping point is usually determined by clinical history, physical exam, and plain radiographs. Once the patient's pain, swelling, overall soft tissue status, and x-rays have reached a stable, nonactive, nonprogressive condition, then definitive treatment can be carried out as needed. Laboratory tests and bone scans were used in the past to determine when it was safe to proceed with definitive treatment for heterotopic ossification but these have largely been abandoned recently.

If range of motion is sufficiently limited by the heterotopic ossification, it can be removed surgically. Preoperative CT scans can be very helpful in mapping out the extent of the bone that needs to be removed and can guide surgical approaches (see HO figure). CT scan can also help determine that the joint surfaces are in adequate condition to allow an attempt at regaining motion. Neurovascular structures are at risk during removal of the heterotopic bone and must be identified and protected throughout the procedure. The bone that is blocking joint range of motion is then removed. If joint range of motion is still insufficient, then joint soft tissue/capsule releases may be necessary. The patient can also have a large amount of intraoperative or postoperative bleeding with these procedures and should be counseled and prepared for the possible need for blood or blood product replacement. Range of motion is started as soon as possible

postoperatively. There is no definitive evidence that any treatments to try to prevent recurrence of heterotopic bone are more beneficial than harmful. However, many surgeons still prefer to use a postoperative anti-inflammatory medication regimen or a single dose of postoperative irradiation in an effort to prevent recurrence [3].

Summary Points

- It can be challenging for care providers to adequately evaluate and optimally treat patients presenting with significant upper extremity neuromuscular involvement.
- It is critical to work with a multidisciplinary team, including the patient, any caregivers, therapists, physicians, surgeons, and any ancillary providers in an effort to allow these patients to achieve maximal function.
- Treatment options for upper extremity neuromuscular disorders typically are instituted for patients from proximal to distal in a sequential fashion, although the elbow is often given special early consideration. At

each stage, the response to the prior treatments is assessed, and once outcome from those treatments is maximized, then further options are considered.
- Surgical options for upper extremity neuromuscular disorders typically involve one or more of the following: nerve transfers, tendon transfers, nerve excisions, tendon/muscle releases, joint releases, and joint fusions.
- Some of the most exciting and innovative treatment options for severe neuromuscular disorders are the recent use of nerve transfers and free muscle/tendon transfers for reanimation of portions of the upper extremity (Figs. 24.1, 24.2, 24.3, 24.4, 24.5, 24.6, 24.7, 24.8, 24.9, and 24.10).

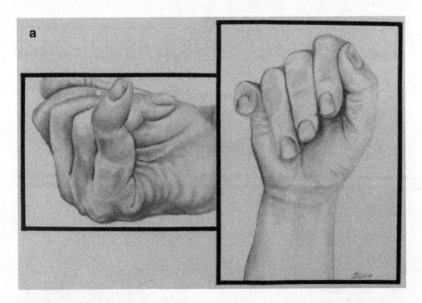

Fig. 24.1 PIP fusion figures: (**a**) illustration of Clinical photos of a patient with rigid swan neck deformity of the small finger. (**b**) illustration of Intraoperative photos of figure-of-8 tension band PIP fusion technique. (**c**) A/P and lateral fluoroscopic X-ray images of PIP fusion using figure-of-8 tension band technique

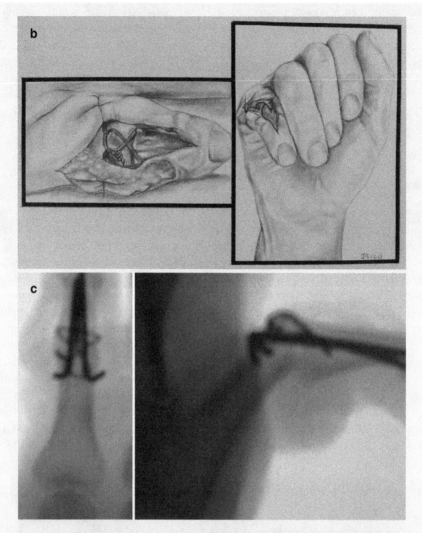

Fig. 24.1 (continued)

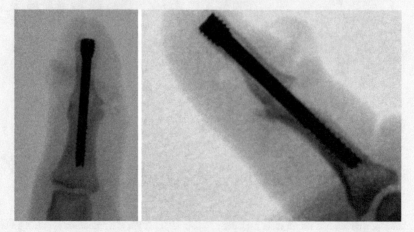

Fig. 24.2 DIP fusion figure: Fluoroscopic X-ray images of DIP fusion using intramedullary headless compression screw

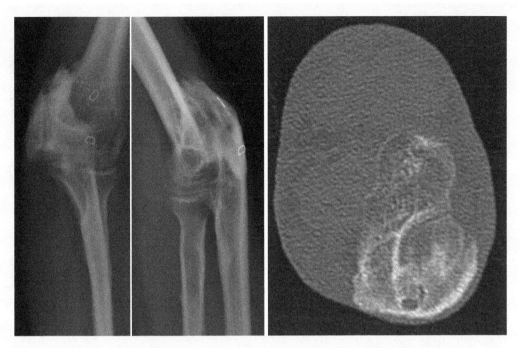

Fig. 24.3 HO figure: X-rays and cross-sectional CT scan demonstrating extent and location of heterotopic ossification about the elbow

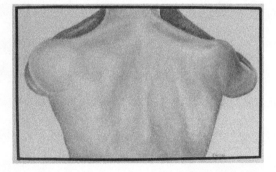

Fig. 24.4 Lateral scapular winging figure: illustration of Clinical photo of a patient with right-sided trapezius palsy demonstrating lateral winging of the right scapula as the patient pushes against a wall

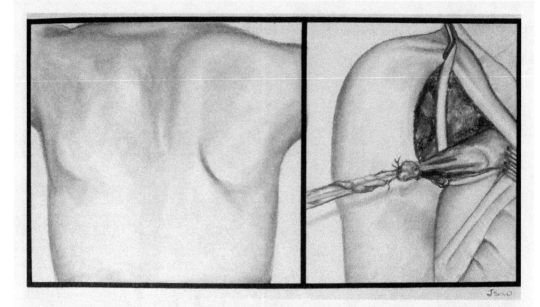

Fig. 24.5 Medial scapular winging and tendon transfer figure: Illustration of Clinical and intraoperative photos of a patient with right-sided serratus anterior palsy demonstrating medial winging of the right scapula as the patient pushes against a wall. The pectoralis major was transferred, with a tendon graft for added length, to the inferior posterior scapula

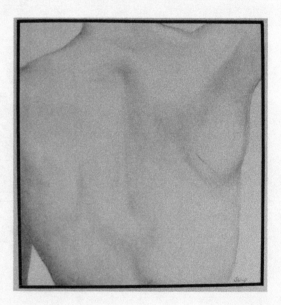

Fig. 24.6 Medial scapular winging postoperative figure: Postoperative clinical photo of same patient after recovery from surgery

Fig. 24.7 Spinal accessory to suprascapular nerve transfer figure: Illustration of intraoperative photo of a patient undergoing spinal accessory to suprascapular nerve transfer

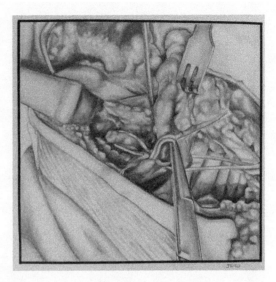

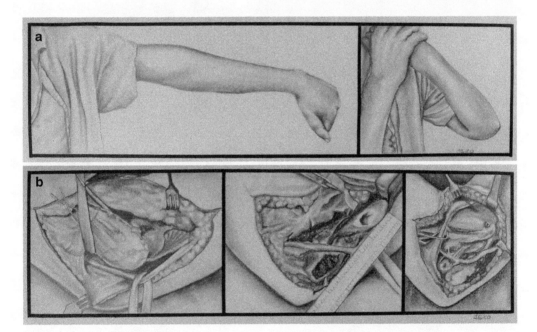

Fig. 24.8 Steindler flexorplasty figures: (**a**) Preoperative photo of patient demonstrating no active elbow flexion but full passive elbow flexion. (**b**) Illustration of Intraoperative photos of surgical procedure. The hand is to the left and the shoulder is to the right in these photos. The flexor-pronator mass is shifted proximally on the humerus and secured with a screw. (**c**) Postoperative photo of patient demonstrating active elbow flexion

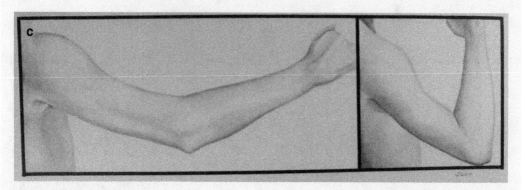

Fig. 24.8 (continued)

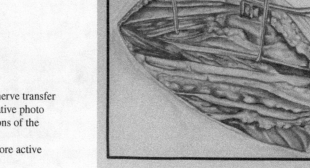

Fig. 24.9 Musculocutaneous nerve transfer figure: Illustration of Intraoperative photo demonstrating transfer of portions of the median and ulnar nerves to the musculocutaneous nerve to restore active elbow flexion

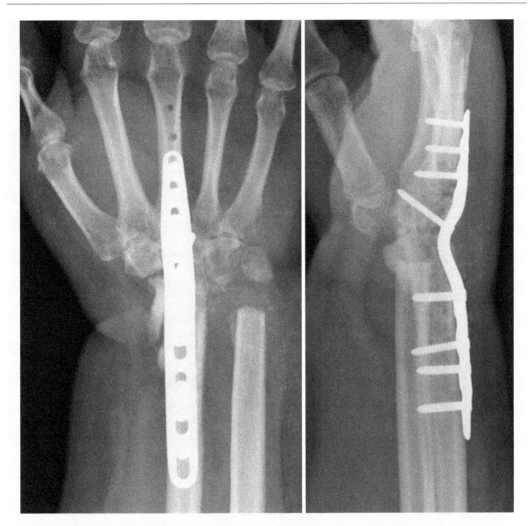

Fig. 24.10 Wrist fusion X-rays figure: Anteroposterior and lateral X-ray views of a patient who underwent total wrist fusion with a plate and screws. The distal ulna was removed as part of the procedure as well

References

1. Buckwalter JA, Einhorn TA, Simon SR. Orthopaedic basic science: biology and biomechanics of the musculoskeletal system. 2nd ed. Rosemont: American Academy of Orthopaedic Surgeons; 2000.
2. Jupiter JB, Ring DC. AO Manual of fracture management: hand and wrist. Stuttgart: Thieme; 2005.
3. Means Jr KR, Graham TJ. Disorders of the forearm axis. In: Wolfe SW, Hotchkiss RN, Pederson WC, Kozin SH, editors. Green's operative hand surgery. 6th ed. Philadelphia: Elsevier; 2011. p. 837–68.
4. Schütz M, Südkamp NP. Revolution in plate osteosynthesis: new internal fixator systems. J Orthop Sci. 2003;8:252–8.
5. Teboul F, Bizot P, Kakkar R, Sedel L. Surgical management of trapezius palsy. J Bone Joint Surg Am. 2004;86-A:1884–90.
6. Kozin SH. The evaluation and treatment of children with brachial plexus birth palsy. J Hand Surg Am. 2011;36:1360–9.
7. Harryman II DT, Walker ED, Harris SL, Sidles JA, Jackins SE, Matsen III FA. Residual motion and function after glenohumeral or scapulothoracic arthrodesis. J Shoulder Elbow Surg. 1993;2:275–85.
8. Anderson KD, Friden J, Lichen RL. Acceptable benefits and risks associated with surgically improving arm function in individuals living with cervical spinal cord injury. Spinal Cord. 2009;47:334–8.
9. Mackinnon SE, Novak CB, Myckatyn TM, Tung TH. Results of reinnervation of the biceps and brachialis muscles with a double fascicular transfer for elbow flexion. J Hand Surg Am. 2005;31:183–9.
10. Kozin SH, D'Addesi L, Chafetz RS, Ashworth S, Mulcahey MJ. Biceps-to-Triceps transfer for elbow extension in person with tetraplegia. J Hand Surg. 2010;35A:968–75.
11. Young JH. Implications of elbow arthrodesis for individuals with paraplegia. Phys Ther. 1993;73:194–201.
12. Davidge KM, Yee A, Kahn LC, Mackinnon SE. Median to radial nerve transfers for restoration of wrist, finger, and thumb extension. J Hand Surg Am. 2013;38:1812–27.
13. Rayan GM, Young BT. Arthrodesis of the spastic wrist. J Hand Surg Am. 1999;24:944–52.
14. Terzis JK, Kostopoulos VK. Free muscle transfer in posttraumatic plexopathies: part III. The hand. Plast Reconstr Surg. 2009;124:1225–36.
15. Goldner JL, Koman LA, Gelberman R, Levin S, Goldner RD. Arthrodesis of the metacarpophalangeal joint of the thumb in children and adults. Adjunctive treatment of thumb-in-palm deformity in cerebral palsy. Clin Orthop Relat Res. 1990;253:75–89.
16. Lomita C, Ezaki M, Oishi S. Upper extremity surgery in children with cerebral palsy. J Am Acad Orthop Surg. 2010;18:160–8.

Surgical Considerations in Neurogenic Bladder

25

Todd A. Linsenmeyer

Introduction

The vast majority of those with spinal cord injury (SCI) and neurologic impairment also have voiding dysfunctions with associated problems [1]. While caring for these individuals, a surgical team may need to modify a bladder management program pre- or postsurgery, such as switching from an intermittent to an indwelling catheter, or may need to anticipate possible unique postsurgical problems such as autonomic dysreflexia. This chapter will review normal anatomy and physiology of the urinary system. In addition, it will describe urological preoperative considerations, various methods of bladder management, and some of the more common potential urological problems in those with neurogenic bladders who are planning to undergo surgery.

Anatomy and Physiology of the Upper and Lower Urinary Tracts

When considering the various types of bladder management, it is important to understand the neuroanatomy and neurophysiology of the urinary tract. Discussions often focus solely on a

T.A. Linsenmeyer, MD
Kessler Institute for Rehabilitation,
West Orange, NJ, USA
e-mail: tlinsenmeyer@kessler-rehab.com

patient's "neurogenic bladder." However, changes in the lower tract such as poor drainage or high bladder pressures often have a direct impact on the kidneys as well. This can have important implications in the postoperative patient with a neurogenic bladder. High bladder pressures with stasis of the upper tracts or vesicoureteral reflux could predispose to postoperative pyelonephritis. Therefore, even though this discussion will treat the kidneys and bladder separately as part of the upper and lower urinary tracts, it is beneficial to consider them as a single unit.

Upper Urinary Tract

The kidney consists of two parts: the renal parenchyma and the collecting system. The renal parenchyma secretes, concentrates, and excretes urine into the collecting system. Peristaltic waves propel urine down the ureters to the bladder. Ureteral dilatation for any reason results in inefficient propulsion of the urine bolus, which can delay drainage proximal to that point. This can result in further dilatation and over time lead to hydronephrosis [2].

The ureters connect to the bladder at the ureterovesical junction. They tunnel obliquely, "sandwiched" between the muscular and submucosal layers of the bladder wall 1–2 cm before opening into the bladder at the ureteral orifices. This submucosal tunnel is designed to allow urine to flow into the bladder and to prevent

© Springer International Publishing Switzerland 2017
A.I. Elkwood et al. (eds.), *Rehabilitative Surgery*, DOI 10.1007/978-3-319-41406-5_25

reflux into the ureter. Any increase in intravesical pressure compresses the submucosal ureter, effectively creating a one-way valve. This configuration is important in preventing reflux [3]. Unfortunately, this same configuration can inhibit urine drainage from the kidneys if there are sustained high intravesical (bladder wall) pressures.

Lower Urinary Tract

Anatomically, the bladder is divided into the detrusor and the trigone. The detrusor is composed of smooth muscle bundles that freely crisscross and interlace with each other. Near the bladder neck, the muscle fibers assume three distinct layers. The circular arrangement of the smooth muscles at the bladder neck allows them to act as a functional sphincter. The trigone is located at the inferior base of the bladder and extends from the ureteral orifices to the bladder neck.

Traditionally, the urethra has been thought to have two distinct sphincters: the internal and the external, or rhabdosphincter. The internal sphincter is not a true anatomic sphincter but does act as a functional sphincter. In both males and females, the term refers to the junction of the bladder neck and proximal urethra, formed from the circular arrangement of connective tissue and smooth muscle fibers that extend from the bladder. This area around the bladder neck is considered to be a functional sphincter because as the bladder fills, the tone of the sphincter increases, which prevents urinary incontinence since the urethral pressure is greater than the intravesical pressure. This internal urethral sphincter *has been described* as being under the control of the autonomic system. This area has a large number of sympathetic alpha-receptors, which cause closure of the internal sphincter when stimulated.

In males, the external sphincter has the bulk of its fibers found at the membranous urethra, but fibers also run up to the bladder neck. In females, striated skeletal muscle fibers circle the upper two-thirds of the urethra. In non-SCI individuals, the external sphincter is under voluntary control. Somatic innervation of the sphincter is from the sacral region (S2–S4) via the pudendal nerve, allowing the sphincter to be closed at will.

Changes to the lower urinary tract frequently occur after SCI. In those with SCI, the distinction between the internal and external sphincter becomes less clear. There may be substantial invasion of the alpha-adrenergic nerve fibers into the smooth and striated muscle in the urethra of individuals with SCI with lower motor neuron lesions. Moreover, those with SCI frequently lose control of their external sphincter. If the sphincter does not relax when the bladder is contracting (detrusor sphincter dyssynergia), high pressures often build in the bladder, which can affect kidney drainage. In those with sacral injuries, there may be less ability of the sphincter to contract, allowing urinary incontinence to occur.

Neuroanatomy of the Lower Urinary Tract

Bladder storage and emptying is a function of interactions among the peripheral parasympathetic, sympathetic, and somatic innervation of the lower urinary tract. Additionally, there is modulation from the central nervous system. The parasympathetic efferent (motor) supply originates from the sacral cord at S2–S4. Sacral efferents travel via the pelvic nerves to provide excitatory input to the bladder. Parasympathetic bladder receptors are called cholinergic because the primary postganglionic neurotransmitter is acetylcholine. These receptors are distributed throughout the bladder. Stimulation causes a bladder contraction.

The sympathetic efferent nerve supply to the bladder and urethra begins in the intermediolateral gray column from T11 through L2 and provides inhibitory input to the bladder. Sympathetic impulses travel a relatively short distance to the lumbar sympathetic paravertebral (sympathetic) ganglia. From here the sympathetic impulses travel over long postganglionic fibers in the hypogastric nerves to synapse at alpha- and beta-adrenergic receptors within the bladder and urethra. The primary postganglionic neurotransmitter for the sympathetic system is norepinephrine.

Sympathetic efferent stimulation facilitates bladder storage through the strategic location of the adrenergic receptors in different parts of the bladder. Beta-3 adrenergic receptors, which cause bladder relaxation when stimulated, predominate in the superior portion (i.e., body) of the bladder. Alpha-receptors have a higher density near the base of the bladder and prostatic urethra; stimulation of these receptors causes smooth muscle contractions of the sphincter and prostate, which increases the outlet resistance of the bladder and prostatic urethra.

After SCI, changes in receptor location, density, and sensitivity may occur. Evidence exists that there is invasion of alpha-receptors into the external striated sphincter so that it responds to alpha stimulation. Moreover, when smooth muscle is denervated, its sensitivity to a given amount of neurotransmitter increases (i.e., denervation supersensitivity). As a result, smaller doses of various pharmacologic agents would be expected to have a much more pronounced effect in those with SCI as compared to those with non-neurogenic bladders [4, 5].

Recently scientists have gained a better understanding of the afferent (sensory) system of the bladder. The most important afferents pass to the sacral cord via the pelvic nerves. These afferents are of two types: small myelinated A-delta and unmyelinated (C) fibers. The small myelinated A-delta fibers respond in a graded fashion to bladder distention and are essential for normal voiding. The unmyelinated (C) fibers have been termed "silent C-fibers" because they do not respond to bladder distention and therefore are not essential for normal voiding. However, these "silent C-fibers" have been found to "wake up" and respond to distention and to stimulate involuntary bladder contractions in animals with suprasacral SCI. This has been further confirmed in studies which showed that two C-fiber neurotoxins, capsaicin and resiniferatoxin (RTX) toxin, dramatically block involuntary bladder contractions. Further work is being done on their potential for clinical use. Botulinum A toxin (BTX A) has been found to inhibit sensory receptors in the bladder. Therefore, it is possible that BTX A quiets the bladder by having its impact on the afferent system and actually helps to quiet the bladder by acting as a C-fiber neurotoxin [6, 7].

Voiding Centers

Facilitation and inhibition of voiding is due to three main centers, the sacral micturition center, the pontine micturition center, and the higher centers (cerebral cortex). Thus, locations of injury can be classified as suprapontine, suprasacral, and sacral in order to make generalizations of voiding dysfunction based on level of injury.

Suprapontine (Higher) Centers

The net effect of the cerebral cortex on micturition is inhibitory to the sacral micturition center. Because suprasacral SCI also disrupts the inhibitory impulses from the cerebral cortex, those with suprasacral SCI frequently have small bladder capacities with involuntary bladder contractions.

Pontine Micturition Center

The pontine micturition center is primarily responsible for coordinating relaxation of the urinary sphincter when the bladder contracts. Suprasacral SCI disrupts the signals from the pontine micturition center, which is why detrusor sphincter dyssynergia is common in those with suprasacral SCI.

Sacral Micturition Centers

The sacral micturition center (S2–S4) is primarily a reflex center in which efferent parasympathetic impulses to the bladder cause bladder contraction and afferent impulses from the bladder to the sacral micturition center provide feedback regarding bladder fullness.

Impact of the Location of Spinal Cord Injury on Voiding

The location of the SCI in relation to the voiding centers is important in predicting the type of voiding dysfunction. The three major locations are classified as suprapontine (higher centers), suprasacral SCI, and sacral SCI. While the exact degree of bladder and sphincter function cannot be predicted based on the level and completeness of injury, generalizations of bladder and sphincter function can be made. It is also important to note that the voiding dysfunction may be very different from expectations due to various factors, such as medications, prostate obstruction, and possible normal bladder function but poor cognition. The following discusses expected bladder and sphincter function based on the suprapontine (higher centers), suprasacral SCI, and sacral SCI.

It is also important to remember that those with injuries above thoracic level T6 are likely to have autonomic dysreflexia. However, the amount of BP (blood pressure) elevation and severity of autonomic dysreflexia cannot be predicted.

Suprapontine Lesions (Higher Centers)

Any suprapontine lesion may cause a voiding dysfunction by damaging afferent or efferent input to and from the upper tracts. Lesions may result from cerebrovascular disease, hydrocephalus, intracranial neoplasms, traumatic brain injury, Parkinson's disease, and multiple sclerosis. Since the higher centers exhibit an overall inhibitory influence on the sacral voiding center, the expected urodynamic finding following a suprapontine lesion is detrusor overactivity without detrusor sphincter dyssynergia (DSD). This is because inhibitory signals from higher centers are unable to inhibit the sacral micturition center. However, the sphincter does relax during voiding because the signals from the pontine micturition center are below the area of injury/dysfunction.

Suprasacral Spinal Cord Lesions

Traumatic suprasacral SCI results in an initial period of spinal shock. During this phase, the bladder has no contractions (detrusor areflexia).

The neurophysiology for spinal shock and its recovery are not known. Usually a person with a suprasacral SCI develops detrusor overactivity. Bladder overactivity usually follows recovery of skeletal muscle reflexes. Involuntary bladder contractions gradually return after 6–8 weeks but have been reported up to 2 years later. Clinically, when people with traumatic suprasacral SCI begin to have detrusor (bladder) overactivity, they may begin having episodes of urinary incontinence and various visceral sensations, such as tingling, flushing, increased lower extremity spasms, or autonomic dysreflexia (T6 and above) with the onset of involuntary bladder contractions. As involuntary bladder contractions become stronger, the post-void residuals (PVRs) decrease.

Detrusor overactivity has the potential to cause several problems. The first is that the high pressures in the bladder can cause stasis of the upper tracts. This usually results in problems over time such as hydronephrosis, renal calculi, and gradual decline in renal function. However acutely, poor drainage of the upper tracts can make it more difficult to treat pyelonephritis. In addition to detrusor overactivity (DO), individuals with suprasacral injuries generally also develop detrusor sphincter dyssynergia (DSD). DSD is defined as intermittent or complete failure of relaxation of the urinary sphincter during a bladder contraction and voiding. It has been reported to occur in 96% of individuals with suprasacral lesions. This is because inhibitory signals from higher centers and signals from the pontine micturition center that coordinate detrusor (bladder) and sphincter function are blocked by the spinal cord injury.

Some individuals develop a "balanced bladder" over time. This refers to the bladder having minimal post-void residual volumes following an involuntary bladder contraction. Unfortunately, because of the DSD, very forceful involuntary contractions are usually required for the development of a balanced bladder. It has been found that high voiding pressures and prolonged duration of the bladder contractions may cause hydronephrosis and renal deterioration. Those with suprasacral injuries at T6 and above are at risk of autonomic dysreflexia with bladder over-distention and/or forceful bladder contractions combined with DSD (see section "Autonomic Dysreflexia" for more information about autonomic dysreflexia).

Sacral Lesions

A variety of lesions can affect the sacral cord or roots. Damage to the sacral cord or roots generally results in a highly compliant acontractile bladder. However, particularly in individuals with partial injuries, the areflexia may be accompanied by decreased bladder compliance resulting in progressive increases in intravesical pressure with filling [8].

The exact mechanism by which sacral parasympathetic decentralization of the bladder causes decreased compliance is unknown.

It has been noted that the external sphincter is not affected to the same extent as the detrusor. This is because the pelvic nerve innervation to the bladder usually arises one segment higher than the pudendal nerve innervation to the sphincter. Also, the nuclei are located in different portions of the sacral cord, with the detrusor nuclei located in the intermediolateral cell column and the pudendal nuclei located in the ventral gray matter. This combination of detrusor areflexia and an intact sphincter helps contribute to bladder overdistention and decompensation.

Preoperative Urologic Evaluation

There are a number of considerations in the preoperative evaluation of a person with a neurogenic bladder. These are listed in Table 25.1.

Prior to a major procedure, it is often important to know the status and function of the upper and lower urinary tracts. This information may already be available for review since it is not uncommon for a person with an SCI to have a yearly urological evaluation of the upper and lower urinary tracts. Unfortunately, history, level of injury, and signs and symptoms alone are not enough to evaluate the lower urinary tracts *to*

Table 25.1 Urological preoperative considerations

Does the person have a neurogenic bladder?

Has there been a recent evaluation of the lower urinary tract (urodynamics and cystoscopy)?

Has there been a recent evaluation of the upper urinary tracts (renal scan and or renal ultrasound)?

Is there urinary tract colonization and/or urinary tract infection?

What is the bacterial culture and sensitivity of the urinary colonization/infection?

What is the type of bladder management and how will it affect intraoperative and postoperative management?

Risk of AD dysreflexia? (T6 and above)

What is the risk of bladder stones? (increased risk with indwelling catheter with recurrent bladder stones or catheter blockage)

determine bladder function and degree of possible sphincter dyssynergia. The gold standard to evaluate the lower tract is water fill urodynamics study. Blood pressure monitoring is done in those with SCI levels at or above T6 to check for autonomic dysreflexia. Urodynamics will objectively evaluate the bladder and sphincter function. In addition it will give a good idea of the accuracy of bladder sensation of fullness. For those with SCI above T6, urodynamics is an excellent way to determine the degree of autonomic dysreflexia and whether or not a person has silent autonomic dysreflexia. Silent autonomic dysreflexia is characterized by a significant elevation in BP due to bladder distention or other noxious stimuli without having any other signs or symptoms (see section "Autonomic Dysreflexia"). Cystograms are used to evaluate for vesicoureteral reflux, and cystoscopy is used to evaluate urethral and bladder anatomy [9].

If further information is needed about the upper tracts, several tests are available depending on what information is needed. Mercaptoacetyltriglycine (MAG3) renal scans are used to evaluate renal function [10].

A Lasix renal scan can be used to help differentiate between a patulous system and extrarenal pelvis versus obstruction. Renal ultrasounds are used to evaluate anatomy. If detailed anatomy is needed, a CT scan of the abdomen and pelvis is helpful. Non-contrast studies are used to evaluate for renal and ureteral calculi. CT scans with and without contrast are also important when evaluating a person with gross hematuria or suspicion of a renal lesion found on another type of imaging study. The major drawback of CT scans is radiation exposure and the potential of an allergic reaction if a contrast agent is used.

Contrast studies are used to evaluate for other potential anatomical problems. It should be noted that serum creatinine is not a useful way to follow renal function. There has to be a 50–80 % decline in renal function before there is a change in the serum creatinine. In addition, those with SCI often have a large amount of loss of muscle mass. Since serum creatinine is dependent on muscle mass, a "normal" serum creatinine in an SCI individual may therefore indicate renal insufficiency.

Preoperatively, a urine analysis with culture and sensitivity is important. Those with neurogenic bladders, especially with indwelling catheters, are often colonized with multiple organisms, so it is important to request that the lab "culture all organisms." Otherwise, the laboratory report result may say something to the effect "more than two organisms, probable contaminant, please repeat" or "less than 10,000 organisms probable contaminant, please repeat." It is helpful to order a urine sample 2 weeks before an elective procedure. This allows enough time to call the lab and repeat the sample if it has been discarded due to multiple organisms. Since most individuals with SCI have bladder colonization, it is helpful to give several days of culture specific antibiotics to help reduce any inflammation in addition to providing a transient sterilization of the urine.

Types of Bladder Management and Surgical Considerations

There are several types of bladder management programs one may encounter preoperatively in those with SCI and neurogenic bladder. The most common are intermittent catheterization, indwelling suprapubic or indwelling urethral catheters, reflex voiding, and Crede/Valsalva voiding. It is important to have some familiarity with the different types of bladder management since decisions may need to be made postoperatively

concerning optimum bladder management. In general it is best to keep the same bladder management postoperatively as a person had preoperatively. However, bladder function or fluid status may temporarily change postoperatively, necessitating a temporary change in bladder management. The following gives an overview of some of the more common types of bladder management. A more detailed description and the reasons for and against the different methods and potential complications can be found in the Consortium for Spinal Cord Medicine Guideline titled "Bladder management for adults with spinal cord injury" [11].

Intermittent Catheterization

Intermittent catheterization involves draining the bladder with a urethral catheter every 4–6 h. Generally a 14 or 16 French straight catheter is used. Men with enlarged prostates will often find it easier to pass a coudé (slightly curved tip) rather than a straight (tip) catheter. It is important to catheterize at a frequency to keep catheterized volumes less than 500 ml. Individuals with spinal cord injuries at or below C6 to C7 are the best candidates for intermittent catheterization because they have adequate hand function to dress and undress and can therefore be independent at performing their own catheterization.

In the hospital setting, the initial order is usually to catheterize a person's bladder every 4 h. Special care needs to be taken not to allow a person's bladder to become overdistended. Overdistension of the bladder is the most common cause of bladder infections due to a relative ischemia of the bladder wall and potential small tears in the bladder mucosa. The small tears can also cause hematuria when the overdistended bladder is drained and there is a return of regular blood flow to the bladder mucosa. This hematuria is usually short lived. In those with SCI at T6 and above, bladder distention is also of particular concern since it can cause potentially life-threatening autonomic dysreflexia. Autonomic dysreflexia often presents as the sudden onset of a severe headache, elevated BP, sweating, and piloerection. However, a sudden severe elevation in BP can also occur without any symptoms and is termed "silent" autonomic dysreflexia (see section "Autonomic Dysreflexia").

Those with suprasacral injuries as discussed above usually have overactive bladders. The bladder overactivity is usually controlled with anticholinergics. Anticholinergics are very helpful at decreasing involuntary contractions and the potential for urinary incontinence and stasis of the upper tract. Therefore, it is important to resume a person's anticholinergic medications postoperatively. It must, however, be kept in mind that anticholinergic medications will slow intestinal peristalsis and increase the likelihood of constipation. When there is a concern of constipation, it is better to give medications to treat or prevent constipation rather than withhold the anticholinergic medication. If a urodynamics study shows that the involuntary contractions are poorly controlled or a person is having significant side effects from the anticholinergics (dry mouth and constipation most common), intravesical instillations of oxybutynin (off-label) or botulinum toxin A injections into the bladder wall are usually effective at controlling the overactivity. Currently the only FDA-approved botulinum toxin to use for neurogenic and non-neurogenic overactive bladders is onabotulinum toxin A (Botox ®).

Indwelling Catheterization (Urethral and Suprapubic Catheterization)

Suprapubic and indwelling urethral catheters are most commonly used in those with suprasacral spinal cord injuries and poor hand function who are unable to catheterize themselves or do not have a willing caregiver who can perform the catheterization. Catheters are also particularly useful in a surgical setting if the person is on a large amount of IV fluid or there is a need to monitor fluid output. As discussed previously, those with suprasacral SCI usually have overactive bladders. They are usually on maintenance anticholinergic medication to quiet their bladder just like those with suprasacral SCI on intermit-

tent catheterization. The above discussion regarding those with overactive bladders and use of anticholinergic medications applies to those with indwelling catheters. In fact, it is even more important to make sure that those with indwelling catheters are on anticholinergic medications since the indwelling catheter will often trigger involuntary bladder contractions.

Currently there is a strong push to maintain a closed system and remove the indwelling catheter as soon as possible because of the increased risk of a catheter-associated urinary tract infection (CAUTI) (see section "Urinary Tract Infection"). This is not an issue with a SP (suprapublic) catheter.

Reflex Voiding

Reflex voiding is primarily used for men with suprasacral SCI who have overactive bladders and who are not able to control their urinary stream. It involves wearing an external condom catheter and a leg bag so that when the bladder has an involuntary contraction and voiding occurs, the urine flows out the bladder and urethra into an external condom catheter that is connected to tubing and a leg bag. This can be switched to a larger bag at night. There is usually some degree of sphincter dyssynergia. Generally, some type of treatment to relax the sphincter is needed to prevent back pressure to the kidneys and autonomic dysreflexia and help improve emptying of the bladder with a bladder contraction. Treatment usually involves giving an alpha-blocker. However, Botox injection into the sphincter (off-label) is sometimes used. In the past, sphincterotomy was frequently used. It is currently not used very often due to its irreversibility, frequent need to be redone, and less experience among urologists at how to perform a sphincterotomy.

Reflex voiding has limited utility in women because there is not an effective external collecting device that a woman can use. An alternative that can be used by men and women is to wear pads or diapers. Most do not like the discomfort of wearing wet pads, inconvenience of changing the pads frequently, and the expense of purchasing the pads, not covered by a number of insurance plans.

The advantages of reflex voiding are no fluid restrictions and not having to undress to catheterize the bladder. The disadvantages are having to wear and change the external condom catheter daily, the potential for skin breakdowns from the condom, and the very embarrassing situation of the external condom catheter coming off and then voiding. This is most likely to happen if the condom twists on itself before voiding and then a person voids, pushing the condom catheter off.

Crede/Valsalva Voiding

Credé/Valsalva voiding is used by those with sacral SCI who have no bladder contractions. It involves the use of intra-abdominal pressure to force the urine out of the bladder. The difference between Credé and Valsalva voiding is that those who use Credé voiding make a fist and push it into their lower abdomen over their bladder to empty their bladder. Valsalva voiding involves taking a deep breath and bearing down to push out the urine, much like trying to have a bowel movement. This method is not recommended for those with sphincter dyssynergia since high pressures are needed within the bladder to push the urine out of the bladder. There is concern that constant frequent bearing down may cause hemorrhoids and hernia or may cause or exacerbate bladder/vaginal prolapse. In general, a person needs to be sitting up in order to have enough intra-abdominal pressure to effectively "bear down" to void. An alpha-blocker is sometimes used to help quiet the sphincter and improve voiding in those who use intra-abdominal pressure to void.

Common Urological Problems Following SCI

In addition to a neurogenic bladder, there are several other urological problems encountered pre- and postoperatively in a person with an SCI (see

Table 25.2 Common urological problems in those with neurogenic bladder

Voiding dysfunction (urinary retention, urinary incontinence, or both), urinary tract infection
Autonomic dysreflexia (T6 and above)
Bladder stones and catheter blockage (especially with an indwelling catheter)

Table 25.2). The most common potential problems are urinary tract infections and the risk of autonomic dysreflexia in those with SCI at or above T6. The following sections will discuss these problems and their management.

Urinary Tract Infections

Bacteria in the urine are common and an important consideration in those with neurogenic bladders. There is a lot of confusion between asymptomatic bacteriuria, which is usually colonization, and a true symptomatic infection. There are often a lot of questions with regard to diagnosis and when to treat and not to treat. The diagnosis of a UTI (urinary tract infection) in those with neurogenic bladder should not be made based solely on the presence of increased bacteria in the urine. There is consensus that three criteria must be met for an individual to be considered as having a UTI: (1) significant bacteriuria, (2) pyuria (increased white blood cells in the urine), and (3) signs and symptoms [12].

Criteria for significant bacteriuria (the number of bacteria that signify that the bacteria are truly from the bladder and not just a contaminant) depend on the method of bladder management being used:

- For those on intermittent catheterization = 10^2 colony forming units (cfu)
- For those using clean-void specimens from catheter-free males who use external condom collecting devices = 10^4 cfu
- For those with specimens from indwelling catheters, any detectable concentration [13]

A UTI implies bacteriuria with bladder wall tissue invasion. This tissue invasion also results in signs and symptoms, which may include one or more of the following: (1) leukocytes (increased white blood cells, or WBCs) in the urine generated by the mucosal lining (on rare occasions gram-positive bacteria do not provoke a WBC response); (2) discomfort or pain over the kidney or bladder, or during urination; (3) onset of urinary incontinence; (4) increased spasticity; (5) autonomic dysreflexia; (6) cloudy urine with increased odor; (7) malaise, lethargy, or sense of unease [12].

In addition to a different set of criteria to define a UTI in those with neurogenic bladder, there is often a difference in the number of different types of bacteria in the urine. Those without a neurogenic bladder or indwelling catheter usually have a single organism, most commonly *E. coli*. However, those with an indwelling catheter frequently have two or more organisms in the bladder [14].

It is also important to note that the bacteria in the urine represent the skin flora, and the flora in SCI individuals is different compared to able-bodied individuals. In one study, Gram-positive cocci and diphtheroids were the predominant isolates from controls with no enteric organisms recovered except *Escherichia coli* in four instances. Among SCI patients, in addition to normal Gram-positive flora, one species of Gram-negative rod was isolated from three patients, two species from five patients, three species from three patients, four species from three patients, and five species from one individual. Skin isolates included various members of Enterobacteriaceae, Pseudomonas, Acinetobacter, and Enterococcus. Average bacterial counts in perineal, penile, and urethral cultures from SCI patients were each 1 log greater than in controls. Bacteria were isolated from 12 of 14 urine cultures obtained from SCI patients immediately after collection of skin cultures. Organisms isolated from urine were present in one or more skin sites in every instance [15].

In another study, 54 identical bacterial isolates were observed both from urine and one or more skin sites in 43 patients. *Escherichia coli*, *Proteus mirabilis*, *Klebsiella pneumoniae*, and *Proteus stuartii* were the most common bacterial isolates [16].

Therefore, these studies show that a urine sample with culture and sensitivities is very important prior to surgery since organisms that colonize the bladder frequently also colonize the person's skin in those with neurogenic bladder.

When and How to Treat UTI in SCI

Prior to surgery, it is important to treat both colonization and active infections. Since multiple organisms with resistance to various antibiotics are frequently found in those with a neurogenic bladder, it is particularly important to get a urine culture and sensitivity prior to surgery. A problem that can be encountered is a lab not culturing the organisms. Because there is more than one type of bacteria in the urine, the lab discards the sample with the note "multiple organisms, probable contaminant, please repeat." Therefore, it is helpful to write on the lab slip "Please culture and obtain sensitivities on all organisms." Though this instruction works relatively well, it is advisable to obtain a pre-procedure urine culture and sensitivity 2 weeks prior to the scheduled procedure. This allows a repeat sample if the first one is discarded. The person can then be treated with culture specific antibiotics, rather than empiric antibiotics.

Traditionally, an able-bodied person is given an antibiotic an hour before the start of surgery. Because of the neurogenic bladder and poor emptying and foreign body in those with indwelling catheters, a pre-procedure antibiotic should be started 3–5 days prior to a procedure. An exception would be a person with a history of *Clostridium difficile*. In that case, an antibiotic can be given the morning of the procedure and a dose post procedure and when appropriate, prophylaxis for *C. difficile*.

Autonomic Dysreflexia

Autonomic dysreflexia (AD) can occur in any SCI individual with injuries at T6 and above. Classically the typical signs are a sudden severe rise in BP, headaches, flushing, and piloerection.

The most dramatic problem associated with autonomic dysreflexia is a sudden severe elevation in blood pressure. Those with an SCI at or above T6 frequently have a baseline systolic blood pressure in the 90–110 mmHg range. Autonomic dysreflexia is frequently defined in adults as a systolic blood pressure greater than 140 mmHg. Another definition is a systolic blood pressure 20–40 mmHg above baseline. Systolic blood pressures elevations more than 15–20 mmHg above baseline in adolescents with SCI or more than 15 mmHg above baseline in children may be a sign of autonomic dysreflexia [9, 17, 18].

However, it has been found that up to 40 % of individuals have "silent" autonomic dysreflexia. Those with silent autonomic dysreflexia have been found to have significant elevations in their baseline blood pressures with none of the other signs of dysreflexia. In addition, those with silent autonomic dysreflexia are not aware themselves that they are having an elevated BP during their episode of autonomic dysreflexia [9]. Therefore, it is essential that all patients with SCI above T6 have frequent BP monitoring immediately before, during, and after a procedure.

Autonomic dysreflexia occurs as a result of any noxious stimulus. The most common causes are bladder distention and bowel problems such as constipation and impaction. Both of these have particular significance in the postsurgical patient since both conditions commonly occur postsurgery. In a person with unexplained autonomic dysreflexia lying on the table, check to see if they are lying on a pressure sore. Rolling off the sore will decrease the noxious stimulus and will immediately allow resolution of the dysreflexia. For a more detailed review on how to manage autonomic dysreflexia, see Consortium for Spinal Cord Medicine (2002) [17, 18].

Prevention of Autonomic Dysreflexia

Bladder overdistention can cause AD in two ways. The first is the noxious stimulus from bladder overdistention. The other way is that in those with overactive bladders from suprasacral SCI, the bladder overdistention causes involuntary bladder contractions. This in turn triggers reflex tightening of the sphincter (DSD), which can then trigger AD in those with injuries at T6 and above.

This has implications in the prevention and treatment of AD. Overdistention can be prevented by limiting fluid intake, increasing the frequency of catheterization, or both. If a person requires intravenous fluids or large intake or is having a postoperative diuresis, indwelling catheter (see discussion below) is helpful. FDA-approved pharmacological treatments to prevent involuntary bladder contractions include anticholinergic medications and intradetrusor injections of botulinum toxin A (Botox) into the bladder. More work is needed to determine the role of beta 3 agonists in neurogenic detrusor overactivity (off-label). Pharmacological treatment to help decrease DSD with alpha-blockers can also be used.

The second most common cause of AD is constipation and fecal impaction. Making sure the person has "empty bowels" before a procedure and making sure a person does not get constipated or impacted is very important for preventing AD. It must be remembered that even though a person may not have sensation, noxious stimuli will still cause AD. Therefore, when performing a procedure with local anesthesia, give the topical anesthetic the same way you would if a person had sensation.

Treatment of Autonomic Dysreflexia (AD)

If autonomic dysreflexia occurs, immediately sit the person up (if the person is supine), loosen any clothing or constrictive devices, monitor the blood pressure and pulse frequently, and quickly survey the individual for possible causes, beginning with the urinary system. Make sure the catheter is not kinked and that the bladder is not overdistended. If it is felt that the catheter is blocked, it needs to be changed. Since passing a new catheter down the urethra into the bladder may exacerbate AD if readily available, consider gently instilling 5–10 cc of

Table 25.3 Autonomic dysreflexia evaluation and management

Once a person is identified to have AD – closely monitor the BP

Sit person up, legs down (if possible)

Evaluate for possible reversible causes – tight clothing, abdominal binder, bladder, or bowel issues

Bladder issues – check for and correct if present (such as overfilled drainage bag, kinked tubing, blocked catheter, overdistended bladder)

Bowel issues – check for and correct if present (such as constipation, fecal impaction)

Consider pharmacological management at any time during the above. In individuals with elevated BP, consider pharmacotherapy while investigating and managing autonomic dysreflexia. Topical nitropaste is a good first choice. The use of antihypertensive drugs in the presence of sustained elevated blood pressure is supported by level 1 (prazosin) and level 2 evidence (nifedipine and prostaglandin E$_2$). If pharmacotherapy has been used, monitor for rebound hypotension after the cause of the AD has been identified and treated.

If no obvious cause of AD or poor response to treatment, hospitalization should be strongly considered.

Note: Be aware that when changing an indwelling catheter or passing a straight catheter, there may be an initial increase in BP. Therefore, instillation of lidocaine jelly into the urethra before passing the catheter may be helpful. This may also be helpful in the rectum prior to fecal disimpaction

For more details on evaluation and management of autonomic dysreflexia, see Consortium for Spinal Cord Medicine (2002) [17, 18]

2 % lidocaine jelly in a prefilled syringe, such as lidocaine hydrochloride 2 % jelly 100 mg/5 mL prior to catheterization. If constipation is suspected, 2 % lidocaine jelly instilled into the rectum prior to digital disimpaction may be helpful to prevent AD. It is may also be helpful to administer a fast-acting pharmacological agent, such as nitropaste to the forehead, to lower the BP prior to catheterization or disimpaction. If the cause of AD cannot be identified or does not respond to treatment, hospital admission should be considered for a more detailed evaluation of possible causes and treatment (Table 25.3) [17–19]. Rarely, a person with severe AD that does not respond to treatment will need spinal anesthesia to block the noxious stimuli.

Pharmacological Treatment for Acute Autonomic Dysreflexia (AD)

Frequently a person has very high BP and pharmacological treatment should be considered at the time of evaluating and treating the cause of the AD. Pharmacotherapy, such as 1/2–1″ of nitropaste, is recommended to treat a person with autonomic dysreflexia and an elevated BP. Nitropaste, which has rapid onset, can be placed on the forehead so it can be easily applied or removed depending on the BP [17, 18]. If further pharmacotherapy is needed, the use of antihypertensive drugs in the presence of sustained elevated blood pressure is supported by level 1 (prazosin) and level 2 evidence (nifedipine and prostaglandin E$_2$) [19]. Nifedipine, nitrates, and captopril are the most commonly used and recommended agents for the management of acute AD episodes and are supported by level 2, 5, and 4 evidence, respectively. However, to date, no RCTs (randomized controlled trials) have been conducted to determine which of these agents is best [17–21].

Nifedipine was used preferentially by 48 % of physicians for minor AD cases and by 58 % of physicians for severe symptomatic AD. Even though nifedipine has been the most commonly used agent in the management of AD in subjects with SCI, its use has declined recently because of concern over the potential for adverse events [22]. There have been no reported serious adverse events from the use of nifedipine in the treatment of AD [20].

Post-autonomic Dysreflexia Management

Once the cause of AD has been identified and treated, the person should be monitored for a rebound hypotension. This is why quick onset short-acting agents should be used. Topical nitropaste applied to the forehead is a good pharmacological agent to use because it has a rapid onset and can also be removed quickly. Conversely, one should also monitor the blood pressure for recurrent elevation in BP after the pharmacological agents have worn off, just in case the precipitating cause of the dysreflexia has not been adequately treated. Long-term management with agents to quiet an overactive bladder or alpha-blockers to help decrease DSD may be considered.

Bladder Stones

After UTIs, bladder stones are the second most common urological problem in those with a neurogenic bladder [23]. More commonly, bladder stones occur in those with indwelling catheters. Since most of these stones are formed from urease-producing organisms, the majority of these stones are calcium phosphate (46.8 %) or struvite (26.7 %). *Proteus mirabilis*, *Providencia stuartii*, and *Klebsiella* species are frequently found in the urine although any stone-forming organism that is a urease producer has the potential to alkalinize the urine and form stones. There should be a strong suspicion of urease-producing organisms if there is a persistent alkaline urine pH (6.5–9.0).

Bladder stones rarely develop in those performing intermittent catheterization. Usually if stones are found, these are due to stones that formed when the catheter was first in place during the acute injury. Occasionally a pubic hair is accidentally pushed up into the bladder during intermittent catheterization and this serves as a nidus to form a bladder stone. These are found to occur in approximately 30 % of those with indwelling catheters. Of interest, those getting recurrent bladder stones seem to be the same group of individuals who got stones initially. It is unusual for the other 70 % of individuals to get bladder stones [24].

Therefore, once an individual is determined to be a bladder stone former, increasing the frequency of catheter changes to once every 1–2 weeks to help prevent catheter blockage is helpful. In addition they should be scheduled for more frequent cystoscopies at approximately every 3–6 months. Consideration should be given for a preoperative cystoscopy to check for bladder stones. Bladder stones can be a problem in a person undergoing a surgical procedure because they can block a catheter. Blockage of the catheter can cause bladder distention, potentially leading to autonomic dysreflexia, hematuria, bacteremia, and possibly sepsis [25]. Therefore, it is important to make sure that a person does not have bladder stones prior to a procedure, especially if the use of an indwelling catheter is expected [24].

Summary

Those with SCI may present with a number of unique urological pre- and postoperative challenges. The first is that most have a neurogenic bladder with a variety of voiding dysfunctions. Since there is no one best way to manage a neurogenic bladder, there are a number of different types of bladder management. Each type of bladder management has its own set of advantages and disadvantages. Sometimes a person has to be temporarily changed from one type of bladder management to another immediately postoperatively. In addition, individuals with neurogenic bladder frequently have a number of potentially preventable intraoperative and postoperative conditions such as autonomic dysreflexia, bacterial colonization of the urinary tract, and possible bladder stones. Of particular concern is that many health-care providers have little or no experience with the recognition, evaluation, and immediate treatment of autonomic dysreflexia that can occur in those with injuries above T6. Therefore, it is incumbent on the surgeon to be familiar with neurogenic bladder and its management and potential problems and to make sure the medical staff working with the SCI patient is familiar with these various issues as well.

References

1. McGuire EJ, Savastano J. Comparative urological outcome in women with spinal cord injury. J Urol. 1986;135:730–1.
2. Griffiths DJ, Notschaele C. Mechanics of urine transport in the upper urinary tract: the dynamics of the isolated bolus. Neurourol Urodyn. 1983;2:155–66.

3. Stephens FD, Lenaghan D. The anatomical basis and dynamics of vesicoureteral reflux. J Urol. 1962;87:669–80.

4. Benson GS, McConnell JA, Wood JG. Adrenergic innervation of the human bladder body. J Urol. 1979;122:189–91.

5. Elbadawi A. Autonomic muscular innervation of the vesical outlet and its role in micturition. In: Hinman Jr F, editor. Benign prostatic hypertrophy. New York: Springer; 1983. p. 330–48.

6. Conte A, Giannantoni A, Proietti S, Giovannozzi S, Fabbrini G, Rossi A, et al. Botulinum toxin A modulates afferent fibers in neurogenic detrusor overactivity. Eur J Neurol. 2012;19:725–32.

7. Apostolidis A, Popat R, Yiangou Y, Cockayne D, Ford AP, Davis JB, et al. Decreased sensory receptors P2X3 and TRPV1 in suburothelial nerve fibers following intradetrusor injections of botulinum toxin for human detrusor overactivity. J Urol. 2005;174:977–83.

8. Herschorn S, Hewitt RJ. Patient perspective of long-term outcome of augmentation cystoplasty for neurogenic bladder. Urology. 1998;52:672–8.

9. Linsenmeyer TA, Campagnolo DI, Chou IH. Silent autonomic dysreflexia during voiding in men with spinal cord injuries. J Urol. 1996;155:519–22.

10. Tempkin A, Sullivan G, Paldi J, Perkash I. Radioisotope renography in spinal cord injury. J Urol. 1985;133:228–30.

11. Consortium for Spinal Cord Medicine. Bladder management for adults with spinal cord injury. A clinical practice guideline for health-care providers. J Spinal Cord Med. 2006;29:527–73.

12. National Institute on Disability and Rehabilitation Research Consensus Statement. The prevention and management of urinary tract infections among people with spinal cord injuries. J Am Paraplegia Soc. 1992;15:194–204.

13. Gribble MJ. The diagnosis and significance of bacteriuria in people with spinal cord injury. NeuroRehabilitation. 1994;4:205–13.

14. Linsenmeyer TA, Harrison B, Oakley A, Kirshblum S, Stock JA, Millis SR. Evaluation of cranberry supplement for reduction of urinary tract infections in individuals with neurogenic bladders secondary to spinal cord injury. A prospective, double-blinded, placebo-controlled, crossover study. J Spinal Cord Med. 2004;27:29–34.

15. Taylor TA, Waites KB. A quantitative study of genital skin flora in male spinal cord-injured outpatients. Am J Phys Med Rehabil. 1993;72:113–77.

16. Hamamci N, Dursun E, Akbas E, Aktepe OC, Àakc AC. A quantitative study of genital skin flora and urinary colonization in spinal cord injured patients. Spinal Cord. 1998;36:617–20.

17. Consortium for Spinal Cord Medicine. Acute management of autonomic dysreflexia: individuals with spinal cord injury presenting to health care facilities. 2nd ed. Washington, DC: Paralyzed Veterans of America; 2001.

18. Consortium for Spinal Cord Medicine. Acute management of autonomic dysreflexia: individuals with spinal cord injury presenting to health-care facilities. J Spinal Cord Med. 2002;25 Suppl 1:S67–88.

19. Krassioukov A, Warburton DE, Teasell R, Eng JJ, Spinal Cord Injury Rehabilitation Evidence Research Team. A systematic review of the management of autonomic dysreflexia after spinal cord injury. Arch Phys Med Rehabil. 2009;90:682–93.

20. Blackmer J. Rehabilitation medicine, 1: autonomic dysreflexia. CMAJ. 2003;169:931–5.

21. Braddom RL, Rocco JF. Autonomic dysreflexia: a survey of current treatment. Am J Phys Med Rehabil. 1991;70:234–41.

22. Dykstra DD, Sidi AA, Anderson LC. The effect of nifedipine on cystoscopy-induced autonomic hyperreflexia in patients with high spinal cord injuries. J Urol. 1987;138:1155–7.

23. Cardenas D, Farrell-Roberts L, Sipski M, Rubner D. Management of gastrointestinal, genitourinary and sexual function. In: Stover SL, DeLisa JA, editors. Spinal cord injury—clinical outcomes from the model systems. Gaithersburg: Aspen Publication; 1995. p. 120–45.

24. Linsenmeyer MA, Linsenmeyer TA. Accuracy of bladder stone detection using abdominal x-ray after spinal cord injury. J Spinal Cord Med. 2004;27:438–42.

25. Linsenmeyer MA, Linsenmeyer TA. Accuracy of predicting bladder stones based on catheter encrustation in individuals with spinal cord injury. J Spinal Cord Med. 2006;29:402–5.

Part IX

Vascular Considerations,
Including Lymphedema

Vascular Considerations in Rehabilitative Surgery

Jonathan Weiswasser, A. Ashinoff, and Lisa F. Schneider

Introduction

Diseases of the vascular system affect both the arterial and venous sides of the circulation. While arterial insufficiency is often considered to be a more serious threat to life and limb, the disability associated with venous disease cannot be discounted, especially given that venous disease is the most commonly encountered vascular disease in Western populations. It is estimated that 200 million people live with peripheral arterial disease (PAD) worldwide [1] and that venous disease alone affects 50% of adults [2]. Due to the variety and breadth of arterial and venous disease processes, this discussion will be limited to peripheral arterial disease and deep venous thrombosis, the two most likely vascular processes that the rehabilitation specialist is likely to encounter. The clinician is referred elsewhere for discussion of cerebrovascular disease, arterial aneurysms, and superficial venous disease.

J. Weiswasser, MD • A. Ashinoff, MD
L.F. Schneider, MD
The Plastic Surgery Center, Institute for Advanced Reconstruction, 535 Sycamore Ave, Shrewsbury, NJ 07702, USA
e-mail: jweiswassermd@theplasticsurgerycenternj.com; rashinoffmd@theplasticsurgerycenternj.com; lschneidermd@theplasticsurgerycenternj.com

Peripheral Arterial Disease

Epidemiology

Several risk factors found primarily in elderly patients have been strongly associated with peripheral arterial disease in addition to coronary artery disease, a connection that should always stay foremost in the specialist's mind. Increasing age, hypertension, diabetes, current or former history of smoking, hypercholesterolemia and hypertriglyceridemia, increased serum C-reactive protein levels, and a history of other cardiovascular disease have all been strongly associated with the development of peripheral arterial disease. Atherosclerosis remains the most common underlying cause of PAD, but other, perhaps more unusual, causes can include vasculitis, aneurysm disease, trauma, and anatomic variants such as popliteal entrapment, cystic adventitial disease, and rare congenital abnormalities. Atherosclerosis continues to be defined by the presence of intimal injury followed by activation of the inflammatory cascade, resulting, ultimately, in macroscopic stenotic or occlusive vessel disease.

History and Physical Exam

The most common complaint among patients with PAD is impairment in walking ability or endurance, also known as *claudication*.

© Springer International Publishing Switzerland 2017
A.I. Elkwood et al. (eds.), *Rehabilitative Surgery*, DOI 10.1007/978-3-319-41406-5_26

Claudication typically manifests as pain that occurs in the calf after walking a set distance that is relieved by rest. While many conditions, such as orthopedic and rheumatologic disorders, may affect one's ability to ambulate, the harbinger of claudication is the onset of discomfort at a relatively repeatable distance. The interval of rest that then allows for further ambulation is also of a typically repeatable interval. Claudication can be further defined by whether the symptoms are in fact life limiting, a variable which helps guide therapy.

Pain that occurs in the feet or toes at rest or when the patient is in a recumbent position defines a more serious progression of disease and is known as *rest pain*. Rest pain often occurs at night, requiring the patient to stand up and ambulate in order to alleviate the often severe discomfort, which typically occurs in the forefoot and toes, representing the distal-most anatomic point in the circulation. A patient who sleeps in a chair or recliner typically should be strongly investigated for the presence of severe PAD.

Gangrene, or the presence of a nonhealing sore or ulcer, represents the most severe form of PAD and requires swift and aggressive treatment in order to avoid loss of limb. Limb-threatening ischemia represents 1–2 % of patients with PAD. The presence of risk factors, especially those that can be attenuated, should be aggressively pursued at the first encounter. It is estimated that more than 90 % of patients referred for evaluation of PAD report a current or former history of smoking and smoking remains the risk factor most amenable to amelioration [3]. The smoking status of every patient should be inquired about at each visit.

The physical examination of the patient suspected of PAD should focus attention on the presence and quality of pulses throughout. The carotid arteries should be auscultated for bruits, and the abdomen palpated for a wide or prominent pulse, which may signify the presence of aneurysmal disease of the aorta. Pulses should be examined in the radial, femoral, popliteal, dorsalis pedis, and anterior tibialis positions on both sides. Weakening or absence of pulses should prompt further evaluation and are important clues as to the level and degree of vascular impairment [4]. The skin should be thoroughly inspected for the presence of ulceration or gangrene. Skin that appears cellulitic in the foot may manifest underlying severe peripheral arterial disease and can be distinguished from an infectious process by raising the foot with the patient supine; if the redness disappears, the patient should be strongly suspected of PAD. Attention to the girth and health of the muscles of the lower extremity may also be useful.

Noninvasive Testing

Foremost in the armamentarium of tests for PAD is the *ankle-brachial index* (ABI), which divides the highest blood pressure recorded at the ankle with the patient supine by the highest blood pressure recorded at the brachial position. The result, expressed as an index, can help confirm the presence or absence of PAD, with any result of less than 0.9 considered abnormal. A result less than 0.4 is considered severe. *Pulse volume recordings* (PVR) are often performed in conjunction with the ABI and provide additional information that may enhance the sensitivity and specificity of the ABI result. Conditions that lead to calcification of the arterial system especially below the knee, such as diabetes, can lead to abnormally elevated ABIs and an erroneous presumption of the absence of PAD. PVRs are particularly useful in this circumstance.

Noninvasive imaging of the vascular tree can be accomplished with the use of *magnetic resonant angiography* (MRA), a relatively new modality that has significantly aided the vascular specialist. MRA can help identify the location and degree of vascular compromise and help guide further treatment. In many cases, MRA may be all that is necessary to plan definitive management. Given the cost of these studies, however, use should be reserved for patients with an abnormal ABI or in whom an anatomic cause of PAD is considered [5]. CT angiography offers similar advantages as MRA, but suffers from the administration of ionizing radiation.

Invasive imaging is considered the gold standard for diagnosis of PAD, but should be employed primarily by the vascular specialist. A discussion of invasive imaging can be found elsewhere.

Treatment

Treatment of the patient with PAD begins with mitigation of risk factors. The cessation of smoking is mandatory. It is incumbent upon the practitioner to refer the patient with a current history of smoking to cessation therapy. Control of other risk factors should include management of hypertension, control of glucose levels in the diabetic, and treatment of other cardiovascular risk factors. Patients with non-life-limiting claudication can safely undergo exercise therapy.

Supervised exercise therapy, which typically has the patient ambulate until pain is encountered in the calf with persistence of ambulation as long as possible *with* the pain, for 30–45 min during three sessions in a week, has demonstrated improvement in endurance over time. This is due to the development of collateral circulation and is the safest method to improve symptoms. Furthermore, the clinician should reassure patients that the pain encountered during such sessions, while possibly severe, will not cause harm. The use of phosphodiesterase inhibitors such as cilostazol has been shown to improve ambulatory distance, whereas other medications such as pentoxifylline have not [6].

The presence of life-limiting claudication, rest pain, or gangrene or ulceration should elicit prompt evaluation of the patient by a vascular specialist. Further management is often invasive and involves endovascular techniques, such as angioplasty or stenting, or open surgical techniques, such as bypass or endarterectomy. Therapy in this regard is guided by several factors including the clinical severity of disease, anatomic considerations, life expectancy, and risk associated with intervention.

Venous Disease and Deep Vein Thrombosis

Deep venous thrombosis (DVT) refers to the development of an occlusive thrombus in one of the deep veins of the extremity, typically the lower extremity. While the occlusion can lead to sequelae of its own, the most feared result of a DVT is the development of a pulmonary embolus (PE), which may be fatal. DVT has an incidence in the general population of about 20 per 100,000 per year, resulting in over 500,000 hospitalizations per year, and represents a significant challenge to the rehabilitation patient and specialist alike [7, 8].

Risk Factors

Several risk factors for the development of DVT have been identified in addition to the classic Virchow's triad of trauma (to a vein wall), stasis (of blood within the vein), and hypercoagulability. Factors such as presence of malignancy, prior venous thromboembolism, inflammatory diseases, hormonal contraceptives or replacement therapy, thrombophilia, prolonged travel, family history, and being postpartum are all considered significant risk factors for the development of DVT.

History and Physical Exam

Most DVT are asymptomatic. Symptoms such as leg swelling or pain, particularly if it occurs unilaterally, should prompt concern. A history of thrombophilia is an essential part of the intake history. The patient should be asked about a personal or family history of factor V Leiden mutation, prothrombin G20210A mutation, antithrombin III deficiency, protein C or S deficiency, and antiphospholipid antibody syndrome (lupus anticoagulant). The physical examination should concentrate on the affected extremity. Signs of DVT include unilateral pitting edema, leg swelling, tenderness, and prominent superficial veins. Although a traditional sign of DVT, a positive Homans' sign, pain elicited in the calf with passive dorsiflexion of the foot, has been discredited as a useful marker for disease [9].

Other diseases that should be considered as part of the differential diagnosis in the case of DVT are lymphedema, cellulitis, superficial thrombophlebitis, leg trauma, ruptured popliteal cyst, tendonitis and other orthopedic conditions, peripheral neuropathy, heart failure, nephrotic syndrome, and cirrhosis.

Testing for DVT

The paradigm for testing depends on clinical suspicion. Initial tests include the D-dimer assay and venous duplex ultrasound. A quantitative D-dimer assay is not specific, so that it cannot confirm the presence of a DVT or PE, but a negative test can effectively rule out either form of thrombus. Often, when clinical suspicion is low, a negative D-dimer assay can avoid any further testing [10]. However, if suspicion is high or the patient is considered high risk, the clinician should consider the use of both modalities. If suspicion persists after negative testing, tests should be repeated after 1 week.

Treatment

Treatment of the detected DVT primarily relies upon aggressive anticoagulation to prevent further propagation of the thrombus. Typically this can be accomplished at home. However, the presence of a massive DVT, pulmonary embolism, high risk of bleeding, or other comorbid conditions may dictate that this be performed in an inpatient setting. Typical initial treatment includes the use of low molecular weight heparin, unfractionated heparin, or fondaparinux for immediate anticoagulation. This is then followed by long-term, oral, vitamin K antagonist treatment, e.g., Coumadin, for a period of time dependent upon whether the DVT was provoked, the underlying cause, and history of prior DVT. This interval must also take into account the patient's risk of bleeding and may vary from 3 months of treatment to lifelong, indefinite anticoagulation.

The vena caval filter should be reserved for patients in whom a DVT is confirmed and anticoagulation is contraindicated, a pulmonary embolus has occurred and the patient has poor functional reserve, or a large iliac thrombus is "floating" in the pelvis. Softer indications include bariatric or neurosurgical procedures and recurrent DVT despite adequate anticoagulation and can include the use of retrievable filters. Vena caval filters may reduce the risk of PE but do not appear to reduce mortality [11]. Consideration for additional therapies, such as catheter-directed thrombolytic therapy, should be made in conjunction with the vascular specialist.

Lymphedema

Epidemiology and Etiologies

Lymphedema is a common disease affecting approximately 140 million people throughout the world [12]. It is an abnormal buildup of fluid that causes swelling, most often in the arms or legs. The condition develops when lymph vessels or lymph nodes are missing, impaired, damaged, or removed. Primary lymphedema develops from birth and has no known cause. Secondary lymphedema can develop after the removal of lymph nodes for cancer. It can also develop after infection, trauma, or radiation. Tissues with lymphedema are at a risk of infection. Chronic lymphedema can lead to recurrent infections and permanent swelling, in some cases impairing function. The effects of lymphedema on a patient's quality of life are substantial and can be devastating [13]. There is an ongoing search for alternative methods for treatment of lymphedema in order to provide a more complete return of function in patients with recurrent lymphedema. No cure currently exists for lymphedema.

Many women who are diagnosed with breast cancer are treated with axillary lymph node dissection [12]. Axillary lymph node dissection (ALND) is associated with an increased risk of lymphedema of the ipsilateral arm. This risk persists throughout the patient's life and is directly linked with the extent of the dissection as well as with postoperative radiation dose [14]. Radiation in addition to ALND is typically used for patients with four or more positive nodes and may also be used in selected patients with one to three positive nodes [15]. Although the rate referenced in the literature for incidence of lymphedema after ALND is typically between 6 and 30%, Petrek et al. [16] reported that 49% of patients developed lymphedema within a 20-year follow-up period, which suggests that inadequate follow-up leads to underestimation of prevalence [16]. A systematic review of all studies addressing incidence of breast cancer-related arm lymphedema revealed that the risk was four times higher in women who underwent ALND relative to sentinel lymph node biopsy (SLNB) [17].

The financial impact of lymphedema is also considerable. A recent study demonstrated significantly higher medical costs within a 2-year period in patients with breast cancer-related lymphedema compared with patients who had breast cancer alone. These costs are likely underestimates given that they were only evaluated for 2 years, and lymphedema is typically a lifelong condition. Patients with lymphedema were also twice as likely within that 2-year period to present with cellulitis or lymphangitis as breast cancer patients without lymphedema were [18]. Lymphedema is also associated with inguinal lymphadenectomy. In a group of 101 patients that suffered complications after modified radical vulvectomy and groin dissection, 28% presented

with lymphedema [19]. In another study of 205 patients who underwent groin dissection for malignant melanoma, 40% developed lymphedema of the operated leg below the knee [20].

Pathophysiology

Lymphedema is the accumulation of lymph fluid in the interstitial space and may be secondary to infection, trauma, or congenital abnormalities [13]. The lymphatic system is composed of superficial and deep lymphatic vessels that collect lymph from the skin, subcutaneous tissue, muscle, bone, and other structures. The lymphatic system is designed to drain fluid and return it to the intravascular circulation. Lymph fluid enters the interstitium, which increases oncotic pressure, thereby drawing water to the interstitium. When this drainage is compromised, fluid collects in the interstitial space, resulting in swelling known as lymphedema. Left untreated, this stagnant, protein-rich fluid causes tissue channels to increase in size and number, reducing the availability of oxygen. This interferes with wound healing and provides a rich culture medium for bacterial growth that can result in infections such as lymphangitis, lymphadenitis, and, in severe cases, skin ulcers [21].

Treatment

Conservative treatment with decongestive therapy has been the primary choice for lymphedema treatment, but has limited benefits. To date, there is no consensus on surgical procedure and protocol. However, refinements in microsurgical techniques and improved methods may lead to the establishment of a standard surgical treatment for treatment of lymphedema [22]. Lymphaticovenous anastomosis (LVA) is a procedure that has the potential to help a certain subset of patients with lymphedema. In this procedure, the distal lymphatics are anastomosed to small superficial veins, creating a "bypass" for the lymphatic fluid into the venous system. This operation has been performed successfully by some surgeons for many years [23–26], but others found the operation had a high rate of variability (Fig. 26.1).

However, recently, indocyanine green (ICG) imaging has allowed for advances in both preoperative selection and intraoperative mapping. ICG imaging can differentiate between patients who still have some degree of functioning lymphatics, evidenced by proximally progressing lines on the extremity, and those who do not, evidenced by a diffuse pattern (personal communication, Barcelona lymphedema group). In those with functioning lymphatics, the ICG imaging provides direct data on the patient to indicate the location of surgery. In a study from MD Anderson Cancer Center, Chang et al. performed a prospective study in 100 patients; symptom improvement was noted by 96 % and quantitative improvement by 74 %. He also noted a significant improvement in identification of lymphatics within the study through the use of preoperative ICG imaging [27].

Another surgical modality for the treatment of lymphedema is free lymph node transfer. In this procedure, lymph nodes from the groin or chest wall are isolated with their blood supply and microsurgically transferred to the axilla or groin. In the axilla, the artery and vein of the pedicle is anastomosed to the thoracodorsal vessels using microsurgical techniques. In the groin, the vessels are anastomosed to the superficial branches of the femoral artery and vein. Corinne Becker in France pioneered this procedure and has published the largest series of patients [28, 29]. In her landmark paper in the Annals of Surgery, she reported a series of 24 patients who underwent groin to axillary lymph node transfer. Ten patients had complete resolution of their lymphedema, and 12 patients had decreased lymphedema of their upper extremity [29] (Fig. 26.2).

For patients who are not candidates or do not wish for LVA or lymph node transfer, e.g., patients with "late stage" lymphedema or advanced fibrotic disease, liposuction may potentially reduce the subjective "weight" and objective circumference of the arm, leading to improvements

in functioning. This can also be performed after LVA or node transfer surgery. Brorson is one of the most prolific authors in this field and has good reported patient outcomes [30, 31]. In a 5-year prospective study of 12 patients from another group, the final volumes of the affected and unaffected arms were virtually equivalent after liposuction, and this reduction was stable with up to 5 years of follow-up. These patients also had significant reductions in anxiety scores ($p < 0.05$) as well as an improvement in overall well-being [32]. The major limitation of this method is the guaranteed continued need for compression garments. If the compression garments are discontinued, the lymphedema is likely to recur [31].

There is a possibility that upper extremity lymphedema may be improved through release of the contracture and interposition of soft tissue. Two patients with severe postmastectomy lymphedema of the upper extremity were treated with a latissimus dorsi muscle flap. Complete disappearance of edema was achieved by 11 months postoperatively in one case and 50 % reduction by 8 months in the other case [33]. The tissue was transposed through the axilla to make a new breast, and there is a distinct possibility that the transposition of healthy, living tissue into the axilla provides a means of improving lymphedema by promoting lymphatic vessel ingrowth. In another larger retrospective review of 38 patients, 23.7 % demonstrated significant improvement in their lymphedema after free flap breast reconstruction, with none demonstrating worsening [34]. Because the tissue was transferred as a free flap directly to the breast, the patients who did not improve may not have had a sufficient amount of tissue transferred to the axilla. In an animal model, lymphatic continuity was noted to be restored with transfer of a rectus abdominis myocutaneous flap, providing an experimental model to explain the lymphedema improvement [35]. Furthermore, even if the lymphedema does not improve, the patient should benefit in terms of shoulder range of motion and improvement in functioning from release of the axillary contracture alone.

a   LVA is performed at multiple sites   **b**   Drainage of lymphatic fluid

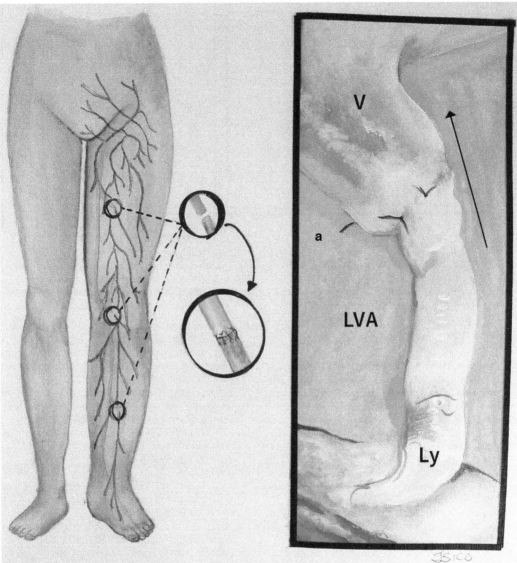

Fig. 26.1 Lymphaticovenous anastomosis (LVA) demonstrated above involves microscopic connections between small peripheral lymphatics and veins in order to allow for an alternate lymphatic drainage pathway. Detail shows close up view of lymphatic-venous anastomosis with the direction of flow indicated by the arrow.

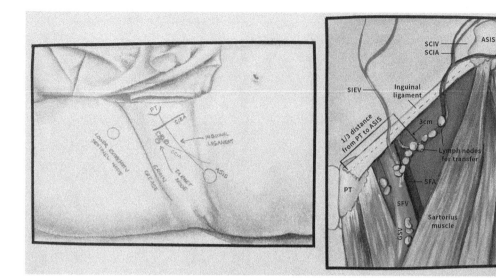

Fig. 26.2 Free lymph node transfers from the lower abdomen are taken from an area above the inguinal ligament bounded by the superficial circumflex iliac artery (SCIA) ad superficial inferior epigastric artery (SIEA). These lymph nodes can be transferred as a free tissue transfer to the contralateral groin or either axillary area.

References

1. Fowkes F, Rudan D, Rudan I, et al. Comparison of global estimates of prevalence and risk factors for peripheral artery disease in 2000 and 2010: a systematic review and analysis. Lancet. 2013;382:1329.
2. Chwala M, Szczekik W, Szczkek M, et al. Varicose veins of the lower extremities, hemodynamics and treatment methods. Adv Clin Exp Med. 2015;24:5–14.
3. Powell J, Edwards R, Worrell P, et al. Risk factors associated with the development of peripheral arterial disease in smokers: a case–control study. Atherosclerosis. 1997;129:41–8.
4. Arain F, Cooper L. Peripheral arterial disease: diagnosis and management. Mayo Clin Proc. 2008;83: 944–9.
5. Menke J, Larsen J. Meta-analysis: accuracy of contrast-enhanced magnetic resonance angiography for assessing steno-occlusions in peripheral arterial disease. Ann Intern Med. 2010;153:325.
6. Bedenis R, Stewart M, Cleanthis M, et al. Cilostazol for intermittent claudication. Cochrane Database Syst Rev. 2014;(10):CD003748.
7. Fowkes F, Price J, Fowkes F. Incidence of diagnosed deep vein thrombosis in the general population: systematic review. Eur J Vasc Endovasc Surg. 2003;25:1.
8. Centers for Disease Control and Prevention. Venous thromboembolism in adult hospitalizations – United States, 2007–2009. MMWR Morb Mortal Wkly Rep. 2012;61:401.
9. Anand S, Wells P, Hunt D, et al. Does this patient have deep vein thrombosis? JAMA. 1998;279:1094.
10. Kearon C, Ginsberg J, Douketis J, et al. A randomized trial of diagnostic strategies after normal proximal vein ultrasonography for suspected deep venous thrombosis: D-dimer testing compared with repeated ultrasonography. Ann Intern Med. 2005;142:490.
11. Young T, Tang H, Hughes R. Vena caval filters for the prevention of pulmonary embolism. Cochrane Database Syst Rev. 2010;(1):CD006212.
12. Paskett ED, Stark N. Lymphedema: knowledge, treatment, and impact among breast cancer survivors. Breast J. 2000;6:373–8.
13. Andersen L, Hojri I, Erlandsen M, Andersen J. Treatment of breast-cancer-related lymphedema with or without manual lymphatic drainage. Acta Oncol. 2000;39:399–405.
14. Marcks P. Lymphedema: pathogenesis, prevention, and treatment. Cancer Pract. 1997;5:32–8.
15. Haffty B, Hunt K, Harris J, Buchholz T. Positive sentinel nodes without axillary dissection: implications for the radiation oncologist. J Clin Oncol. 2011;29:4479–81.
16. Petrek J, Peters M, Senie R, Peterrosen P. Lymphedema in a cohort of breast carcinoma survivors 20 years after diagnosis. Cancer. 2001;92:1368–77.
17. Disipio T, Rye S, Newman B, Hayes S. Incidence of unilateral arm lymphoedema after breast cancer: a systematic review and meta-analysis. Lancet Oncol. 2013;14:500–15.
18. Shih Y, Xu Y, Cormier J, Giordano S, Ridner S, Buchholz T, Perkins GH, Elting L. Incidence, treatment costs, and complications of lymphedema after breast cancer among women of working age: a 2-year follow-up study. J Clin Oncol. 2009;27:2007–14.
19. Gaarenstroom KN, Kenter GG, Trimbos JB, Agous I, Amant F, Peters AAW, Vergote I. Postoperative com-

plications after vulvectomy and inguinofemoral lymphadenectomy using separate groin incisions. Int J Gynecol Cancer. 2003;13:522–7.

20. Karakousis C, Rose B, Driscoll D, Walsh D. Groin dissection in malignant melanoma. Ann Surg Oncol. 1994;1:271–7.

21. Woods M. The experience of manual lymph drainage as an aspect of treatment for lymphoedema. Int J Palliat Nurs. 2003;9:336–42.

22. Suami H, Chang DW. Overview of surgical treatments for breast cancer related lymphedema. Plast Reconstr Surg. 2010;126:1853–63.

23. O'Brien BM, Sykes P, Threlfall GN, Browning FS. Microlymphaticovenous anastomoses for obstructive lymphedema. Plast Reconstr Surg. 1977;60:197–211.

24. O'Brien BM, Mellow CG, Khazanchi RK, Dvir E, Kumar V, Pederson WV. Long term results after microlymphaticovenous anastomoses for the treatment of obstructive lymphedema. Plast Reconstr Surg. 1990;85:562–72.

25. Koshima I, Inagawa K, Urushibara K, Moriguchi T. Supermicrosurgical lymphaticovenular anastomosis for the treatment of lymphedema in the upper extremities. Plast Reconstr Surg. 2000;16:437–42.

26. Campisi C, Davini D, Bellini C, et al. Lymphatic microsurgery for the treatment of lymphedema. Microsurgery. 2006;26:65–9.

27. Chang DW, Suami H, Skoracki R. A prospective analysis of 100 consecutive lymphovenous bypass cases for treatment of extremity lymphedema. Plast Reconstr Surg. 2013;132:1305–14.

28. Becker C, Vasile JV, Levine JL, Batista BN, Studinger RM, Chen CM, Riquet M. Microlymphatic surgery for the treatment of iatrogenic lymphedema. Clin Plast Surg. 2012;39:385–98.

29. Becker C, Assouad J, Riquet M, Hidden G. Postmastectomy lymphedema: long-term results following microsurgical lymph node transplantation. Ann Surg. 2006;243:313–5.

30. Brorson H. Liposuction in arm lymphedema treatment. Scand J Surg. 2003;92:287–95.

31. Brorson H. Liposuction normalizes – in contrast to other therapies – lymphedema-induced adipose tissue hypertrophy. Handchir Mikrochir Plast Chir. 2012;44:348–54.

32. Schaverien MV, Munro KJ, Baker PA, Munnoch DA. Liposuction for chronic lymphoedema of the upper limb: 5 years of experience. J Plast Reconstr Aesthet Surg. 2012;65:935–42.

33. Kambayashi J, Ohshiro T, Mori T. Appraisal of myocutaneous flapping for treatment of postmastectomy lymphedema: case report. Acta Chir Scand. 1990;156:175–7.

34. Chang DW, Kim S. Breast reconstruction and lymphedema. Plast Reconstr Surg. 2010;125:19–23.

35. Slavin SA, Van den Abbeele AD, Losken A, Swartz MA, Jain RK. Return of lymphatic function after flap transfer for acute lymphedema. Ann Surg. 1999;229:421–7.

Part X

Future Directions

Spinal Cord and Peripheral Nerve Regeneration Current Research and Future Possibilities

Wise Young and Hilton M. Kaplan

Abbreviations

Akt	Oncogene of transforming retrovirus AKT8 (also Akt1 and PKB)
ATF-2	Activating transcription factor 2
ATF-3	Activating transcription factor 3
BBI	Brain-to-brain interface
BDNF	Brain-derived neurotrophic factor
chABC	Chondroitinase ABC
cAMP	Cyclic adenosine monophosphate
Caspr	Contactin-associated protein
CE	Conformité Européenne
CNS	Central nervous system
CSPG	Chondroitin-6-sulfate proteoglycan
DREADDS	Designer Receptors Exclusively Activated by Designer Drugs
DRG	Dorsal root ganglia
EMG	Electromyography
FDA	Food and Drug Administration
FLAMES	Floating light-activated microelectrical stimulators
GFAP	Glial fibrillary acidic protein
GHBP	Glial hyaluronate-binding protein
HSPG	Heparin sulfate proteoglycan
IGF-1	Insulin-like growth factor-1
IL-1	Interleukin-1
IN-1	IgM antibody that inhibits axonal growth
KSPG	Keratin sulfate proteoglycan (KSPG)
MAG	Myelin-associated glycoprotein
mTOR	Mammalian target of rapamycin
NED	Neural Enhancement Divide
NEP1-40	Peptide 1–40 of Nogo that inhibits NgR
NG2	Neural/glial antigen 2 (includes CSPG4)
NGC	Nerve guidance conduit
NgR	Nogo receptor
NgR1	Nogo receptor 1
NgR3	Nogo receptor 3
NMES	Neuromuscular electrical stimulation
Nogo	Neuronal growth inhibitory molecule in myelin
Nogo-A	The A version of Nogo
Nogo-A/Nogo-B	Nogo-A and Nogo-B genes
NS2.0	Nervous System 2.0

W. Young, MD, PhD (✉) • H.M. Kaplan, MBBCh, FCSSA, PhD
Rutgers, The State University of New Jersey, New Brunswick, NJ, USA
e-mail: wisey@mac.com; hilton.kaplan@rutgers.edu

© Springer International Publishing Switzerland 2017
A.I. Elkwood et al. (eds.), *Rehabilitative Surgery*, DOI 10.1007/978-3-319-41406-5_27

NTR	Neurotrophin receptor (p75 receptor)
OmgP	Oligodendroglial myelin glycoprotein
p75	75 KD protein
PC12	Pheochromocytoma 12
PDGF	Platelet-derived growth factor
PDK1/2	Phosphoinositide-dependent protein kinase 1 and 2
PI3K	Phosphoinositol 3 kinase
PIP2	Phosphoinositol phosphate 2
PIP3	Phosphoinositol phosphate 3
PKA	Phosphokinase A
PKB	Phosphokinase B (also Akt) a serine/threonine protein kinase
PNS	Peripheral nervous system
PTEN	Phosphatase tensin homologue
Rheb1	Ras homologue enriched in brain 1
RhoA	Rho A
RhoK	Rho kinase
RPTPsigma	Receptor protein tyrosine phosphatase sigma
SCI	Spinal cord injury
STAT3	Signal transducer and activator of transcription 3
TSC1/2	Tuberous sclerosis 1 and 2
UCSD	University of California San Diego

Introduction

Our nervous system is remarkable. It not only monitors and controls every part of our bodies but it does so in complex and often elegant ways that exceed our wildest imagination. For example, we know not just the positions but velocities of all our body parts not only relative to ourselves but to the outside world and also our expectations. If you have ever stepped on a moving walkway that is not operating, you may experience a strange feeling and even stumble because you expect the walkway to propel you forward and it does not. The information pouring in through our peripheral nerve system (PNS), vestibular, visual, and olfactory system combine to allow our brain and spinal cord or central nervous system (CNS) to interact smoothly with our environment.

While the brain has been recognized for its momentous processing capabilities, until a few decades ago, we thought the spinal cord to be just a conduit for signals between the brain and the body. We now know that this is wrong and that in addition to substantial processing capabilities, the spinal cord in fact has the ability to learn and interpret information for the brain. So in essence, the spinal cord is a "brain" as well.

The brainstem connects the spinal cord with the brain. It contains the autonomic centers for respiratory and cardiac systems that modulate our breathing and the beating of our hearts, in response to feedback they receive regarding blood pressure, acid, and gas levels (oxygen and carbon dioxide). From second to second, brainstem neurons continually adjust our respiration and cardiac output to maintain our bodies in homeostatic balance, in the face of continually changing physiologic needs and without any conscious effort at all. These brainstem systems connect to the autonomic nervous system that controls skin blood flow and sweating to affect body temperature, mediates vasoconstriction of large blood vessels in the legs that allow you to stand up without fainting, and regulates metabolism.

Another spectacular example of the spinal cord's independent functionality is seen in "walking circuits" [133]. Over the past two decades, researchers have discovered spinal circuits that, when stimulated, create all the complexities of walking, involving the coordinated control of agonist and antagonist muscle pairs in each limb to create the timed flexion and extension of hip, knee, and ankle joints, and all in reciprocal coordination with the other limb! When we walk, we don't think of moving our muscles in the sequences of hip flexors, quadriceps, anterior tibialis, gastrocnemius, hamstring, and gluteus maximus on the left and then on the right. Our brain simply tells the spinal cord to walk, and the central pattern generator located in our lumbosacral spinal cord instructs our legs and postural muscles to walk, hop, skip, trot, gallop, or run. Initially described by Miller and Scott in a feline model, this mechanism is now being used to help humans learn to walk again and rebuild their muscles after spinal cord injury (SCI) [227, 228, 338]. Our automated walking patterns may in fact be "simply" ingrained in highly tuned spinal circuits, so that our brains really only need to change the gain on these (inhibit or stimulate them) to influence pace and provide more detailed control for more specific tasks such as dealing with perturbations (e.g., tripping), climbing stairs or rocks, or walking on an uneven terrain or across a beach. The same is true when we micturate, defecate, and ejaculate. In fact, our brain does not control these activities explicitly, as we all know, when we need to go to the bathroom and our brain has a hard time inhibiting the urgency.

In 1906, Santiago Ramón y Cajal opined that "once the development has ended, the founts of growth and regeneration of axons and dendrites dried up irrevocably," as translated by Raoul May [140, 262]. This opinion by Cajal, the revered "father of neuroscience," influenced many generations of investigators. For much of the last and current century, scientists assumed that the central nervous system not only does not but cannot regenerate. In contrast, scientists assume that peripheral nerves can and do regenerate. For the last three decades, regeneration research focused on why the central nervous system cannot regenerate while the peripheral nervous system can.

We hope the following will show that these ideas are too simplistic and misrepresent the ability of both the CNS and the PNS to recover from injury. In the case of CNS injuries, clinicians are deeply pessimistic about the possibility of recovery and often express this pessimism to their patients. In the case of PNS injuries, clinicians are sometimes overoptimistic in their prediction of recovery and do not express the limitations of recovery, particularly after delayed or long gap repairs. Finally, the future of repairing both the spinal cord and peripheral nerves is bright. Scientists are considering not only restoring function to normal but propose even improving function beyond normal. Combinations of advanced technology may enable patients to perform better in some respects than before injury.

Spinal Cord Regeneration

Three theories dominate neuroscience today concerning why the central nervous system cannot regenerate while the peripheral nervous system can. The first is axon growth inhibitory effects of the myelin-associated protein Nogo [283, 296]. The second is glial scar, i.e., that astrocytes form a barrier to axonal growth [268, 273]. The third emphasizes extracellular matrix proteins produced by glial cells, particularly chondroitin proteoglycans [35, 80, 86, 109, 214]. All three theories are based on the assumption that the spinal cord cannot regenerate and that peripheral nerve can regenerate without difficulty. This assumption has unfortunately become a self-fulfilling prophecy. Despite much evidence indicating that the spinal cord can regenerate, investigators chose spinal cord models that cannot regenerate to substantiate their assumption and ignored evidence that the spinal cord can regenerate. Recent research indicates that axons can regrow in the spinal cord despite glial scars, Nogo, and chondroitin proteoglycans and that peripheral nerves do not regenerate as well as usually assumed [357].

Early Studies of Spinal Cord Regeneration

In the nineteenth century, several European investigators studied injured animal spinal cords. In 1874, Eichhorst and Naunyn crushed the spinal cords of rabbits and dogs and described many nerve fibers that "infiltrated with neuroglial tissue after three to five weeks" [91]. They saw modest improvement of function. In 1876, Schiefferdecker severely criticized the study by Eichhorst and Naunyn [281]. He found no evidence of regeneration or functional return in dogs up to 300 days after spinal cord transection, claiming that they needed to transect the spinal cord and that any apparently recovered function was due to residual axons or reflexes.

In 1906, Ramon y Cajal largely resolved the issue by transecting the spinal cord of young cats and dogs and found that large numbers of severed intraspinal fibers sprouted new processes with growth cones similar to those observed in transected peripheral nerves [262]. After several weeks, however, the growth slowed and became abortive. He and his colleagues proposed that central nerve fibers commenced regeneration like the peripheral nerve but, for reasons that were not clear, did not continue across the transection site and did not make functional connections in the opposite stump [263]. In contrast, he described robust regeneration of peripheral nerves. The matter of regeneration rested there for several decades.

In the 1920s and 1930s, several investigators reported regeneration in the spinal cord of tadpoles, newts, and young rainbow trout [138, 139, 210]. As Sugar and Gerard pointed out in 1940, regeneration in the central nervous system of nonmammalian vertebrates was generally accepted by the 1920s [204, 311]. Many investigators studied regeneration in lower vertebrates in hopes of finding differences between mammalian and nonmammalian spinal cords that would explain the inability of the former to regenerate [30, 61]. After World War II, when the advent of antibiotics and better bladder care allowed long-term survival of many spinal-injured patients, many investigators began to study treatments to regenerate mammalian spinal cords.

By 1980, the field had divided into those who believed in regeneration and those who did not [344]. The latter dominated. In 1980, Guth et al. reported that enzyme therapy does not regenerate transected rat spinal cords [119]. In that study, they found that if they left even a small strand of spinal cord in the ventral side of the spinal cord, some of the rats recovered walking. So, they proposed a "string" test, recommending that investigators slip a string under the spinal cord and pull it up to confirm transection. The string test ensures a gap between cut ends of the spinal cord and requires transection of the anterior spinal artery, which caused ischemic necrosis of the stumps. A gap and ischemia virtually guarantees no regeneration. Some investigators even sought to find ways to eliminate dorsal root sensory fiber growth so that they could study "true central axonal growth" [315]. Those who did not believe used models to ensure growth does not occur.

In the mid-1980s, several scientists began putting bridges into the spinal cord in the belief that axons need something to grow on. In 1984, de la Torre put a collagen matrix bridge into the spinal cord and found that central neurites and catecholaminergic axons extended across the bridge into the distal stump, albeit without functional recovery [76]. In 1985, Reier et al. began to use a variety of neural tissues to bridge the SCI site, finding that fibers would grow into fetal tissues used in this way, and may even extend beyond, but without functional recovery [266].

Other investigators, such as David and Aguayo and Carlstedt et al., were fascinated by the growth of fibers out of and into the spinal cord [49, 50, 74]. When peripheral nerves were inserted into the spinal cord, fibers grew out of the spinal cord to travel long distances in the peripheral nerve. Based on these results, David and Aguayo hypothesized that spinal fibers are able to grow long distances in peripheral nerve, but that something in the central nervous system environment prevented their growth in the spinal cord. The hypothesis initiated a worldwide search for axonal growth inhibitors.

Go or Nogo?

In 1990, Savio and Schwab reported that lesioned corticospinal tract axons regenerate in demyelinated rat spinal cords [277]. Schnell and Schwab found that corticospinal axons will regenerate in rats treated with an implanted hybridoma secreting an IgM antibody (IN-1) against myelin [283]. This finding initiated intensive efforts to identify the responsible myelin protein [11, 18, 102, 106, 136, 137, 280, 288, 289, 324]. Schwegler et al. confirmed that demyelination allows regeneration in the spinal cord [296]. Others showed that the IN-1 stimulates regeneration and plasticity [36, 39, 42, 102, 117, 170, 182, 261, 272, 287, 290–293, 314, 322, 323, 327, 334, 336, 362]. Immunization of animals against myelin promoted axon growth [300].

In 1998, Schwab et al. isolated a myelin protein that inhibited axonal growth [57, 307]. Called Nogo, the molecule belongs to the reticulon family of proteins [12, 57, 115, 143, 241]. Antibodies against Nogo enhanced regeneration and reorganization of the brain and spinal cord [196, 211, 233, 337]. Discovery and characterization of the Nogo receptor soon followed [17, 37, 77, 100, 146–148, 218, 252]. The Nogo receptor (NgR) provided insights into how Nogo may work. Several myelin proteins bind the Nogo receptor, which acts through the intracellular messenger rho A (RhoA) and rho kinase (RhoK), to regulate microtubule formation essential for axon growth [13, 17]. Increasing intracellular messenger cyclic adenosine monophosphate (cAMP) inactivates RhoA and blocks effects of Nogo and other growth inhibitors. Fournier et al. found that RhoK inhibition enhances axon regeneration in chick dorsal root ganglia (DRGs) [101]. NgR activation not only inhibits neurite growth but cell spreading as well [244]. NgR blockade promotes recovery after SCI [193, 194].

Nogo turned out to be more complicated than anybody suspected. First, there are three Nogo proteins: A, B, and C. Genetic knockout of Nogo-A promotes sprouting [302]. Only Nogo-A binds NgR, but Nogo-C delays regeneration, and adult mice lacking both Nogo-A and Nogo-B sprout corticospinal tracts and recover more function than mice that lack Nogo-A alone [171]. Nogo-A interacts with Nogo-B and -C, as the well as paranodal axonal protein Caspr [84, 240]. Second, neurons express Nogo-A not only on their surfaces but in nuclear chromatin, cytoplasm, and postsynaptic zones [154, 199]. Nogo-A expression increases with neuronal activity [160, 222]. Schwann cells also express Nogo-A [255]. Third, Nogo affects more than just neuronal growth. Nogo-A modulates experimental autoimmune encephalomyelitis, regulates hippocampal neuronal architecture, inhibits angiogenesis, and redistributes protein disulfide isomerase [98, 328, 353, 363]. Nogo-B suppresses tumors and induces apoptosis in cancer cells, regulates hepatic fibrosis, is necessary for macrophage infiltration, and interferes with mitochondria-endoplasmic reticulum interactions [258, 312, 359, 365].

NgR turned out to be complicated as well. NgR exists in a complex with p75 receptor (NTR), the low-affinity neurotrophin receptor

[331]. The NgR/NTR receptor complex binds at least three known axon growth inhibitory proteins: Nogo-A, OMgP, and MAG [45, 186]. However, multiple receptors mediate the effects of these growth-inhibiting proteins. For example, MAG inhibition of neurite outgrowth may not require NgR [348]. For DRG neurons, NgR mediates most MAG inhibition because it is reversed by phosphatidyl-specific phospholipase C, which cleaves glycosylphosphatidylinositol anchors, or NEP1-40, a peptide inhibitor of NgR. However, gangliosides mediate MAG inhibition in cerebellar granular neurons because sialidase or ganglioside synthesis inhibitors block MAG effects [221, 343]. Finally, NgR is a family of receptors and NgR1 is the one that binds Nogo.

Genetic results have been mixed. Mice lacking Nogo-A have increased sprouting, enhanced motor coordination and balance, and more spontaneous locomotor activity after spinal cord transection, but the effects were strain dependent [82, 302, 341]. Genetic knockouts result in less regeneration than blocking Nogo or Nogo receptor [317]. Genetic knockout of NgR1 impairs cognitive outcomes, but inhibition of NgR1 enhances cognitive function after brain injury [126, 319]. NgR1 knockout and NgR1 decoy treatment (administering a soluble NgR1 receptor that binds Nogo so that it cannot bind NgR on cells) improve recovery in SCI [320, 332]. Kim et al. reported Nogo-A/Nogo-B knockout mice sprouted corticospinal tracts rostral to spinal cord transection sites and recovered locomotor function [172].

Glial Scar

For many years, scientists knew that "glial scars" formed in brain and spinal cord but did not think that they prevented regeneration [23, 256, 257]. For example, in 1979, Reier described regenerative optic nerve axons that penetrated "extremely dense" glial scars in Xenopus tadpoles and concluded that mature hypertrophic astrocytes do not represent a major obstacle to axonal outgrowth [264]. Matthews et al. described axons crossing the glial limitans into glial scar in transected rat spinal cords [215]. In 1981, Guth et al. found "extensive regeneration" of intrinsic spinal cord and dorsal root fibers in transected spinal cords of hibernating squirrels, concluding that mammalian spinal cord neurons have considerable regenerative potential and that "mechanical impediments such as collagenous and glial scarring, cyst formation, and cavitation" cannot be the sole explanation of why regeneration in mammalian CNS is abortive [120]. In 1983, Shreyer and Jones reported that corticospinal axons, in many cases, grow past both thermal lesions and sharp sections of the spinal cord despite glial scars [286].

By the mid-1980s, much evidence suggested that glial scars block regeneration. In 1986, Borgens et al. found that dorsal column axons seldom grew into a glial scar of a transected spinal cord [31]. Smith et al. showed that a critical period exists after injury during which reactive glia will not support axon growth [303]. In 1984, Kastner assessed axonal growth through astrocytes in fish, finding that astrocytes without orthogonal arrays of particles allow axons to grow through, but astrocytes with such arrays will not [346]. In 1988, Houle et al. described foci of dense confluent neuropil crossing the injury site of chronically injured spinal cord, wherever openings of glial scar occur, suggesting that glial scar does obstruct axonal growth [142, 268]. However, Dahl et al. described axons growing through old multiple sclerosis plaques, concluding that reactive astrocytes do not constitute non-permissible substrate for axon growth [67]. Mansour et al. suggested that astrocytes expressing glial hyaluronate-binding protein (GHBP) permit axon growth [212].

In 1990, Rudge and Silver studied neurite outgrowth into astroglial scars in vitro [273]. They found that glial scars stimulated minimal neurite outgrowth compared to other cells or tissues and proposed the glial scar theory. Bovolenta et al. found that growing neurites avoid anisomorphic reactive gliosis but neonatal glia stimulate neurite outgrowth and concluded that astrocytes both stimulate and inhibit axonal growth [33, 34].

Many subsequent investigators studied glial scars to understand how they form. For example, Guilian et al. examined the effects of microglia-derived cytokines on brain gliosis, finding that the proinflammatory cytokine interleukin-1 (IL-1) is a potent microglial mitogen and regulates microglial components of the glial scar and that IL-1 supported neuronal growth through the glial scar [112]. Frisen et al. observed that pheochromocytoma-12 (PC12) cells do not adhere to spinal cord sections taken rostral to a dorsal funiculus section even though no myelin is present in these areas, suggesting that glial scars lack critical cellular adhesion molecules [103]. In 1997, Davies et al. found that transplanted dorsal root ganglion neurons grow long distances in myelinated white matter tracts but stop at cuts of the spinal cord where a glial scar is present, suggesting that the main obstacle to regeneration is the glial scar and not myelin-based inhibition of axon growth [75].

A popular approach to glial scars is to bridge them with fetal tissues and peripheral nerves, even though such transplants stimulate gliosis and even glial scars [2, 9, 64, 73, 142, 164, 217, 265, 267, 279]. Some investigators reported that axons seldom entered into scar without accompanying astrocytes, suggesting that astrocytes guide axonal growth [24, 95, 121, 123]. Gliosis is essential for repair of the blood-brain barrier [269]. In 2005, Hermanns et al. reported that iron chelation and a collagen synthesis inhibitor reduced scar formation in spinal cord [131]. Klapka et al. subsequently reported that iron chelation and cAMP delayed fibrous scarring, promoted corticospinal tract growth, and improved functional recovery in SCI [173].

Proteoglycans

In 1991, McKeon et al. found that neurite outgrowth in glial scars correlated inversely with expression of inhibitory molecules on reactive astrocytes, particularly chondroitin sulfate proteoglycans (CSPG) independently of glial fibrillary acidic protein (GFAP) production [220, 330]. In 1994, Levine et al. described increased expression of the neural/glial antigen 2 (NG2) family of CSPG after brain injury [191]. Proliferating NG2-positive cells clustered around the lesion, peaked at 7 days, and then declined. Concurrently, microglia activated and increased in number, monocytes invaded the injury site, and an astrocyte scar formed. He proposed that these NG2-positive cells prevent axonal growth in the central nervous stem. In the same year, Jones et al. showed that macrophages and oligodendrocyte progenitor cells express NG2 [157].

In 2002, Bradbury et al. reported that a bacterial enzyme called chondroitinase ABC (ChABC), that broke down CSPG in injured spinal cords, promotes functional recovery after SCI in rats [35]. Many investigators subsequently confirmed beneficial effects of treatments that break down or reduce CSPG production [32, 79, 93, 113, 116, 125, 152, 161, 195, 360, 361]. In 2006, Barritt et al. reported that ChABC promotes sprouting in intact and injured spinal cords [16]. In 2007, Cafferty et al. found functional regeneration through astrocytic scar genetically modified to digest CSPG [44]. In 2009, Nakamae et al. found ChABC promotes corticospinal tract growth in organotypic cocultures [234]. Lee et al. showed that thermostabilized ChABC enhanced axonal sprouting and improved recovery [189]. In 2011, Carter et al. showed that delayed ChABC treatment reverses atrophy of rubrospinal neurons [55]. Wang et al. found that ChABC therapy and rehabilitation promotes forelimb recovery of rats with chronic SCI [333]. Zhao et al. transfected animals with ChABC expressing lentiviral vectors and found better recovery [367]. In 2012, Starkey et al. showed that ChABC promoted compensatory sprouting of remaining corticospinal axons and improved forelimb function after unilateral pyramidotomy [308]. In 2015, Mondello et al. found that 4 weeks of ChABC treatment promoted earlier recovery in cats after SCI [232].

Some beneficial effects of ChABC may be due to mechanisms other than regeneration. Garcia-Alias et al. found that ChABC injected into C5 spinal cord lesions improved forelimb functional recovery by increasing plasticity [108]. Orlando et al., however, showed that full digestion of motor cortex CSPG by ChABC aggravated motor deficits, suggesting that too much plasticity is not beneficial [246]. Milbreta et al. found that ChABC altered astrocytic and vascular structure in injured spinal cords [226]. ChABC also promotes remyelination [185].

Krautstrunk et al. found increased keratin sulfate proteoglycan (KSPG) in injured spinal cords and proposed that KSPG contributes to poor growth of corticospinal tract axons in injured spinal cords [178]. Ito et al. found that mice deficient in N-acetylglucosamine 6-O-sulfotransferase-1 lack 5D4 reactive keratin sulfate in the CNS and that contusions of these mice at the T10 spinal cord level resulted in better locomotor recovery than in control mice [151]. Ishikawa et al. recently showed that combination of keratin sulfate and chondroitin sulfate digestion followed by rehabilitation is better than either alone or without rehabilitation [150].

In 2005, Sapieha et al. reported that the receptor protein tyrosine phosphatase sigma (RPTPsigma) inhibits retinal ganglionic axon growth [275]. In 2010, Duan and Giger proposed that KSPG inhibits axon growth by binding RPTPsigma [86]. Fry et al. soon showed that mice deficient in RPTPsigma regenerate their corticospinal tracts [104]. Coles et al. found that RPTPsigma acts bimodally in sensory neurons, with KSPG inhibiting growth while heparin sulfate proteoglycan (HSPG) promotes growth [63]. In the meantime, Dickendesher et al. reported that NgR1 and NgR3 are receptors of KSPG [80]. In 2014, Zhou et al. showed that reducing RPTPsigma with lentiviral shRNA promotes neurite outgrowth and improves recovery in rat spinal cord contusion [369]. Xu et al. showed that RPTPsigma inhibition enhanced corticospinal and serotonergic axonal growth [352]. Dyck et al. showed that KSPG binding of RPTPsigma inhibits neural stem cell growth, attachment, survival, proliferation, and differentiation [88]. Lang et al. found that blocking RPTPsigma improves connections and functional recovery [183].

One, Some, or All of the Above?

Several key negative studies encouraged many investigators to believe that none of the growth inhibitors are solely or even primarily responsible for regeneration failure in SCI. In 2003, Jones et al. studied axon growth through CSPG, NG2, brevican, neurocan, versican, and phosphacan deposits at interfaces of NGF-secreting fibroblast transplants in injured spinal cords [158]. Many axons penetrated this inhibitory milieu to the fibroblast grafts, including dorsal column sensory fibers, rubrospinal, and nociceptive axons. The axons grew on NG2 especially when the cell adhesion molecules L1 and laminin were present. They concluded that local permissive molecules can balance or exceed inhibitory signals from KSPG. In 2007, Hossain-Ibrahim et al. studied SCI in mice that do not express NG2 [141]. In theory, these animals should show better regeneration, but they did not differ from wild-type mice in their regenerative response or recovery after SCI. They concluded that NG2 is not a major inhibitor of axonal regeneration after SCI. In the same year, Lu et al. found that axons readily penetrated glial scars and deposits of KSPG and NG2 in chronically injured spinal cord transplanted with bone marrow stromal cells, especially in the presence of NT-3 [205]. In 2010, Lee et al. systematically deleted Nogo, MAG, or OMgP [190]. Deleting one of the three inhibitors enhanced corticospinal or serotonergic axonal sprouting without behavioral improvement. However, deleting all three inhibitors was not synergistic. They concluded that Nogo, MAG, and OMgP modulate axon sprouting but do not play a central role in CNS axon regeneration failure.

Many investigators consequently believe that multiple growth inhibitors must be blocked and that growth factors should be provided for regeneration to occur. For example, Schwab et al. gave NT-3 alongside the Nogo antibody IN-1 [36, 114, 284, 285, 327]. Others used IN-1 with acidic FGF-fibrin and with fetal transplants [117, 287]. Liu et al. used recombinant adenovirus to introduce multiple therapeutic genes [197]. In 2013, Hunanyan et al. found that combination of ChABC and AAV-NT3 was synergistic in promoting neural plasticity of descending spinal pathways after SCI [145]. Karimi-Abdolrezaee et al. showed that ChABC and growth factors enhanced endogenous neural precursor differentiation and functional recovery after SCI [168, 169]. In 2014, Alluin et al. found that ChABC, neurotrophins, and locomotor training enhanced sprouting of corticospinal and serotonergic fibers,

attenuated astrogliosis and inflammation, and improved walking recovery in rats [5]. The authors noted that growth factors increase KSPG production by astrocytes [304].

Interestingly, ChABC is synergistic with many therapies but not with Nogo receptor blockade [368]. For example, Nakamae et al. found that ChABC and NEP1-40 (a Nogo receptor blocker) each improved corticospinal tract growth, but the combination did not have synergistic effects [235]. ChABC is synergistic with many cellular transplant therapies, including immature astrocytes, Schwann cells, and olfactory ensheathing glia [43, 97, 99]. Kanno et al. found that Schwann cells genetically modified to secrete neurotrophin and chondroitinase promote axonal regeneration and locomotion in rats [166].

Bridging: Many investigators use peripheral nerve, scaffolding, or other bridges, to bypass the lesion site, although it is questionable whether bridging alone can completely avoid myelin-based inhibitors, glial scar, and inhibitory extracellular matrices at spinal cord interface to the bridges [181]. For example, Guest et al. used channels containing Schwann cells to recruit axons and direct the axonal growth to spinal cord below the injury site [118]. However, while the axons grew into the channel, they were reluctant to grow out of the channel into the spinal cord. Liu et al. used collagen tubes to bridge spinal cord directly to nerve roots, showing that many spinal cord neurons sent axons into these tubular implants to reinnervate muscle [198]. Kaneko et al. used a nanofibrous hydrogel combined with a honeycomb collagen sponge to repair completely transected spinal cords and improve locomotor recovery [165]. Most of these therapies, however, achieved only modest regeneration of long tracts with limited and often nonfunctional locomotor recovery.

None of the Above

Some investigators claim to have achieved regeneration in the spinal cord even though they did not address any of the known inhibitors and obstacles to regeneration. In 2005, Tsai et al. reported corticospinal tract regeneration into lumbar gray matter, correlating with loco-motor recovery, after complete transection and repair with peripheral nerve grafts, fibroblast growth factor, and fibrin glue, together with spinal fusion [321]. Novikova et al. reported regeneration after neurotransplants combined with brain-derived neurotrophic factors (BDNF) [242]. Oudega et al. combined insulin-like growth factor-1 (IGF-1) and platelet-derived growth factor (PDGF) alongside Schwann cell grafts [247].

The best regenerative therapies appear to be ones that do not involve blockade of any of the growth inhibitors. In 2012 Lu et al. from the Tuszynski laboratory at the University of California, San Diego (UCSD), published two papers reporting massive regeneration in the spinal cords of rats [206, 207]. The first study examined rats treated with cAMP injections into the brainstem, bone marrow stromal cell grafts in the lesion site, and virally induced BDNF expression beyond the injury site [208]. This combinatorial therapy resulted in massive motor axon regeneration beyond both C5 hemisection and T3 complete transection sites, formation of many synapses with neurons below the injury site, but paradoxically worse locomotor func-tion. The second study assessed long-distance connectivity of axons grown from neural stem cells transplanted into transected spinal cords [207]. The neural stem cells were grafted into transection sites in fibrin containing a cocktail of growth factors. Many thousands of axons from grafted neural stem cells grew out both rostrally and caudally, penetrating glial scars and areas of NG2 deposits, extending long distances, and making synapses with neurons to the brain and lower spinal cord. Host fibers entered the graft and made synapses with the neural stem cells. Interestingly, the rats showed some improve-ment in hind limb movement although they could not walk. Lu et al. subsequently showed similar results with induced pluripotent human stem cells [209].

In 2010, Liu et al. reported that conditional deletion of the phosphatase tensin (PTEN) homo-logue gene upregulated mammalian target of rapamycin (mTOR) and allowed remarkable regeneration of corticospinal tracts in mice [200]. Unlike the Lu studies where cells had been trans-planted into the spinal cord and various manipu-lations might have altered the microenvironment of the spinal cord, the conditional deletion of PTEN occurred only in the motor cortex, the ori-gin of the corticospinal axons that grew across the injury site. The axons grew across transec-tion, hemisection, and crush injury sites without regard for the presence of myelin, glial scar, or inhibitory extracellular matrix glycoproteins. Recently, Du et al. from the Liu laboratory reported that PTEN deletion promotes regrowth of the corticospinal tract 1 year after injury in mice, suggesting that this treatment would be effective in chronic SCI [85]. However, despite many axons making synapses in neurons below the injury site, the mice did not recover walking. In 2014, Danilov et al. showed that conditional genetic deletion of PTEN enhances corticospinal regeneration and motor functional recovery after cervical SCI in mice [72].

The mechanism by which PTEN inhibits axonal growth is complicated. PTEN normally acts by converting phosphoinositol phosphate 3 (PIP3) to PIP2. Phosphoinositol 3 kinase (PI3K) converts PIP2 to PIP3, which in turn activates phosphoinositide-dependent protein kinase 1 and 2 (PDK1/2) to activate protein kinase B (PKB or Akt). Akt in turn inhibits tuberous scle-rosis 1 and 2 (TSC1/2) to inhibit Ras homologue enriched in brain 1 (Rheb1). Rheb1 normally activates mTOR, which acts through several intracellular messengers to regulate protein syn-thesis and cell growth. Thus, in the absence of PTEN, PIP3 accumulates and activates Akt. Akt inhibits TSC1/2, which normally inhibits Rheb1, thereby disinhibiting Rheb1 to activate mTOR. This pathway can be influenced by many drugs. Thus, for example, lithium directly activates Akt, and this may be one of the mecha-nisms by which lithium stimulates spinal cord and peripheral nerve regeneration [56, 81, 105, 310, 355, 356]. Rapamycin is a potent inhibitor of mTOR. Lu et al. [207] found treating rats with rapamycin reduced axonal outgrowth in his experiments.

All By Itself

The currently accepted dogma is that the spinal cord cannot regenerate. This dogma arose from early studies of spinal cord transection models, which did more than just divide the spinal cord. First, because spinal cords are under tension, the stumps separate and a gap is almost invariably present after transection. Second, unless care is taken to preserve the anterior spinal artery, transections eliminate crucial blood supply and causes severe ischemia of spinal cord stumps and cystic necrosis at the injury site. Third, scientists seldom closed the dura after transection, allowing fibroblasts from surrounding tissues to migrate into the injury site, resulting in a fibrous scar. Axons will not grow readily across gaps, in necrotic and cystic spinal cord, or through fibrous scars. It is little wonder that most scientists did not think that the spinal cord can regenerate – but they did not consider that most SCIs do not involve cutting or transection of the spinal cord. A vast majority of human spinal cord injuries involve crush or contusion.

In 1995, Anghelescu et al. administered large doses of the glucocorticoid methylprednisolone or saline to rabbits after an experimental crush injury of the spinal cord [7]. Both treated and control groups of animals showed histological evidence of severe injury, including necrosis, vacuolization, cavitation, myelinic and axonal fragmentation, demyelination, and mesenchyme-glial scar reactions. However, in both treated and untreated groups, they observed large numbers of regenerated axons growing into the "dense scar of the injured cord." Damaged fibers die back some distance from the injury site and grow back to the injury site. The growing axons were clearly not deterred by the inhibitory effects of myelin in the white matter, physical presence of glial scar, or deposits of chondroitin proteoglycans that surround the injury site. This study was largely ignored because it was published in an obscure journal and showed no difference due to treatment with methylprednisolone.

In 1997, the Multicenter Animal Spinal Cord Injury Study, involving eight leading SCI laboratories in the United States, reported that large numbers of spinal axons grow into the injury site of contused spinal cords, the type of injury that is the most common form of human SCI [19]. In 610 rat spinal cords contused with a 10-g weight dropped 12.5, 25.0, or 50.0 mm onto spinal cord exposed by T9–10 laminectomies, over 80 % of the spinal cords showed many axons growing into the injury site. In fact, the more severe the injury, the more axons grew into the injury site. Many were myelinated by Schwann cells entering from dorsal roots. A subsequent study by Hill et al. suggested that both ascending and descending spinal axons grew into and out of the injury site, including reticulospinal and corticospinal axons, despite the gliosis, myelin, and chondroitin proteoglycans around the injury site [132].

Since a majority of spinal cord injuries involve crush or contusions of the spinal cord, the observation of axon growth into the injury site and beyond in animal models of these injury mechanisms suggests that spontaneous regeneration may occur in many human SCI cases. This may explain why over 90 % of people will recover substantial function after even severe complete SCI, including independent walking [83]. Even after the so-called complete SCI, many people will recover 1–2 segmental levels of motor or sensory function [254, 345].

Perhaps it is time to reconsider the dogma that the spinal cord cannot regenerate and consider the possibility that some observed recovery in human spinal cord may be due to regrowth of long tracts across compressed or contused injury sites. The dogma was established over a century ago using models of SCI that are not clinically relevant. The weight of evidence in support of the ability of the spinal cord to regenerate is overwhelming.

Peripheral Nerve Effects on Spinal Cord Regeneration

Scientists have long known that prior injury of a peripheral nerve increases both rates of regeneration and numbers of regenerated fibers in the peripheral nerve. In 1983, Bisby et al. [26] noted that a prior crush injury of a sciatic nerve increased axon growth rates by 68 % after a second injury 7 days later to the nerve. In 1985, Bisby and Keen found that a conditioning injury stimulated small diameter unmyelinated axons containing substance P-like immunoreactivity to grow faster [27, 28]. Jenq et al. found that a conditioning injury not only increased the rate but also the number of regenerated fibers [153]. Bajrovic et al. showed that prior injuries enhanced the ability of axons to grow across acellular segments of crushed nerves [10]. These effects can be achieved by inflaming or compressing nerves [68–70]. Conditioning lesions resulted in faster growth initiation and initially faster axon growth, reduced long neurite extension, and fewer neuritic branches [184].

Do peripheral nerve lesions alter central axonal growth? In 1984, Oblinger and Lasek reported that peripheral axotomy did not affect regenerative properties of the central branch of DRG neurons [243]. Many investigators consequently thought that conditioning effects were limited to peripheral nerves. In 1989, Ebner et al. found that peripheral nerve damage facilitated functional innervation of embryonic brain grafts in adult sensory cortex [89]. In 1995, Woolf et al. reported that peripheral axotomy massively reorganized central terminals of primary afferents in the dorsal gray horn [347]. Then, in 1999, Neumann and Woolf showed that peripheral nerve lesions stimulated central axonal growth of DRGs across dorsal column lesions made 2 weeks later [236]. In the same year, Chong et al. cut and anastomosed L4, L5, and L6 dorsal roots of rats and found that injuring the ipsilateral sciatic nerve greatly increased the number of dorsal root axons penetrating and growing in the dorsal column [59]. In 2002, Neumann et al. showed that intraganglionic administration of cAMP induced regeneration of sensory axons in injured spinal cord [237]. In 2005, Neumann et al. showed that peripheral nerve injury after SCI stimulates central regeneration [238].

Many investigators have studied the mechanisms by which conditioning peripheral nerve injuries enhance DRG neurons to regenerate. In 1999, Lazar et al. found that peripheral nerve injuries modulated macrophage and microglial responses to axonal injury and proposed that these responses may contribute to the regeneration in the spinal cord [187]. Delcroix et al. showed that peripheral nerve injury upregulated activating transcription factor 2 (ATF-2) in nociceptive DRG neurons and may be responsible for neuropathic pain [78]. In 2006, Seijffers et al. found that ATF-3 promotes neurite outgrowth of DRG neurons and that peripheral nerve lesions but not central lesions induced ATF-3 expression in DRG neurons and subsequently showed that ATF-3 expression increased the intrinsic growth state of DRG neurons [297, 298]. In 2005, Qiu et al. showed that sciatic nerve transection caused transient phosphorylation and activation of the transcription factor signal transducer and activator of transcription 3 (STAT3) in DRG neurons [260]. Blocking STAT3 prevented the effects of the conditioning lesion. Interestingly, we recently showed that lithium directly blocks STAT3 in neural stem cells and suppresses astrogliogenesis and also reduces severe neuropathic pain in patients with chronic SCI [354, 371].

Neuronal cAMP levels regulate growth cone behavior. In 1997, Ming et al. found that Netrin-1, a well-known chemoattractant for neurons, guides growth cones by increasing cAMP [229, 305]. The growth cones of Xenopus spinal neurons showed chemorepulsive responses in the presence of a competitive analog of cAMP or an inhibitor of protein kinase A (PKA). Song et al. showed that changing cAMP switched turning directions of nerve growth cones and that a gradient of brain-derived neurotrophic factor (BDNF) triggers attraction of the growth cones to the higher BDNF concentrations but that the presence of a competitive analog to cAMP or inhibition of PKA induces repulsion [305]. In 2003, Qiao et al. reported that PKA activation inhibits RhoA, the protein that is known to mediate inhibition of axonal growth [259]. Increasing neuronal cAMP levels blocks inhibition of axonal regeneration by MAG and myelin [46, 47].

The Importance of Rehabilitation

Despite rivers of axons crossing the injury site and making synaptic connections above and below the injury site in the studies by Liu et al. and Lu et al., animals recovered relatively little function after complete transections [85, 200, 206, 207]. Interestingly, none of these studies did any rehabilitation of the rats. The reason for the lack of recovery is evident. The rats do not know how to use any of the new pathways that have regenerated. Without activity, synapses do not consolidate. Much evidence suggests that motor recovery does not occur without exercise [94, 274]. Rehabilitation was essential for recovery.

In 2009, Garcia-Alias et al. found that ChABC treatment opens a window of opportunity for task-specific rehabilitation after SCI [107]. Rats received a C4 dorsal funiculus, followed by ChABC or penicillinase control therapy and different types of rehabilitation. The rats recovered functions that are specific for the rehabilitation they received and rehabilitation for certain function may be deleterious for other function. For example, locomotor training resulted in locomotor recovery and worse skilled forelimb reach behaviors. In 2014, Zhang et al. showed that combining treadmill training with semaphorin3A inhibition helped rewire central pattern generators and improved locomotion in rats [366]. In 2015, Ishikawa et al. showed that a combination of keratin sulfate digestion or ChABC and rehabilitation promoted anatomical plasticity in injured rat spinal cords [150].

ChABC increases plasticity of the motor cortex, respiratory motor system, and lumbosacral spinal cord after SCI [96, 108, 150, 224, 245, 246, 335]. Likewise, blockade or deletion of Nogo and NGR1 increases plasticity [38, 295, 301, 306, 318]. For example, Zenmar et al. reported that anti-Nogo or anti-NgR1 antibodies increased long-term potentiation of pyramidal cells induced by stimulating horizontal fibers [364]. These treatments may extend the period of time during which rehabilitation improves functional recovery.

Clinical experience also suggests that locomotor training early after SCI improves recovery [20, 177, 370]. Walking activates multisegmental monosynaptic responses [65, 87, 129, 175, 176]. The functionally isolated spinal cord is plastic and has the capacity to generate locomotor patterns with appropriate afferent input, to undergo periods of spontaneous activity, and to make decisions to generate successful postural and locomotor tasks [127, 219, 271].

Electrical stimulation provides activity needed for synaptic consolidation [358]. In 2007, Brus-Ramer et al. reported that electrical stimulation of spared corticospinal axons augments ipsilateral spinal motor circuits after injury [40]. This effect is not mediated by the corpus callosum but through latent or newly sprouted connections by the spared motor cortex [41]. In 2010, Carmel et al. showed chronic electrical stimulation of the spared motor corticospinal tract after spinal cord hemisection induced outgrowth of spared axons into spinal cord below the hemisection to restore skilled paw placement on the impaired side [51–54].

Epidural stimulation of the spinal cord has recently become popular because of reports that such stimulation restores voluntary, standing, and locomotor function [6, 90, 128, 278]. Animal studies show that such epidural stimulation can not only improve locomotion but improves urethral relaxation during voiding and reduces hyperalgesia and neuropathic pain [3, 276, 325]. Several investigators have empirically developed criteria for optimal electrode placement and stimulation parameters for rats, monkeys, and humans [4, 278, 299]. Epidural and functional electrical stimulation does not replace rehabilitation. Electrical stimulation may increase the rate and extent of functional recovery associated with intensive directed rehabilitation.

The data strongly affirms the old maxim, "use it or lose it." Brain and spinal cord cannot afford to maintain unused circuits. Regenerated connections, if not used, will fade and disconnect. Exercise and directed rehabilitation is essential for functional recovery. We must not judge regeneration without rehabilitation harshly.

Peripheral Nerve Regeneration

Peripheral nerve injury is increasing in both incidence and severity, as populations increase together with concomitant increases in traffic and industrial accidents, violence, and battlefield injuries. It has been estimated that global nerve repair and regeneration costs will increase from $4.5 billion in 2013 to $7.8 billion in 2018 [213]. The current gold standard of care involves *autologous repairs*: direct repair (gaps of ~0–1 cm), nerve autografts (replacement nerves from elsewhere in the patient, usually the sensory, sural nerve; for gaps of ~1–10 cm), or vascularized nerve autografts (for gaps ~10+cm) [25, 62, 316].

Autologous Repairs and Timing

In contrast to the belief that spinal cords cannot regenerate, scientists and clinicians have long agreed that peripheral nerves will regrow, make synaptic connections with muscles and sensory organs, and are remyelinated by Schwann cells. Recovery takes place over many months and is consistent with distance and slow rate of axonal growth (~1 mm/d). Thus, unlike the field of spinal cord regeneration, the field of peripheral nerve regeneration has not been stymied by the dogma that regeneration cannot occur. In clinical practice, a vast majority (90%) of patients with peripheral nerve injuries are treated by primary nerve repair, elective delayed nerve repair, or primary surgical exploration [216].

Animal studies suggested that the critical period for peripheral nerve repair is 1–2 months. In 1988, Bolesta et al. reported that immediate repair of rabbit sciatic nerve had the best results, but 1–6 months delay resulted in 25–50% less function [29]. In 1989, Gattuso et al. compared immediate and delayed repair of peripheral nerves using freeze-thawed autologous skeletal muscle grafts in rat at 3, 5, 7, 14, 28, and 56 days after transection [110]. A delay of 56 days was found to be incompatible with useful recovery, but myelinated nerve fiber number and diameters of nerves repaired in 3–28 days did not differ significantly from immediate repaired nerves. In 1994, Baranowski et al. compared DRG neurons in rats that were repaired immediately or 3 months after sural nerve transection [15]. The number of surviving DRG neurons was 60% after both immediate and delayed repair, suggesting that loss of sensory neurons is not the reason.

In 1995, Lawson and Glasby used freeze-thawed muscle grafts to repair 3-cm gaps in median nerves in sheep. Five were repaired immediately (A) and 5 after 4 weeks. Peak nerve conduction velocities were significantly slower in repaired nerves; mean fiber diameters were 5.06, 3.90, and 8.58 μm in the immediate, delayed, and control groups. Short delays of 3 days have little effect [253]. In 2013, Wu et al. standardized a rat model of delayed sciatic nerve repair, showing that the compound action potentials were worse only after 6-, 8-, and 12-week delays [349].

Clinical experience confirms poor results in delayed nerve repairs [135, 144, 174]. In 2010, Mohseni et al. in Iran reported that early primary repairs have the best results with all 60 patients showing some recovery and 25/65 (38%) having excellent results, compared to poor recovery and 7/25 (28%) failures with delayed primary repair and 5/15 (33%) failures after delayed nerve graft [231]. In 2014, George and Boyce reviewed 28 studies (1577) of peroneal nerve repairs [111]. Good results were obtained in 45% of cases: 80% for neurolysis, 37% for primary repair, and 36% for nerve graft. Excluding neurolysis, good outcomes were obtained in 44% of repairs performed within 6 months and 12% of repairs done after 12 months. These results do not seem better than recovery from SCI.

Many investigators focused on changes in the distal stump or end organs. In 1985, Pellegrino and Spencer pointed out that Schwann cells undergo atrophy in distal stumps that have been denervated for long periods [250]. In 2005, Midha et al. attempted to protect the distal stump by cross-suturing the quadriceps motor nerve (motor) or re-suturing of the saphenous nerve (sensory) for 8 weeks [225]. More myelinated axons innervated motor- than sensory-protected or unprotected nerve. They concluded that even a 2-month denervation of distal nerve is deleterious to regeneration and that protecting the distal stump with another nerve improves subsequent reinnervation and regeneration. Ronkko et al. showed no difference in the capacity of the distal stump to receive growing axons after 2- or 6-month denervation in rats [270]. In 2013, Jonsson et al. in Sweden compared immediate

(0)-, 1-, 3-, or 6-month delays in nerve graft repair of transected sciatic nerves [159]. The number of regenerating motoneurons and myelinated axons in the distal nerve stump declined dramatically in the 3- and 6-month groups with greater muscle atrophy and neuromuscular junction changes. Key changes of muscles include fragmentation of the neuromuscular junction [350]. Electrical stimulation accelerates peripheral nerve regeneration up to 1 month after injury but not in nerves that were repaired more than a month after injury, possibly due to fibrosis in the distal stump [92, 124, 340, 351].

Nerve Guidance Conduits and Neurotrophic Devices

Despite being the current gold standard, autografts have significant drawbacks, including the surgical procedure to harvest a donor nerve, with its associated morbidity; limited options for matching length and size of donor nerves to the injured nerve; and sensory-mixed mismatching, i.e., the mismatches that results from donor nerves typically being *sensory*, when most of the defects they must repair are typically *mixed* (motor and sensory). Therefore, many clinicians have sought alternatives as far back as 1880 [149]. Kaplan et al. reported that this effort has accelerated in the past five decades, with published studies on the subject almost doubling over the past two decades [167]. Although solutions for bridging short nerve gaps have been somewhat effective, repairs of long nerve gaps (5–30+ cm) remain less effective and are a key research challenge.

Nerve guidance conduits (NGCs) are an alternative to autograft repairs. These conduits generally consist of a tube filled with axon growth supporting material and neurotrophic factors. Kaplan et al. and Windebank's group have both noted that testing of NGCs has been limited mostly to the rat sciatic nerve injury model [8, 167]. As Kaplan et al. pointed out: "(1) The preponderance of nerve regeneration data is now in a single species, which is likely to skew treatment outcomes and lead to inappropriate evaluation of

risks and benefits. (2) The rat is a particularly poor model for the repair of human critical gap defects due to both its small size and its species-specific neurobiological regenerative profile: The real mismatch is that the rat model is used to test NGCs over 1–1.5 cm gaps, while they are ultimately supposed to work clinically in 5–30 cm gaps. (3) Translation from rat to human has proven unreliable for nerve regeneration, as for many other applications."

Clinicians currently used several NGCs to repair nerves, including decellularized allografts (decellularized nerves from human cadavers, e.g., Avance® made by AxoGen, Alachua, FL), vein and other biologic conduits (type I collagen, e.g., Neuragen® made by Integra Life Sciences, Plainsboro, NJ), and synthetic conduits (such as woven polyglycolic acid, e.g., Neurotube® made by Synovis Micro Companies Alliance, Birmingham, AL) [313]. Allografts or synthetic conduits avoid the morbidity of harvesting a donor nerve but are less effective in supporting regeneration. Disadvantages of vein conduits and other biologic NGCs include collapsing, kinking, lack of neurotrophic support, and promotion of scarring (e.g., some components such as collagen promote fibroblast activity). Synthetic NGCs can be designed to avoid the disadvantages of biologic NGCs, but currently synthetic NGCs cannot match the performance of autografts and allografts and offer only limited functional recovery.

To date, few synthetic NGCs have achieved US Food and Drug Administration (FDA) or Conformité Européenne (CE) approvals for clinical use (only 4 by 2014) and almost exclusively for repair of short gaps (≤4 cm; one ≤6.35 cm) [71, 248]. New NGCs must address two major issues. First, chemical and mechanical properties of the conduit wall must be optimized to facilitate handling, to be suturable, to have appropriate stiffness and flexibility, and to resist compression and kinking for longer nerve gap repairs and for crossing moving joints of the finger, elbow, shoulder, or knee. Second, effective biological enhancement strategies must be incorporated into synthetic NGCs, to create a biological milieu within the conduit that supports and directs nerve growth.

Each of the three main components of the NGC, i.e., the wall, the filler, and bioactive moieties, must be optimized. This requires testing variants of each alone and in combinations, to identify designs that will support nerve regeneration while inhibiting scar infiltration, be kink and compression resistant while offering superior handling and suturability, and will allow nutrient and waste exchange while retarding the ingress of fibrous tissue. In vivo studies are critical for preclinical testing. Most academic laboratories rely on rat sciatic nerve injury models to test NGCs. The sizes of rats limit the nerve gap to 1–2 cm and the sciatic nerve injury model, so commonly used does not expose NGCs to significant mechanical forces or bending. Furthermore, rats have a strong regenerative potential compared to human patients, who are often old and suffer from diseases that compromise healing and regeneration, such as diabetes.

Variations of neuroregenerative potential between species further complicate interpretation of preclinical results [282]. A "critical nerve gap" is a nerve gap over which no recovery will occur without some form of nerve grafting or bridging [71, 316]. The critical nerve gap is ~1.5 cm for rats, ~3 cm for rabbits, and ~4 cm for pigs and humans. These differences exist despite the fact that longitudinal axonal growth rates are similar across most species, at approximately 1 mm/d (potentially due to the primitive and phylogenetically common ancestry of the neurite lengthening machinery involved) [122]. This phenomenon may be explained by differing rates of fibrin degradation across species: Early on in the nerve repair process, an acellular fibrin-extracellular matrix cable is laid down between the proximal and distal stumps [21, 71, 134, 342]. In rats, this occurs within 1 week of repair and is followed by cellular infiltration. Schwann cells, endothelial cells, and fibroblasts migrate into the cable from both the proximal and distal nerve stumps. The Schwann cells proliferate and align to form parallel cables (the "glial bands of Büngner"), which provide neurotrophic and structural support for axonal regeneration. The fibrin cable is a critical component of this process and, due to variable thicknesses and degradation rates across species,

is believed to define the maximum gap length over which healing can occur. Its degradation time is about 2 weeks in the rat, and up to 4 weeks in the human, leading to critical nerve gaps of ~1.5 cm in a rat sciatic nerve model and ~4 cm in humans [163, 251].

Into the Future

Why just restore function? Why not exceed normal function? These questions generate quandaries of such proportions that they are fit for an entire ethical textbook and certainly cannot be done justice here. We leave the reader to consider for themselves the risks and benefits of what is now already achievable, and the future possibilities, some examples of which we explore here. Author Kaplan proposes that we are nearing and, in some cases, are already capable of achieving, what he coins "Nervous System 2.0" (NS2.0) and the "Neural Enhancement Divide" (NED) – which is that inflection point where instead of restoring the nervous system, we begin to improve on it!

NED: The End or the Beginning?

Ethical issues abound when we can make some individuals better than "normal." Arguably, the first example ever is that of the bilateral lower limb amputee runner Oscar Pistorius. In the 2008 Olympics, Oscar's team lobbied furiously to allow him to run in the Olympics rather than in the Para-Olympics but to no avail as it was widely considered unfair to Pistorius as he would be *disadvantaged*. That year, at the Para-Olympics, he won his races spectacularly. In 2012, after much lobbying once again, the team managed to gain entry to the Olympics, and Oscar went on to beat all the "able-bodied" athletes, running on 2 C-legs. This time, there was an outcry that he might have been unfairly *advantaged* by his prosthetics.

Although we have not reached the NED yet, the time is coming for our nerve regenerative and restorative capabilities to do so. Is it reasonable to add infrared or X-ray vision to retinal implants?

Is it fair to literally provide "superhuman" strength through implantable extra muscles or mechanical actuators that may be implanted or at least part of wearable exoskeletons? Is it reasonable to provide unlimited computing power through visual system digital overlays or interfaces directly with the brain? The list is inexhaustible.

Recently, much discussion has revolved around the relatively easy and cheap use of the CRISPR/Cas system for modifying our genetic code [130, 155, 188]. First described by Jinek et al. in mid-2012, the publication of this technique – that offers such great promise – still precedes any adequate ethical or legal framework to contain it [155]. Is it safe or ethical for researchers to be able to readily change the DNA of almost any organism? How will this impact our futures and, existentially, the evolution of all species? Two sides to this argument have arisen. One school believes that we should use the utmost caution and aggressively control genetic modifications, while at the other extreme, there are those who believe that our acquiring the capability to modify genetic code, and *modifying our own code, is in fact part of evolution itself*!

Whichever school of thought you subscribe to, the NED is fast approaching and it is inevitable.

Nervous System 2.0

Regeneration and/or restoration of function beyond the NED, to create a *super/augmented/enhanced* NS2.0, will no doubt be achieved through both biologic mechanisms (as discussed above, and many of which are yet to be elucidated still) and through – or in combination with – neural prosthetic mechanisms.

Loeb defines neural prosthetics as "the subset of neural control concerned with replacing and repairing neural function via electronic interfaces" [202]. In his fascinating chapter, "We Made the Deaf Hear. Now What?", he describes how when cochlear implants were first being developed (circa 1975), many expert auditory neurophysiologists believed that a functional auditory prosthesis could not be achieved [201].

The biophysics of electrically excitable tissues had been well established already for about 50 years, and clinical experiments had already demonstrated that sounds could be perceived through electrical stimulation. Their concerns were, instead, based on their beliefs of how the CNS might process and perceive the wide variety of temporospatial patterns generated by the electrical activity of so many auditory neurons. Human hearing covers frequencies from 20 to 20,000 Hz (cycles/s). It was believed by some that computing, interpreting, and stimulating signals that covered approximately 20,000 frequency possibilities, each with their own varying temporal, spatial, and intensity profiles, were an impossible task, which was furthermore, significantly compounded by the varied perceptions of sounds by different patient types (e.g., previously hearing vs. congenitally deaf).

On the other hand, around the same time, researchers who were starting to work on retinal implants generally felt confident that success could be achieved relatively more easily, because of our ability to gather useful information from images containing as little as $4 \times 4 = 16$ pixels (vs. 20,000 frequencies for hearing) [66].

So for many years, it was commonly believed that retinal implants would be more easily achievable than cochlear implants, but in fact the exact opposite has proven true: While auditory neurophysiologists were struggling with the best ways to approach cochlear nerve stimulation, in an unrelated but serendipitous effort, AT&T were struggling with the best ways to carry wide frequency bands of data over copper telephone wires. The work they did showed clearly that we could understand conversation with as few as just eight bands of averaged frequencies across the speech region of the *audible* frequency spectrum (20–6000 Hz).

Suddenly cochlear implants with just eight electrodes could prove extremely useful. It also taught us the importance of miniaturizing the cochlear implant electrodes sufficiently to achieve the lower frequencies required, as these are tonotopically mapped along the basilar membrane toward its narrowest tip in the cochlea's "snail shell." Today, cochlear implants with

16–24 electrodes are becoming the standard, offering even music appreciation! While, on the other hand, visual prosthesis researchers are still working to elicit small and reproducible phosphenes, and attempting to achieve stable long-term visual percepts. Much of the recent research is still conducted using arrays with very limited numbers of electrodes, e.g., the A16 (4×4 electrodes) and Argus II (6×10 electrodes) by Second Sight Medical Products Inc. (Sylmar, California, USA) [66] and a 9×9 research array proposed by Monash University [192].

These examples of two neural prosthetics highlight two important points for a future NS2.0. Firstly, unexpected developments in seemingly unrelated fields can hasten the understanding and development in neural prosthetics, driving the NED and ultimately making NS2.0 capabilities possible that we have yet to envision. Secondly, unexpected and poorly understood neurophysiological phenomena can retard the NED, prohibiting us from even just restoring normal function to our nervous system 1.0. Clearly, the NED will be achieved for varying neural functions throughout the future of humanity, some in coming decades, and others over many centuries to come, as Loeb describes in his chapter, "Neuroprosthetic Interfaces – The Reality Behind Bionics and Cyborgs" [202].

NS2.0 Possibilities

In Michio Kaku's enlightening book, *Physics of the Impossible: A Scientific Exploration into the World of Phasers, Force Fields, Teleportation, and Time Travel*, Kaku explores physical possibilities and categorizes them into three classes of impossibilities: Class I Impossibilities are impossible today but might be possible within this century; Class II Impossibilities are those that sit at the very edge of our understanding and might be realized on a scale of millennia, if at all; and Class III Impossibilities are technologies that violate our known laws of physics and would involve a fundamental shift in these laws if they ever proved possible [162].

Taking Kaku's lead, Kaplan would like to propose considering NS2.0 possibilities in a similar fashion, by categorizing them into three classes of *possibilities* (rather than impossibilities). As our understanding of neurobiology is progressing on a different timescale to the laws of physics, I would propose here that *Class I Possibilities* are those that are almost possible today and might be possible within the next three decades; *Class II Possibilities* are those that still sit at the edge of our understanding and might be realized beyond three decades to centuries; *Class III Possibilities* are technologies that could have great utility, but on which no substantial research achievements have yet been made.

The following are just some examples of current technologies that may ultimately lead to future NS2.0 technologies.

Class I Possibilities (Within 30 Years)

Advanced Tissue Regeneration We have discussed in detail above the many advances that are being researched in terms of spinal cord and peripheral nerve regeneration from a biological point of view. Tapping into the inherent regenerative capabilities of the human body will continue to yield remarkable advances over the coming decades, particularly together with the influence of other emerging fields such as DREADDs (Designer Receptors Exclusively Activated by Designer Drugs) [58, 249]. While open to debate, we believe that these Class I Possibilities will vastly improve the degrees of *partial* recovery that we are currently seeing in both the CNS and the PNS.

However, true and *full* regeneration of the brain, spinal cord, and peripheral nerves remain Class II Possibilities. Loeb refers to the opportunity for "Augmented Plastic Recovery," based on the relatively recent acceptance in neuroscience that adult brains are in fact capable of substantial reorganization and of regenerating some neurons [156, 202, 223]. While traditionally patients with strokes, traumatic brain injuries, and SCIs have been taught to live with their disabilities, the emphasis over the past two decades has grown to include recovery of function. Intense exercise and training programs are now part of standard physical therapy treatments for these patients, often enhanced by robotic aids that adjust the levels of support and challenge the patient receives in real time [326]. Loeb explains that electrical stimulation of muscle and nerves produces patterned electrical activity that projects back to the spinal cord and brain, where it may provide neurotrophic effects.

Embedded Sensory-Motor Activity for Prosthetic Limbs Nghiem et al. have recently reviewed methods of providing a sense of touch for prosthetic hands [239]. One such technique that shows great promise for not only sensory activity but for prosthetic motor activity as well is "targeted reinnervation," as originally described by Kuiken and Dumanian et al. in 2004 [179, 180, 202]. This involves rerouting the major nerve trunks of the upper limb (radial, median, and ulnar) into the anterior chest wall during or after an amputation, instead of burying them in stump muscles as is traditionally done to minimize the risks of neuroma and/or phantom limb pains. In the anterior chest wall, these nerves are anastomosed to the nerves to the chest wall muscles (pectoralis major and serratus anterior) and to the nerves that supply sensation to the overlying skin. Now, after healing, the reinnervated chest wall targets are mapped out for motor function via electromyography (EMG) recording patterns over the chest wall during attempted upper limb movements and for sensory function by determining upper limb sensations experienced during electrical stimulation of the chest skin via surface or wirelessly implanted electrodes at a grid of sites over the chest wall. Within an afternoon, this mapping procedure provides a data set that can drive and receive sensory input from a prosthetic device, without any patient learning required at all. This paradigm shift in how we control and sense prosthetic limbs has bypassed centuries of work on controlling prosthetics through patient or machine-learning techniques!

Another exciting development is the robotic finger pulp developed by Loeb et al. [339]. This award-winning biomimetic "finger tip" comprises several electrodes along a rigid "phalynx" of plastic, embedded in an electrically conductive gel surrounded by a silicon "skin." Small changes in the amount of gel between the electrodes can

be measured electrically with such sensitivity that tiny vibrations of a slipping cup, for example, can be detected and adjusted for, so that a robotic hand with these fingers can pick up a Styrofoam cup without crushing it or dropping it or determine if a piece of fruit is ripe without bruising it. Clearly, these techniques are still approaching restoration of our nervous system's function, but over the coming decades, it could be feasible to insert a cam into the motor pathway so large movements at the chest level can be converted into minute movements of the arm or vice versa; that tremors may be removed if necessary, etc. Similarly, one could now "sense" how hot a kiln is inside, or pick up a giant metal beam, or …

Superhuman Strength Through implantable extra muscles or mechanical actuators that may be implanted or at least part of wearable exoskeletons or through robotic arms as discussed above, superhuman strength may certainly become a reality. Surgical feasibility for implanting an additional muscle has already occurred, and exoskeletons with EMG pickup and electrical stimulation capabilities exist [60, 329]. Refining these technologies is a matter of time.

Unlimited Computing Power Through Visual System Digital Overlays One example of this possibility may be the combination of a Google Glass-type computer with a retinal implant of sufficient resolution to scroll a text overlay initially and to provide a high-resolution detailed virtual environment overlay ultimately.

Floating Light-Activated Microelectrical Stimulators (FLAMES) Neural stimulation and recording are usually performed using fine wire microelectrodes. Not only are these inserted traumatically, causing damage to the spinal cord, brain, or peripheral nerves, but their rigidity, relatively large size (on the order of 100s of microns), and fixed, tethered nature lead to scarring, with increasing thresholds for stimulation and decreasing signal-to-noise ratio for recording. Furthermore, the fine cables that connect to the driving electronics break easily. Together, these events severely limit the functional lifespan of implantable electrodes, in some cases to just weeks to months. FLAMES are a new technology that may solve some of these issues by providing wireless neural stimulation in submillimeter devices of ~150 μm in thickness [1]. Once implanted, a near-infrared laser beam transfers energy to the devices through the tissues to wirelessly activate the devices via their photo-diodes and generate stimulus current. To date, prototype testing in a rat model has demonstrated successful intraspinal stimulation resulting in forelimb movement.

Fetal Pacemaker Currently if a fetus requires a pacemaker, in utero surgery is performed at great risk. Loeb et al. have developed a prototype inject-able microstimulator to avoid the associated risks and have tested it in vivo [14, 203]. This device is injected through the mother's abdomen and the soft cartilaginous sternum of the fetus, under ultra-sound guidance, and the distal corkscrew electrode is then screwed into the myocardium where it remains until a definitive pacemaker can be implanted after birth. It is powered by a small bat-tery with or without inductive charging if needed. Over the coming decades, this is likely to translate into clinical use, and the idea could potentially be applied to other applications, such as in utero dia-phragm pacing or neuromuscular electrical stimu-lation (NMES) for cerebral palsy, as examples.

Long-Distance Brain-Brain Communication Stocco et al. have recently described a collabora-tive problem-solving effort by humans using a brain-to-brain interface (BBI) [309]. BBIs combine neuroimaging and neurostimulation to exchange information between brains directly in neural code. This has now been explored both in vivo and in humans. Currently, the techniques are slow and have limited accuracy or utility. Over the coming decades, we believe these problems could be solved to make true BBIs a reality with extraordinary capabilities, both civilian and military, including truly watching or controlling a surgical procedure remotely or providing detailed thoughts and infor-mation to an "avatar" for execution.

Class II Possibilities (30 Years to Centuries)

Class II Possibilities are rare by definition, but a few are listed here for discussion.

Infrared or X-Ray Vision Extending the capabil-ities of the retinal implants referred to above that will 1 day be of sufficient resolution to provide a high-resolution detailed virtual environment overlay, one can easily live imagine inputs from IR cameras or X-ray devices.

Complete Spinal Cord Injury Recovery No doubt this will ultimately be achievable. At that stage, many of the prosthetic devices we are discussing here as "futuristic" will no longer be needed and will ultimately become obsolete technology.

Unlimited Computing Power Through Interfaces Directly with the Brain (Cognitive Neural Prostheses) A prosthesis that can enhance higher cognitive functions such as memory and learning will have to receive neural data from parts of the brain, process this data and integrate new data as needed, and then activate the brain's recipient areas with the transformed data. This will require highly sophisticated neural interfaces and a detailed understanding of the transforma-tions needed and that will be acceptable to the recipient areas. Research into some of these vari-ous aspects has recently begun [22, 202].

Class III Possibilities (No Substantial Achievements Yet)

Body Transplants or Brain Transplants? Today, a patient with a debilitating musculoskeletal neu-rodegenerative disorder awaits a body transplant in Russia [48, 230]. This has been ethically approved by the responsible institution's review committee, because since it cannot be performed, he will die. If it is performed, his new body will keep his head and brain alive as a quadriplegic. But in the future, once we can regenerate spinal cords and peripheral nerves completely, a brain transplant into a healthy body may be feasible.

Concluding Thought

In this chapter, we have laid out the current understanding of the detailed science behind spi-nal cord and peripheral nerve regeneration and a possible framework for considering where it might all go from here. The former is the current state of the art, while the latter is merely informed speculation and ideas. We hope this will excite you as much as this field excites us!

References

1. Abdo A, Sahin M, Freedman DS, Cevik E, Spuhler PS, Unlu MS. Floating light-activated microelectrical stimulators tested in the rat spinal cord. J Neural Eng. 2015;8:056012.

2. Abrous N, Guy J, Vigny A, Calas A, Le Moal M, Herman JP. Development of intracerebral dopaminergic grafts: a combined immunohistochemical and autoradiographic study of its time course and environmental influences. J Comp Neurol. 1988;273:26–41.

3. AbudF EM, Ichiyama RM, Havton LA, Chang HH. Spinal stimulation of the upper lumbar spinal cord modulates urethral sphincter activity in rats after spinal cord injury. Am J Physiol Renal Physiol. 2015;308:F1032–40.

4. Alam M, Garcia-Alias G, Shah PK, Gerasimenko Y, Zhong H, Roy RR, Edgerton VR. Evaluation of optimal electrode configurations for epidural spinal cord stimulation in cervical spinal cord injured rats. J Neurosci Methods. 2015;247:50–7.

5. Alluin O, Delivet-Mongrain H, Gauthier MK, Fehlings MG, Rossignol S, Karimi-Abdolrezaee S. Examination of the combined effects of chondroitinase ABC, growth factors and locomotor training following compressive spinal cord injury on neuroanatomical plasticity and kinematics. PLoS One. 2014;9:e111072.

6. Angeli CA, Edgerton VR, Gerasimenko YP, Harkema SJ. Altering spinal cord excitability enables voluntary movements after chronic complete paralysis in humans. Brain. 2014;137:1394–409.

7. Anghelescu N, Petrescu A, Alexandrescu I. Therapy study on the experimental injury of spinal cord. IV. High doses of methyl-prednisolone. Rom J Neurol Psychiatry. 1995;33:241–9.

8. Angius D, Wang H, Spinner RJ, Gutierrez-Cotto Y, Yaszemski MJ, Windebank AJ. A systematic review of animal models used to study nerve regeneration in tissue-engineered scaffolds. Biomaterials. 2012;33:8034–9.

9. Azmitia EC, Whitaker PM. Formation of a glial scar following microinjection of fetal neurons into the hippocampus or midbrain of the adult rat: an immunocytochemical study. Neurosci Lett. 1983;38:145–50.

10. Bajrovic F, Remskar M, Sketelj J. Prior collateral sprouting enhances elongation rate of sensory axons regenerating through acellular distal segment of a crushed peripheral nerve. J Peripher Nerv Syst. 1999;4:5–12.

11. Bandtlow C, Schiweck W, Tai HH, Schwab ME, Skerra A. The Escherichia coli-derived Fab fragment of the IgM/kappa antibody IN-1 recognizes and neutralizes myelin-associated inhibitors of neurite growth. Eur J Biochem. 1996;241:468–75.

12. Bandtlow CE, Schwab ME. NI-35/250/nogo-a: a neurite growth inhibitor restricting structural plasticity and regeneration of nerve fibers in the adult vertebrate CNS. Glia. 2000;29:175–81.

13. Bandtlow CE. Regeneration in the central nervous system. Exp Gerontol. 2003;38:79–86.

14. Bar-Cohen Y, Loeb GE, Pruetz JD, Silka MJ, Guerra C, Vest AN, Zhou L, Chmait RH. Preclinical testing and optimization of a novel fetal micropacemaker. Heart Rhythm. 2015;12:1683–90.

15. Baranowski AP, Priestley JV, McMahon SB. The consequence of delayed versus immediate nerve repair on the properties of regenerating sensory nerve fibers in the adult rat. Neurosci Lett. 1994;168:197–200.

16. Barritt AW, Davies M, Marchand F, Hartley R, Grist J, Yip P, McMahon SB, Bradbury EJ. Chondroitinase ABC promotes sprouting of intact and injured spinal systems after spinal cord injury. J Neurosci. 2006;26:10856–67.

17. Barton WA, Liu BP, Tzvetkova D, Jeffrey PD, Fournier AE, Sah D, Cate R, Strittmatter SM, Nikolov DB. Structure and axon outgrowth inhibitor binding of the Nogo-66 receptor and related proteins. EMBO J. 2003;22:3291–302.

18. Bartsch U, Bandtlow CE, Schnell L, Bartsch S, Spillmann AA, Rubin BP, Hillenbrand R, Montag D, Schwab ME, Schachner M. Lack of evidence that myelin-associated glycoprotein is a major inhibitor of axonal regeneration in the CNS. Neuron. 1995;15:1375–81.

19. Beattie MS, Bresnahan JC, Komon J, Tovar CA, Van Meter M, Anderson DK, Faden AI, Hsu CY, Noble LJ, Salzman S, Young W. Endogenous repair after spinal cord contusion injuries in the rat. Exp Neurol. 1997;148:453–63.

20. Behrman AL, Harkema SJ. Physical rehabilitation as an agent for recovery after spinal cord injury. Phys Med Rehabil Clin N Am. 2007;18:183–202.

21. Belkas SJ, Shoichet SM, Midha R. Peripheral nerve regeneration through guidance tubes. Neurol Res. 2004;26:151–60.

22. Berger TW, Glanzman DL. Toward replacement parts for the brain: implantable biomimetic electronics as neural prostheses. Cambridge: MIT Press; 2005.

23. Bernstein JJ, Bernstein ME. Effect of glial-ependymal scar and teflon arrest on the regenerative capacity of goldfish spinal cord. Exp Neurol. 1967;19:25–32.

24. Bignami A. The role of astrocytes in CNS regeneration. J Neurosurg Sci. 1984;28:127–32.

25. Birch R, Dunkerton M, Bonney G, Jamieson AM. Experience with the free vascularized ulnar nerve graft in repair of supraclavicular lesions of the brachial plexus. Clin Orthop Relat Res. 1988;237:96–104.

26. Bisby MA, Pollock B. Increased regeneration rate in peripheral nerve axons following double lesions: enhancement of the conditioning lesion phenomenon. J Neurobiol. 1983;14:467–72.

27. Bisby MA, Keen P. The effect of a conditioning lesion on the regeneration rate of peripheral nerve axons containing substance P. Brain Res. 1985;336: 201–6.

28. Bisby MA, Keen P. Regeneration of primary afferent neurons containing substance P-like immunoreactivity. Brain Res. 1986;365:85–95.

29. Bolesta MJ, Garrett Jr WE, Ribbeck BM, Glisson RR, Seaber AV, Goldner JL. Immediate and delayed neurorrhaphy in a rabbit model: a functional, histologic, and biochemical comparison. J Hand Surg Am. 1988;13:352–7.

30. Borgens RB, Roederer E, Cohen MJ. Enhanced spinal cord regeneration in lamprey by applied electric fields. Science. 1981;213:611–7.

31. Borgens RB, Blight AR, Murphy DJ, Stewart L. Transected dorsal column axons within the guinea pig spinal cord regenerate in the presence of an applied electric field. J Comp Neurol. 1986;250:168–80.

32. Bottai D, Scesa G, Cigognini D, Adami R, Nicora E, Abrignani S, Di Giulio AM, Gorio A. Third trimester NG2-positive amniotic fluid cells are effective in improving repair in spinal cord injury. Exp Neurol. 2014;254C:121–33.

33. Bovolenta P, Wandosell F, Nieto-Sampedro M. Neurite outgrowth over resting and reactive astrocytes. Restor Neurol Neurosci. 1991;2:221–8.

34. Bovolenta P, Wandosell F, Nieto-Sampedro M. CNS glial scar tissue: a source of molecules which inhibit central neurite outgrowth. Prog Brain Res. 1992;94: 367–79.

35. Bradbury EJ, Moon LD, Popat RJ, King VR, Bennett GS, Patel PN, Fawcett JW, McMahon SB. Chondroitinase ABC promotes functional recovery after spinal cord injury. Nature. 2002;416:636–40.

36. Bregman BS, Kunkel-Bagden E, Schnell L, Dai HN, Gao D, Schwab ME. Recovery from spinal cord injury mediated by antibodies to neurite growth inhibitors. Nature. 1995;378:498–501.

37. Brittis PA, Flanagan JG. Nogo domains and a Nogo receptor: implications for axon regeneration. Neuron. 2001;30:11–4.

38. Broggini T, Nitsch R, Savaskan NE. Plasticity-related gene 5 (PRG5) induces filopodia and neurite growth and impedes lysophosphatidic acid- and nogo-A-mediated axonal retraction. Mol Biol Cell. 2010;21:521–37.

39. Brosamle C, Huber AB, Fiedler M, Skerra A, Schwab ME. Regeneration of lesioned corticospinal tract fibers in the adult rat induced by a recombinant, humanized IN-1 antibody fragment. J Neurosci. 2000;20:8061–8.

40. Brus-Ramer M, Carmel JB, Chakrabarty S, Martin JH. Electrical stimulation of spared corticospinal axons augments connections with ipsilateral spinal motor circuits after injury. J Neurosci. 2007;27:13793–801.

41. Brus-Ramer M, Carmel JB, Martin JH. Motor cortex bilateral motor representation depends on subcortical and interhemispheric interactions. J Neurosci. 2009;29:6196–206.

42. Buffo A, Zagrebelsky M, Huber AB, Skerra A, Schwab ME, Strata P, Rossi F. Application of neutralizing antibodies against NI-35/250 myelin-associated neurite growth inhibitory proteins to the adult rat cerebellum induces sprouting of uninjured purkinje cell axons. J Neurosci. 2000;20:2275–86.

43. Bunge MB. Novel combination strategies to repair the injured mammalian spinal cord. J Spinal Cord Med. 2008;31:262–9.

44. Cafferty WB, Yang SH, Duffy PJ, Li S, Strittmatter SM. Functional axonal regeneration through astrocytic scar genetically modified to digest chondroitin sulfate proteoglycans. J Neurosci. 2007;27:2176–85.

45. Cafferty WB, Duffy P, Huebner E, Strittmatter SM. MAG and OMgp synergize with Nogo-A to restrict axonal growth and neurological recovery after spinal cord trauma. J Neurosci. 2010;30:6825–37.

46. Cai D, Shen Y, De Bellard M, Tang S, Filbin MT. Prior exposure to neurotrophins blocks inhibition of axonal regeneration by MAG and myelin via a cAMP-dependent mechanism. Neuron. 1999;22:89–101.

47. Cai D, Qiu J, Cao Z, McAtee M, Bregman BS, Filbin MT. Neuronal cyclic AMP controls the developmental loss in ability of axons to regenerate. J Neurosci. 2001;21:4731–9.

48. Canavero S. HEAVEN: The head anastomosis venture Project outline for the first human head transplantation with spinal linkage (GEMINI). Surg Neurol Int. 2013;4 Suppl 1:S335–42.

49. Carlstedt T, Cullheim S, Risling M, Ulfhake B. Mammalian root-spinal cord regeneration. Prog Brain Res. 1988;8:225–9.

50. Carlstedt T. Reinnervation of the mammalian spinal cord after neonatal dorsal root crush. J Neurocytol. 1988;17:335–50.

51. Carmel JB, Berrol LJ, Brus-Ramer M, Martin JH. Chronic electrical stimulation of the intact corticospinal system after unilateral injury restores skilled locomotor control and promotes spinal axon outgrowth. J Neurosci. 2010;30:10918–26.

52. Carmel JB, Kimura H, Berrol LJ, Martin JH. Motor cortex electrical stimulation promotes axon outgrowth to brain stem and spinal targets that control the forelimb impaired by unilateral corticospinal injury. Eur J Neurosci. 2013;37:1090–102.

53. Carmel JB, Kimura H, Martin JH. Electrical stimulation of motor cortex in the uninjured hemisphere after chronic unilateral injury promotes recovery of skilled locomotion through ipsilateral control. J Neurosci. 2014;34:462–6.

54. Carmel JB, Martin JH. Motor cortex electrical stimulation augments sprouting of the corticospinal tract and promotes recovery of motor function. Front Integr Neurosci. 2014;8:51.

55. Carter LM, McMahon SB, Bradbury EJ. Delayed treatment with chondroitinase ABC reverses chronic atrophy of rubrospinal neurons following spinal cord injury. Exp Neurol. 2011;228:149–56.

56. Chalecka-Franaszek E, Chuang DM. Lithium activates the serine/threonine kinase Akt-1 and sup-

presses glutamate-induced inhibition of Akt-1 activity in neurons. Proc Natl Acad Sci U S A. 1999;96:8745–50.

57. Chen MS, Huber AB, van der Haar ME, Frank M, Schnell L, Spillmann AA, Christ F, Schwab ME. Nogo-A is a myelin-associated neurite outgrowth inhibitor and an antigen for monoclonal antibody IN-1. Nature. 2000;403:434–9.

58. Chen X, Choo H, Huang XP, Yang X, Stone O, Roth BL, Jin J. The first structure-activity relationship studies for designer receptors exclusively activated by designer drugs. ACS Chem Neurosci. 2015;6: 476–84.

59. Chong MS, Woolf CJ, Haque NS, Anderson PN. Axonal regeneration from injured dorsal roots into the spinal cord of adult rats. J Comp Neurol. 1999;410:42–54.

60. Chuang DC, Chen KT. The possibility and potential feasibility of putting an extra functioning free muscle transplant onto a normal limb: experimental rat study. Plast Reconstr Surg. 2011;128:853–9.

61. Clemente CD. Regeneration in the vertebrate central nervous system. Int Rev Neurobiol. 1964;6:257–301.

62. Colen KL, Choi M, Chiu DT. Nerve grafts and conduits. Plast Reconstr Surg. 2009;124(6 Suppl):e386–94.

63. Coles CH, Shen Y, Tenney AP, Siebold C, Sutton GC, Lu W, Gallagher JT, Jones EY, Flanagan JG, Aricescu AR. Proteoglycan-specific molecular switch for RPTPsigma clustering and neuronal extension. Science. 2011;332:484–8.

64. Connor JR, Bernstein JJ. Astrocytes in rat fetal cerebral cortical homografts following implantation into adult rat spinal cord. Brain Res. 1987;409:62–70.

65. Courtine G, Harkema SJ, Dy CJ, Gerasimenko YP, Dyhre-Poulsen P. Modulation of multisegmental monosynaptic responses in a variety of leg muscles during walking and running in humans. J Physiol. 2007;582:1125–39.

66. Dagnelie G. Retinal implants: emergence of a multidisciplinary field. Curr Opin Neurol. 2012;25:67–75.

67. Dahl D, Perides G, Bignami A. Axonal regeneration in old multiple sclerosis plaques. Immunohistochemical study with monoclonal antibodies to phosphorylated and non-phosphorylated neurofilament proteins. Acta Neuropathol. 1989;79:154–9.

68. Dahlin LB. Stimulation of regeneration of the sciatic nerve by experimentally induced inflammation in rats. Scand J Plast Reconstr Surg Hand Surg. 1992;26:121–5.

69. Dahlin LB, Kanje M. Conditioning effect induced by chronic nerve compression. An experimental study of the sciatic and tibial nerves of rats. Scand J Plast Reconstr Surg Hand Surg. 1992;26:37–41.

70. Dahlin LB, Thambert C. Acute nerve compression at low pressures has a conditioning lesion effect on rat sciatic nerves. Acta Orthop Scand. 1993;64:479–81.

71. Daly W, Yao L, Zeugolis D, Windebank A, Pandit A. A biomaterials approach to peripheral nerve regeneration: bridging the peripheral nerve gap and

enhancing functional recovery. J R Soc Interface. 2012;9:202–21.

72. Danilov CA, Steward O. Conditional genetic deletion of PTEN after a spinal cord injury enhances regenerative growth of CST axons and motor function recovery in mice. Exp Neurol. 2015;266:147–60.

73. Das GD, Ross DT. Neural transplantation: autoradiographic analysis of histogenesis in neocortical transplants. Int J Dev Neurosci. 1986;4:69–79.

74. David S, Aguayo AJ. Axonal elongation into peripheral nervous system "bridges" after central nervous system injury in adult rats. Science. 1981;214: 931–3.

75. Davies SJ, Fitch MT, Memberg SP, Hall AK, Raisman G, Silver J. Regeneration of adult axons in white matter tracts of the central nervous system. Nature. 1997;390:680–3.

76. de la Torre JC, Hill PK, Gonzalez-Carvajal M, Parker Jr JC. Evaluation of transected spinal cord regeneration in the rat. Exp Neurol. 1984;84:188–206.

77. Dechant G, Barde YA. The neurotrophin receptor p75(NTR): novel functions and implications for diseases of the nervous system. Nat Neurosci. 2002;5: 1131–6.

78. Delcroix JD, Averill S, Fernandes K, Tomlinson DR, Priestley JV, Fernyhough P. Axonal transport of activating transcription factor-2 is modulated by nerve growth factor in nociceptive neurons. J Neurosci. 1999;19:RC24.

79. Deng WP, Yang CC, Yang LY, Chen CW, Chen WH, Yang CB, Chen YH, Lai WF, Renshaw PF. Extracellular matrix-regulated neural differentiation of human multipotent marrow progenitor cells enhances functional recovery after spinal cord injury. Spine J. 2014;14:2488–99.

80. Dickendesher TL, Baldwin KT, Mironova YA, Koriyama Y, Raiker SJ, Askew KL, Wood A, Geoffroy CG, Zheng B, Liepmann CD, Katagiri Y, Benowitz LI, Geller HM, Giger RJ. NgR1 and NgR3 are receptors for chondroitin sulfate proteoglycans. Nat Neurosci. 2012;15:703–12.

81. Dill J, Wang H, Zhou F, Li S. Inactivation of glycogen synthase kinase 3 promotes axonal growth and recovery in the CNS. J Neurosci. 2008;28:8914–28.

82. Dimou L, Schnell L, Montani L, Duncan C, Simonen M, Schneider R, Liebscher T, Gullo M, Schwab ME. Nogo-A-deficient mice reveal strain-dependent differences in axonal regeneration. J Neurosci. 2006;26: 5591–603.

83. Dobkin B, Apple D, Barbeau H, Basso M, Behrman A, Deforge D, Ditunno J, Dudley G, Elashoff R, Fugate L, Harkema S, Saulino M, Scott M. Spinal cord injury locomotor trial, g. weight-supported treadmill vs over-ground training for walking after acute incomplete SCI. Neurology. 2006;66:484–93.

84. Dodd DA, Niederoest B, Bloechlinger S, Dupuis L, Loeffler JP, Schwab ME. Nogo-A, −B, and -C are found on the cell surface and interact together in many different cell types. J Biol Chem. 2005;280:12494–502.

85. Du K, Zheng S, Zhang Q, Li S, Gao X, Wang J, Jiang L, Liu K. Pten deletion promotes regrowth of corticospinal tract axons 1 year after spinal cord injury. J Neurosci. 2015;35:9754–63.
86. Duan Y, Giger RJ. A new role for RPTPsigma in spinal cord injury: signaling chondroitin sulfate proteoglycan inhibition. Sci Signal. 2010;3:pe6.
87. Dy CJ, Gerasimenko YP, Edgerton VR, Dyhre-Poulsen P, Courtine G, Harkema SJ. Phase-dependent modulation of percutaneously elicited multisegmental muscle responses after spinal cord injury. J Neurophysiol. 2010;103:2808–20.
88. Dyck SM, Alizadeh A, Santhosh KT, Proulx EH, Wu CL, Karimi-Abdolrezaee S. Chondroitin sulfate proteoglycans negatively modulate spinal cord neural precursor cells by signaling through LAR and RPTPsigma and modulation of the Rho/ROCK pathway. Stem Cells. 2015;33:2550–63.
89. Ebner FF, Erzurumlu RS, Lee SM. Peripheral nerve damage facilitates functional innervation of brain grafts in adult sensory cortex. Proc Natl Acad Sci U S A. 1989;86:730–4.
90. Edgerton VR, Harkema S. Epidural stimulation of the spinal cord in spinal cord injury: current status and future challenges. Expert Rev Neurother. 2011;11:1351–3.
91. Eichhorst H, Naunyn B. Ueber die Regeneration und Veränderungen im Rückenmarke nach streckenweiser totaler Zerstörung desslben. Naunyn Schmiedebergs Arch Exp Pathol Pharmakol. 1874;2:225–53.
92. Elzinga K, Tyreman N, Ladak A, Savaryn B, Olson J, Gordon T. Brief electrical stimulation improves nerve regeneration after delayed repair in Sprague Dawley rats. Exp Neurol. 2015;269:142–53.
93. Esmaeili M, Berry M, Logan A, Ahmed Z. Decorin treatment of spinal cord injury. Neural Regen Res. 2014;9:1653–6.
94. Fakhoury M. Spinal cord injury: overview of experimental approaches used to restore locomotor activity. Rev Neurosci. 2015;26:397–405.
95. Fallon JR. Neurite guidance by non-neuronal cells in culture: preferential outgrowth of peripheral neurites on glial as compared to nonglial cell surfaces. J Neurosci. 1985;5:3169–77.
96. Fawcett JW. The extracellular matrix in plasticity and regeneration after CNS injury and neurodegenerative disease. Prog Brain Res. 2015;218:213–26.
97. Filous AR, Miller JH, Coulson-Thomas YM, Horn KP, Alilain WJ, Silver J. Immature astrocytes promote CNS axonal regeneration when combined with chondroitinase ABC. Dev Neurobiol. 2010;70:826–41.
98. Fontoura P, Ho PP, DeVoss J, Zheng B, Lee BJ, Kidd BA, Garren H, Sobel RA, Robinson WH, Tessier-Lavigne M, Steinman L. Immunity to the extracellular domain of Nogo-A modulates experimental autoimmune encephalomyelitis. J Immunol. 2004;173:6981–92.
99. Fouad K, Schnell L, Bunge MB, Schwab ME, Liebscher T, Pearse DD. Combining Schwann cell bridges and olfactory-ensheathing glia grafts with chondroitinase promotes locomotor recovery after complete transection of the spinal cord. J Neurosci. 2005;25:1169–78.
100. Fournier AE, Gould GC, Liu BP, Strittmatter SM. Truncated soluble Nogo receptor binds Nogo-66 and blocks inhibition of axon growth by myelin. J Neurosci. 2002;22:8876–83.
101. Fournier AE, Takizawa BT, Strittmatter SM. Rho kinase inhibition enhances axonal regeneration in the injured CNS. J Neurosci. 2003;23:1416–23.
102. Frank M, Schaeren-Wiemers N, Schneider R, Schwab ME. Developmental expression pattern of the myelin proteolipid MAL indicates different functions of MAL for immature Schwann cells and in a late step of CNS myelinogenesis. J Neurochem. 1999;73:587–97.
103. Frisen J, Haegerstrand A, Fried K, Piehl F, Cullheim S, Risling M. Adhesive/repulsive properties in the injured spinal cord: relation to myelin phagocytosis by invading macrophages. Exp Neurol. 1994;129:183–93.
104. Fry EJ, Chagnon MJ, Lopez-Vales R, Tremblay ML, David S. Corticospinal tract regeneration after spinal cord injury in receptor protein tyrosine phosphatase sigma deficient mice. Glia. 2010;58:423–33.
105. Fu R, Tang Y, Ling ZM, Li YQ, Cheng X, Song FH, Zhou LH, Wu W. Lithium enhances survival and regrowth of spinal motoneurons after ventral root avulsion. BMC Neurosci. 2014;15:84.
106. Fuss B, Pott U, Fischer P, Schwab ME, Schachner M. Identification of a cDNA clone specific for the oligodendrocyte-derived repulsive extracellular matrix molecule J1-160/180. J Neurosci Res. 1991;29:299–307.
107. Garcia-Alias G, Barkhuysen S, Buckle M, Fawcett JW. Chondroitinase ABC treatment opens a window of opportunity for task-specific rehabilitation. Nat Neurosci. 2009;12:1145–51.
108. Garcia-Alias G, Truong K, Shah PK, Roy RR, Edgerton VR. Plasticity of subcortical pathways promote recovery of skilled hand function in rats after corticospinal and rubrospinal tract injuries. Exp Neurol. 2015;266:112–9.
109. Gates MA, Fillmore H, Steindler DA. Chondroitin sulfate proteoglycan and tenascin in the wounded adult mouse neostriatum in vitro: dopamine neuron attachment and process outgrowth. J Neurosci. 1996;16:8005–18.
110. Gattuso JM, Glasby MA, Gschmeissner SE, Norris RW. A comparison of immediate and delayed repair of peripheral nerves using freeze-thawed autologous skeletal muscle grafts – in the rat. Br J Plast Surg. 1989;42:306–13.
111. George SC, Boyce DE. An evidence-based structured review to assess the results of common peroneal nerve repair. Plast Reconstr Surg. 2014;134:302e–11.
112. Giulian D, Li J, Li X, George J, Rutecki PA. The impact of microglia-derived cytokines upon gliosis in the CNS. Dev Neurosci. 1994;16:128–36.

113. Goldshmit Y, Frisca F, Pinto AR, Pebay A, Tang JK, Siegel AL, Kaslin J, Currie PD. Fgf2 improves functional recovery-decreasing gliosis and increasing radial glia and neural progenitor cells after spinal cord injury. Brain Behav. 2014;4:187–200.

114. Gonzenbach RR, Zoerner B, Schnell L, Weinmann O, Mir AK, Schwab ME. Delayed anti-nogo-a antibody application after spinal cord injury shows progressive loss of responsiveness. J Neurotrauma. 2012;29:567–78.

115. GrandPre T, Nakamura F, Vartanian T, Strittmatter SM. Identification of the Nogo inhibitor of axon regeneration as a Reticulon protein. Nature. 2000;403:439–44.

116. Grimpe B, Silver J. A novel DNA enzyme reduces glycosaminoglycan chains in the glial scar and allows microtransplanted dorsal root ganglia axons to regenerate beyond lesions in the spinal cord. J Neurosci. 2004;24:1393–7.

117. Guest JD, Hesse D, Schnell L, Schwab ME, Bunge MB, Bunge RP. Influence of IN-1 antibody and acidic FGF-fibrin glue on the response of injured corticospinal tract axons to human Schwann cell grafts. J Neurosci Res. 1997;50:888–905.

118. Guest JD, Rao A, Olson L, Bunge MB, Bunge RP. The ability of human Schwann cell grafts to promote regeneration in the transected nude rat spinal cord. Exp Neurol. 1997;148:502–22.

119. Guth L, Albuquerque EX, Deshpande SS, Barrett CP, Donati EJ, Warnick JE. Ineffectiveness of enzyme therapy on regeneration in the transected spinal cord of the rat. J Neurosurg. 1980;52:73–86.

120. Guth L, Barrett CP, Donati EJ, Deshpande SS, Albuquerque EX. Histopathological reactions and axonal regeneration in the transected spinal cord of Hibernating squirrels. J Comp Neurol. 1981;203:297–308.

121. Guth L, Barrett CP, Donati EJ, Anderson FD, Smith MV, Lifson M. Essentiality of a specific cellular terrain for growth of axons into a spinal cord lesion. Exp Neurol. 1985;88:1–12.

122. Gutmann E, Guttmann L, Medawar PB, Young JZ. The rate of regeneration of nerve. J Exp Biol. 1942;19:14–44.

123. Hall S, Berry M. Electron microscopic study of the interaction of axons and glia at the site of anastomosis between the optic nerve and cellular or acellular sciatic nerve grafts. J Neurocytol. 1989;18:171–84.

124. Han N, Xu CG, Wang TB, Kou YH, Yin XF, Zhang PX, Xue F. Electrical stimulation does not enhance nerve regeneration if delayed after sciatic nerve injury: the role of fibrosis. Neural Regen Res. 2015;10:90–4.

125. Hanada M, Tsutsumi K, Arima H, Shinjo R, Sugiura Y, Imagama S, Ishiguro N, Matsuyama Y. Evaluation of the effect of tranilast on rats with spinal cord injury. J Neurol Sci. 2014;346:209–15.

126. Hanell A, Clausen F, Bjork M, Jansson K, Philipson O, Nilsson LN, Hillered L, Weinreb PH, Lee D,

McIntosh TK, Gimbel DA, Strittmatter SM, Marklund N. Genetic deletion and pharmacological inhibition of Nogo-66 receptor impairs cognitive outcome after traumatic brain injury in mice. J Neurotrauma. 2010;27:1297–309.

127. Harkema SJ. Plasticity of interneuronal networks of the functionally isolated human spinal cord. Brain Res Rev. 2008;57:255–64.

128. Harkema S, Gerasimenko Y, Hodes J, Burdick J, Angeli C, Chen Y, Ferreira C, Willhite A, Rejc E, Grossman RG, Edgerton VR. Effect of epidural stimulation of the lumbosacral spinal cord on voluntary movement, standing, and assisted stepping after motor complete paraplegia: a case study. Lancet. 2011;377:1938–47.

129. Harkema S, Behrman A, Barbeau H. Evidence-based therapy for recovery of function after spinal cord injury. Handb Clin Neurol. 2012;109:259–74.

130. Hendel A, Bak RO, Clark JT, Kennedy AB, Ryan DE, Roy S, Steinfeld I, Lunstad BD, Kaiser RJ, Wilkens AB, Bacchetta R, Tsalenko A, Dellinger D, Bruhn L, Porteus MH. Chemically modified guide RNAs enhance CRISPR-Cas genome editing in human primary cells. Nat Biotechnol. 2015;33(9):985–9.

131. Hermanns S, Reiprich P, Muller HW. A reliable method to reduce collagen scar formation in the lesioned rat spinal cord. J Neurosci Methods. 2001;110:141–6.

132. Hill CE, Beattie MS, Bresnahan JC. Degeneration and sprouting of identified descending supraspinal axons after contusive spinal cord injury in the rat. Exp Neurol. 2001;171:153–69.

133. Hinckley CA, Alaynick WA, Gallarda BW, Hayashi M, Hilde KL, Driscoll SP, Dekker JD, Tucker HO, Sharpee TO, Pfaff SL. Spinal locomotor circuits develop using hierarchical rules based on motorneuron position and identity. Neuron. 2015;87:1008–21.

134. Hoffman-Kim D, Mitchel JA, Bellamkonda RV. Topography, cell response, and nerve regeneration. Annu Rev Biomed Eng. 2010;12:203–31.

135. Holst HI. Primary peripheral nerve repair in the hand and upper extremity. J Trauma. 1975;15:909–11.

136. Holz A, Frank M, Copeland NG, Gilbert DJ, Jenkins NA, Schwab ME. Chromosomal localization of the myelin-associated oligodendrocytic basic protein and expression in the genetically linked neurological mouse mutants ducky and tippy. J Neurochem. 1997;69:1801–9.

137. Holz A, Schwab ME. Developmental expression of the myelin gene MOBP in the rat nervous system. J Neurocytol. 1997;26:467–77.

138. Hooker D. Studies on regeneration in the spinal cord. III. Reestablishment of anatomical and physiological continuity after transection in frog tadpoles. J Comp Neurol (Philadelphia). 1925;38:315–47; p [1 v.].

139. Hooker D. Spinal-cord regeneration in the young rainbow fish, Lebistes reticulatus. Jour Comp Neur (Philadelphia). 1932;56(Hooker D):277–97. p [1 v.].

140. Horner PJ, Gage FH. Regenerating the damaged central nervous system. Nature. 2000;407:963–70.

141. Hossain-Ibrahim MK, Rezajooi K, Stallcup WB, Lieberman AR, Anderson PN. Analysis of axonal regeneration in the central and peripheral nervous systems of the NG2-deficient mouse. BMC Neurosci. 2007;8:80.

142. Houle JD, Reier PJ. Transplantation of fetal spinal cord tissue into the chronically injured adult rat spinal cord. J Comp Neurol. 1988;269:535–47.

143. Huber AB, Schwab ME. Nogo-A, a potent inhibitor of neurite outgrowth and regeneration. Biol Chem. 2000;381:407–19.

144. Hudson AR, Hunter D. Timing of peripheral nerve repair: important local neuropathological factors. Clin Neurosurg. 1977;24:391–405.

145. Hunanyan AS, Petrosyan HA, Alessi V, Arvanian VL. Combination of chondroitinase ABC and AAV-NT3 promotes neural plasticity at descending spinal pathways after thoracic contusion in rats. J Neurophysiol. 2013;110:1782–92.

146. Hunt D, Mason MR, Campbell G, Coffin R, Anderson PN. Nogo receptor mRNA expression in intact and regenerating CNS neurons. Mol Cell Neurosci. 2002;20:537–52.

147. Hunt D, Coffin RS, Anderson PN. The Nogo receptor, its ligands and axonal regeneration in the spinal cord; a review. J Neurocytol. 2002;31:93–120.

148. Hunt D, Coffin RS, Prinjha RK, Campbell G, Anderson PN. Nogo-A expression in the intact and injured nervous system. Mol Cell Neurosci. 2003;24:1083–102.

149. IJpma FF, Van De Graaf RC, Meek MF. The early history of tubulation in nerve repair. J Hand Surg Eur Vol. 2008;33:581–6.

150. Ishikawa Y, Imagama S, Ohgomori T, Ishiguro N, Kadomatsu K. A combination of keratan sulfate digestion and rehabilitation promotes anatomical plasticity after rat spinal cord injury. Neurosci Lett. 2015;593:13–8.

151. Ito Z, Sakamoto K, Imagama S, Matsuyama Y, Zhang H, Hirano K, Ando K, Yamashita T, Ishiguro N, Kadomatsu K. N-acetylglucosamine 6-O-sulfotransferase-1-deficient mice show better functional recovery after spinal cord injury. J Neurosci. 2010;30:5937–47.

152. Jahan N, Hannila SS. Transforming growth factor beta-induced expression of chondroitin sulfate proteoglycans is mediated through non-Smad signaling pathways. Exp Neurol. 2015;263:372–84.

153. Jenq CB, Jenq LL, Bear HM, Coggeshall RE. Conditioning lesions of peripheral nerves change regenerated axon numbers. Brain Res. 1988;457: 63–9.

154. Jin WL, Liu YY, Liu HL, Yang H, Wang Y, Jiao XY, Ju G. Intraneuronal localization of Nogo-A in the rat. J Comp Neurol. 2003;458:1–10.

155. Jinek M, Chylinski K, Fonfara I, Hauer M, Doudna JA, Charpentier E. A programmable dual-RNA-guided DNA endonuclease in adaptive bacterial immunity. Science. 2012;337:816–21.

156. Johansson CB, Momma S, Clarke DL, Risling M, Lendahl U, Frisen J. Identification of a neural stem cell in the adult mammalian central nervous system. Cell. 1999;96:25–34.

157. Jones LL, Yamaguchi Y, Stallcup WB, Tuszynski MH. NG2 is a major chondroitin sulfate proteoglycan produced after spinal cord injury and is expressed by macrophages and oligodendrocyte progenitors. J Neurosci. 2002;22:2792–803.

158. Jones LL, Sajed D, Tuszynski MH. Axonal regeneration through regions of chondroitin sulfate proteoglycan deposition after spinal cord injury: a balance of permissiveness and inhibition. J Neurosci. 2003;23:9276–88.

159. Jonsson S, Wiberg R, McGrath AM, Novikov LN, Wiberg M, Novikova LN, Kingham PJ. Effect of delayed peripheral nerve repair on nerve regeneration. Schwann cell function and target muscle recovery. PLoS ONE. 2013;8:e56484.

160. Josephson A, Trifunovski A, Scheele C, Widenfalk J, Wahlestedt C, Brene S, Olson L, Spenger C. Activity-induced and developmental downregulation of the Nogo receptor. Cell Tissue Res. 2003;311:333–42.

161. Joy MT, Vrbova G, Dhoot GK, Anderson PN. Sulf1 and Sulf2 expression in the nervous system and its role in limiting neurite outgrowth in vitro. Exp Neurol. 2015;263:150–60.

162. Kaku M. Physics of the impossible: a scientific exploration into the world of phasers, force fields, teleportation, and time travel. 1st ed. New York: Doubleday; 2008.

163. Kalbermatten DF, Kingham PJ, Mahay D, Mantovani C, Pettersson J, Raffoul W, Balcin H, Pierer G, Terenghi G. Fibrin matrix for suspension of regenerative cells in an artificial nerve conduit. J Plast Reconstr Aesthet Surg. 2008;61:669–75.

164. Kallioinen MJ, Heikkinen ER, Nystrom S. Histopathological and immunohistochemical changes in neurosurgically resected epileptic foci. Acta Neurochir (Wien). 1987;89:122–9.

165. Kaneko A, Matsushita A, Sankai Y. A 3D nanofibrous hydrogel and collagen sponge scaffold promotes locomotor functional recovery, spinal repair, and neuronal regeneration after complete transection of the spinal cord in adult rats. Biomed Mater. 2015;10(1):015008.

166. Kanno H, Pressman Y, Moody A, Berg R, Muir EM, Rogers JH, Ozawa H, Itoi E, Pearse DD, Bunge MB. Combination of engineered schwann cell grafts to secrete neurotrophin and chondroitinase promotes axonal regeneration and locomotion after spinal cord injury. J Neurosci. 2014;34:1838–55.

167. Kaplan HM, Mishra P, Kohn J. The overwhelming use of rat models in nerve regeneration research may compromise designs of nerve guidance conduits for humans. J Mater Sci Mater Med. 2015; 26(8):226.

168. Karimi-Abdolrezaee S, Eftekharpour E, Wang J, Schut D, Fehlings MG. Synergistic effects of transplanted adult neural stem/progenitor cells, chondroitinase, and growth factors promote functional repair and plasticity of the chronically injured spinal cord. J Neurosci. 2010;30:1657–76.

169. Karimi-Abdolrezaee S, Schut D, Wang J, Fehlings MG. Chondroitinase and growth factors enhance activation and oligodendrocyte differentiation of endogenous neural precursor cells after spinal cord injury. PLoS One. 2012;7:e37589.

170. Kartje GL, Schulz MK, Lopez-Yunez A, Schnell L, Schwab ME. Corticostriatal plasticity is restricted by myelin-associated neurite growth inhibitors in the adult rat. Ann Neurol. 1999;45:778–86.

171. Kim JE, Bonilla IE, Qiu D, Strittmatter SM. Nogo-C is sufficient to delay nerve regeneration. Mol Cell Neurosci. 2003;23:451–9.

172. Kim JE, Li S, GrandPre T, Qiu D, Strittmatter SM. Axon regeneration in young adult mice lacking Nogo-A/B. Neuron. 2003;38:187–99.

173. Klapka N, Hermanns S, Straten G, Masanneck C, Duis S, Hamers FP, Muller D, Zuschratter W, Muller HW. Suppression of fibrous scarring in spinal cord injury of rat promotes long-distance regeneration of corticospinal tract axons, rescue of primary motoneurons in somatosensory cortex and significant functional recovery. Eur J Neurosci. 2005;22:3047–58.

174. Kline DG, Hackett ER. Reappraisal of timing for exploration of civilian peripheral nerve injuries. Surgery. 1975;78:54–65.

175. Knikou M, Angeli CA, Ferreira CK, Harkema SJ. Flexion reflex modulation during stepping in human spinal cord injury. Exp Brain Res. 2009;196:341–51.

176. Knikou M, Angeli CA, Ferreira CK, Harkema SJ. Soleus H-reflex modulation during body weight support treadmill walking in spinal cord intact and injured subjects. Exp Brain Res. 2009;193:397–407.

177. Kose N, Muezzinoglu O, Bilgin S, Karahan S, Isikay I, Bilginer B. Early rehabilitation improves neurofunctional outcome after surgery in children with spinal tumors. Neural Regen Res. 2014;9:129–34.

178. Krautstrunk M, Scholtes F, Martin D, Schoenen J, Schmitt AB, Plate D, Nacimiento W, Noth J, Brook GA. Increased expression of the putative axon growth-repulsive extracellular matrix molecule, keratan sulphate proteoglycan, following traumatic injury of the adult rat spinal cord. Acta Neuropathol. 2002;104:592–600.

179. Kuiken TA, Dumanian GA, Lipschutz RD, Miller LA, Stubblefield KA. The use of targeted muscle reinnervation for improved myoelectric prosthesis control in a bilateral shoulder disarticulation amputee. Prosthet Orthot Int. 2004;28:245–53.

180. Kuiken TA, Miller LA, Lipschutz RD, Lock BA, Stubblefield K, Marasco PD, Zhou P, Dumanian GA. Targeted reinnervation for enhanced prosthetic arm function in a woman with a proximal amputation: a case study. Lancet. 2007;369:371–80.

181. Kumar P, Choonara YE, Modi G, Naidoo D, Pillay V. Multifunctional therapeutic delivery strategies for effective neuro-regeneration following traumatic spinal cord injury. Curr Pharm Des. 2015;21:1517–28.

182. Lang DM, Rubin BP, Schwab ME, Stuermer CA. CNS myelin and oligodendrocytes of the Xenopus spinal cord – but not optic nerve – are nonpermissive for axon growth. J Neurosci. 1995;15:99–109.

183. Lang BT, Cregg JM, DePaul MA, Tran AP, Xu K, Dyck SM, Madalena KM, Brown BP, Weng YL, Li S, Karimi-Abdolrezaee S, Busch SA, Shen Y, Silver J. Modulation of the proteoglycan receptor PTPsigma promotes recovery after spinal cord injury. Nature. 2015;518:404–8.

184. Lankford KL, Waxman SG, Kocsis JD. Mechanisms of enhancement of neurite regeneration in vitro following a conditioning sciatic nerve lesion. J Comp Neurol. 1998;391:11–29.

185. Lau LW, Keough MB, Haylock-Jacobs S, Cua R, Doring A, Sloka S, Stirling DP, Rivest S, Yong VW. Chondroitin sulfate proteoglycans in demyelinated lesions impair remyelination. Ann Neurol. 2012;72:419–32.

186. Lauren J, Airaksinen MS, Saarma M, Timmusk T. Two novel mammalian Nogo receptor homologs differentially expressed in the central and peripheral nervous systems. Mol Cell Neurosci. 2003;24:581–94.

187. Lazar DA, Ellegala DB, Avellino AM, Dailey AT, Andrus K, Kliot M. Modulation of macrophage and microglial responses to axonal injury in the peripheral and central nervous systems. Neurosurgery. 1999;45:593–600.

188. Ledford H. CRISPR, the disruptor. News feature. Nature. 2015;522:20–4.

189. Lee H, McKeon RJ, Bellamkonda RV. Sustained delivery of thermostabilized chABC enhances axonal sprouting and functional recovery after spinal cord injury. Proc Natl Acad Sci U S A. 2010;107:3340–5.

190. Lee JK, Geoffroy CG, Chan AF, Tolentino KE, Crawford MJ, Leal MA, Kang B, Zheng B. Assessing spinal axon regeneration and sprouting in Nogo-, MAG-, and OMgp-deficient mice. Neuron. 2010;66:663–70.

191. Levine JM. Increased expression of the NG2 chondroitin-sulfate proteoglycan after brain injury. J Neurosci. 1994;14:4716–30.

192. Lewis PM, Ackland HM, Lowery AJ, Rosenfeld JV. Restoration of vision in blind individuals using bionic devices: a review with a focus on cortical visual prostheses. Brain Res. 2015;1595:51–73.

193. Li S, Strittmatter SM. Delayed systemic Nogo-66 receptor antagonist promotes recovery from spinal cord injury. J Neurosci. 2003;23:4219–27.

194. Li SX, Kim JE, Liu BP, Li MW, Ji BX, Pepinsky B, Relton J, Strittmatter SM. Inhibition of Nogo-66 receptor with its soluble ectodomain promotes axonal regeneration and functional recovery after spinal cord injury. J Neurotrauma. 2003;20:1057.

195. Li ZW, Li JJ, Wang L, Zhang JP, Wu JJ, Mao XQ, Shi GF, Wang Q, Wang F, Zou J. Epidermal growth factor receptor inhibitor ameliorates excessive astrogliosis and improves the regeneration microenvironment and functional recovery in adult rats following spinal cord injury. J Neuroinflammation. 2014;11:71.

196. Liebscher T, Schnell L, Schnell D, Scholl J, Schneider R, Gullo M, Fouad K, Mir A, Rausch M, Kindler D, Hamers FP, Schwab ME. Nogo-A antibody improves regeneration and locomotion of spinal cord-injured rats. Ann Neurol. 2005;58:706–19.

197. Liu Y, Himes BT, Moul J, Huang W, Chow SY, Tessler A, Fischer I. Application of recombinant adenovirus for in vivo gene delivery to spinal cord. Brain Res. 1997;768:19–29.

198. Liu S, Peulve P, Jin O, Boisset N, Tiollier J, Said G, Tadie M. Axonal regrowth through collagen tubes bridging the spinal cord to nerve roots. J Neurosci Res. 1997;49:425–32.

199. Liu YY, Jin WL, Liu HL, Ju G. Electron microscopic localization of Nogo-A at the postsynaptic active zone of the rat. Neurosci Lett. 2003;346:153–6.

200. Liu K, Lu Y, Lee JK, Samara R, Willenberg R, Sears-Kraxberger I, Tedeschi A, Park KK, Jin D, Cai B, Xu B, Connolly L, Steward O, Zheng B, He Z. PTEN deletion enhances the regenerative ability of adult corticospinal neurons. Nat Neurosci. 2010;13:1075–81.

201. Loeb GE. We made the deaf hear. Now what? In: Berger TW, Glanzman DL, editors. Toward replacement parts for the brain: implantable biomimetic electronics as neural prostheses. Cambridge: MIT Press; 2005. p. 3–13.

202. Loeb GE. Neuroprosthetic interfaces – The reality behind bionics and cyborgs. In: Schleidgen S, Jungert M, Bauer R, Sandow V, editors. Human nature and self-design. Paderborn, Germany: Mentis Verlag GmbH; 2011.

203. Loeb GE, Zhou L, Zheng K, Nicholson A, Peck RA, Krishnan A, Silka M, Pruetz J, Chmait R, Bar-Cohen Y. Design and testing of a percutaneously implantable fetal pacemaker. Ann Biomed Eng. 2013;41:17–27.

204. de Nó Lorente R. La regeneración de la medula espinal en las larvas de batracio. Trab Lab Invest Biol Univ Madrid. 1921;19:147–83.

205. Lu P, Jones LL, Tuszynski MH. Axon regeneration through scars and into sites of chronic spinal cord injury. Exp Neurol. 2007;203:8–21.

206. Lu P, Tuszynski MH. Growth factors and combinatorial therapies for CNS regeneration. Exp Neurol. 2008;209:313–20.

207. Lu P, Wang Y, Graham L, McHale K, Gao M, Wu D, Brock J, Blesch A, Rosenzweig ES, Havton LA, Zheng B, Conner JM, Marsala M, Tuszynski MH. Long-distance growth and connectivity of neural stem cells after severe spinal cord injury. Cell. 2012;150:1264–73.

208. Lu P, Blesch A, Graham L, Wang Y, Samara R, Banos K, Haringer V, Havton L, Weishaupt N, Bennett D, Fouad K, Tuszynski MH. Motor axonal regeneration after partial and complete spinal cord transection. J Neurosci. 2012;32:8208–18.

209. Lu P, Woodruff G, Wang Y, Graham L, Hunt M, Wu D, Boehle E, Ahmad R, Poplawski G, Brock J, Goldstein LS, Tuszynski MH. Long-distance axonal growth from human induced pluripotent stem cells after spinal cord injury. Neuron. 2014;83:789–96.

210. MacCreight J. The regeneration of the spinal cord in adult Triturus viridescens. Univ Pittsburgh Bull. 1931;28:7.

211. Maier IC, Ichiyama RM, Courtine G, Schnell L, Lavrov I, Edgerton VR, Schwab ME. Differential effects of anti-Nogo-A antibody treatment and treadmill training in rats with incomplete spinal cord injury. Brain. 2009;132:1426–40.

212. Mansour H, Asher R, Dahl D, Labkovsky B, Perides G, Bignami A. Permissive and non-permissive reactive astrocytes: immunofluorescence study with antibodies to the glial hyaluronate-binding protein. J Neurosci Res. 1990;25:300–11.

213. Markets and Markets Report. Nerve repair & regeneration market by xenografts (conduits, protectors), neuromodulation [internal (spinal cord, deep brain), external (transcranial magnetic)], surgery [direct nerve repair, grafting, stem cell] – Global trend & forecast to 2018. By: marketsandmarkets.com. Report Code: BT 2105. Sep 2013.

214. Matsui F, Oohira A. Proteoglycans and injury of the central nervous system. Congenit Anom (Kyoto). 2004;44:181–8.

215. Matthews MA, St Onge MF, Faciane CL, Gelderd JB. Axon sprouting into segments of rat spinal cord adjacent to the site of a previous transection. Neuropathol Appl Neurobiol. 1979;5:181–96.

216. McAllister RM, Gilbert SE, Calder JS, Smith PJ. The epidemiology and management of upper limb peripheral nerve injuries in modern practice. J Hand Surg Br. 1996;21:4–13.

217. McEvoy RC, Leung PE. Transplantation of fetal rat islets into the cerebral ventricles of alloxan-diabetic rats. Amelioration of diabetes by syngeneic but not allogeneic islets. Diabetes. 1983;32:852–7.

218. McGee AW, Strittmatter SM. The Nogo-66 receptor: focusing myelin inhibition of axon regeneration. Trends Neurosci. 2003;26:193–8.

219. McKay WB, Ovechkin AV, Vitaz TW, Terson de Paleville DG, Harkema SJ. Long-lasting involuntary motor activity after spinal cord injury. Spinal Cord. 2011;49:87–93.

220. McKeon RJ, Schreiber RC, Rudge JS, Silver J. Reduction of neurite outgrowth in a model of glial scarring following CNS injury is correlated with the expression of inhibitory molecules on reactive astrocytes. J Neurosci. 1991;11:3398–411.

221. Mehta NR, Lopez PH, Vyas AA, Schnaar RL. Gangliosides and Nogo receptors independently mediate myelin-associated glycoprotein inhibition of neurite outgrowth in different nerve cells. J Biol Chem. 2007;282:27875–86.

222. Meier S, Brauer AU, Heimrich B, Schwab ME, Nitsch R, Savaskan NE. Molecular analysis of Nogo expression in the hippocampus during development and following lesion and seizure. FASEB J. 2003;17:1153–5.

223. Merzenich MM, Kaas JH, Wall J, Nelson RJ, Sur M, Felleman D. Topographic reorganization of somatosensory cortical areas 3B and 1 in adult monkeys following restricted deafferentation. Neuroscience. 1983;8:33–55.

224. Miao QL, Ye Q, Zhang XH. Perineuronal net, CSPG receptor and their regulation of neural plasticity. Sheng Li Xue Bao. 2014;66:387–97.

225. Midha R, Munro CA, Chan S, Nitising A, Xu QG, Gordon T. Regeneration into protected and chronically denervated peripheral nerve stumps. Neurosurgery. 2005;57:1289–99.

226. Milbreta U, von Boxberg Y, Mailly P, Nothias F, Soares S. Astrocytic and vascular remodeling in the injured adult rat spinal cord after chondroitinase ABC treatment. J Neurotrauma. 2014;31:803–18.

227. Miller S, Scott PD. A model of the spinal locomotor generator in the cat [proceedings]. J Physiol. 1977;269:20P–2.

228. Miller S, Scott PD. The spinal locomotor generator. Exp Brain Res. 1977;30:387–403.

229. Ming GL, Song HJ, Berninger B, Holt CE, Tessier-Lavigne M, Poo MM. cAMP-dependent growth cone guidance by netrin-1. Neuron. 1997;19:1225–35.

230. Mohney G. Doctor aims to perform head transplant in 2017, Experts remain skeptical. ABC News post. 2015. Retrieved Dec 22, 2015, from: http://abcnews.go.com/Health/doctor-aims-perform-head-transplant-2017-experts-remain/story?id=33775323.

231. Mohseni MA, Pour JS, Pour JG. Primary and delayed repair and nerve grafting for treatment of cut median and ulnar nerves. Pak J Biol Sci. 2010;13:287–92.

232. Mondello SE, Jefferson SC, Tester NJ, Howland DR. Impact of treatment duration and lesion size on effectiveness of chondroitinase treatment post-SCI. Exp Neurol. 2015;267:64–77.

233. Mullner A, Gonzenbach RR, Weinmann O, Schnell L, Liebscher T, Schwab ME. Lamina-specific restoration of serotonergic projections after Nogo-A antibody treatment of spinal cord injury in rats. Eur J Neurosci. 2008;27:326–33.

234. Nakamae T, Tanaka N, Nakanishi K, Kamei N, Sasaki H, Hamasaki T, Yamada K, Yamamoto R, Mochizuki Y, Ochi M. Chondroitinase ABC promotes corticospinal axon growth in organotypic cocultures. Spinal Cord. 2009;47:161–5.

235. Nakamae T, Tanaka N, Nakanishi K, Kamei N, Sasaki H, Hamasaki T, Yamada K, Yamamoto R, Izumi B, Ochi M. The effects of combining chondroitinase ABC and NEP1-40 on the corticospinal axon growth in organotypic co-cultures. Neurosci Lett. 2010;476:14–7.

236. Neumann S, Woolf CJ. Regeneration of dorsal column fibers into and beyond the lesion site following adult spinal cord injury. Neuron. 1999;23:83–91.

237. Neumann S, Bradke F, Tessier-Lavigne M, Basbaum AI. Regeneration of sensory axons within the injured spinal cord induced by intraganglionic cAMP elevation. Neuron. 2002;34:885–93.

238. Neumann S, Skinner K, Basbaum AI. Sustaining intrinsic growth capacity of adult neurons promotes spinal cord regeneration. Proc Natl Acad Sci U S A. 2005;102:16848–52.

239. Nghiem BT, Sando IC, Gillespie RB, McLaughlin BL, Gerling GJ, Langhals NB, Urbanchek MG, Cederna PS. Providing a sense of touch to prosthetic hands. Plast Reconstr Surg. 2015;135:1652–63.

240. Nie DY, Zhou ZH, Ang BT, Teng FY, Xu G, Xiang T, Wang CY, Zeng L, Takeda Y, Xu TL, Ng YK, Faivre-Sarrailh C, Popko B, Ling EA, Schachner M, Watanabe K, Pallen CJ, Tang BL, Xiao ZC. Nogo-A at CNS paranodes is a ligand of Caspr: possible regulation of K(+) channel localization. EMBO J. 2003;22:5666–78.

241. Niederost BP, Zimmermann DR, Schwab ME, Bandtlow CE. Bovine CNS myelin contains neurite growth-inhibitory activity associated with chondroitin sulfate proteoglycans. J Neurosci. 1999;19:8979–89.

242. Novikova L, Novikov L, Kellerth JO. Effects of neurotransplants and BDNF on the survival and regeneration of injured adult spinal motoneurons. Eur J Neurosci. 1997;9:2774–7.

243. Oblinger MM, Lasek RJ. A conditioning lesion of the peripheral axons of dorsal root ganglion cells accelerates regeneration of only their peripheral axons. J Neurosci. 1984;4:1736–44.

244. Oertle T, van der Haar ME, Bandtlow CE, Robeva A, Burfeind P, Buss A, Huber AB, Simonen M, Schnell L, Brosamle C, Kaupmann K, Vallon R, Schwab ME. Nogo-A inhibits neurite outgrowth and cell spreading with three discrete regions. J Neurosci. 2003;23:5393–406.

245. Orlando C, Raineteau O. Integrity of cortical perineuronal nets influences corticospinal tract plasticity after spinal cord injury. Brain Struct Funct. 2015;220(2):1077–91.

246. Orlando C, Raineteau O. Integrity of cortical perineuronal nets influences corticospinal tract plasticity after spinal cord injury. Brain Struct Funct. 2015;220:1077–91.

247. Oudega M, Xu XM, Guenard V, Kleitman N, Bunge MB. A combination of insulin-like growth factor-I and platelet-derived growth factor enhances myelination but diminishes axonal regeneration into Schwann cell grafts in the adult rat spinal cord. Glia. 1997;19:247–58.

248. Pabari A, Lloyd-Hughes H, Seifalian AM, Mosahebi A. Nerve conduits for peripheral nerve surgery. Plast Reconstr Surg. 2014;133:1420–30.

249. Pei Y, Dong S, Roth BL. Generation of designer receptors exclusively activated by designer drugs (DREADDs) using directed molecular evolution. Curr Protoc Neurosci. 2010;Chapter 4:Unit 4.33.

250. Pellegrino RG, Spencer PS. Schwann cell mitosis in response to regenerating peripheral axons in vivo. Brain Res. 1985;341:16–25.

251. Pettersson J, Kalbermatten D, Mcgrath A, Novikova LN. Biodegradable fibrin conduit promotes long-term regeneration after peripheral nerve injury in adult rats. J Plast Reconstr Aesthet Surg. 2010;63:1893–9.

252. Pignot V, Hein AE, Barske C, Wiessner C, Walmsley AR, Kaupmann K, Mayeur H, Sommer B, Mir AK, Frentzel S. Characterization of two novel proteins, NgRH1 and NgRH2, structurally and biochemically homologous to the Nogo-66 receptor. J Neurochem. 2003;85:717–28.

253. Piskin A, Altunkaynak BZ, Citlak A, Sezgin H, Yaziotaciota O, Kaplan S. Immediate versus delayed primary nerve repair in the rabbit sciatic nerve. Neural Regen Res. 2013;8:3410–5.

254. Possover M. Recovery of sensory and supraspinal control of leg movement in people with chronic paraplegia: a case series. Arch Phys Med Rehabil. 2014;95:610–4.

255. Pot C, Simonen M, Weinmann O, Schnell L, Christ F, Stoeckle S, Berger P, Rulicke T, Suter U, Schwab ME. Nogo-A expressed in Schwann cells impairs axonal regeneration after peripheral nerve injury. J Cell Biol. 2002;159:29–35.

256. Prendergast J, Stelzner DJ. Increases in collateral axonal growth rostral to a thoracic hemisection in neonatal and weanling rat. J Comp Neurol. 1976;166:145–61.

257. Prendergast J, Stelzner DJ. Changes in the magnocellular portion of the red nucleus following thoracic hemisection in the neonatal and adult rat. J Comp Neurol. 1976;166:163–71.

258. Qi B, Qi Y, Watari A, Yoshioka N, Inoue H, Minemoto Y, Yamashita K, Sasagawa T, Yutsudo M. Pro-apoptotic ASY/Nogo-B protein associates with ASYIP. J Cell Physiol. 2003;196:312–8.

259. Qiao J, Huang F, Lum H. PKA inhibits RhoA activation: a protection mechanism against endothelial barrier dysfunction. Am J Physiol Lung Cell Mol Physiol. 2003;284:L972–80.

260. Qiu J, Cafferty WB, McMahon SB, Thompson SW. Conditioning injury-induced spinal axon regeneration requires signal transducer and activator of transcription 3 activation. J Neurosci. 2005;25:1645–53.

261. Raineteau O, Z'Graggen WJ, Thallmair M, Schwab ME. Sprouting and regeneration after pyramidotomy and blockade of the myelin-associated neurite growth inhibitors NI 35/250 in adult rats. Eur J Neurosci. 1999;11:1486–90.

262. Ramón y Cajal S. Notas preventivas sobre la degeneración y regeneración de las vías nerviosas centrales. Trab Lab Invest Biol Univ Madrid. 1906;4:295–301.

263. RamónyCajal S. Degeneration and regeneration of the nervous system. London: Oxford Univ. Press; 1928.

264. Reier PJ. Penetration of grafted astrocytic scars by regenerating optic nerve axons in Xenopus tadpoles. Brain Res. 1979;164:61–8.

265. Reier PJ, Perlow MJ, Guth L. Development of embryonic spinal cord transplants in the rat. Brain Res. 1983;312:201–19.

266. Reier PJ. Neural tissue grafts and repair of the injured spinal cord. Neuropathol Appl Neurobiol. 1985;11:81–104.

267. Reier PJ, Bregman BS, Wujek JR. Intraspinal transplantation of embryonic spinal cord tissue in neonatal and adult rats. J Comp Neurol. 1986;247:275–96.

268. Reier PJ, Houle JD. The glial scar: its bearing on axonal elongation and transplantation approaches to CNS repair. Adv Neurol. 1988;47:87–138.

269. Risling M, Linda H, Cullheim S, Franson P. A persistent defect in the blood–brain barrier after ventral funiculus lesion in adult cats: implications for CNS regeneration? Brain Res. 1989;494:13–21.

270. Ronkko H, Goransson H, Siironen P, Taskinen HS, Vuorinen V, Roytta M. The capacity of the distal stump of peripheral nerve to receive growing axons after two and six months denervation. Scand J Surg. 2011;100:223–9.

271. Roy RR, Harkema SJ, Edgerton VR. Basic concepts of activity-based interventions for improved recovery of motor function after spinal cord injury. Arch Phys Med Rehabil. 2012;93:1487–97.

272. Rubin BP, Spillmann AA, Bandtlow CE, Hillenbrand R, Keller F, Schwab ME. Inhibition of PC12 cell attachment and neurite outgrowth by detergent solubilized CNS myelin proteins. Eur J Neurosci. 1995;7:2524–9.

273. Rudge JS, Silver J. Inhibition of neurite outgrowth on astroglial scars in vitro. J Neurosci. 1990;10:3594–603.

274. Sandrow-Feinberg HR, Houle JD. Exercise after spinal cord injury as an agent for neuroprotection, regeneration and rehabilitation. Brain Res. 1619;2015:12–21.

275. Sapieha PS, Duplan L, Uetani N, Joly S, Tremblay ML, Kennedy TE, Di Polo A. Receptor protein tyrosine phosphatase sigma inhibits axon regrowth in the adult injured CNS. Mol Cell Neurosci. 2005;28:625–35.

276. Sato KL, Johanek LM, Sanada LS, Sluka KA. Spinal cord stimulation reduces mechanical hyperalgesia and glial cell activation in animals with neuropathic pain. Anesth Analg. 2014;118:464–72.

277. Savio T, Schwab ME. Lesioned corticospinal tract axons regenerate in myelin-free rat spinal cord. Proc Natl Acad Sci U S A. 1990;87:4130–3.

278. Sayenko DG, Angeli C, Harkema SJ, Edgerton VR, Gerasimenko YP. Neuromodulation of evoked muscle potentials induced by epidural spinal-cord stimulation in paralyzed individuals. J Neurophysiol. 2014;111:1088–99.

279. Sceats Jr DJ, Friedman WA, Sypert GW, Ballinger Jr WE. Regeneration in peripheral nerve grafts to the cat spinal cord. Brain Res. 1986;362:149–56.

280. Schaeren-Wiemers N, Schaefer C, Valenzuela DM, Yancopoulos GD, Schwab ME. Identification of new oligodendrocyte- and myelin-specific genes by a differential screening approach. J Neurochem. 1995;65:10–22.

281. Schiefferdecker P. Ueber Regeneration, Degeneration und Architectur des Rèuckenmarkes. Berlin: Gedruckt bei G. Reimer; 1876. p. 76.

282. Schmidt CE, Leach JB. Neural tissue engineering: strategies for repair and regeneration. Annu Rev Biomed Eng. 2003;5:293–347.

283. Schnell L, Schwab ME. Axonal regeneration in the rat spinal cord produced by an antibody against myelin-associated neurite growth inhibitors. Nature. 1990;343:269–72.

284. Schnell L, Schneider R, Kolbeck R, Barde YA, Schwab ME. Neurotrophin-3 enhances sprouting of corticospinal tract during development and after adult spinal cord lesion. Nature. 1994;367:170–3.

285. Schnell L, Hunanyan AS, Bowers WJ, Horner PJ, Federoff HJ, Gullo M, Schwab ME, Mendell LM, Arvanian VL. Combined delivery of Nogo-A antibody, neurotrophin-3 and the NMDA-NR2d subunit establishes a functional 'detour' in the hemisected spinal cord. Eur J Neurosci. 2011;34:1256–67.

286. Schreyer DJ, Jones EG. Growing corticospinal axons by-pass lesions of neonatal rat spinal cord. Neuroscience. 1983;9:31–40.

287. Schulz MK, Schnell L, Castro AJ, Schwab ME, Kartje GL. Cholinergic innervation of fetal neocortical transplants is increased after neutralization of myelin-associated neurite growth inhibitors. Exp Neurol. 1998;149:390–7.

288. Schwab ME. Myelin-associated inhibitors of neurite growth and regeneration in the CNS. Trends Neurosci. 1990;13:452–6.

289. Schwab ME, Schnell L. Channeling of developing rat corticospinal tract axons by myelin-associated neurite growth inhibitors. J Neurosci. 1991;11:709–21.

290. Schwab ME. Regeneration of lesioned CNS axons by neutralization of neurite growth inhibitors: a short review. J Neurotrauma. 1992;9 Suppl 1:S219–21.

291. Schwab ME, Bartholdi D. Degeneration and regeneration of axons in the lesioned spinal cord. Physiol Rev. 1996;76:319–70.

292. Schwab ME. Structural plasticity of the adult CNS. Negative control by neurite growth inhibitory signals. Int J Dev Neurosci. 1996;14:379–85.

293. Schwab ME, Brosamle C. Regeneration of lesioned corticospinal tract fibers in the adult rat spinal cord under experimental conditions. Spinal Cord. 1997; 35:469–73.

294. Schwab ME, Strittmatter SM. Nogo limits neural plasticity and recovery from injury. Curr Opin Neurobiol. 2014;27:53–60.

295. Schwegler G, Schwab ME, Kapfhammer JP. Increased collateral sprouting of primary afferents in the myelin-free spinal cord. J Neurosci. 1995;15:2756–67.

296. Seijffers R, Allchorne AJ, Woolf CJ. The transcription factor ATF-3 promotes neurite outgrowth. Mol Cell Neurosci. 2006;32:143–54.

297. Seijffers R, Mills CD, Woolf CJ. ATF3 increases the intrinsic growth state of DRG neurons to enhance peripheral nerve regeneration. J Neurosci. 2007;27:7911–20.

298. Sharpe AN, Jackson A. Upper-limb muscle responses to epidural, subdural and intraspinal stimulation of the cervical spinal cord. J Neural Eng. 2014;11:016005.

299. Sicotte M, Tsatas O, Jeong SY, Cai CQ, He Z, David S. Immunization with myelin or recombinant Nogo-66/MAG in alum promotes axon regeneration and sprouting after corticospinal tract lesions in the spinal cord. Mol Cell Neurosci. 2003;23:251–63.

300. Siegel CS, Fink KL, Strittmatter SM, Cafferty WB. Plasticity of intact rubral projections mediates spontaneous recovery of function after corticospinal tract injury. J Neurosci. 2015;35:1443–57.

301. Simonen M, Pedersen V, Weinmann O, Schnell L, Buss A, Ledermann B, Christ F, Sansig G, van der Putten H, Schwab ME. Systemic deletion of the myelin-associated outgrowth inhibitor Nogo-A improves regenerative and plastic responses after spinal cord injury. Neuron. 2003;38:201–11.

302. Smith GM, Miller RH, Silver J. Changing role of forebrain astrocytes during development, regenerative failure, and induced regeneration upon transplantation. J Comp Neurol. 1986;251:23–43.

303. Smith GM, Strunz C. Growth factor and cytokine regulation of chondroitin sulfate proteoglycans by astrocytes. Glia. 2005;52:209–18.

304. Song HJ, Ming GL, Poo MM. cAMP-induced switching in turning direction of nerve growth cones. Nature. 1997;388:275–9.

305. Spejo AB, Oliveira AL. Synaptic rearrangement following axonal injury: old and new players. Neuropharmacology. 2015;96:113–23.

306. Spillmann AA, Bandtlow CE, Lottspeich F, Keller F, Schwab ME. Identification and characterization of a bovine neurite growth inhibitor (bNI-220). J Biol Chem. 1998;273:19283–93.

307. Starkey ML, Bartus K, Barritt AW, Bradbury EJ. Chondroitinase ABC promotes compensatory sprouting of the intact corticospinal tract and recovery of forelimb function following unilateral pyramidotomy in adult mice. Eur J Neurosci. 2012;36:3665–78.

308. Stocco A, Prat CS, Losey DM, Cronin JA, Wu J, Abernethy JA, et al. Playing 20 Questions with the mind: Collaborative problem solving by humans using a Brain-to-Brain Interface. PLoS One. 2015;10:e0137303.

309. Su H, Yuan Q, Qin D, Yang X, Wong WM, So KF, Wu W. Lithium enhances axonal regeneration in peripheral nerve by inhibiting glycogen synthase kinase 3beta activation. Biomed Res Int. 2014;2014:658753.

310. Sugar O, Gerard RW. Spinal cord regeneration in the rat. J Neurophysiol. 1940;3:1–19.

311. Sutendra G, Dromparis P, Wright P, Bonnet S, Haromy A, Hao Z, McMurtry MS, Michalak M, Vance JE, Sessa WC, Michelakis ED. The role of Nogo and the mitochondria-endoplasmic reticulum unit in pulmonary hypertension. Sci Transl Med. 2011;3:88ra55.

312. Szynkaruk M, Kemp SW, Wood MD, Gordon T, Borschel GH. Experimental and clinical evidence for use of decellularized nerve allografts in peripheral nerve gap reconstruction. Tissue Eng Part B Rev. 2013;19:83–96.

313. Tatagiba M, Brosamle C, Schwab ME. Regeneration of injured axons in the adult mammalian central nervous system. Neurosurgery. 1997;40:541–7.

314. Tator CH, Rivlin AS. Elimination of root regeneration in studies of spinal cord regeneration. Surg Neurol. 1983;19:255–9.

315. Taylor GI, Ham FJ. The free vascularized nerve graft. A further experimental and clinical application of microvascular techniques. Plast Reconstr Surg. 1976;57:413–26.

316. Teng FY, Tang BL. Why do Nogo/Nogo-66 receptor gene knockouts result in inferior regeneration compared to treatment with neutralizing agents? J Neurochem. 2005;94:865–74.

317. Tennant KA. Thinking outside the brain: structural plasticity in the spinal cord promotes recovery from cortical stroke. Exp Neurol. 2014;254:195–9.

318. Tong J, Liu W, Wang X, Han X, Hyrien O, Samadani U, Smith DH, Huang JH. Inhibition of Nogo-66 receptor 1 enhances recovery of cognitive function after traumatic brain injury in mice. J Neurotrauma. 2013;30:247–58.

319. Tong J, Ren Y, Wang X, Dimopoulos VG, Kesler HN, Liu W, He X, Nedergaard M, Huang JH. Assessment of Nogo-66 receptor 1 function in vivo after spinal cord injury. Neurosurgery. 2014;75:51–60.

320. Tsai EC, Krassioukov AV, Tator CH. Corticospinal regeneration into lumbar grey matter correlates with locomotor recovery after complete spinal cord transection and repair with peripheral nerve grafts, fibroblast growth factor 1, fibrin glue, and spinal fusion. J Neuropathol Exp Neurol. 2005;64:230–44.

321. van de Meent H, Schwab ME. Regeneration of the lesioned spinal cord. Neurorehabilitation. 1998;10:119–29.

322. Vanek P, Thallmair M, Schwab ME, Kapfhammer JP. Increased lesion-induced sprouting of corticospinal fibres in the myelin-free rat spinal cord. Eur J Neurosci. 1998;10:45–56.

323. Varga ZM, Schwab ME, Nicholls JG. Myelin-associated neurite growth-inhibitory proteins and suppression of regeneration of immature mammalian spinal cord in culture. Proc Natl Acad Sci U S A. 1995;92:10959–63.

324. Vasudeva VS, Abd-El-Barr M, Chi J. Lumbosacral spinal cord epidural stimulation enables recovery of voluntary movement after complete motor spinal cord injury. Neurosurgery. 2014;75:N14–5.

325. Volpe BT, Krebs HI, Hogan N, Edelstein L, Diels C, Aisen M. A novel approach to stroke rehabilitation. Neurology. 2000;54:1938–44.

326. von Meyenburg J, Brosamle C, Metz GA, Schwab ME. Regeneration and sprouting of chronically injured corticospinal tract fibers in adult rats promoted by NT-3 and the mAb IN-1, which neutralizes myelin-associated neurite growth inhibitors. Exp Neurol. 1998;154:583–94.

327. Walchli T, Pernet V, Weinmann O, Shiu JY, Guzik-Kornacka A, Decrey G, Yuksel D, Schneider H, Vogel J, Ingber DE, Vogel V, Frei K, Schwab ME. Nogo-A is a negative regulator of CNS angiogenesis. Proc Natl Acad Sci U S A. 2013;110:E1943–52.

328. Wall A, Borg J, Palmcrantz S. Clinical application of the Hybrid Assistive Limb (HAL) for gait training-a systematic review. Front Syst Neurosci. 2015;9:48.

329. Wang X, Messing A, David S. Axonal and nonneuronal cell responses to spinal cord injury in mice lacking glial fibrillary acidic protein. Exp Neurol. 1997;148:568–76.

330. Wang KC, Kim JA, Sivasankaran R, Segal R, He Z. P75 interacts with the Nogo receptor as a co-receptor for Nogo, MAG and OMgp. Nature. 2002;420:74–8.

331. Wang X, Duffy P, McGee AW, Hasan O, Gould G, Tu N, Harel NY, Huang Y, Carson RE, Weinzimmer D, Ropchan J, Benowitz LI, Cafferty WB, Strittmatter SM. Recovery from chronic spinal cord contusion after Nogo receptor intervention. Ann Neurol. 2011;70:805–21.

332. Wang D, Ichiyama RM, Zhao R, Andrews MR, Fawcett JW. Chondroitinase combined with rehabilitation promotes recovery of forelimb function in rats with chronic spinal cord injury. J Neurosci. 2011; 31:9332–44.

333. Wanner M, Lang DM, Bandtlow CE, Schwab ME, Bastmeyer M, Stuermer CA. Reevaluation of the growth-permissive substrate properties of goldfish optic nerve myelin and myelin proteins. J Neurosci. 1995;15:7500–8.

334. Warren PM, Alilain WJ. The challenges of respiratory motor system recovery following cervical spinal cord injury. Prog Brain Res. 2014;212:173–220.

335. Weibel D, Cadelli D, Schwab ME. Regeneration of lesioned rat optic nerve fibers is improved after neutralization of myelin-associated neurite growth inhibitors. Brain Res. 1994;642:259–66.

336. Weinmann O, Schnell L, Ghosh A, Montani L, Wiessner C, Wannier T, Rouiller E, Mir A, Schwab ME. Intrathecally infused antibodies against Nogo-A penetrate the CNS and downregulate the endogenous neurite growth inhibitor Nogo-A. Mol Cell Neurosci. 2006;32:161–73.

337. Wenger N, Moraud EM, Raspopovic S, Bonizzato M, DiGiovanna J, Musienko P, Morari M, Micera S, Courtine G. Closed-loop neuromodulation of spinal sensorimotor circuits controls refined locomotion after complete spinal cord injury. Sci Transl Med. 2014;6:255ra133.

338. Wettels N, Fishel JA, Loeb GE. Multimodal tactile sensor. In: Balasubramanian R, Santos VJ, editors. The human hand as an inspiration for robot hand development, Springer Tracts in Advanced Robotics (STAR) series. Springer: Heidelberg; 2014.

339. Willand MP, Holmes M, Bain JR, de Bruin H, Fahnestock M. Sensory nerve cross-anastomosis and electrical muscle stimulation synergistically enhance functional recovery of chronically denervated muscle. Plast Reconstr Surg. 2014;134:736e–45.

340. Willi R, Aloy EM, Yee BK, Feldon J, Schwab ME. Behavioral characterization of mice lacking the neurite outgrowth inhibitor Nogo-A. Genes Brain Behav. 2009;8:181–92.

341. Williams LR, Longo FM, Powell HC, Lundborg G, Varon S. Spatial-temporal progress of peripheral nerve regeneration within a silicone chamber: parameters for a bioassay. J Comp Neurol. 1983;218:460–70.

342. Williams G, Wood A, Williams EJ, Gao Y, Mercado ML, Katz A, Joseph-McCarthy D, Bates B, Ling HP, Aulabaugh A, Zaccardi J, Xie Y, Pangalos MN, Walsh FS, Doherty P. Ganglioside inhibition of neurite outgrowth requires Nogo receptor function: identification of interaction sites and development of novel antagonists. J Biol Chem. 2008;283:16641–52.

343. Windle WF. Recollections of research in spinal cord regeneration. Exp Neurol. 1981;71:1–5.

344. Wirz M, Dietz V. European Multicenter Study of Spinal Cord Injury, N. Recovery of sensorimotor function and activities of daily living after cervical spinal cord injury: the influence of age. J Neurotrauma. 2015;32:194–9.

345. Wolburg H, Kästner R. Is the architecture of astrocytic membrane crucial for axonal regeneration in the central nervous system? Naturwissenschaften. 1984;71:484–5.

346. Woolf CJ, Shortland P, Reynolds M, Ridings J, Doubell T, Coggeshall RE. Reorganization of central terminals of myelinated primary afferents in the rat dorsal horn following peripheral axotomy. J Comp Neurol. 1995;360:121–34.

347. Worter V, Schweigreiter R, Kinzel B, Mueller M, Barske C, Bock G, Frentzel S, Bandtlow CE. Inhibitory activity of myelin-associated glycoprotein on sensory neurons is largely independent of NgR1 and NgR2 and resides within Ig-Like domains 4 and 5. e5218. 2009;4.

348. Wu P, Spinner RJ, Gu Y, Yaszemski MJ, Windebank AJ, Wang H. Delayed repair of the peripheral nerve: a novel model in the rat sciatic nerve. J Neurosci Methods. 2013;214:37–44.

349. Wu P, Chawla A, Spinner RJ, Yu C, Yaszemski MJ, Windebank AJ, Wang H. Key changes in denervated muscles and their impact on regeneration and reinnervation. Neural Regen Res. 2014;9:1796–809.

350. Xu C, Kou Y, Zhang P, Han N, Yin X, Deng J, Chen B, Jiang B. Electrical stimulation promotes regeneration of defective peripheral nerves after delayed repair intervals lasting under one month. PLoS One. 2014;9:e105045.

351. Xu B, Park D, Ohtake Y, Li H, Hayat U, Liu J, Selzer ME, Longo FM, Li S. Role of CSPG receptor LAR phosphatase in restricting axon regeneration after CNS injury. Neurobiol Dis. 2015;73:36–48.

352. Yang YS, Harel NY, Strittmatter SM. Reticulon-4A (Nogo-A) redistributes protein disulfide isomerase to protect mice from SOD1-dependent amyotrophic lateral sclerosis. J Neurosci. 2009;29:13850–9.

353. Yang ML, Li JJ, So KF, Chen JY, Cheng WS, Wu J, Wang ZM, Gao F, Young W. Efficacy and safety of lithium carbonate treatment of chronic spinal cord injuries: a double-blind, randomized, placebo-controlled clinical trial. Spinal Cord. 2012;50:141–6.

354. Yick LW, So KF, Cheung PT, Wu WT. Lithium chloride reinforces the regeneration-promoting effect of chondroitinase ABC on rubrospinal neurons after spinal cord injury. J Neurotrauma. 2004;21:932–43.

355. Young W. Review of lithium effects on brain and blood. Cell Transplant. 2009;18:951–75.

356. Young W. Spinal cord regeneration. Cell Transplant. 2014;23:573–611.

357. Young W. Electrical stimulation and motor recovery. Cell Transplant. 2015;24:429–46.

358. Yu J, Fernandez-Hernando C, Suarez Y, Schleicher M, Hao Z, Wright PL, DiLorenzo A, Kyriakides TR, Sessa WC. Reticulon 4B (Nogo-B) is necessary for macrophage infiltration and tissue repair. Proc Natl Acad Sci U S A. 2009;106:17511–6.

359. Yu Z, Yu P, Chen H, Geller HM. Targeted inhibition of KCa3.1 attenuates TGF-beta-induced reactive astrogliosis through the Smad2/3 signaling pathway. J Neurochem. 2014;130:41–9.

360. Yuan J, Zou M, Xiang X, Zhu H, Chu W, Liu W, Chen F, Lin J. Curcumin improves neural function after spinal cord injury by the joint inhibition of the intracellular and extracellular components of glial scar. J Surg Res. 2015;195:235–45.

361. Zagrebelsky M, Buffo A, Skerra A, Schwab ME, Strata P, Rossi F. Retrograde regulation of growth-associated gene expression in adult rat Purkinje cells by myelin-associated neurite growth inhibitory proteins. J Neurosci. 1998;18:7912–29.

362. Zagrebelsky M, Schweigreiter R, Bandtlow CE, Schwab ME, Korte M. Nogo-A stabilizes the architecture of hippocampal neurons. J Neurosci. 2010;30:13220–34.

363. Zemmar A, Weinmann O, Kellner Y, Yu X, Vicente R, Gullo M, Kasper H, Lussi K, Ristic Z, Luft AR, Rioult-Pedotti M, Zuo Y, Zagrebelsky M, Schwab ME. Neutralization of Nogo-A enhances synaptic plasticity in the rodent motor cortex and improves motor learning in vivo. J Neurosci. 2014;34:8685–98.

364. Zhang D, Utsumi T, Huang HC, Gao L, Sangwung P, Chung C, Shibao K, Okamoto K, Yamaguchi K, Groszmann RJ, Jozsef L, Hao Z, Sessa WC, Iwakiri Y. Reticulon 4B (Nogo-B) is a novel regulator of hepatic fibrosis. Hepatology. 2011;53:1306–15.

365. Zhang L, Kaneko S, Kikuchi K, Sano A, Maeda M, Kishino A, Shibata S, Mukaino M, Toyama Y, Liu M,

Kimura T, Okano H, Nakamura M. Rewiring of regenerated axons by combining treadmill training with semaphorin3A inhibition. Mol Brain. 2014;7:14.

366. Zhao RR, Muir EM, Alves JN, Rickman H, Allan AY, Kwok JC, Roet KC, Verhaagen J, Schneider BL, Bensadoun JC, Ahmed SG, Yanez-Munoz RJ, Keynes RJ, Fawcett JW, Rogers JH. Lentiviral vectors express chondroitinase ABC in cortical projections and promote sprouting of injured corticospinal axons. J Neurosci Methods. 2011;201:228–38.

367. Zhao RR, Fawcett JW. Combination treatment with chondroitinase ABC in spinal cord injury – breaking the barrier. Neurosci Bull. 2013;29:477–83.

368. Zhou HX, Li XY, Li FY, Liu C, Liang ZP, Liu S, Zhang B, Wang TY, Chu TC, Lu L, Ning GZ, Kong XH, Feng SQ. Targeting RPTPsigma with lentiviral shRNA promotes neurites outgrowth of cortical neurons and improves functional recovery in a rat spinal cord contusion model. Brain Res. 2014;1586:46–63.

369. Zhu H, Feng YP, Young W, You SW, Shen XF, Liu YS, Ju G. Early neurosurgical intervention of spinal cord contusion: an analysis of 30 cases. Chin Med J (Engl). 2008;121:2473–8.

370. Zhu Z, Kremer P, Tadmori I, Ren Y, Sun D, He X, Young W. Lithium suppresses astrogliogenesis by neural stem and progenitor cells by inhibiting STAT3 pathway independently of glycogen synthase kinase 3 beta. PLoS One. 2011;6:e23341.

Erratum to: Rehabilitative Surgery: A Comprehensive Text for an Emerging Field

Andrew I. Elkwood, Matthew Kaufman, and Lisa F. Schneider

Erratum to
A.I. Elkwood et al. (eds.), *Rehabilitative Surgery*,
DOI 10.1007/978-3-319-41406-5

In the original version of front matter, Foreword in Book Front matter was missing.

In the original version for chapter 20, the author name Matthew Pontell, MD, Department of Surgery, Drexel University College of Medicine, Philadelphia, PA, USA was missing which has been included.

The above mentioned corrections also updated in Table of Contents.

The updated online version of the original book can be found under
DOI 10.1007/978-3-319-41406-5

© Springer International Publishing Switzerland 2017
A.I. Elkwood et al. (eds.), *Rehabilitative Surgery*, DOI 10.1007/978-3-319-41406-5_28

Index

A

Acetaminophen, 26–27
Acute burn management
    care of, 181–182
    epidemiology, 179
    infection, 182
    inhalational injury, 182
    reconstruction by anatomical site, 184–186
    rule of nines, 180–181
    surgery
        burn reconstructive ladder, 183
        escharotomy and fasciotomy, 182
        excision and grafting, 182–183
        principles, 182–183
        tissue expansion, 183–184
    wound and triage, 179–181
Adjacent tissue transfer, 183
Advanced Balancing Combined Digital
        Extension Flexion Grip (ABCDEFG)
        Reconstruction, 244
Advanced Trauma Life Support (ATLS), 221–222
Air-fluidized (AF) beds, 160
Allograft, 182–183
Allotransplantation, hand
    donor and recipient selection, 278
    donor limb procurement, 278
    maintenance immunosuppression, 278–279
    recipient surgery, 278
American Association of Hip and Knee Surgeons
        (AAHKS), 300
American Burn Association, 179, 180
American College of Surgeons (ACS), 221
American Spinal Injury Association (ASIA) score, 98
Amion, 182
Amputation *vs.* limb salvage
    financial considerations, 231–233
    litigation and outcomes, 231
    orthopedic care, 222–226
    overall outcomes, 230–231
    pathologic process, 221
    plastic surgery care, 226–230
    psychosocial aspects, 230
    traumatic etiologies, 221–222
    vascular etiologies, 221
Amyotrophic lateral sclerosis (ALS), 120, 125

Anesthesia
    autonomic dysreflexia (*see* Autonomic dysreflexia
        (AD))
    emergence, 23
    induction, 22–23
    intraoperative monitoring, 22
    maintenance, 23
    peripheral nerve reconstruction, 25–26
    postoperative considerations
        acute pain management, 26–28
        long-term care, 26
        postanesthesia care, 26
    preoperative evaluation
        cardiovascular system, 20–21
        genitourinary system, 21
        musculoskeletal system, 21
        psychological issues, 22
        respiratory system, 21
        thermal regulation, 21–22
    SCI, 19
    spinal and epidural *vs.* regional, 24
Aneurysmal subarachnoid hemorrhage (SAH), 55–56
Antiseizure medications, 51
Antiseptic technique, 9
Arteriovenous malformations (AVM), 56
Arthritis and avascular necrosis, 299–300
Arthrofibrosis, 300–302
Athletic pubalgia
    clinical presentation and physical examination,
        268–269
    diagnostic imaging, 269
    MRI grading, 269
    pathophysiology, 267–268
    surgical and postoperative management, 269–270
Atrophic nonunion, 298–299
Autonomic dysreflexia (AD), 154, 339
    acute management of, 19–20, 22
    bladder stones, 342
    evaluation and management, 341
    pharmacological treatment, 341
    post-autonomic dysreflexia management, 341–342
    prevention, 340
    symptomatic manifestations, 19
    treatment, 24–25, 340–341
Avascular necrosis (AVN), 300

© Springer International Publishing Switzerland 2017
A.I. Elkwood et al. (eds.), *Rehabilitative Surgery*, DOI 10.1007/978-3-319-41406-5